Hospital

Abingdon VA
'24210

CRC Handbook
of
Hospital Acquired
Infections

Editor

Richard P. Wenzel, M.D.
Associate Professor of Medicine
Hospital Epidemiologist
University of Virginia Medical Center
Charlottesville, Virginia

CRC Press, Inc.
Boca Raton, Florida

Library of Congress Cataloging in Publication Data

Main entry under title:

CRC handbook of hospital acquired infections.

   Bibliography: p.
   Includes index.
   1. Nosocomial infections—Prevention. I. Wenzel,
Richard P. [DNLM: 1. Cross infection—Prevention and
control—Handbooks. WX167 C106]
RA969.C16   614.4'4   80-11716
ISBN O-8493-0202-1

Direct all inquiries to CRC Press, Inc., 2000 N.W. 24th Street, Boca Raton, Florida 33431.

© 1981 by CRC Press, Inc.

International Standard Book Number 0-8493-0202-1

Library of Congress Card Number 80-11716
Printed in the United States

PREFACE

Almost 40 million Americans are hospitalized annually; and 5 to 10% acquire an infection which was not present or incubating at the time when they were admitted. It has become increasingly obvious that such hospital acquired infections contribute significantly to patients' morbidity and mortality and that they severely tax the economy of our nation. As a result, a new specialty of medicine/infectious diseases is evolving — Infection Control, and the primary missions of the physician epidemiologist and infection control practitioner (ICP) are to minimize infections in hospitalized patients and to help optimize patient care. Health care in hospitals is obviously a major priority of U.S. citizens, as illustrated by the current debate in Congress on national health care proposals. Furthermore, the legal aspects of medical care are increasingly visible. At the same time, within our own ranks, the Joint Commission for the Accreditation of Hospitals (JCAH) has urged a review and revision of common hospital policies and procedures on an annual basis. Thus, infection control has emerged in response to the needs and demands of health care consumers. Such response is being witnessed in efforts to improve surveillance of nosocomial infections (including use of the computer), in a critical review of the proper use of the microbiology laboratory, a reassessment of antibiotic usage, and in an examination of the relative merits of common antiseptics and disinfectants in hospitals. Improved skills for investigating outbreaks of hospital associated infections using appropriate statistics have begun to show the medical value and cost effectiveness of hospital epidemiology and infection control as an important subspecialty. In addition, resources for answering questions and solving problems on site are available on both local and national levels. Thus, it seemed appropriate to focus on the state of the art, existing infection control problems, and current information available to cope with them. The result is the *Handbook of Hospital Acquired Infections.*

This book was conceived and written for the practitioner — nurse, physician, technologist, etc. — who is actively involved in infection control. Although the novice may find it of considerable value, the book was written with the experienced practitioner very much in mind. Sections and chapters were designed to answer questions which seem to be most frequently asked of us in infection control. Hopefully the book will be a guide for practitioners with problems. Certainly, the field of infection control is young, and the data are limited, but the authors of this text have tried to state clearly where the facts end and where the biases begin. The book is also meant to stimulate the talented people in our field who have worked diligently, and who now seek new challenges in their expanding role as sophisticated surveillance experts, teachers, administrators, and investigators. It is likely that the unusually rapid and exciting evolution of our role in patient care is the result of their idealism, energies, tenaciousness, and wisdom.

I wish to acknowledge the highest cooperation of all authors in the Handbook. They are friends as well as colleagues and gave up valuable time from their original pursuits and from their families to contribute to this work. Expert secretarial assistance was provided by Patti Miller, Stella King, and Debbie Crickenberger.

Richard P. Wenzel, M.D.
January 1981

THE EDITOR

Dr. Richard P. Wenzel received his B.S. degree at Haverford College and his M.D. degree at Thomas Jefferson University in Philadelphia. After a medical residency, infectious diseases fellowship, and chief residency at the University of Maryland Medical School, he spent 2 years as a naval medical officer in a virus research laboratory at Camp LeJeune, N.C. For the past 8 years, he has been at the University of Virginia Medical Center in Charlottesville where he is an Associate Professor of Medicine and the Hospital Epidemiologist.

Author of 100 scientific publications, Dr. Wenzel is Board Certified in Internal Medicine and in Infectious Diseases. He is Editor-in-Chief of *Infection Control* and on the Editorial Board of the *American Journal of Infection Control* and *Antimicrobial Agents and Chemotherapy.* He is the recipient of the Wellcome Prize and Medal and the Louis Livingston Seaman Award for work performed while in the military on acute respiratory infections and malaria in Vietnam, respectively.

Collaborating with the State Health Department in Virginia, Dr. Wenzel coordinates a statewide program for the surveillance and reporting of hospital acquired infections. He directs a certificate program for the training of practitioners in infection control and a fellowship program for training future hospital epidemiologists. In 1978, the APIC-Virginia Chapter presented him with an award for his contributions to the Association of Practitioners of Infection Control. In 1980, after reviewing Dr. Wenzel's physician training fellowship, the Board of Visitors at the University of Virginia approved a Masters of Science degree program in Hospital Epidemiology — Infection Control.

CONTRIBUTORS

Robert C. Aber, M.D.
Assistant Professor of Medicine and
Hospital Epidemologist
Chief, Division of Infectious
Diseases
Department of Medicine
The Milton S. Hershey Medical
Center
The Pennsylvania State University
Hershey, Pennsylvania

Nuzhet Osman Atuk, M.D.
Professor of Medicine
University of Virginia School of
Medicine
Charlottesville, Virginia

Karen J. Axnick, R.N.
Supervisor, Infection Control
Department
Stanford University Hospital
Stanford, California

Michael R. Britt, M.D.
Medical Director
Utah Professional Review
Organization
Utah/PSRO
Salt Lake City, Utah

Carole De Mille, R.N.*
Department of Medicine
Massachusetts General Hospital
Boston, Massachusetts

Harvey A. Elder, M.D.
Chief, Hospital Epidemiology
Loma Linda University Medical
Center
Associate Professor of Medicine
Loma Linda University School of
Medicine
Loma Linda, California

Richard A. Garibaldi, M.D.
Associate Professor of Medicine
University of Utah College of
Medicine
Hospital Epidemiologist
University of Utah Medical Center
and Veterans Administration
Hospital
Salt Lake City, Utah

Julia S. Garner, R.N., M.N.
Chief, Consultation Activity
Hospital Infections Branch
Bureau of Epidemiology
Center for Disease Control
Atlanta, Georgia

Richard L. Guerrant, M.D.
Head, Division of Geographic
Medicine
Associate Professor of Medicine
Department of Medicine
University of Virginia School of
Medicine
Charlottesville, Virginia

James M. Hughes, M.D.
Assistant Chief
Enteric Diseases Branch
Bacterial Diseases Division
Bureau of Epidemiology
Center for Disease Control
Atlanta, Georgia

Ella Hunt, R.N.
Department of Medicine
University of Virginia Medical
Center
Charlottesville, Virginia

Robert M. Jackson, M.D.
State Health Commissioner
South Carolina Department of
Health and Environmental Control
Columbia, South Carolina

* Deceased, January, 1979

Thomas F. Keys, M.D.
Associate Professor of Medicine
Hospital Epidemiologist
Mayo Clinic
Rochester, Minnesota

Darrell A. Leonhardt, M.P.H.
Analyst, Hospital Epidemiology
Loma Linda University Medical
Center
Loma Linda, California

Dennis G. Maki, M.D.
Ovid O. Meyer Associate Professor
of Medicine
Head, Infectious Disease Section
University of Wisconsin Medical
School
Hospital Epidemiologist
University of Wisconsin Hospitals
and Clinics
Madison, Wisconsin

George F. Mallison, M.P.H.
Assistant Director
Bacterial Diseases Division
Center for Disease Control
Atlanta, Georgia

Gerald L. Mandell, M.D.
Professor of Medicine
Head, Division of Infectious Disease
University of Virginia School of
Medicine
Charlottesville, Virginia

Stanley M. Martin, M.S.
Chief, Statistical Services Branch
Bacterial Diseases Division
Bureau of Epidemiology
Center for Disease Control
Atlanta, Georgia

C. Glen Mayhall, M.D.
Associate Professor of Medicine
Hospital Epidemiologist
Division of Infectious Diseases
Medical College of Virginia
Virginia Commonwealth University
Richmond, Virginia

John E. McGowan, Jr., M.D.
Hospital Epidemiologist
Grady Memorial Hospital
Associate Professor of Medicine and
Preventive Medicine
Emory University School of
Medicine
Atlanta, Georgia

Grayson B. Miller, Jr., M.D.
Director, Division of Epidemiology
State Epidemiologist
Virginia State Department of Health
Richmond, Virginia

Joel L. Nitzkin, M.D., D.P.A.
Director, Monroe County Health
Department
Rochester, New York

Harry Charles Nottebart, Jr., J.D.,
M.D.
Director, Bureau of Communicable
Diseases
Virginia State Department of Health
Richmond, Virginia

Charles A. Osterman, R.N.
Epidemiology Nursing Supervisor
Division of Hospital Epidemiology
Department of Nursing
University of Virginia Medical
Center
Charlottesville, Virginia

Jay P. Sanford, M.D.
Professor of Medicine
Dean, School of Medicine
Uniformed Services University of the
Health Sciences
Bethesda, Maryland

William Schaffner, M.D.
Professor of Medicine and
Preventive Medicine
Hospital Epidemiologist
Vanderbilt University School of
Medicine
Nashville, Tennessee

Timothy R. Townsend, M.D.
 Assistant Professor of Pediatrics
 Hospital Epidemiologist
 The Johns Hopkins Hospital
 Baltimore, Maryland

James M. Veazey, Jr., M.D.
 Assistant Professor Medicine
 Albany Medical College
 Hospital Epidemiologist
 Albany Medical Center Hospital
 Albany, New York

Richard P. Wenzel, M.D.
 Associate Professor of Medicine
 Hospital Epidemiologist
 University of Virginia Medical
 Center
 Charlottesville, Virginia

TABLE OF CONTENTS

THE BEGINNING

IDENTIFYING AND REPORTING INFECTIONS

MICROBIOLOGIC CONSIDERATIONS

ORGANIZATION FOR INFECTION CONTROL

MEDICAL-LEGAL POLICIES

INVESTIGATING AN EPIDEMIC

RESOURCES FOR THE INFECTION CONTROL PRACTITIONER

The Beginning

PERSPECTIVES IN INFECTION CONTROL

Jay P. Sanford

INTRODUCTION

"There is some fear lest hospitals, as they have been hitherto, may not have generally increased, rather than diminished, the rate of mortality."[1] This admonition of Florence Nightingale is as applicable today as it was in 1860. The purpose of this Handbook is to serve as a source of information to provide individuals involved in hospital associated (nosocomial) infection control programs with an understanding of the problems and with rational guidelines toward their identification and prevention. Infection control had its origin more than 100 years ago. A brief review of the observations and problems which these pioneers faced will provide some consolation for the frustrations currently encountered in the establishment of effective infection control programs.

HISTORY

Preantibiotic Era

In 1847 Ignaz Philipp Semmelweis, then an obstetrician in the First Division clinic of the Lying-In Hospital in Buda (now Budapest, Hungary), which was under the direction of Johann Klein, made a series of careful clinical observations which formed the basis for his recognition of the epidemiology and control of puerperal sepsis or childbed fever.[2] At that time, 8.3% of women admitted to the maternity service died of puerperal sepsis. Semmelweis observed that the mortality was four times higher on the First Division than it was on the Second Division, although conditions, such as overcrowding and poor ventilation, were similar on both divisions. He began to keep notes on the activities of the two clinics and observed that medical students were trained on the First Division, while only midwives were trained on the Second Division. He reasoned that students must be bringing to their patients in labor something which did not affect midwives. Following the death of a close friend from a wound infection incurred in performing an autopsy on a woman who had died of puerperal fever, he hypothesized that the students who came directly to the First Division from the dissecting rooms must be carrying the infection back to the women they were examining. He then required his students to wash their hands between the dissecting room and the clinic, but this proved ineffective. He then required them to wash their hands in a solution of chlorinated lime. The mortality figures in the First Division fell to 2.3%, slightly below those of the Second Division. In 1850 when Semmelweis came up for promotion, Klein, who was extremely jealous of Semmelweis' success, refused to support the proposal, and Semmelweis departed, accepting a position at the University of Pest. There his method reduced that clinic's high mortality from puerperal sepsis to 0.85%. Unfortunately, there was virtually no acceptance of his observations by the medical community. Semmelweis grew morose, claiming through the press that his colleagues were participating in a "massacre". In 1861 he published *The Etiology, Concept and Prophylaxis of Puerperal Fever.* After waiting 13 years, he wrote, "I find that the amount of progress has not been made which is necessary for the welfare of mankind." He became more depressed, haunted by the belief that thousands had died because of his failure to disseminate and implement his observations. In 1865 he was admitted to an insane assylum, dying 6 weeks later of erysipelas.

Just before Semmelweis' death, Lister first attempted the use of carbolic acid in the

Table 1
CHANGING PATTERN OF LIFE-THREATENING MICROBIAL
DISEASES

Etiological agents or circumstances	Fatal infections observed on the medical service[a]	
	1938—1940	1957—1958
Streptococcus pneumoniae, Staphylococcus pyogenes, Mycobacterium tuberculosis	40	4
S. aureus	15	15
Aerobic Gram-negative bacilli	9	22
"Mycotic"	2	9
Hospital associated origin of infection	7%	54%

[a] Study based upon 200 necropsy patients in each time interval. Infection judged to be the or a major contributory factor to mortality.

prevention and treatment of infection in compound fractures and wounds.[3] In his memoirs Sir Alexander Ogston, Professor of Surgery at the University of Aberdeen, noted "Unforgettable was the incredulity with which we heard the first announcement that Lister has discovered a means of avoiding suppuration and blood poisoning in operation wounds. It was unbelievable that it could be true ... we shook our heads and agreed that he was risking a great reputation."[4] Despite the efficacy of carbolic acid spray, it should be appreciated that in Lister's writings, the nature of septic poison was not clearly stated, and the broad view that wound infection was caused by germs was based more on speculation than observation.

Antibiotic Era

The introduction of penicillin into clinical practice in 1941 was followed by a wave of premature optimism that infections, particularly those acquired in hospitals, could now be readily cured. Interest in infection control practices rapidly waned.

The almost simultaneous world-wide appearance of penicillinase-producing staphylococci, especially those of phage type 80/81 in newborn nurseries in the mid-1950s, resulted in a rebirth of the awareness of the need for establishment of infection control programs in hospitals.[5] Unfortunately the awareness and enthusiasm were not always directed toward rationally proven means of infection control, e.g., practices such as "fogging" of rooms with phenolic disinfectants or the extensive culturing of walls and floors to detect the source of the organisms were instituted as dogma. It was considerably later that these practices were subjected to critical evaluation and found not to be of value in reducing the prevalence of hospital acquired staphylococcal disease.

During the past 25 years, the pattern of life-threatening bacterial illnesses encountered in the urban areas of the world has undergone progressive change.[6] This change is depicted as well by the data of Rogers in 1959 as by any subsequent observations (see Table 1).[7] Note that the overall prevalence of infection as the primary or as a major contributory cause of death only decreased from 33 to 24% after the introduction of numerous effective antibiotics. Concomitantly there were striking increases in the prevalence of infections caused by aerobic Gram-negative bacilli and by fungal organisms.

MAGNITUDE OF THE PROBLEM

In 1976, 83 hospitals participated in the National Nosocomial Infections Study

Table 2
ESTIMATED YEARLY NUMBER OF NOSOCOMIAL
INFECTIONS IN THE U.S.

	Infections[a]				
Pathogen	Bacteremia	Respiratory	Genitourinary	Other	Total
Bacteria[b]	185.6	238.8	773.3	628.1	1825.8
Fungus	7.9	10.8	52.8	124.6	196.1
Parasite	—	0.5	—	—	0.5
Virus[c]	—	0.5	—	5.3	5.8
Total	194	251	826	758	2029

[a] Numbers in thousands.
[b] Includes mycobacteria.
[c] Includes rickettsia.

(NNIS). These NNIS hospitals conducted nosocomial infection surveillance on more than 1.3 million hospitalized patients, approximately 3.4% of all patients hospitalized in the U.S.[8] Nosocomial infections were recognized and reported in 3.6% of discharges. Adjusting for under reporting, up to 5.5% of hospitalized patients acquire a nosocomial infection. Projecting to a national incidence, over 2 million nosocomial infections are estimated to occur yearly (see Table 2).[8] Dixon has estimated that more than 6 million days are attributable to prolongation of stay for nosocomial infections (see Table 3). The incremental cost attributable to this prolongation in stay, without considering physician fees or loss of productive activity, is estimated at more than $1 billion for 1977 (see Table 3).

The information collected in these studies illustrates several important considerations which will be discussed in detail in subsequent chapters. From Table 2, it should be noted that hospital associated infections are not limited to those caused by bacteria, but that fungi, parasites, and viruses can be incriminated. Furthermore, nosocomial infections may involve various organ systems or anatomic sites, the genitourinary tract (38%) and lower respiratory tract (20%) being the most common sites of infection.

In addition to costs, nosocomial infections represent important and potentially preventable causes of death. Data from the Special Study Group on Gram-Negative Rod Bacteremia, which were based upon compilations from the literature and on input from the Center for Disease Control (CDC) NNIS hospitals, the rate of Gram-negative bacteremia was estimated to be 1.97 per 1000 hospital admissions in 1972.[9] More recently Scheckler has reported an incidence of Gram-negative bacteremia of 1.8 per 1000 admissions in a community hospital during 1970 through 1973.[10] Application of this figure to the approximately 37 million patients discharged annually from U.S. hospitals provides an estimate of 66,600 cases. In Scheckler's study, septicemia-related mortality was 20.3%. Based on these calculations, which may represent underestimates, there would have been approximately 13,500 deaths attributable to Gram-negative bacillary bacteremia in 1976. Based on data such as these, are we still participating in a "massacre" as described by Semmelweis in his paranoid state?

From the experiences of Semmelweis and Lister, the assumption is made that many if not most hospital associated infections are preventable. Eickhoff has pointed out that there is some evidence suggesting that the potential for prevention of nosocomial infection may not be as great as thought.[11] McGowan et al., studying nosocomial bacteremia at Grady Memorial Hospital, reported that only 32 of 91 episodes of nosocomial bacteremia were procedure related, i.e., related to urinary catheters, respiratory,

Table 3

ESTIMATED DIRECT HOSPITAL COSTS ATTRIBUTABLE TO TREATMENT OF PERSONS WITH NOSOCOMIAL INFECTIONS IN THE U.S. IN 1977[a]

Measure of cost	Infections							
	Bacteremia	Upper respiratory	Lower respiratory	Enteric	Genitourinary	CNS	Other	Total
Estimated prolongation of stay per patient (days)	7	0.5	4	2	1.2	5	4.2	—
Estimated per day cost (dollars)	175	143	208	175	143	175	143	—
Total prolongation of hospital stay (thousands of days)	1354	6	950	9	991	23	3114	6450
Total cost (millions of dollars)	237	0.8	198	1.6	142	4	445	1028

[a] Costs attributable to physicians' fees or loss of productive activity are not included in the estimates.

Table 4
CLASSES OF MICROORGANISMS
INCRIMINATED IN ENDEMIC OR EPIDEMIC
NOSOCOMIAL INFECTIONS

Class of agent	Specific organism[a]
Viruses	Herpes virus: cytomegalovirus, EB virus, herpes virus type 1
	Myxovirus: influenza, parainfluenza, respiratory syncytial virus, rubeola
	Varicella-zoster
	Hepatitis B
	Rubella
Chylamidia	*C. trachomatis*
Bacteria	Gram-positive cocci: *Streptococcus pyogenes*, *S. pneumoniae*, *S. aureus*
	Gram-positive bacilli: Clostridia
	Gram-negative bacilli: virtually all aerobes and anaerobes, including *Legionella pneumophila*,
	Mycobacterium: Mycobacterium tuberculosis, *M. fortuitum* complex
	Nocardia:
Fungi	
Protozoa	*Toxoplasma gondii*
	Pneumocystis carnii

[a]   The list is not inclusive, only illustrative.

I.V. therapy, or total parenteral hyperalimentation.[12] Furthermore, no deviation from established protocols could be identified in 25 of the 32 procedure-related bacteremias. To counterbalance this pessimistic view, there are several reports which suggest that surveillance programs which emphasize in-service education and awareness are effective.[13,14] The implementation of a program of infection surveillance and control at the Milwaukee County General Hospital resulted in a decrease in prevalence of nosocomial infection from 14% in 1970 before the program to 7.6% in 1972.[13]

The CDC has a large study in progress, the Study on the Efficacy of Nosocomial Infection Control (SENIC) which will be of enormous potential, since it may provide evidence for the relative efficacy of many currently recommended procedures.[15]

THE PARASITE

A compilation of microorganisms which have produced disease in the hospital setting is extremely long; Table 4 is a partial list. There are generalizations which can be made with respect to microorganisms which are likely to cause endemic or epidemic nosocomial infections; the organisms are likely to be ubiquitous in distribution, either being common within the environment or belonging to the indigenous microflora of the host; the organisms are likely to be resistant to commonly employed antimicrobial agents.

The combination of improved identification of microorganisms by diagnostic laboratories and increased frequency of their isolation from clinical specimens has resulted in a striking increase in the recognition of heretofore unappreciated organisms as serious human pathogens. For example, in the past, the procedures for the identification of aerobic Gram-negative bacilli were designed primarily to enable rapid detection of *Salmonella* sp. and *Shigella* sp. from fecal specimens and *Klebsiella pneumoniae* from sputum, lumping of the remaining organisms as "coliforms". Today, members of four families of aerobic Gram-negative bacilli as well as a large miscellaneous group (Enterobacteriaceae, *Aeromonas*, *Pseudomonas*, Comamonas, and the miscellaneous organisms, *Acinetobacter*, Eikenella, *Alcaligenes*, *Achromobacter*, *Flavobacterium*, and *Moraxella*) have all been incriminated as potential human pathogens.

It may well be asked why serious generalized infections by such organisms have become increasingly common. These bacteria owe much to their antibiotic multiresistance, and the selective effect of indiscriminate antibiotic treatment is often to blame for giving them a chance. However, the main cause lies with the host.

The causative agents are present both in the exogenous environment to which patients and personnel are exposed and in the endogenous environment of the GI tract. Many of the causative organisms not only are ubiquitous, but are psychrophilic or cryophilic. The growth of pseudomonads and aeromonads in moist environments or water is well recognized by microbiologists, but often is overlooked when the hospital environment is being assessed. For example, refrigerators, ice machines, faucet aerators, and sink drains in intensive care units may be the source of more pseudomonads than a patient with *Pseudomonas* pneumonia. Great concern may be directed toward the isolation of such a patient, whereas no one is concerned with these other sources with which personnel have frequent contact. As another example, the patient with leukemia, who is profoundly neutropenic as a consequence of his treatment is placed in protective isolation, along with his vases of flowers which often are heavily contaminated with pseudomonads. Although personnel may wear gloves while handling the patient, they seldom do so while handling the flowers. It is important to recognize that hospital associated infections do not necessarily represent breaks in technique on the part of hospital personnel.

Endogenous sources or organisms also must be considered. Infection around arteriovenous cannulae is an important cause of morbidity in patients treated by intermittent hemodialysis.[16] A bacteriological survey of patients and staff by means of routine culture of shunt, nasal, throat, axillary, chest, and perineal swabs showed that the majority of infections were caused by *Staphylococcus aureus*. Bacteriophage typing of the isolates showed that auto-infection was responsible for 81%, while cross-infection from patient to patient was found in 19%. Transfer from staff to patient was not demonstrated.

MODES OF TRANSMISSION

Recognizing these reservoirs (exogenous and endogenous), the modes of transfer to susceptible hosts are multiple. Vehicles such as water, milk, food, aerosols, or inanimate objects, have all been incriminated on occasion in direct spread.

Most bacteria and the hepatitis viruses are transmitted primarily by contact spread; *Streptococcus pneumoniae*, respiratory viruses, *Mycobacterium tuberculosis* and *Aspergillus* are spread by the airborne route.

Maki, as well as others, have studied hand carriage of nosocomial pathogens by medical personnel.[17] Some 44% of personnel randomly sampled carried Gram-negative bacilli, and 11% carried *Staphylococcus aureus*. Culturing serially showed that all persons, at various times, carried Gram-negative bacilli, and two thirds carried *S. aureus*. However, carriage of both Gram-negative bacilli and *S. aureus* was typically transient.

Table 5
PHARYNGEAL COLONIZATION WITH AEROBIC
GRAM-NEGATIVE BACILLI

Study group	Number of subjects	Cultures containing Gram-negative bacilli[a] (%)
Normal subjects		
Nonhospital associated	82	2
Hospital associated	47	2
Patients		
Psychiatry service	20	0
Moderately ill	81	16
Moribund	23	57

[a] Results based upon single culture surveys.

THE HOST

The normal host defense mechanisms may be summarized as:

1. Protection provided by normal antimicrobial flora
2. Anatomical barriers and secretions
3. Inflammatory response
4. Immune response: humoral and cellular
5. Reticuloendothelial system

The administration of "broad-spectrum" antimicrobial agents may suppress components of the normal host microbial flora and allow for the emergence of aerobic Gram-negative bacilli, clostridia, or fungi. Alterations in the balance of interbacterial antagonism may be partially responsible for this occurrence.[18] In addition, there are other host factors which prevent or minimize colonization of various areas with Gram-negative bacilli which are modified independently of antibiotics. The mechanisms underlying such "colonization immunity" remain to be defined, but there is clear evidence that patients who become "very ill" or moribund commonly become colonized with Gram-negative bacilli without having received antibiotics, (see Table 5).[19,20]

Anatomical barriers may be circumvented by means beyond those which mechanically transgress their integrity. For example, ventilatory equipment which incorporates nebulizers into its design will deliver aerosols of $5\mu g$ or less to the patient. Such equipment is designed to enable delivery of moisture to the level of the respiratory bronchioles and alveoli. If the fluid being nebulized is contaminated, the contaminating organisms also will be delivered to these areas, thereby bypassing the protective mechanism of the mucociliary apparatus. In a discussion of both the inflammatory and immune responses, the influence of the milieu in which the cells are to function must be considered. Most in vitro observations and those in animals involve normal environments. It has been shown that the severe hypophosphatemia which may accompany parenteral hyperalimentation precludes normal neutrophil function.[21] Newberry et al. have shown that both the responsiveness to phytohemagglutinin and the induction of interferon production by lymphocytes in response to Newcastle disease virus are suppressed when lymphocytes are placed in uremic serum.[22,23] Likewise, the responsiveness of normal lymphocytes to phytohemagglutinin is suppressed in the presence of serum obtained from patients with jaundice.[24]

The critical role which devitalized tissue, foreign materials, or implants may have in altering host defenses is an area which is often overlooked, even by the surgeon whose activities are dependent upon such materials. The interrelating influence of devitalized tissue and foreign bodies on susceptibility of wounds to developing infection is well demonstrated by the studies of Altemeier and Furste.[25] They observed that the minimal lethal dose of *Clostridium perfringens* for guinea pigs was decreased 1000-fold when associated with crushed muscle and 1 million-fold when sterile dirt was added to the crushed muscle. Suture material also can act as a foreign body. In humans, a minimum of 1 to 5 million staphylococci are required to produce visible suppuration after intradermal injection, whereas only 100 to 10,000 organisms are required if they are introduced into the skin as a buried silk suture.[26] The same general phenomenon is encountered with all bacteria.

The role of multiple host factors in a system as complex as the human is more difficult to assess accurately, but there are observations which clearly imply their importance. In a prospective study of 213 patients admitted to a medical intensive care unit, cultures of the oropharynx obtained from 95 patients (45%) revealed aerobic Gram-negative bacilli. Most factors associated with colonization were the presence of underlying respiratory tract disease, antimicrobial therapy, coma, hypotension, tracheal intubation, acidosis, azotemia, and either leukocytosis or leukopenia.[27] Nosocomial respiratory infections occurred in 23% of colonized patients, but in only 3.3% of noncolonized patients. In a study designed to assess factors which predispose to the development of bacteriuria during indwelling urethral catheterization, Garibaldi and associates found that bacteriuria was most common patients who were female, elderly, and who had critical underlying illnesses.[28]

Host factors not only predispose to the development of aerobic Gram-negative bacillary bacteremia, but also are the most important determinants of the outcome of the disease. In the now classic studies of McCabe and Jackson, when the severity of the host's underlying disease was quantitated on a crude basis according to the anticipated duration of survival if the patient had not developed bacteremia, a marked difference in survival from Gram-negative bacillary bacteremia was observed.[29] In patients with "rapidly fatal disease", whose anticipated survival was less than 1 year (almost exclusively patients with acute leukemia, chronic leukemia in blastic crisis, far advanced cancer, or massive burns), only 9% survived Gram-negative bacillary bacteremia. In patients with "ultimately fatal disease" (estimated to be fatal within 5 years, i.e., patients with severe lupus erythematosus, myeloma, severe liver disease, or endstage renal disease), survival rate improved to 34%. In patients with nonfatal underlying disease, the survival rate was 89%. The importance of such classification in assessing factors such as antimicrobial therapy is illustrated by the observations of Bryant et al. (see Table 6).[30] From Table 6, it is apparent that valid conclusions regarding many aspects of treatment can be reached only when the importance of the variation in host factors is recognized and either controlled or appropriately matched.

Although infections could not occur in the absence of the offending microorganisms, host factors exert the major role in determining not only the occurrence of infection and disease, but also the outcome of such disease.

INFECTION CONTROL PROGRAM

The goal of infection control is the control of infection. Surveillance, audits, and teaching are essential, but are merely means to the end. For individuals interested in the control of hospital associated infections, it is essential not to lose sight of the goal. Begin to question, is this procedure or practice effective and place emphasis on documentation of effectiveness as measured by outcome.

Table 6
EFFECT OF APPROPRIATE
ANTIBIOTIC THERAPY ON
MORTALITY OF GRAM-NEGATIVE
BACILLARY BACTEREMIA[a]

| Disease category | Therapy (number died of total) (%) | |
	Appropriate	Inappropriate
Rapidly fatal	41/ 49 (84)	17/20 (85)
Ultimately fatal	62/149 (42)	32/48 (67)
Nonfatal	25/253 (10)	22/71 (31)

[a]   Includes data from Reference 3.

REFERENCES

1. **Nightingale, F.**, *Notes on Nursing* (D. Appleton & Co., 1860, unabridged republication), Dover Publications, New York, 1969, 10.
2. **Semmelweis, I. P.**, Vortrag uber die genesis des puerperal fiebers, vom 15 May 1850, in *Milestones in Microbiology*, Brock, T. D., Ed., American Society of Microbiology, Washington, D. C., 1961, 80.
3. **Lister, J.**, On a new method of treating compound fractures, abscess, and so forth. With observations on the conditions of suppuration, *Lancet*, 1, 326, 357, 387, 507, and 2, 95, 1867.
4. **Ogston, W. H., Cowan, H. H., and Smith, H. E.**, Alexander Ogston KCVO, Aberdeen University Press, Scotland, 1943.
5. Proceedings of the National Conference on Hospital-Acquired Staphylococcal Disease, U.S. Department of Health, Education and Welfare, Communicable Disease Center, Atlanta, Ga., 1958.
6. **Finland, M.**, Changing ecology of bacterial infections as related to antibacterial therapy, *J. Infect. Dis.*, 122, 419, 1970.
7. **Rogers, R. E.**, The changing pattern of life threatening microbial disease, *N. Engl. J. Med.*, 261, 677, 1959.
8. **Dixon, R. E.**, Effect of infections on hospital care, *Ann. Intern. Med.*, 89 (2), 749, 1978.
9. **Wolff, S. M. and Bennett, J. V.**, Gram-negative rod bacteremia, *N. Engl. J. Med.*, 291, 733, 1974.
10. **Scheckler, W. E.**, Septicemia and nosocomial infections in a community hospital, *Ann. Intern. Med.*, 89 (2), 754, 1978.
11. **Eickhoff, T. C.**, Standards for hospital infection control, *Ann. Intern. Med.*, 89 (2), 829, 1978.
12. **McGowan, J. E., Jr., Parrott, P. L., and Duty, V. P.**, Nosocomial bacteremia: potential for prevention of procedure related cases, *JAMA*, 237, 2727, 1977.
13. **Shoji, K. T., Axnick, K., and Rytel, M. W.**, Infections and antibiotic use in a large municipal hospital 1970-1972: a prospective analysis of the effectiveness of a continuous surveillance program, *Health Lab. Sci.*, 11, 283, 1974.
14. **Britt, M. R., Schleupner, C. J., and Matsumija, S.**, Severity of underlying disease as a predictor of nosocomial infection: utility in the control of nosocomial infection, *JAMA*, 239, 1047, 1978.
15. Center for Disease Control, Infection Surveillance and Control Programs in U.S. Hospital: An Assessment, 1976, Morbidity and Mortality Weekly Report 27, 139, 1978.
16. **Martin, A. M., Clunie, G. J. A., Tonkin, R. W., and Robson, J. S.**, The etiology and management of shunt infections in patients on intermittent hemodialysis, in *Dialysis and Renal Transplantation*, Kerr, D.N.S., Ed., Excerpta Medica Foundation, Int. Congr. Series No. 155, Bosten and Stols, Maastricht, The Netherlands, 1968, 67.
17. **Maki, D. G.**, Control of colonization and transmission of pathogenic bacteria in the hospital, *Ann. Intern. Med.*, 89 (2), 777, 1978.

18. **Sprunt, K. and Redman, W.**, Evidence suggesting importance of role of interbacterial inhibition in maintaining balance of normal flora, *Ann. Intern. Med.*, 68, 579, 1968.
19. **Stratford, B., Gallus, A. S., Matthiesson, A. M., and Dixson, S.**, Alteration of the superficial bacterial flora in severely ill patients, *Lancet*, 1, 68, 1968.
20. **Johanson, W. G., Jr., Pierce, A. K., and Sanford, J. P.**, Changing pharyngeal flora bacterial flora of hospitalized patients, *N. Engl. J. Med.*, 281, 1137, 1969.
21. **Craddock, P. R., Yawata, Y., van Santen, L., Gilbustadt, S., Silvis, S., and Jacob, H. S.**, Acquired phagocyte dysfunction. A complication of the hypophosphatemia of parenteral hyperalimentation, *N. Engl. J. Med.*, 290, 1403, 1974.
22. **Newberry, W. M. and Sanford, J. P.**, Defective cellular immunity in renal failure: depression of reactivity of lymphocytes to phytohemagglutinin by renal failure serum, *J. Clin. Invest.*, 50, 1262, 1971.
23. **Sanders, C. V., Jr., Luby, J. P., Sanford, J. P., and Hull, A. R.**, Suppression of interferon response in lymphocytes from patients with uremia, *J. Lab. Clin. Med.*, 77, 768, 1971.
24. **Newberry, W. M., Shorey, J. W., Sanford, J. P., and Combes, B.**, Depression of lymphocyte reactivity to phytohemagglutinin by serum from patients with liver disease, *Cell. Immunol.*, 6, 87, 1973.
25. **Altemeier, W. A. and Furste, W. L.**, Studies in virulence of *Clostridium welchii*, *Surgery*, 25, 12, 1949.
26. **Elek, S. D. and Conen, P. E.**, The virulence of *Staphylococcus pyogenes* for man: a study of the problem of wound infection, *Br. J. Exp. Pathol.*, 38, 573, 1957.
27. **Johanson, W. G., Jr., Pierce, A. K., Sanford, J. P., and Thomas, G. D.**, Nosocomial respiratory infections with Gram-negative bacilli, *Ann. Intern. Med.*, 77, 710, 1972.
28. **Garibaldi, R. A., Burke, J. P., Dickman, M. L., and Smith, C. B.**, Factors predisposing to bacteriuria during indwelling urethral catheterization, *N. Engl. J. Med.*, 291, 215, 1974.
29. **McCabe, W. R. and Jackson, G. G.**, Gram-negative bacteremia. I. Etiology and ecology, *Arch. Intern. Med.*, 110, 847, 1962.
30. **Bryant, R. E., Hood, A. F., Hood, C. F., and Koenig, M. G.**, Factors affecting mortality of gram-negative rod bacteremia, *Arch. Intern. Med.*, 127, 120, 1971.

THE EFFECTIVE PHYSICIAN EPIDEMIOLOGIST

William Schaffner

INTRODUCTION

"An ounce of prevention is worth a pound of cure."

Folk Saying

"It may seem a strange principle to enunciate as the very first requirement in a hospital that it should do the sick no harm."

Florence Nightingale

The position of hospital physician epidemiologist is of recent vintage, and its functions are still somewhat ill-defined. The designation often evokes puzzlement that goes beyond the universal difficulties with its spelling. When hospitals first were encouraged to establish infection control programs, it soon became apparent that it was desirable for a physician to provide leadership within each institution. Originally called "infection control officers", this term was discarded because it suggested a police function. Instead, the more neutral term "hospital epidemiologist" was selected. The choice was a happy one. The title evokes a studious and nonthreatening image; it also emphasizes the incumbent's concern for the entire population of patients, staff, and visitors encompassed by the hospital.

Two personal characteristics are basic to an effectively functioning hospital epidemiologist. First, the individual should be dedicated to the concept of prevention. It is a truism to say that the goal of an infection control program is to prevent as many hospital associated infections as possible. However, this orientation is somewhat foreign to many clinicians who are trained primarily in the diagnosis and treatment of established disease. Thus, the personal satisfactions of the job come not from healing the sick, but from the hope that one's efforts have kept some persons well, a considerably more ephemeral reward. Further, in order to prevent infection, the epidemiologist must deal less with individuals and more with groups of persons. For example, the clinician will be very concerned with the specific details of a *Klebsiella* pneumonia which occurred while his or her patient was in the medical intensive care unit. In contrast, the focus of the epidemiologist will be on the entire group of patients and personnel in the intensive care unit in order to determine how the *Klebsiella* strain is being transmitted in the unit and what means are available to interrupt its spread. Sustaining an interest in groups of mostly uninfected persons rather than individual ill patients is not easy. Nevertheless, without it, one cannot aspire to success as a hospital epidemiologist.

Secondly, the epidemiologist ought to be a person who has the interpersonal skills necessary to implement improved infection control practices in the institution. This function calls for the delicate diplomatic techniques of a "change agent". The most critical features of an infection control program directly involve patient care practices, often the behavior of physicians. Skill in the arts of education, persuasion, and even gentle, but firm, coercion are highly valued in successful hospital epidemiologists.

Professional Background

Most epidemiologists are clinicians in active practice at the hospital. Although microbiologists and pathologists are sometimes selected, they generally enjoy less credibility on the patient care divisions where most of the "action" is. The author has met effective hospital epidemiologists of all clinical specialities. Subspecialty training in infectious diseases is not a prerequisite, but a "special" fondness for infectious illness, microbes, and antibiotic therapy seems to be a common characteristic. In addition, whatever the physician's clinical practice, a broad professional awareness must be cultivated. Nosocomial infections respect no specialty and occur on all patient divisions: the nursery, the postpartum floor, the surgical recovery room, the medical ward, etc. The epidemiologist's inquisitiveness should be equal to the inventiveness of microorganisms in finding ecologic niches in our hospitals.

TRAINING IN HOSPITAL EPIDEMIOLOGY

Obviously, there is much to infection control which is not taught in medical school. One can begin to acquire additional sophistication in the two traditional ways, by reading and attending courses. The literature related to the occurrence, transmission, and control of nosocomial infections is voluminous and scattered throughout many journals. Thus, the importance of this volume and a recently published text by Bennett and Brachman cannot be overestimated.[1] For the first time, both the novice and the seasoned epidemiologist have summaries of the scientific and practical issues in the field readily at hand. The selected bibliography at the end of this chapter offers opportunities for further reading.

Numerous short courses on infection control are now being given around the country. These offerings vary in quality, but have the advantages of brevity (usually 1 or 2 days) and modest expense. They also present the opportunity to question the speakers informally about one's own problems. There are, as yet, almost no courses available which are specifically designed for the needs of physician-epidemiologists. An exception is a course held periodically at the University of Virginia in Charlottesville. Inquiries should be directed to the editor of this book. The most comprehensive course, 8 days in duration, is given at the Center for Disease Control (CDC). Although designed primarily for nurses, physicians may enroll. Send inquiries to the CDC in Atlanta regarding the course "Surveillance, Prevention, and Control of Nosocomial Infections". Beginners may also have the opportunity to visit more experienced hospital epidemiologists in their area to inspect functioning infection control programs.

ADMINISTRATIVE RELATIONSHIPS

The hospital epidemiologist usually chairs the institution's Infection Control Committee. Therefore, there still is a tendency for hospital administrators to regard this position as similar to chairing other hospital committees, i.e., the chair rotates to a new physician each year, and it represents service donated to the hospital. The positions are not analogous. To be effective, the hospital epidemiologist must spend a regular period of time in the hospital each week supervising diverse infection control activities. Suspected outbreaks of infection and other problems will make additional visits necessary. The new epidemiologist will undertake a learning program to become knowledgable in infection control theory and practice. Thus, the position should not rotate, but be considered a long-term committment. It is only over time that the epidemiologist will be able to develop a credible "image" among the professional staff. Also, the implementation of infection control initiatives is a long-term process; continuity is essential.

For all these reasons, the hospital epidemiologist should be paid for performing these tasks. This concept is being accepted by an ever-increasing number of hospitals.

In addition to the epidemiologist's compensation, a budget is required to pay for nurse-epidemiologists, secretarial support, books and journal subscriptions, travel to meetings and courses, and the telephone (long-distance calls provide immediate, inexpensive, expert consultative advice). The administrative details vary considerably from hospital to hospital, and it is important that the specific arrangements be clearly understood by all parties at the outset. Because circumstances change, an annual review of the budget is helpful in planning the coming year's activities.

FUNCTIONS

The subsequent chapters provide detailed discussions of the many facets of a hospital infection control program for which the epidemiologist is expected to provide leadership. The following comments are of a more anecdotal nature.

The beginning hospital epidemiologist is likely to discover that infection control practices in his or her institution have been somewhat neglected and that much needs to be done. Priorities are essential; everything cannot be done at once. It is vitally important to focus on those selected patient care procedures which are widely recognized to be proven risk factors for nosocomial infections. Foremost among these are hospital policies regarding:

1. I.V. catheter insertion and care
2. Bladder catheter insertion and care
3. Cleaning of inhalation therapy machines

In addition, some method of surveillance of nosocomial infections should be instituted.

As a second order of priority, the following are suggested:

1. Review of disinfection and sterilization procedures in all hospital units
2. The acceptance of a standard patient isolation policy
3. Reduce or eliminate routine bacteriological monitoring of the inanimate environment and hospital personnel

As a third priority: everything else. Ironically, many questions arise from this relatively low-priority area (handling of soiled linen is a favorite). Some questions can be answered quickly; others should be deferred in order that their solution not drain scarce resources better devoted to higher priority issues. This may be the first test of an epidemiologist's diplomatic skills.

The epidemiologist becomes a problem seeker and solver, an ombudsperson for good infection control practices throughout the institution. One device to develop a "feel" for the hospital is to make "infection control rounds" with the nurse-epidemiologist on different units each week. The various patient care divisions are natural targets, but other areas (the laboratories, surgical suite, radiology, laundry, kitchen, solid waste disposal area, etc.) ought not be neglected. In so doing, the infection control team soon will develop a more intimate acquaintance with people and practices throughout the hospital than any chief of service or administrator. In turn, the team will develop recognition as an important resource to be contacted when questions arise. The discussions which occur with the staff during rounds can have an educational impact which should not be underestimated.

A strong skeleton of the hospital's infection control program will grow out of the work on the high-priority issues and the solutions to the questions discussed on rounds.

A written infection control manual will flesh out the program with contributions coming from all departments. Because infection control is the proper concern of all persons working in the institution, it is important that the supervisors of all units provide their own first drafts for the sections of the manual which pertain to their activities. The infection control practitioners (ICP) can provide helpful guidance during this procedure. We have found that this process focuses the hospital staff on the goal of preventing infections.

A word of caution, however. Infection control manuals do not prevent infections; guard against a paper-oriented program. The manual ought to describe precisely what actually is done on each unit. Again, resist the urge to cover all areas at once; begin with those areas where the risk of acquiring nosocomial infections is high (e.g., intensive care units) and move deliberately to areas of lesser risk. Our manual required over 2 years to compile. Each section ought to be reviewed by the epidemiologist, and if less-than-adequate practices are revealed, this presents a marvelous opportunity to begin the process of change.

> "Habit is . . . not to be flung out of the window by any man, but coaxed downstairs a step at a time."
>
> Mark Twain

The persuasive talents of the epidemiologist are needed to convince physicians to change established habits of practice. Presentations to the entire medical staff and hospital committees supported by literature citations and graphs or tables of appropriate local surveillance data are useful. Conversations with leaders on the attending staff or with recalcitrant physicians can gain valued support for your suggestions (or at least soften the opposition). This gradual method of winning endorsement is recommended for changes which directly involve the way individual doctors care for individual patients. The adoption of policies requiring closed drainage of bladder catheters or of changing I.V. infusion sites every 48 to 72 hr would be examples.

> "It is easier to get forgiveness than permission."
>
> Anonymous

On the other hand, there are instances where direct, incisive action can result in rapid policy change. The comparatively ineffective disinfectants, mercurochrome and aqueous benzalkonium chloride, were removed from Vanderbilt University Hospital after only a single administrator was convinced the policy was appropriate. The diplomatic focus was shifted to the individual patient care units where appropriate substitutions and education in their use were provided for the nursing staff. A great deal of debate among the medical staff was avoided; only two or three passionate users of these agents had to be placated after the fact.

A word about the microbiology laboratory: the technologists in the laboratory provide data essential to the infection control effort. The closer the relationship between the infection control team and the laboratory, the better. Visit it often; talk with the technologists. Occasional in-service education presentations by the epidemiologist will be greatly appreciate and help ensure their cooperation. In turn, the epidemiologist will learn more clinical microbiology, painlessly.

The Infection Control Committee is an administrative structure required by the Joint Commission on Accreditation of Hospitals (JCAH). After chairing such a committee for 10 years, I am still tinkering with how best to use this device. Its precise function will, in all likelihood, evolve along lines determined by the inclinations of the epidemiologist. Our committee functions best as a sounding board and as an arbiter of policy. The members freely offer practical suggestions on the implications of changes in hospital procedures under discussion. They also raise questions for further investigation. The committee does not bog down in discussions of infections in individual patients (that is the function of the ICP and epidemiologist). The formal motions passed by the committee go to the Hospital Medical Board for final endorsement. These formal notifications are the culmination of extensive work by the infection control nurse and epidemiologist on the "front lines" in the hospital and by discussion in the committee. In this way, the committee has earned credibility with the Board, submitting only proposals that already have earned a consensus of acceptance in the hospital community.

> "Soap and water and common sense are the best disinfectants."
>
> Sir William Osler

Lastly, I would emphasize the educational function of personal example. Every day, during his or her clinical practice, the epidemiologist has the opportunity to "bear witness" for infection control. I ostentatiously wash my hands before and after every patient contact. This time-honored ablution remains the most effective means of interrupting the spread of microorganisms in the hospital, especially Gram-negative bacilli which cause the majority of contemporary nosocomial infections. The epidemiologist must practice what is preached, or who else shall?

THE EPIDEMIOLOGIST AFIELD

The epidemiologist will soon find that, in this institution devoted to the healing arts, he or she has become the single person most committed to prevention. This committment can extend beyond an interest in infectious diseases. In cooperation with the Employee Health Service, screening programs for a number of chronic noninfectious diseases may be established. These include hypertension, carcinoma of the breast, and diabetes, among others. These efforts are usually well received by the employees and help to demonstrate that their employer, the hospital, is interested in their welfare. My first success was in securing the removal of all cigarette machines from the hospital. This was an appropriate concern for, after all, the title was not "infection control officer", but hospital epidemiologist!

> "It is better to avert a malady with care than to use physic after it has appeared."
>
> Shao Tze

BIBLIOGRAPHY

Bennett, J. V. and Brachman, P. S., Eds., *Hospital Infections,* Little, Brown, Boston, 1979.

Barrett-Connor, E., Brandt, S. L., Simon, H. J., and Dechairo, D. C., Eds., *Epidemiology for the Infection Control Nurse,* C. V. Mosby, St. Louis, 1978.

American College of Surgeons, *Manual on Control of Infection in Surgical Patients,* Lippincott, Philadelphia, 1976.

Brachman, P. S. and Eickhoff, T. C., Eds., *Proceedings of the International Conference on Nosocomial Infections,* American Hospital Association, Chicago, 1970.

Craig, C. P. and Reifsnyder, D. N., Eds., *Departmental Procedures for Infection Control Programs,* Medical Economics, Oradell, N.J., 1977.

Kunin, C. M., *Detection, Prevention, and Management of Urinary Tract Infection,* 2nd ed., Lea & Febiger, Philadelphia, 1979.

Samuels, T. M., Swidler, H. J., and Hawkins, P. A., *Infection Control in Hospitals. An Annotated Bibliography 1963-1973,* The 3M Company, Medical Products Division, St. Paul, Minn., 1975.

Samuels, T. M., Hawkins, P. A., and Carver, E. J., *Infection Control in Hospitals. An Annotated Bibliography 1974-June 1976,* Vol. 2, The 3M Company, Medical Products Division, St. Paul, Minn, 1976.

Center for Disease Control Publications,* Morbidity and Mortality Weekly Report, National Nosocomial Infections Study Surveillance Reports, Atlanta, Ga.

Hospital Infection Control (periodical), published monthly by American Health Consultants, 67 Peachtree Park Drive, NE, Atlanta, Ga., 30309.

American Journal of Infection Control (periodical), published by C. V. Mosby, 11830 Westline Industrial Drive, St. Louis, Mo., 63141.

The Journal of Hospital Infection (British periodical), Academic Press, 111 Fifth Avenue, New York, 10003.

Infection Control (periodical), published by Charles B. Slack, 6900 Grove Road, Thorofare, N.J., 08086.

Castle, M., *Hospital Infection Control. Principles and Practice,* John Wiley & Sons, New York, 1980.

* You will be placed on mailing list on request, no charge.

THE INFECTION CONTROL PRACTITIONER

C. A. Osterman

INTRODUCTION

The infection control practitioner (ICP) is the backbone of any infection control program.[1] While a program is more complete and more effective when it includes a physician with specific responsibility for infection control, many programs function quite well without benefit of such a "luxury". The reverse is not true. This chapter will examine the development of the unique role and responsibilities of the ICP, and it will review what a hospital should seek in hiring a practitioner and what the prospective ICP should expect upon entry into the field of hospital infection control.

HISTORICAL

The relatively new field of hospital infection control had its beginning in England in the late 1950s when Dr. Brendan Moore, Director of the Public Health Laboratory in Exeter, had a nurse in Torbay Hospital appointed as "infection control sister".[2,3] A year later, a second sister was appointed at the Exeter Hospital through Dr. Moore's efforts. The mission of the two nurses was to improve efforts to combat and control the widespread problem of hospital acquired staphylococcal infection. Dr. Moore had already witnessed a number of such epidemics in English hospitals and had been consulted to investigate and control them. Since 1955, he had been preparing detailed quarterly reports for his Control of Infection Committee which in his estimation were no more than retrospective chronicles of hospital infected patients and were achieving very little in terms of controlling infection.[4] His growing disenchantment with this method of "hospital infection control" led him to the concept of the full-time ("whole time") sister. Such persons had been suggested by others, though most authors generally underestimated the time requirements for effective infection control.[5] Dr. Moore also thought that senior sisters, experienced clinical nurses who enjoyed the respect of their colleagues in the hospitals, would not only aid colleagues in their observations, but would also gain the staff's compliance with "control efforts". Thus, in 1959, the first infection control nurse came into existence.

While many other significant events may be cited as earlier infection control efforts, i.e., the development of antibiotics two decades earlier or Dr. Ignaz Semelweiss's discovery of the cause of puerperal sepsis a century earlier, none is seen as having triggered the development of a whole new professional subspecialty as did those fateful events in England some 25 years ago. Ironically, to Dr. Moore (Association for Practitioners in Infection Control [APIC] Boston Conference of 1978), " . . . those events did not seem all that significant at the time . . . ".

Although growth of the subspecialty has perhaps been most dramatic in North America, it is directly attributable to the "seeds" planted in the "soil" of the hospitals in Great Britain. The U.S. followed England's lead into the field of infection control in 1963 with the appointment of the first infection control nurse (ICN), Kathryn Wenzel (Owen), R.N., at Stanford University, Stanford, Calif. She described her new role as one of case finding of patients who became infected while in the hospital.[1] No doubt her publication contributed to the rapid influx of nurses into a new area of interest.

CHANGING ROLE

The new role for nurses which Kathryn Wenzel (Owen) and others have pioneered has evolved into a multifaceted and diverse one. Obvious signs of growth included the increasing number of individuals entering the field in proportions which soon warranted the formation of a professional organization to answer their particular interests, the APIC (see chapter entitled Association for Practitioners in Infection Control). Additional signs were the educational programs, such as Center for Disease Control (CDC) courses on infection control (see chapter entitled "The Center for Disease Control") and the courses of the Virginia State Health Department — University of Virginia Training Program[6] (initially sponsored by the CDC as a pilot project), which address the practitioner's basic and continuing educational needs, and efforts by APIC to develop certification requirements for practitioners which will ultimately determine "standards of practice" for all who practice infection control.

Traditionally, the ICPs role has been predominantly filled by registered nurses and by women.* Nurses, by virtue of their training and experience, are well suited for the practice of infection control in the hospital, being intimately involved in patient care and policy formulation. A large majority of individuals in the field today (85 to 90%) are indeed R.N.s. However, as the field is growing, there is also a trend of "non-nurses" (medical technologists, sanitarians, pharmacists, etc.) entering infection control. They bring with them varied backgrounds and valuable talents, as well as new perspectives on dealing with the changing problems of controlling infections. For example, emphasis of nursing education is primarily on patient care and is generally weak in the areas of microbiology and pharmacology, with education in the area of statistics generally nonexistent; the medical technologist's education, on the other hand, is generally strong on all phases of microbiology, pathology, and biochemistry, with little or no emphasis on patient contact. While the pharmacists' education may include facets of both the nurses' and the medical technologists' education, by far the strongest emphasis is placed on a thorough understanding of the pharmacology, indications, and efficacy of drugs. Even those in fields not traditionally involved in hospital health care, e.g., biostatistics and data processing (see chapters entitled "The Computers and Infection Surveillance" and "Choosing the Correct Statistical Tests") must be added to the growing list of resource individuals whose special education and talents are needed to aid in optimal analysis of data collected through surveillance and research. In a field far too complex to be left in the hands of one discipline, it is certainly appropriate to encourage others to participate in the search for solutions to health care problems.

Subtle signs that have accompanied such changes in the ICPs role may be witnessed in the transition that the ICPs title has undergone. Beginning as "infection control sister/nurse", it later became the "nurse-epidemiologist". Early efforts to eliminate the connotation nurse from the title by adopting "infection control officer" were equally unsatisfactory because of the association of the term officer with a policeman's or military image. The evolution continued and the title of "infection control practitioner" or "infection control coordinator" has been widely supported by both nurses and nonnurses alike.

As a result of the widening scope of the field of hospital epidemiology, today a growing number of physicians are also entering and practicing in the field of infection control. Although technically they too are infection control "practitioners" they fulfill a different role already addressed (see chapter entitled "The Effective Physician Epi-

---

* The pronoun "he" as used in this chapter refers to all practitioners and is used with no sexual bias or chauvenistic intent.

demiologist"). Physicians are mentioned here primarily in order to present the proper perspective of their role in relation to that of the ICP, i.e., to direct the overall infection control program. The addition of a physician to an infection control program definitely influences and alters the role of the ICP from what it would have been in his absence. A physician brings "clout" to a program, making possible accomplishments that might not otherwise be likely, particularly in the area of policy or procedure changes which directly affect the medical staff. The ICP alone might not be able to gain the cooperation of the medical staff as readily as a physician can. Unquestionably, the physician and ICP must be a compatible pair if they are to be an effective team.

The role of today's ICP is a continually changing one responding to newly identified needs in the entire health care field. This then demands that the practitioner be motivated by a professional commitment to investigative research, a desire to bring that research to practical application in the hospital, and a desire to share knowledge gained with others in the field to maximize the usefulness of that information in the broadest sense. Motivation and interest are the two principle drives required of the practitioner.

DIVERSITY OF RESPONSIBILITIES

An Investigator ("Super-Sleuth")

Initially the role which was given those early "sisters" was quite simple in scope, although a formidable challenge to nurses in times when physicians were not all accustomed to nor very tolerant of having their actions reviewed by anyone, much less by nurses. They were charged with the responsibility of finding, documenting, and reporting to Dr. Moore all patients with staphylococcal infections in the hospital, so that control measures (isolation, etc.) could be promptly instituted; their job was essentially surveillance, case finding, and reporting. The same three elements are still basic to infection control today, though many others have been added. Without some form of surveillance, it is impossible to know what or where the infection problems are occurring in the hospital. It may also be difficult to impossible to know when or where clustering of infections is occurring which may signal a common source outbreak. Surveillance provides data on infection rates, necessary in any effort to bring about changes in policies or procedures to improve infection control in the hospital. Data are essential to demonstrate the size of a problem in the appraisal of whether or not changes are indicated (see chapter entitled "Surveillance and Reporting of Hospital Acquired Infection").

Educator/Teacher

The early English sisters had relatively little autonomy in carrying out their infection control responsibilities compared to their modern counterparts on the other side of the Atlantic. The former had to conduct their surveillance diligently and report their findings, without concerning themselves with many of the tasks which have since become the responsibility of the ICP. Even then, those sisters had to assert themselves when encountering a physician who balked at their insistance on his abiding by the control measures which they were responsible for implementing.

There is little doubt that the sisters conducted some teaching of basic infection control principles, such as handwashing and aseptic and isolation techniques in the course of their rounds. However, it must be borne in mind that although there were fewer principles established at that time, it must nevertheless have demanded at least as much of their time devoted to this important aspect of infection control as that demanded of today's practitioner. Infection control awareness was probably not so widespread as it is today, as a result of the presence of so many infection control programs. However, the challenge of the ICP of today is to find innovative and imaginative ways to teach the current infection control concepts to all the various departments in a modern hospital and then reteach them as newer concepts are developed through research. Every infection control program should include the following educational goals: new employee orientation classes on infection control, on-going in-service education at all levels to all departments, and participation in the education of nursing and medical students, as well as the education of all the health care specialties in institutions having such programs. In addition, in teaching hospitals having large support service departments, each of these must be taught their specific roles in relation to infection control at a level of understanding, including maintenance and volunteer services. The practitioner's educational efforts should also include patient and family teaching when appropriate. In the meanwhile, the ICP must continue to seek self education and growth to maintain knowledge and expertise.

Consultant

As the "resident expert" on infection control matters, the ICP is a resource person to the entire hospital staff and possesses unique knowledge or has access to additional resources to assist with problems. This role requires that the ICP maintain up-to-date files of well-organized resource material. The practitioner is in close contact with the hospital's staff which then becomes better acquainted with the ICP. The interaction often provides an opportunity for the staff members to raise related questions or to bring information to the attention of the practitioner before a "problem" surfaces. It is also an excellent opportunity for the ICP to do a little public relations work by dispensing some genuine praise. It may take the form of a simple expression of gratitude for their "cooperation in the face of shortages of staff" . . . or praising their "dedicated adherence to isolation policies" . . . or reviewing the monthly nosocomial infection report, "noting their unit's continuing low infection rates" and crediting them with "obviously doing something *right* ". All too often the practitioner is seen as a *correction* officer, remanding to the staff on faulty practices. Such a perception by hospital personnel can easily lead to resentment toward the practitioner and the program itself.

Liaison

The hospital's Infection Control Committee must rely on the ICP for the information which it must analyze, discuss, and act upon. Once particular action has been recommended by the committee, that information must then be disseminated to the hospital's staff if the committee's recommendations are to become a reality in practice. As a member of the Infection Control Committee, accountable to the chairman of that committee or to the hospital epidemiologist, the ICP performs a liaison role as the eyes, ears, voice, and "shoeleather epidemiologist" of the Infection Control Committee. Suffice it to say, that the practitioner will do well to cultivate a keen sense of tactfulness and diplomacy, particularly when acting in the role of liaison. Infection control issues can sometimes touch "sensitive nerves" in otherwise friendly individuals, resulting in unpleasant confrontations and defensive, negative reactions or attitudes which may be destructive to the overall infection control program. Under no circumstances must the ICP confuse *authority* delegated by the Infection Control Committee with *license* to interfere with sound medical practice or patient care. Instead the practitioner should strive to foster an atmosphere of openness in the hospital, by demonstrating assurance that confidences shared with him will neither be aired publicly nor "swept under the rug", but rather that information will be brought to the attention of proper parties concerned in a professional manner.

The ICP must also promote the concept that documentation of all the facts pertinent to a nosocomial infection does not have to be viewed as necessarily incriminating; on the contrary, nondocumentation may be far more incriminating, suggesting a desire to obscure the facts. Fear of the potential implications of documenting a nosocomial infection in their patients leads some physicians and nurses not to record the presence of infections, making the job of the ICP more difficult. Underdocumentation may also surround high-risk procedures which the patient may have undergone, further adding to the ICPs difficulties in conducting accurate surveillance.

Agent of Change

As new technology is added to health care, frequently the new hazards of infection posed by new equipment or procedures may not yet be known. Therefore, the hospital must rely on the practitioner to obtain such information from the available resources and promptly begin urging appropriate changes. The ICP, however, is not only an agent of change when assuring proper cleaning and handling of equipment, but also in a number of other more subtle ways. For example, in every teaching situation, the practitioner has an opportunity to influence attitudes and biases which may impede the progress of his infection control program. With *data* (gathered through surveillance), the ICP may be able to demonstrate that a certain procedure or piece of equipment is associated with a high rate of infection, warranting reevaluation. Concomitantly the practitioner must recognize the need for changes in his own attitude, approach, or conviction, when new evidence points in that direction. Flexibility should be the by-word, for rigid adherence to outmoded concepts may also bring about a change — a change in practitioners in that particular hospital!

As yet, few hospitals have a product/materials management individual on the staff, and they have in the past relied primarily on the purchasing agent to evaluate new or different products for the hospital. Since the purchasing agent's principle area of expertise is generally cost and supply, the products purchased by a hospital may not necessarily be the *best* products from a medical, nursing, or infection control standpoint. Instead a product which *costs less* may be the one purchased. Therefore, the ICP must play a role in reviewing (evaluating) new products for the hospital, as well as reevaluating products in use for possible replacement with better ones available. In the process of doing this, the practitioner must keep the above responsibilities in mind, i.e., balancing the various interests. If the purchase agent recommends a product which is low in price, but neglects the staff's interests, i.e., how the product will function, the hospital may purchase a product which is awkward or impossible to use properly, which could increase the risk of infection to the patient (such a product may in fact also prove to be more costly through increased breakage and waste due to its awkwardness). On the other hand, a product which is convenient and practical to use, and perhaps acceptable in terms of infection control may be exorbitantly priced. In all instances, the practitioner should insist on independent, controlled study information from the sales representative which shows the product to be in fact better compared to the product currently in use. Figure 1 illustrates the form which is in use at the University of Virginia Hospital in an effort to determine documented advantages of new products. Unfortunately, in far too many instances in the past, no such data have been available to the practitioner to make a decision based on sound scientific evidence. Instead, the ICP has had only promotional material available from the product manufacturer for the evaluating process. In some instances, this situation may be made worse by ill-conceived, poorly designed, or uncontrolled studies (in some cases), paid for by the manufacturer, being presented as "evidence" of a product's merit or efficacy. Such material should be viewed by the ICP in the same context as an advertise-

(Front)

UNIVERSITY OF VIRGINIA HOSPITAL
PRODUCT EVALUATION FORM

TO: All Sales Representatives

FROM: Assistant Director, Hospital

This sheet is provided in order for you to have your product considered for hospital-wide use. Please attach any supplemental literature only if published in a refereed journal.

Name of Product: _____ Vendor: _____
The product is specifically designed to do the following: _____

Packaging Quantities: ___/per/___   Approx. Unit Cost $ _____
Shelf Life _____
Is product: ( ) Disposable; ( ) Autoclavable; ( ) Gas sterilizable; Other: _____

Unique features of Item which make it superior to currently available items: Reference: (refereed Journal only)

1 _____   1 _____
2 _____   2 _____
3 _____   3 _____

Are there unique risks for patients or hospital personnel in using this product? _____
Specify: _____

Signed: _____ Sales Representative

Date: _____

(Back)

Infection Control Recommendations: _____

Purchasing: _____

Nursing: _____

Other: _____

Final Disposition   Date

( ) Approved for trial

( ) Accepted for use

( ) Rejected

( ) No decision

FIGURE 1. The above form is employed at the University of Virginia Hospital to screen products. The process begins in an assistant director's office, to whom the product is first presented by the vendor. The form is then routed to the various departments (shown on the back of the form) for input to determine if a clinical trial of the product is indicated.

ment. Therefore, the practitioner should demand accurate data from the sales representatives to avoid possibly selecting a product based on the salesman's charm or the emotional impact which the promotion of a product may have.

Patient Advocate

The patient has little voice in the affairs of the hospital or in the details of his own care. As a lay person, he has little or no insight into the intricacies of his care, and therefore he requires a spokesman to keep his best interests in mind. This is not to imply that the doctor and nurse in charge of his immediate care to not have his best interest in mind, but rather to point out that in the overall planning, development, and establishment of hospital policies or procedures, the patient has no personal representative. Therefore, the ICP, who should be included in all policy and procedure development from an infection control standpoint, should be conscious of his role as the patient's representative. Additionally, whenever the practitioner is called upon to make recommendations regarding infection control policies or procedures, he must bear in mind that while he has a patient advocacy responsibility, he also has responsibility to the hospital itself. Hence, while the ICP is advocating protection of the patients' interests, he must simultaneously be advocating protection of the hospital's and the staff's interests; no simple task, to be sure! Presumably the interests of all three are compatible, however, they may not be so under all circumstances and may also not run parallel with each other. Thus, the practitioner may find himself under "crossfire". In such an unlikely situation, the practitioner must follow his own conscience as to where the priorities should fall regarding whose interests should take precedent over others on certain issues. It would be presumptuous of this author to attempt to advise the practitioner on such a matter of individual ethical or moral conscience.

Research

There are many opportunities for the practitioner to conduct small-scale research or review within the hospital which does not require great funds or demand tremendous manpower. With resources at hand, the ICP may choose to review cumulative data, e.g., on postsurgical wound infections associated with certain surgical procedures over a 1- or 2-year (or more) period in his own hospital; or the impact of a new piece of equipment used in surgery, and to identify possible reasons for the subsequent increase or decrease in infection rates. Other possibilities for research might be to determine what, if any, may be the impact of a reduction in surveillance on the hospital's infection rates, or what may be the level of accuracy of the surveillance efforts. There is no limit to the number of possible questions to which the practitioner may wish to find answers. Research possibilities are often limited only by the inquisitive imagination of the ICP (see chapter entitled "Designing a Study to Answer Infection-Control Questions"). In teaching institutions, the opportunities may be greater than in smaller hospitals, for there are always students anxiously seeking to assist with or conduct their own research projects. Other research may be directed toward finding new and innovative methods of getting the "infection control message" across more effectively, through teaching programs, more effective use of data or the presentation of it, or through use of better visual aid material. Whether a program is sophisticated or modest, the practitioner should actively seek to devote some portion of time to research, no mater how modest an allotment may be feasible.

SELECTION OF THE ICP

Currently there are conflicting views on the qualifications necessary for selection of medical personnel for the ICP position. With respect to R.N.s, some contend that only nurses with baccalaureate degree preparation are properly qualified, others disagree. "Diploma graduates" are in a steadily declining minority today, as most hospital schools of nursing are replaced by university baccalaureate degree programs. Theoretically it would seem to be superfluous to discuss the role of the diploma nurse in the field of infection control. However, there are still a large number of diploma nurses actively practicing. There is little question that nurses filling the role of ICP will be prepared exclusively in a university setting in the future, *when such programs become widely available!* In the meantime, the assumption that preparation in a baccalaureate program in nursing automatically prepares one for the role of ICP would be false. Baccalaureate nursing programs are only now beginning to reinclude infection control concepts in the basic curriculum[7] as the result of new emphasis placed on infection control in hospitals by the Joint Commission on Accreditation of Hospitals (JCAH).

How then can the prospective employer select the most suitable, "best" candidate for the position of ICP? While limiting discussion here primarily to consideration of a nurse, for the sake of brevity, the suggestions outlined may equally apply to consideration of a nonnurse. First the employer should look for motivation, dedication, and commitment. Other desirable qualities include the following: clinical skill/experience, curiosity, self-confidence, tact, tenacity, and a somewhat compulsive nature. While few individuals will probably possess all of these qualities simultaneously or in equal measure, they may all at times be required of the practitioner to some extent and should therefore be considered part of the necessary qualifications. Assessment should be possible to the extent that these can be considered accurate from an individual's complete academic/employment record available to any potential employer.

Thus far, the section has dealt only with the selection of a "new" ICP, untrained and inexperienced in infection control. However, as the field is expanding, the number of "seasoned" practitioners is increasing. Although training programs in infection control are not widely available as yet, their number are sure to increase in the near future, and with this increase will come greater availability of trained and experienced practitioners seeking positions. Additionally, certification of ICPs will hopefully assist in assessing an individual's professional capabilities in the area of infection control. With this in mind, the employer must decide the level of support, both professional as well as financial, with which the hospital intends to provide the practitioner, for there is every indication that if these important requirements are not furnished, the ICP will indeed move on to "greener pastures". The employer has a right to know what the potential practitioner has to offer, as does the ICP have a right to know what the employer wants and is willing to offer in return. Conflict and dissatisfaction are bound to arise, if for example, the hospital has led the practitioner to believe that expansion and growth of the infection control program are real commitments and goals of the hospital, when in fact, the hospital is merely complying with regulatory agencies' "basic" requirements.

The following guidelines (see Tables 1 to 6) are offered to assist with the selection of one or more ICPs for a hospital, building a new infection control program, adding to an existing program, or to assist with efforts to promote practitioners within an existing/growing program. The tables were generated for review by the Virginia State Health Department. No attempt is made at suggesting salary ranges, as these vary from one locality to the next and rapidly grow obsolete due to inflationary pressures. However, comparison salary ranges may be determined in each locality by noting the equivalent salary and responsibility "steps" offered here, as compared to equivalent positions presently established outside the field of infection control. It should further be noted that while the tables provide guidelines on levels of expertise/responsibilities for each hierarchial step, there is some degree of overlap between one step and the next higher one.

Table 1
STEP 1 — STAFF ICP (STAFF NURSE EQUIVALENT)

Minimum Requirements

Enter field as: G.N.   — graduate nurse, graduated from an accredited school in state where employed with an elective in epidemiology, and infection control course[6a]

A.D.   — associate degree in nursing, licensed in state in which to be employed, plus 2 years in nursing field, and infection control course[a]

R.N.   — diploma, graduated from accredited school, licensed in state where to be employed, plus 1 year clinical practice after graduation, and infection control course[a]

R.N.   — B.S., graduated from accredited school, licensed in state where to be employed, and infection control course[a]

R.PH.   — B.S., registered pharmacist, graduated from an accredited school, licensed in state where to be employed, and infection control course[a]

M.T.   — B.S., medical technologist, graduated from accredited school, licensed in state where to be employed (member, American Society of Clinical Pathologists ([ASCP]), and infection control course[a]

B.S.   — in environmental health science, graduated from an accredited school, licensed in state where to be employed, and infection control course[a]

[a]   University of Virginia course or its equivalent, i.e., CDC course 1200-G, etc.

Table 2
STEP 2 — ICP "A" (HEAD NURSE "A" EQUIVALENT)

Minimum Requirements

	A.D.	— in nursing, graduated from accredited school, licensed in state where employed, plus 2 years in clinical nursing field, and infection control course,[a] plus 1 year in Step 1 (See Table 1)
Or enter with		4 years in nursing field plus infection control course[a]
	R.N.	— diploma, graduated from accredited school, licensed in state where employed, plus infection control course,[a] plus one year in Step 1
Or enter with		2 years in nursing field plus infection control course[a]
	R.N.	— B.S., graduated from accredited school, licensed in state where employed, plus infection control course,[a] plus 1 year in Step 1
Or enter with		1 year in nursing field, plus infection control course[a]
	R.Ph.	— B.S., graduated from accredited school, licensed in state where employed, plus infection control course,[a] plus 1 year in Step 1
Or enter with		3 years in pharmacy and infection control course[a]
	P.H.N.	— B.S., public health nurse, graduated from accredited school (with appropriate public health courses), licensed in state where employed plus infection control course,[a] plus 1 year in Step 1
Or enter with		2 years in public health nursing field, plus infection control course,[a] or B.S. in epidemiology and infection control course[a]
	M.T.	— medical technologist, B.S. and ASCP, graduated from an accredited school, licensed in state where employed, and infection control course,[a] plus 2 years in Step 1
Or enter with		3 years in laboratory and infection control course[6a]
	B.S.	— environmental health science, graduated from accredited school licensed (sanitarian, etc.) in state where employed, and infection control course,[a] plus 2 years in Step 1
Or enter with		3 years in health allied field and infection control course[a]

[a]   University of Virginia course or its equivalent, i.e., CDC course 1200-G, etc.

Table 3
STEP 3 — ICP "B" (Head Nurse "B" EQUIVALENT)

A.D.	— in nursing, graduated from accredited school, licensed in state where employed, and 6 years in clinical nursing field plus infection control course[a]
Or	2 years in Step 1, plus 2 years in Step 2
R.N.	— diploma, graduated from accredited school, licensed in state where employed, plus 5 years in clinical nursing field, and infection control course[a]
Or	1 year in Step 1 and 2 years in Step 2
R.N.	— B.S., graduated from accredited school licensed in state where employed, plus 4 years in clinical nursing field, and infection control course[a]
Or	1 year in Step 1 and 2 years in Step 2
R.Ph.	— B.S., registered pharmacist, graduated from accredited school licensed in state where employed, and 5 years in pharmacy, plus infection control course[a]
Or	2 years in Step 1 and 2 years in Step 2
P.H.N.	— B.S., public health nurse, graduated from accredited school (with appropriate public health courses), licensed in state where employed, plus 5 years in public health field, and infection control course[a]
Or	1 year in Step 1 and 2 years in Step 2
M.T.	— medical technologist, B.S. and ASCP, graduated from an accredited school, licensed in state where employed, plus 5 years in laboratory, and infection control course[a]
Or	2 years in Step 1 and 2 years in Step 2
B.S.	— In environmental health science, graduated from an accredited school, licensed in state where employed, plus 5 years employed in allied health field, and infection control course[a]
Or	2 years in Step 1 and 2 years in Step 2

[a]   University of Virginia course or its equivalent, i.e., CDC course 1200-G, etc.

Table 4

STEP 4 — GENERAL EPIDEMIOLOGY/INFECTION CONTROL INSTRUCTOR (GENERAL NURSING INSTRUCTOR EQUIVALENT)

Minimum Requirements

A.D.	— in nursing, graduated from accredited school, licensed in state where employed, plus 10 years in nursing field, plus infection control course,[a] and 2 years in *hospital* epidemiology
Or	7 years in nursing field, and infection control course,[a] and 5 years in *hospital* epidemiology or equivalent post-graduate education
R.N.	— diploma or B.S., graduated from accredited school, licensed in state where employed, plus 10 years in nursing field (9 for B.S.), plus infection control course[a], and 2 years in *hospital* epidemiology
Or	M.A. in nursing and infection control course[a], plus 2 years in *hospital* epidemiology
Or	5 years in nursing and infection control course,[a] plus 5 years in *hospital* epidemiology
R.Ph.	— B.S., registered pharmacist, graduated from accredited school, licensed in state where employed, plus 10 years in pharmacy, and infection control course[a]
Or	M.Ph. and infection control course,[a] plus 2 years in *hospital* epidemiology
Or	5 years in pharmacy and infection control course,[a] plus 5 years in *hospital* epidemiology
P.H.N.	— B.S., public health nurse, graduated from accredited school (with appropriate courses in public health), licensed in state where employed, plus 10 years in public health nursing, and infection control course[a]
Or	M.P.H. and infection control course,[a] plus 2 years in *hospital* epidemiology
Or	5 years in public health nursing, and infection control course,[a] plus 5 years in *hospital* epidemiology
M.T.	— B.S. and ASCP, medical technologist, graduated from an accredited school, licensed in state where employed, plus 10 years in laboratory, and infection control course,[a] plus 2 years in *hospital* epidemiology
Or	5 years in laboratory and infection control course,[a] plus 5 years in *hospital* epidemiology
B.S.	— in environmental health science, graduated from accredited school, licensed in state where employed and 10 years in allied health field, plus infection control course,[a] plus 3 years in *hospital* epidemiology
Or	M.A. in environmental health science and infection control course,[a] plus 2 years in *hospital* epidemiology
Or	5 years in allied health field, plus 5 years in *hospital* epidemiology

[a]   University of Virginia course or its equivalent, i.e., CDC course 1200-G, etc.

Table 5
STEP 5 — EPIDEMIOLOGY/INFECTION CONTROL SUPERVISOR (NURSING SUPERVISOR EQUIVALENT)

Minimum Requirements

R.N.   — diploma or B.S., graduated from an accredited school, licensed in state where employed, plus 10 years (9 years for B.S.) in nursing field and infection control course,[a] plus 5 years in *hospital* epidemiology

Or   M.A. in nursing and infection control course,[a] plus 5 years in *hospital* epidemiology

M.A.   — In epidemiology, graduated from accredited school, licensed in state where employed, plus 5 years in *hospital* epidemiology and infection control course[a]

Or   2 years in epidemiology and infection control course, plus 3 years in *hospital* epidemiology

M.P.H.   — In epidemiology, graduated frm accredited school, licensed in state where employed (where applicable), and infection control course,[a] plus 5 years in *hospital* epidemiology

M.A.   — In microbiology, graduated from accredited school, licensed in state where employed (ASCP), and infection control course,[a] plus 5 years in *hospital* epidemiology

M.Ph.   — pharmacist, graduated from accredited school, licensed in state where employed, and infection control course,[a] plus 5 years in *hospital* epidemiology

[a]   University of Virginia course or its equivalent, i.e., CDC Course 1200-G, etc.

Table 6
GENERAL LEVELS OF EXPERTISE AND RESPONSIBILITY FOR ICPs

Step 1 (Staff ICP)	Surveillance; assist with investigations (under supervision); implement directives for infection control
Step 2 (ICP "A")	Surveillance; assist with or conduct investigations (as directed); continually update hospital personnel on new information regarding infection control; collect data/information for statistical reports (under supervision); assist with data analysis
Step 3 (ICP "B")	Surveillance and analysis of data; able to conduct investigations (under supervision); assist in planning of teaching programs as well as teaching; compile monthly reports (under supervision); consultation on problems (as directed)
Step 4 (Instructor)	Surveillance and analysis of data; assist with statistical evaluations; assist in directing investigations, recognize areas requiring further investigation, and initiate such programs; assist with research (as directed)
Step 5 (Supervisor)	Supervise and coordinate all activities of the division as directed by hospital (physician) epidemiologist; assist in planning and conduct of research projects Plan and assign methods of conducting investigations; assignment of routine surveillance and analysis of nosocomial infections (may also be delegated to Step 4 or Step 3 practitioner, depending on situation); assume responsibility for completeness and accuracy of reports; provide expert consultation on infection control problems, isolation, communicable diseases, relative safety and efficacy of certain hospital products (in or out of the hospital), i.e., other hospitals, etc., serve as a role model to subordinates Responsibility for professional development of infection control staff members and personal continued growth in theory and practice

REFERENCES

1. Wenzel, K., The role of the infection control nurse, *Nurs. Clin. North Am.,* 1, 89, 1970.
2. Gardner, A. M. N., Stamp, M., Bowgen, J. A., and Moore, B., The infection control sister. A new member of the control of infection team in general hospitals, *Lancet,* ii, 710, 1962.
3. Moore, B., The infection control sister in British hospitals, *Int. Nurs. Rev.,* 17, 84, 1970.
4. Moore, B., Surveillance of hospital infection, Proc. Int. Conf. Nosocomial Infections, Center for Disease Control, Atlanta, Ga., August 3 to 6, 1970, 272.
5. May, H. B., Hospital Coccal Infections, *Association of Clinical Pathologists,* 1958, 36.
6. Wenzel, R. P., Osterman, C. A., Townsend, T. R., Veazey, J. M., Jr., Servis, K. H., Miller, L. S., Craven, R. B., Miller, G. B., Jr., and Jackson, R. S., The development of a statewide program for surveillance and reporting of hospital-acquired infections, *J. Infec. Dis.,* 140, 741, 1979.
7. Dunn, H., The infection control nurse-participant in the sequence of events, Proc. 1st North American Eastern Conference on Infection Control, A.P.I.C., Toronto, Canada, 1973, 15.

Identifying and Reporting Infections

SURVEILLANCE AND REPORTING OF HOSPITAL ACQUIRED INFECTIONS

Richard P. Wenzel

INTRODUCTION

A hospital acquired or nosocomial infection is one that was not present or incubating at the time that a patient entered the hospital. In general, infections are not considered nosocomial unless the onset of the infection occurred after 72 hr from the time the patient was admitted. There are exceptions, however, since it is possible that a patient could acquire a new infection on the second day, e.g., having undergone a common hospital procedure on admission. On the other hand, it is also possible that the infection may not become apparent until after the patient is discharged. In the latter instance, the infection would not be identified unless all patients were followed in a type of postdischarge surveillance or were readmitted for the infectious complication to the same hospital.

Approximately 40 million people are hospitalized in the U.S. each year; and of those admitted, 5 to 10% will acquire a nosocomial infection. Of all hospital acquired infections identified, 30 to 40% are urinary tract infections, 25% are postoperative wound infections, and 15% are pneumonias. Fifteen percent are infections of the bloodstream, and the remainder are infections at various other sites, including the skin, spinal fluid, eye, peritoneum, etc. The overall mortality for hospital acquired bloodstream or pulmonary infections has been reported as high as 75%, but many patients die as a result of their underlying illnesses. Although the exact role of bacteremia in relationship to subsequent deaths is undefined in most series of hospital acquired bloodstream infections, the best estimates are that approximately 25% of patients with a hospital acquired bloodstream infection die as a direct result of infection, apart from the underlying illnesses.[1,2,2a,2b] In this context, it should be noted that patients with urinary tract infections and postoperative wound infections occasionally develop secondary bloodstream infections which may place them at increased morbidity and mortality than would be expected with the primary infection alone.

The economic burden of hospital acquired infections has been estimated to be over 1 billion dollars each year in the U.S. This estimate is based on the assumptions that there are an additional 5 to 10 days of hospitalization for each infection and that excess hospitalization costs are at least $100/day. The financial losses are borne by the taxpayers who must support the rising cost of health insurance, due in part, to hospital acquired infections.

Some of the recent "pressures" for good infection control might be summarized as follows:

1. Since 1976 the Joint Commission for Accreditation of Hospitals (JCAH) has forced hospitals to meet increasingly demanding standards for infection control.
2. There is a growing awareness of the medical-legal aspects of nosocomial infections.
3. Approximately 80% of patients' bills are paid for by third-party groups, and it is possible that in the future, third-party payers will be closely observing the progress of control of hospital acquired infections, not only because of their economic burden, but also because of their easy identification.

4.   Various peer groups such as the Professional Standards Review Organization (PSRO) are likely to identify hospital infections as an important area for audit.
5.   There is increasing concern about the use and perhaps overuse of antibiotics in hospitalized patients. Such concern will very likely manifest itself in a review of the use of antibiotics for hospital acquired infections.

Thus, the incentives for infection control are medical, economic, legal, and administrative. In addition, the medical profession in general and infection control practitioners (ICPs) in particular must be sensitive to the needs of patients, who, as informed consumers, are demanding excellence in the delivery of their health care.

DEFINITIONS FOR SURVEILLANCE

In order to assess the priorities for infection control, some method is necessary to determine the extent and consequences of infections acquired by patients after entering hospitals. Surveillance is the beginning of infection control, since it is the method by which ICPs begin to identify the major problems for subsequent solutions. Surveillance could be defined as the routine and orderly collection of information for the purpose of defining endemic or "background" rates. Within the hospital, the goal of surveillance is to define the endemic rates of nosocomial infection. Thus, an epidemic would be identified when the infection rates rose above an expected threshold.

It should be emphasized all rates include a numerator and denominator and that the denominator includes all patients at risk. Furthermore, the time period for the numerator and the denominator must be the same, e.g., all patients infected during the month divided by all patients at risk during the month. The infection rate for the entire hospital and rates by site, service, pathogen, and location have been the traditional starting points for surveillance. Some "short-cuts" are commonly used by practitioners in calculating infection rates. For example, establishing service-specific infection rates within the hospital; most epidemiologists by convention utilize the readily available admission or discharge data in the denominator. In the latter situation, since the denominator would not include all patients present during a given time period, it could be argued that such a convention would inflate infection rates. Nevertheless, the practice seems reasonable, since the addition of the total number of patients admitted earlier, but present on the first day of the new surveillance period (and theoretically at risk of infection), is usually not significant enough to alter the final infection rate over an extended period. With respect to the overall hospital infection rate, the numerator is usually the number of infections rather than the number of patients infected. The information obtained allows the epidemiologist to define infection rates by site. Occasionally, however, chiefs of services who are not keenly interested in epidemiologic data become concerned that rates are exaggerated, since several seriously ill patients have numerous infections, whereas the number of different patients infected are fewer. As a result of such political considerations, some epidemiologists have begun reporting two infection rates — one with the total number of infected patients and another with the total number of infections as a numerator.

An important goal of surveillance — and perhaps its major role — is to identify specific risks for patients undergoing common hospital procedures. With the information obtained, the risk and benefit for many hospital procedures can be weighed and decisions made in a more rational way than have been made in the past. Such procedures include not only specific surgical operations, but also nonsurgical procedures, such as Foley bladder catheterizations, hyperalimentation therapy, and respiratory assistance. The numerator includes the total number of infections associated with the procedure, and the denominator the total number of procedures being surveyed during the same time period.

Ideally, all professional personnel should be aware of the risks of procedures performed on their services. Eventually, the risk of infection following procedures could be defined for specific hospital populations, e.g., the risk of urinary tract infections following catheterization in patients with diabetes, lymphoma, lupus erythematosis, etc. In addition, such risks within certain age brackets could also be identified. Hopefully, the resulting refinements would improve decision making and eventually health care itself.

STARTING POINT

It is imposible for ICPs to review data from all patients hospitalized on a daily basis. Some sampling of the patient population is therefore necessary, and a most reasonable group to select would be those considered to be at high risk for acquiring a hospital infection. An important question therefore is the starting point; and the most efficient method so far identified for surveillance is one in which the program begins with a review of the nursing care plan or Kardex® (see Figure 1), since it contains the patients' diagnoses, procedures, and nursing observations.[3] The case finding "clues" listed in the Kardex® (see Table 1) can be used to select high-risk patients for chart review and to eliminate others. Once there is a method for the selection of charts, then, in order to have an operational system, simple definitions for infections at any given site are utilized (see Table 2).

Each of the standard wards in the hospital are surveyed on a weekly basis, with the exception of the obstetrics ward which is reviewed twice a week. In intensive care areas also, all charts are reviewed twice a week. From the data of the study of surveillance systems, it would appear that another reasonable starting point for some hospitals would be the microbiology laboratory (see Table 3). If this system is preferred, the laboratory should be visited daily, and charts of patients with positive cultures obtained after admission should then be surveyed.

When infections are identified as nosocomial by any surveillance system, the names of patients can be organized on line listings by site and location. These lists should include the patient's history number, dates of admission and infection, ward location, diagnoses, and predisposing factors, such as surgical procedures, hyperalimentation, and respiratory assistance (see Table 4). At the end of the month, line lists are organized into a summary report.

INFECTION RATES

The number of infections per 100 admissions for a university hospital is illustrated in Table 5. There were over 8000 hospital acquired infections identified by continual surveillance for approximately a 6-year period. Although there is an overall infection rate of 7% at the University of Virginia Hospital, specifically higher rates were found on the burn service and on the service housing newborn patients requiring intensive care. General surgical services have approximately a 10% infection rate overall, whereas the medical, pediatric, and neurology services have rates of approximately 5%. Lower rates were found on the obstetrics and gynecology services, as well as those found on otolaryngology and ophthalmology.

Specific rates of infection by site indicate that for every 100 admissions to the burn unit, there were 34 nosocomial bloodstream infections. Such data show the greatly increased risk the thermal injury patient has as a result of his primary skin defenses

EXAMPLE OF
UNIVERSITY OF VIRGINIA
MEDICAL CENTER
TREATMENT RECORD

JOHN DOE WM
00-00-00 S 45Y S-5028A
TCV-SGY MARR. 7-25-80

ADDRESSOGRAPH PLATE

PHYSICIAN

ALLERGIES (WRITTEN IN RED INK) PEN

DATE ORDERED / INITIALS	TREATMENTS, NURSING ORDERS.	DATES HR.
7-29	TURN, DEEP BREATHE, COUGH	
	q 2h	
7-30	INCISION CARE WITH H_2O_2	
	q 4h	
7-29	FOLEY CARE BID	
7-29	CHEST TUBE DRAINAGE	
	q 2h	
7-31	Nasal O_2 @ 2L PRN	

SERVICE

HISTORY #

STAT-SINGLE ORDERS

DATE ORDERED / INITIALS	TREATMENTS, NSG ORDERS, SPECIMENS	DATE DONE	TIME DONE	INITS	DATE ORDERED / INITIALS	TREATMENTS, NSG ORDERS, SPECIMENS	DATE DONE	TIME DONE	INITS
7/28 DM	U/A PU-OP	7-28	1pm	JH					
7/30 DM	HL # 23	7-31	1am	OW					
7/31 DM	URINE CULTURE	7-31	9am	BU					
7/31 DM	SPUTUM CULTURE	8-1	1am	LM					

NAME

ROOM

* SEE FLOW SHEET / PROGRESS NOTE

NO. OF FORMS IN USE (PENCIL)

FIGURE 1A. Example of treatment record.

39

ADDRESSOGRAPH

DIAGNOSIS: CAD, COPD, ASEVD

SURGERY: 7/29 CABG X 1

CARE CATEGORY:

ACTIVITY: BED REST, BR PRIVILEGES WITH ASSISTANCE

TRANSPORTATION: STRETCHER [X] CHAIR [ ] WALK [ ]

CARE STATUS: INDEPENDENT [ ] ASSIST [ ] TOTAL [ ]

DIET: FULL LIQUID

STATUS: INDEPENDENT [X] ASSIST [ ] FEED. [ ]

IV SITE CHANGE:

VITAL SIGNS: TPR q 2h

BP q 1h

WEIGHTS: q day

PRECAUTIONS:

MISC.: CALL HO IF TEMP ↑ 30°C

FAMILY CONTACTS

NAME	RELATIONSHIP	PHONE NO.
JANE DOE	MOTHER	296-0114

INSERT

FIGURE 1B. Example of treatment record.

Table 1
CASE FINDING CLUES IN THE NURSING CARE
PLAN (KARDEX®) WHICH ALERT THE NURSE-
EPIDEMIOLOGIST TO POTENTIAL HOSPITAL
ACQUIRED INFECTIONS

Diagnoses or conditions
    Leukemia, lymphoma, carcinoma, granulocytopenia, collagen vas-
    cular diseases, sarcoid, and widespread dematoses (diagnoses
    often requiring steroid therapy)
    Burns
    Organ transplantation
    Hepatitis (check of earlier transfusions)

Operations or procedures
    All surgery requiring general anesthesia
    Tracheostomies
    CNS shunts
    Bladder catheterization
    Hyperalimentation
    Respiratory assistance therapy
    Special wound or decubitus care

Note: All patients hospitalized for 3 weeks or more.

being damaged. There is a similarly great risk of secondary wound infections (63 per 100 admissions) for burned patients also (see Table 5). Another group of patients with unusually high rates of infections are newborns in the special care unit. Their overall infection rate is 28.55%, with 6 hospital acquired bloodstream infections and 5 hospital acquired pneumonias for every 100 admissions. Obviously this is a selected group of newborns, many of whom are premature and all of whom are of high risk of subsequent infections.

Overall rates reported for other hospitals are illustrated in Table 6. It should be emphasized that both incidence and prevalence rates were used, the methods of surveillance varied, and the types of hospitals and therefore of patients surveyed varied among the reports. One can only compare hospitals within the same category and only when the same systems of surveillance are employed.

In 70% of all hospital acquired infections, Gram-negative rods are recovered. Most frequently isolated are *Escherichia coli*, *Klebsiella pneumoniae*, and *Pseudomonas aeruginosa*. *Staphylococcus aureus* is the most common single organism isolated from postoperative wound infections, representing approximately 25% of cultured wounds. Since one goal of surveillance reporting is to inform the hospital personnel of the risk of infection in patients on a given service, it is desirable to review the site, service, and site pathogen data continually with ward personnel. One of the most propitious times is when the monthly report is distributed by the ICP throughout the hospital. The site pathogen data at the University of Virginia Hospital is illustrated in Table 7 and compares data with the information reported and by hospitals participating in the Virginia statewide surveillance program and by hospitals submitting data to the National Nosocomial Infection Study (NNIS) of the Center for Disease Control (CDC) and/or to private industry.[20]

The purpose of presenting site-pathogen data (see Table 7) is to permit ICPs a yardstick by which to compare their hospital's surveillance data. Specifically the question is, "What is the rate (risk) that a patient admitted to a hospital will develop an infection at a given site with a specific organism?" The data show that between 2 and

Table 2
DEFINITIONS OF INFECTION FOR ICPS PERFORMING SURVEILLANCE

Infection site	Criteria for infection	Comments	Reporting refinements
Blood	Positive culture	Must rule out contaminant	State if primary or secondary to an infection at another site
Urine	$\geq 10^5$ colonies of bacteria per 1 mℓ	Lower counts are accepted if associated with compatible symptoms and pyuria	Note if current or prior bladder catheterization
Postoperative wounds	Pus at the incision site	Deep postoperative wounds and cellulitis are classified separately	Note if stitch abscess, in contrast to a more involved infection
Other wounds	Presence of pus	Includes decubiti tracheostomy site	
Burns	$\geq 10^6$ organisms per 1g of biopsied tissue; alternatively, new inflammation or new pus not present on admission	Considerably greater success rate for skin grafts if placed over burn sites with bacterial counts $\leq 10^5$/g tissue	Note the antibiogram, since antiobiotic resistance often originates in the burn unit.
Pulmonary	New infiltrate on chest X-ray not present on admission associated with new sputum production	Clinical picture must be compatible; other entities, e.g., atelectasis and pulmonary embolus with infarction ruled out	Note if pneumonia associated with assisted ventilation
Intestinal	Positive culture for pathogen or unexplained diarrhea for ≥ 2 days	Pathogen is defined as salmonella, shigella, pathogenic *Escherichia coli*	List any antibiotics patient is receiving
Miscellaneous (hepatitis, upper respiratory infections, peritonitis, etc.)	Clinical picture	—	Note if associated temporally with any hospital procedure

Table 3

COMPARISON OF THE STANDARD WEEKLY SURVEILLANCE SYSTEM EMPLOYED AT THE UNIVERSITY OF VIRGINIA HOSPITAL WITH OTHER SURVEILLANCE METHODS

Surveillance method	Approximate sample size	Time required per week (hr)	Average number of nosocomial infections detected	Relative efficiency (%)	Number of nosocomial infections missed in the study period
Standard weekly surveillance (University of Virginia)	65% chart review	16—25[a]	22[b]	100[c]	1 compared to antibiotic review; 1 compared to fever chart review; 7 compared to combined fever-antibiotic review; 0 compared to chest X-ray review; 2 compared to bacteriology report review
Antibiotic usage	36% chart review	16	12	57	10
Fever (temperature$\geq$37.8°C)	16% chart review	9	9	56	8
Combined fever, antibiotic usage	Not noted	15	14	70	13
Bacteriology reports	Not noted	26	17	77	15
Second week follow-up			28	93	4
Positive chest X-ray for pneumonia	388 films reviewed per week	10	2	7	25

[a] Initially required 22 to 25 hr, but by eliminating the duplication of paperwork this time is now 16 hr per week.

[b] Average weekly total. The total number of infections identified in weekly comparisons of surveillance systems can be obtained by adding the number detected by the respective surveillance system plus the number missed.

[c] This is an arbitrary figure for comparison. The percentages below are derived by dividing the number of infections obtained for the individual surveillance method by the number obtained by the standard weekly surveillance.

Table 4
UNIVERSITY OF VIRGINIA MEDICAL CENTER
LINE LISTING OF NOSOCOMIAL INFECTIONS

Name _____

Month of: _____

Site _____

Year: 198__

History #	Ward	Service/ date adm.	Diagnoses/ operation	Date surgery	I.V.s #>10	F	TC	HA.	Tr	R	Br	SC	Other	Date of infection site	Dates for previous neg. data	Comments: 1) specific procedures 2) organisms recovered
															U/A(WBC) ___ CXR ___ BC ___ CSF ___ CULT ___	
															U/A(WBC) ___ CXR ___ BC ___ CSF ___ CULT ___	
															U/A(WBC) ___ CXR ___ BC ___ CSF ___ CULT ___	

The column group "Dates of procedure" spans F, TC, HA., Tr, R, Br, SC, Other.

Note: The illustration is an example of the type of line lists which can be used to store data obtained from routine surveillance of nosocomial infections. Only one infection site, e.g., bloodstream infections, is recorded on any one sheet which contains space for ten infections. Line lists by site are easily reviewed. In addition, the line lists by site help to prevent the recording of the same infection twice. The ICP carries the line lists of the previous week's surveillance data onto the wards.

Key: I.V.s>10, yes or no response; F = Foley; TC = Texas Catheter; HA = hyperalimentation units prior to infection; Tr = tracheotomy; R = respirator; Br = bronchoscopy; SC = straight in and out catheter.
UA(WBC) = urine analysis (white blood cells); CXR = chest X-ray; BC = blood culture; CSF = cerebrospinal fluid; CULT = culture.

Table 5

NOSOCOMIAL INFECTION RATES BY SITE AND SERVICE
UNIVERSITY OF VIRGINIA HOSPITAL — SEPTEMBER 1972 to JUNE 1978

| Unit | ADM[a] | INF[b] | Rate per 100 | POW[c] | BLD[d] | PUL[e] | Urinary tract infection | | Other |
							F[f]	NF[g]	
Burn unit	126	212	168.25	80 (63.49)	43 (34.13)	12 (9.52)	38 (30.16)	20 (15.87)	23 (18.25)
NICU[h]	543	155	28.55	1 (0.19)	33 (6.08)	29 (5.34)	— (—)	21 (3.87)	93 (17.13)
Plastic surgery[a]	6,245	730	11.69	480 (7.69)	68 (1.08)	205 (3.28)	90 (1.44)	58 (0.94)	141 (2.26)
General surgery	11,422	1,271	11.10	493 (4.32)	175 (1.53)	214 (1.87)	199 (1.74)	100 (0.88)	90 (0.78)
Orthopedics	8,685	908	10.45	168 (1.93)	28 (0.32)	60 (0.69)	506 (5.83)	136 (1.57)	89 (1.02)
TCV surgery[i]	5,839	598	10.24	166 (2.84)	65 (1.11)	201 (3.44)	69 (1.18)	33 (0.57)	68 (1.16)
Urology	5,396	476	8.82	100 (1.85)	28 (0.52)	27 (0.50)	208 (3.85)	85 (1.56)	28 (0.52)
Neurosurgery	7,058	681	9.65	118 (1.67)	43 (0.61)	98 (1.39)	199 (2.82)	77 (1.09)	133 (1.88)
Medicine	27,518	1,746	6.34	4 (0.01)	354 (1.30)	277 (1.01)	224 (0.81)	292 (1.06)	472 (1.72)
Neurology	5,209	253	4.86	2 (0.04)	19 (0.36)	51 (0.98)	92 (1.77)	41 (0.78)	47 (0.90)
Pediatrics	11,860	560	4.72	2 (0.02)	127 (1.07)	47 (0.40)	22 (0.19)	57 (0.48)	305 (2.57)
Gynecology	6,164	256	4.15	120 (1.95)	20 (0.32)	19 (0.31)	39 (0.63)	32 (0.52)	26 (0.42)
Obstetrics	8,729	194	2.22	110 (1.26)	16 (0.18)	2 (0.02)	8 (0.09)	10 (0.11)	23 (0.26)
Otolaryngology	5,539	99	1.79	42 (0.76)	6 (0.11)	22 (0.40)	6 (0.11)	7 (0.13)	15 (0.27)

	ADM	INF							
Ophthalmology	2,477	7	0.28	—	—	1 (0.04)	2 (0.08)	3 (0.12)	1 (0.04)
Total	112,810	8,146	7.22	1,886	1,121	1,265	1,702	972	1,554
% of all inf	—	—	—	23.1	13.7	15.5	20.8	11.9	19
Rate per 100 ADM	—	—	—	1.67	0.99	1.12	1.51	0.86	1.38

a Includes burn patients through 1976.

a ADM = Total number admissions.
b INF = Total number infections.
c POW = Postoperative wound infection.
d BLD = Bloodstream infection.
e PUL = Pulmonary infection.
f F = Foley catheter-related urinary tract infection.
g NF = Non-Foley catheter-related urinary tract infection.
h NICU = Newborn intensive care unit.
i TCV = Thoracic cardiovascular surgery.

Table 6

EXAMPLES OF OVERALL NOSOCOMIAL INFECTION RATES REPORTED IN THE LITERATURE

Type of hospital	Identity of hospital	Infection rate (%)	Year reported	Primary method of surveillance	Ref.
University teaching	Boston City	13.5	1964	2—3 week prospective	4
	Boston City	15.5	1968	Prevalence survey employing physicians	5
	University of Kentucky	6.1	1967	Daily review of bacteriology laboratory reports	6
	Johns Hopkins	4.0	1968	Twice weekly visits to head nurses on wards; daily review of bacteriology laboratory reports	7
	University of Minnesota	5.2	1969	Reports of ward nurse	8
	Grady	11.5	1970	1-week retrospective chart prevalence survey	9
	University of Virginia	6—7	1976	Review of nursing Kardex® weekly to select high-risk patients for chart survey	3,10
Community teaching	Springfield Hospital Medical Center	5.4	1971	Daily visits to ward nurses and daily review of bacteriology laboratory reports	11
	Graduate Hospital	10.8	1975	Prospective surveillance by infection control nurse	12
Community	Six different hospitals throughout U.S.	1.4	1969	Twice weekly ward rounds; review of bacteriology laboratory reports; patient-infection forms used	13
	Two Oklahoma City area hospitals	4	1974	Daily ward rounds by ICP, 4-month study	14
	18 small midwestern hospitals	7.2	1976	1-day prospective bed-to-bed prevalence survey	15

County	Milwaukee County	14, 9.5, 7.6 in successive years	1974	Point prevalence studies, 1970, 1971, 1972, respectively	16
Public health	Public Health Service Hospital, Staten Island	7.8	1969	1-month prevalence	17
Military teaching	Walter Reed	6.9	1976	Review of bacteriology laboratory reports	18
Military non-teaching	Letterman	5.0	1976		
	Moncrief	1.5	1977	Prospective daily survey beginning with review of nursing Kardex® to select high-risk patients	19

26 patients per 10,000 admissions will develop an *E. coli* bloodstream infection (see Table 7A), and that 51 to 84 patients per 10,000 admissions will develop an *E. coli* urinary tract infection (see Table 7B). Furthermore, *E. coli* is the most common isolate from the sputum of patients with hospital acquired pneumonia (see Table 7C), whereas *S. aureus* is the most frequent isolate from patients with postoperative wound infections (see Table 7D). A new problem might be identified if the site-pathogen rates rose above an earlier recorded figure.

In the past, the infection rates by the site and service have been stressed. It is now obvious that while they are important starting points, they are less helpful in bringing about real change in infection control practices than procedure-related rules. Examples of surgical operation-related risks are illustrated in Table 8A (Univesity of Virginia) and compared to earlier reports (Table 8B). By convention, many surgeons have categorized infection rates after surgery into four categories: clean, clean contaminated, contaminated, and dirty.[21] As a result, many operations were grouped into the four categories, but the specific operation-rated risk was not reported. Although this was important in beginning to obtain in-patient data, it is not sufficient for the epidemiologist trying to identify high-risk procedures.

Furthermore, with refined reporting, one should be able to define the risk of infection following only surgery for appendicitis without rupture, uncomplicated (no strangulation) herniorrhaphies (see Table 8A), various types of arterial bypasses (see Tables 8A and 8B), specific additional procedures related to cholecystectomy, excision of an intervertebral disk, or craniotomy (see Table 8B). Only when the specific operation is identified, can one make a decision whether or not the rate obtained by surveillance seems reasonable, unusually high, or unusually low.

The risks following two common hospital procedures are illustrated in Table 9A and 9B. As can be seen, 17% of over 5000 patients catheterized at the University of Virginia Hospital acquired a urinary tract infection. Rates varied from a high of 60% on orthopedic service, where spinal cord injury patients are cared for, to 1% on obstetrics, where hospitalization time is brief and rates are underestimated. The mean and median time of infection after catheterization varied among services, but unusually high rates did not always correlate with length of time of catheterization before infection. Such data are the starting points for individual services to begin to review their own techniques and perhaps improve rates in subsequent time periods. Eventually, with refinements the risk of infection by day of catheterization will be available for each service.

Similar data are illustrated in Table 9B for the rate of pneumonia following use of respirators. Seven percent of almost 3100 patients surveyed who were receiving respirator assistance developed a nosocomial pneumonia. The mean time of pneumonia after being placed on a respirator was 14 days, with mean intervals ranging from 4 days for patients on gynecology to 7 days for burn unit patients and 37 days for pediatric (not newborn) patients.

With still more refined surveillance, data could be generated which will be the basis of decision making in the clinical area such as which antibiotics will be most effective in treating a nosocomial infection at a specific site. This information could be organized by ward location as well, since intensive care areas are the birthplace of antibiotic resistance within the hospital and will have a greater prevalence of antibiotic resistant organisms.

Table 10 shows data relating location in the hospital, risk of bloodstream infection, and risk of aminoglycoside resistant organisms at the University of Virginia in 1977. It is obvious that there is a particularly high risk of acquiring a Gram-negative rod bloodstream infection in the intensive care areas generally, and the greatest risk was in the burn unit. Once a patient developed a Gram-negative rod bloodstream infection,

Table 7A

CAUSES OF HOSPITAL ACQUIRED BLOODSTREAM INFECTIONS
UNIVERSITY OF VIRGINIA (1973—1976, 1977—JUNE 1978), VIRGINIA STATEWIDE
HOSPITALS PROGRAM, THE NNIS SURVEY, AND BAC-DATA

Organism	Number (percent of isolates)[a]		Rate/10,000 admissions				
			University of Virginia		Virginia Statewide Program	NNIS[20]	Bac-Data[22]
	1973—76	1977—6/78	1973—76	1977—78	1975—77[b]	1/74—6/74	7/77—6/78[c]
Escherichia coli	101(16)	80(17)	13	26	6	2.5	3.7
Klebsiella pneumoniae	86(14)	56(12)	11	18	3	—	2.2
Staphylococcus aureus	72(11)	64(13)	9	21	5	2.1	3.5
Pseudomonas aeruginosa	62(10)	36(8)	8	12	2	—	—
Bacteroides fragilis	26(4)	14(3)	3	5	1	—	—
Enterobacter cloacae	26(4)	26(5)	3	8	0.02	—	—
Proteus mirabilis	24(4)	7(1.5)	3	2	1	—	—
β-Hemolytic Streptococcus	23(4)	4(1)	3	1	0.03	—	—
Staphylococcus epidermidis	21(3)	27(6)	3	9	2	—	3.2
Candida albicans	21(3)	20(4)	3	7	0.1	—	—
Enterobacter aerogenes	16(3)	14(3)	2	5	0.06	—	—
Alpha Streptococcus	15(2)	10(2)	3	2	0.5	—	0.8
Serratia marcescens	12(2)	27(6)	2	9	1	—	—
Candida sp.	12(2)	1(0.2)	2	0.3	—	0.6	—
Klebsiella sp.	10(2)	0(0)	1	0	1	1.9	—
Enterococcus	9(1)	21(4)	1	7	2	1.0	0.9
Bacteroides spp.	9(1)	2(0.5)	1	0.7	1	0.8	—
Acinetobacter anitratum	7(1)	8(2)	1	3	0.02	—	—

Table 7A (continued)
CAUSES OF HOSPITAL ACQUIRED BLOODSTREAM INFECTIONS UNIVERSITY OF VIRGINIA (1973—1976, 1977—JUNE 1978), VIRGINIA STATEWIDE HOSPITALS PROGRAM, THE NNIS SURVEY, AND BAC-DATA

Organism	Number (percent of isolates)[a]		Rate/10,000 admissions				
			University of Virginia		Virginia Statewide Program	NNIS[20]	Bac-Data[22]
	1973—76	1977—6/78	1973—76	1977—78	1975—77[b]	1/74—6/74	7/77—6/78[c]
Streptococcus faecalis	8(1)	0(0)	1	0	2	—	—
Candida tropicalis	6(1)	4(1)	1	1	2	—	—
Citrobacter freundii	5(1)	2(0.5)	1	0.7	0.06	—	0.06
Anaerobic Streptococcus	5(1)	0(0)	1	0	0.03	—	—
Streptococcus pneumoniae	5(1)	3(0.7)	1	1	1	0.2	0.3
Proteus morganii	4(1)	1(0.2)	1	0.3	0.06	—	—
Micrococcus sp.	3(0.5)	1(0.2)	4	0.3	—	—	—
Enterobacter agglomerans	2(0.3)	3(0.7)	0.3	1	0.06	—	—
Aeromonas hydrophilia	2(0.3)	0(0)	0.3	0	—	—	—
Candida kruseii	2(0.3)	0(0)	0.3	0	—	—	—
Enterobacter spp.	2(0.3)	0(0)	0.3	0	1	—	—
Candida stellatoides	2(0.3)	0(0)	0.3	0	—	—	—
Proteus rettgeri	2(0.3)	0(0)	0.3	0	0.02	—	—
Proteus vulgaris	2(0.3)	1(0.2)	0.3	0.3	—	—	—
Torulopsis glabrata	2(0.3)	0(0)	0.3	0	—	—	—
Pseudomonas sp.	2(0.3)	4(1)	0.3	1	1.2	1.3	—
Enterobacter liquifaciens	2(0.3)	0(0)	0.3	0	—	—	—
Haemophilus influenzae	2(0.3)	0(0)	0.3	0	0.04	—	0.1

Bacteroides corrodens	1(0.2)	0(0)	0.2	0	—	—	—
Clostridium perfringens	1(0.2)	1(0.2)	0.2	0.3	0.04	—	—
Clostridium spp.	1(0.2)	0(0)	0.2	0	—	—	0.4
Gram-negative anaerobe	1(0.2)	2(0.5)	0.2	0.7	—	—	—
Haemophilus parainfluenzae	1(0.2)	0(0)	0.2	0	—	—	—
Listeria monocytogenes	1(0.2)	0(0)	0.2	0	—	—	—
Moraxella lacunata	1(0.2)	0(0)	0.2	0	—	—	—
Proprionibacterium sp.	1(0.2)	0(0)	0.2	0	—	—	—
Pseudomonas maltophilia	1(0.2)	5(1)	0.2	2	0.04	—	—
Salmonella enteriditis	1(0.2)	0(0)	0.2	0	0.08	—	—
Streptococcus viridans	1(0.2)	0(0)	0.2	0	—	—	—
Veillonella spp.	1(0.2)	0(0)	0.2	0	—	—	—
Diphtheroids spp.	1(0.2)	0(0)	0.2	0	—	—	—
Klebsiella ozaenae	1(0.2)	1(0.2)	0.2	0.3	—	—	—
Acinetobacter spp.	1(0.2)	0(0)	0.2	0	—	—	—
Corynebacterium spp.	1(0.2)	2(0.5)	0.2	0.7	0.1	—	0.3
Proteus sp.	1(0.2)	1(0.2)	0.2	0.3	—	0.6	—
Alkalifaciens dispar	1(0.2)	0(0)	0.2	0	—	—	—
Alkalifaciens spp.	1(0.2)	0(0)	0.2	0	—	—	—
Bacillus sp.	1(0.2)	2(0.5)	0.2	0.7	—	—	—
Flavobacterium spp.	1(0.2)	0(0)	0.2	0	0.06	—	—
Peptococcus	1(0.2)	1(0.2)	0.2	0.3	—	—	—
Proprionibacterium sp.	1(0.2)	0(0)	0.2	0	—	—	—
Pseudomonas cepacia	1(0.2)	0	0.2	0	—	—	—
Yeast	—	3(0.7)	—	1	—	—	0.06
Providencia stuartii	—	2(0.5)	—	0.7	—	—	—
Gram-negative rods (unidentified)	—	1(0.2)	—	0.3	—	—	—
Serratia liquifaciens	—	2(0.5)	—	0.7	—	—	—
Nonhemolytic streptococcus	—	1(0.2)	—	0.3	—	—	—
Gram-positive cocci (unidentified)	—	6(1)	—	2	—	—	—

Table 7A (continued)
CAUSES OF HOSPITAL ACQUIRED BLOODSTREAM INFECTIONS UNIVERSITY OF VIRGINIA (1973—1976, 1977—JUNE 1978), VIRGINIA STATEWIDE HOSPITALS PROGRAM, THE NNIS SURVEY, AND BAC-DATA

Organism	Number (percent of isolates)[a]		Rate/10,000 admissions				
			University of Virginia		Virginia Statewide Program	NNIS[20]	Bac-Data[22]
	1973—76	1977—6/78	1973—76	1977—78	1975—77[b]	1/74—6/74	7/77—6/78[c]
Coccobacillus (unidentified)	—	2(0.5)	—	0.7	—	—	—
Pseudomonas flourescens	—	1(0.2)	—	0.3	—	—	—
Candida parapsilosis	—	1(0.2)	—	0.3	—	—	—
Acinetobacter calcoasceticus	—	2(0.5)	—	0.7	—	—	—
Fusobacterium	—	1(0.2)	—	0.3	—	—	—
β Nonhemolytic streptococcus	—	2(0.5)	—	0.7	—	—	—
Streptococcus (non-B, non-D)	—	2(0.5)	—	0.7	—	—	—
β *Streptococcus* group B	—	2(0.5)	—	0.7	—	—	0.1
Bacterium spp. (unidentified)	—	2(0.5)	—	0.7	—	—	—
Pseudomonas stutzeri	—	1(0.2)	—	0.3	—	—	—

[a]   Total isolates surveyed 1973—76 = 634;
       Total isolates surveyed 1977—June 1978 = 483;
       Refers only to total number of organisms isolated at the University of Virginia Laboratory.
[b]   Sixty hospitals in Virginia of varying sizes submitting data.
[c]   Based on 14 hospitals widely dispersed in the U.S.; total discharges = 171,900.

Table 7B

CAUSES OF HOSPITAL ACQUIRED URINARY TRACT INFECTIONS UNIVERSITY OF VIRGINIA (1973—1976, 1977—JUNE 1978), NNIS, AND BAC-DATA

Organism	Number (percent of isolates)[a]		Rate/10,000 admissions			
			University of Virginia		NNIS[20]	Bac-Data[22]
	1973—76	1977—6/78	1973—76	1977—78	1/74—6/74	7/77—6/78*
Escherichia coli	593(30)	257(29)	77	84	51	48.4
Pseudomonas aeurginosa	145(7)	50(6)	19	16	—	—
P. spp.	136(7)	81(9)	18	26	18	—
Proteus mirabilis	135(7)	32(4)	18	10	—	—
Candida albicans	117(6)	36(4)	15	12	—	—
Klebsiella spp.	111(6)	62(7)	14	20	16	—
K. pneumoniae	104(5)	48(5)	14	16	—	12.9
P. sp.	91(5)	51(6)	12	17	20.6	—
Enterococcus spp.	89(4)	45(5)	12	15	21	17.9
C. sp.	74(4)	6(0.7)	10	10	6.3	—
Enterobacter aerogenes	37(2)	12(1.4)	5	4	—	—
Staphylococcus epidermidis	37(2)	25(3)	5	8	—	6
Enterobacter spp.	36(2)	14(1.6)	5	5	6.4	—
Serratia sp.	35(2)	6(0.7)	5	2	3.3	—
E. cloacae	34(2)	13(1.5)	4	4	—	—
Alpha Streptococcus Group D	29(1)	0(0)	4	0	—	—
Staphylococcus aureus	21(1)	10(1)	3	3	2.6	2.4
Serratia marcescens	20(1)	58(7)	3	19	—	—
Citrobacter diversans	2(0.1)	1(0.2)	0.3	0.3	—	—
Candida tropicalis	1(0.05)	6(0.7)	0.2	2	—	—
Moraxella lacunata	1(0.05)	0(0)	0.2	0	—	—
Pseudomonas cepacia	1(0.05)	0(0)	0.2	0	—	—

Table 7B (continued)

CAUSES OF HOSPITAL ACQUIRED URINARY TRACT INFECTIONS UNIVERSITY OF VIRGINIA (1973—1976, 1977—JUNE 1978), NNIS, AND BAC-DATA

Organism	Number (percent of isolates)[a]		Rate/10,000 admissions			
			University of Virginia		NNIS[20]	Bac-Data[22]
	1973—76	1977—6/78	1973—76	1977—78	1/74—6/74	7/77—6/78[e]
Acinetobacter lowffi	1(0.05)	0(0)	0.2	0	—	—
Flavobacterium sp.	1(0.05)	0(0)	0.2	0	—	—
Sarcina sp.	1(0.05)	0(0)	0.2	0	—	—
Gaffkya tetragena	1(0.05)	0(0)	0.2	0	—	—
Haemophilus sp.	1(0.05)	0(0)	0.2	0	—	—
H. vaginalis	1(0.05)	0(0)	0.2	0	—	—
Providencia alkalifaciens	1(0.05)	0(0)	0.2	0	—	—
E. agglomerans	—	1(0.2)	—	0.3	—	—
Alcaligenes faecalis	—	2(0.3)	—	0.7	—	—
Yeast	—	36(4)	—	12	—	4.5
Nonhemolytic streptococcus	—	6(0.7)	—	2	—	—
Klebsiella/Enterobacter spp.	—	15(2)	—	5	—	—
Streptococcus pneumoniae	—	1(0.2)	—	0.3	—	—
Gram-positive rods (unidentified)	—	3(0.4)	—	1	—	—
Staphylococcus micrococcus	—	2(0.3)	—	0.7	—	—
Torulopsis glabrata	—	1(0.2)	—	0.3	—	—
Streptococcus spp.	17(1)	0(0)	2	0	—	—
Citrobacter freundii	12(1)	1(0.2)	2	0.3	—	—
Proteus morganii	10(0.5)	2(0.3)	1	0.7	—	—

P. vulgaris	9(0.5)	1(0.2)	1	0.3	—	—
Providencia spp.	9(0.5)	0(0)	1	0	—	—
Acinetobacter spp.	9(0.5)	0(0)	1	0	—	—
Ac. anitratum	8(0.4)	1(0.2)	1	0.3	—	—
Micrococcus spp.	8(0.4)	2(0.3)	1	0.7	—	—
Alpha streptococcus	8(0.4)	0(0)	1	0	—	0.8
Hafnia sp.	7(0.4)	0(0)	1	0	—	—
Providencia stuartii	7(0.4)	2(0.3)	1	0.7	—	—
β Streptococcus	6(0.3)	4(0.5)	1	1	—	1.2
Corynebacterium spp.	6(0.3)	0(0)	1	0	—	1.4
Enterobacter hafnia	5(0.3)	0(0)	1	0	—	—
E. liquifaciens	5(0.3)	0(0)	1	0	—	—
K. ozaenae	4(2)	1(0.2)	1	0.3	—	—
Serratia liquifaciens	4(0.2)	0(0)	1	0	—	—
Citrobacter sp.	3(0.2)	0(0)	0.4	0	—	—
Pseudomonas fluorescens	2(0.1)	0(0)	0.3	0	—	—
Lactobacillus spp.	2(0.1)	0(0)	0.3	0	—	—
Proteus rettgeri	2(0.1)	4(0.5)	0.3	1	—	—
Alkalafaciens dispar	2(0.1)	0(0)	0.3	0	—	—
Not speciated	3(0.4)					

a Total isolates surveyed 1973—76 = 2001.
   Total isolates surveyed 1977—June 1978 = 901.
   Refers only to total number of organisms isolated at the University of Virginia Laboratory.
* Based on 14 hospitals widely dispersed in the U.S.; total discharges = 171,900.

Table 7C
ORGANISMS ISOLATED FROM SPUTUM OF PATIENTS WITH HOSPITAL ACQUIRED PNEUMONIAS
UNIVERSITY OF VIRGINIA (1973—1976, 1977—JUNE 1978), NATIONAL NOSOCOMIAL INFECTIONS STUDY, AND BAC-DATA

| Organism | Number (percent of isolates)[f] | | Rate/10,000 admissions | | | |
| | | | University of Virginia | | NNIS[20] | Bac-Data[22] |
	1973—76	1977—6/78	1973—76	1977—78[e]	1/74—6/74	7/77—6/78[h]
Escherichia coli	46(11)	28(11)	6	9	6	7.3
Pseudomonas spp.	46(11)	4(2)	6	1	6	—
Haemophilus influenzae	30(7)	3(1)	4	1	—	3.5
Staphylococcus aureus	30(7)	24(9)	4	8	6.2	6.3
Klebsiella pneumoniae	28(7)	26(10)	4	8	—	10.4
P. aeruginosa	26(6)	27(11)	9	3	—	—
Streptococcus pneumoniae	26(6)	18(7)	3	6	3	2.4
Klebsiella spp.	19(5)	2(0.8)	3	0.7	8	—
Proteus mirabilis	15(4)	22(9)	2	7	—	—
Proteus sp.	15(4)	2(0.8)	2	0.7	3.6	—
Candida albicans	13(3)	2(0.8)	2	0.7	—	—
Neisseria spp.	13(3)	4(2)	2	1	—	—
Enterobacter aerogenes	11(3)	7(3)	2	2	—	—
Enterobacter spp.	11(3)	2(0.8)	2	0.7	5	—
Alpha Streptococcus	10(2)	4(2)	1	1	—	0.4
Acinetobacter anitratum	8(2)	6(2)	1	2	—	—
E. cloacae	7(2)	11(4)	1	4	—	—
Staphylococcus epidermidis	7(2)	3(1)	1	0.1	—	0.3
Candida sp.	6(1)	0(0)	1	0	2.4	—

β Hemolytic Streptococcus Group A	5(1)	0(0)	1	0	—	—
Acinetobacter spp.	5(1)	0(0)	1	0	—	—
P. morganii	4(1)	2(0.8)	1	0.7	—	—
Serratia sp.	4(1)	0(0)	1	0	1.6	—
S. marcescens	4(1)	9(4)	1	3	—	—
Providencia stuartii	3(1)	0(0)	0.4	0	—	—
Streptococcus Group D	3(1)	0(0)	0.4	0	1.0	—
Alpha Hemolytic Streptococcus	3(1)	0(0)	0.4	0	—	—
Citrobacter sp.	2(0.5)	0(0)	0.3	0	—	—
H. parainfluenzae	1(0.2)	0(0)	0.3	0	—	—
Listeria monocytogenes	1(0.2)	0(0)	0.2	0	—	—
Bacillus subtilis	1(0.2)	0(0)	0.2	0	—	—
Citrobacter diversans	1(0.2)	2(0.8)	0.2	0.7	—	—
C. freundii	1(0.2)	0(0)	0.2	0	—	—
Proteus vulgaris	1(0.2)	0(0)	0.2	0	—	—
E. agglomerans	—	1(.4)	—	0.3	—	—
Yeast	—	7(3)	—	2	—	2.5
Pseudomonas maltophilia	—	3(1)	—	1	—	—
Gram positive (unidentified)	—	1(0.4)	—	3	—	—
β Streptococcus (non-group A)		5(2)		2		0.8
Klebsiella/Enterobacter spp.		10(4)		3		
Corynebacterium spp.		1(0.4)		0.3		
S. liquifaciens		1(0.4)		0.3		
Gram-negative rods		3(1)		1		
Hemophilia spp.		9(4)		3		
β Streptococcus group A		4(2)		1		

Table 7C (continued)
ORGANISMS ISOLATED FROM SPUTUM OF PATIENTS WITH HOSPITAL
ACQUIRED PNEUMONIAS
UNIVERSITY OF VIRGINIA (1973—1976, 1977—JUNE 1978), NATIONAL
NOSOCOMIAL INFECTIONS STUDY, AND BAC-DATA

Organism	Number (percent of isolates)[f]		Rate/10,000 admissions			
	1973—76	1977—6/78	University of Virginia		NNIS[20]	Bac-Data[22]
			1973—76	1977—78[g]	1/74—6/74	7/77—6/78[h]
Lactobacillus spp.	1 (0.4)		—	0.3		—
Staphylococcus micro-coccus	2 (0.9)		—	0.7		—
P. putida	1 (0.4)		—	0.3		—

[f] Total isolates surveyed 1973—76 = 723.
Total isolates surveyed 1977—June 1978 = 258.
Refers only to total number of organisms isolated at the University of Virginia Laboratory.
[g] Sixty hospitals in Virginia of varying sizes submitting data.
[h] Based on 14 hospitals widely dispersed in the U.S.; total discharges = 171,900.

Table 7D

ORGANISMS ISOLATED FROM THE PURULENT DRAINAGE OF PATIENTS WITH POSTOPERATIVE WOUND INFECTIONS
UNIVERSITY OF VIRGINIA (1973—76, 1977—MAY 1978), NATIONAL NOSOCOMIAL INFECTIONS STUDY, AND BAC-DATA

| Organism | Number (percent of isolates)[i] | | Rate/10,000 admissions | | | |
| | | | University of Virginia | | NNIS[20] | Bac-Data[22] |
	1973—76	1977—5/78	1973—76	1977—78[j]	7/74—6/74	7/77—6/78[k]
Staphylococcus aureus	158(24)	73(21)	20	25	20	14.8
Escherichia coli	70(11)	40(12)	9	14	15.5	11.2
Pseudomonas aeruginosa	47(7)	37(11)	6	13	—	—
β Streptococcus	36(6)	14(4)	5	5	—	0.6
Pseudomonas spp.	34(5)	1(0.3)	4	0.3	7	—
Proteus mirabilis	29(4)	24(7)	4	8	—	—
Enterobacter cloacae	28(4)	11(3)	4	4	—	—
Enterococci	28(4)	29(8)	4	10	9	—
St. epidermidis	25(4)	18(5)	3	6	—	9.8
α Streptococcus	24(4)	8(2)	3	3	—	1.9
Klebsiella pneumoniae	22(3)	20(6)	3	7	—	3.6
Klebsiella sp.	15(2)	1(0.3)	2	0.3	5.5	—
Candida sp.	12(2)	0(0)	2	0	0.8	—
E. aerogenes	11(2)	0(0)	2	0	—	—
Acinetobacter anitratum	10(2)	4(1)	1	1	—	—
P. morganii	10(2)	8(2)	1	3	—	—
Serratia marcescens	9(1)	13(4)	1	5	—	—
Streptococcus spp.	9(1)	4(1)	1	1	5.2	—
Enterobacter sp.	9(1)	0(0)	1	0	4.2	—
Serratia sp.	6(1)	0(0)	1	0	1	—
Micrococcus sp.	5(1)	1(0.3)	1	0.3	—	—

Table 7D (continued)
ORGANISMS ISOLATED FROM THE PURULENT DRAINAGE OF PATIENTS WITH POSTOPERATIVE WOUND INFECTIONS UNIVERSITY OF VIRGINIA (1973—76, 1977—MAY 1978), NATIONAL NOSOCOMIAL INFECTIONS STUDY, AND BAC-DATA

Organism	Number (percent of isolates)[c]		Rate/10,000 admissions			
			University of Virginia		NNIS[20]	Bac-Data[22]
	1973—76	1977—5/78	1973—76	1977—78[d]	7/74—6/74	7/77—6/78[x]
P. vulgaris	5(1)	0(0)	1	0	—	—
Corynebacterium spp.	5(1)	0(0)	1	0	—	1
Providencia stuartii	5(1)	3(0.9)	1	1	—	—
Proteus sp.	5(1)	6(2)	1	2	7.6	—
Bacteroides fragilis	3(0.5)	5(1.5)	0.4	2	—	—
Bacteroides sp.	3(0.5)	2(0.6)	0.4	0.7	4.3	—
C. albicans	3(0.5)	3(0.9)	0.4	1	—	—
Citrobacter diversans	2(0.3)	0(0)	0.3	0	—	—
Lactobacillus spp.	2(0.3)	1(0.3)	0.3	0.3	—	—
Neisseria sp.	2(0.3)	0(0)	0.3	0	—	—
Clostridium perfringens	2(0.3)	4(1)	0.3	1	—	—
Acinetobacter spp.	2(0.3)	0(0)	0.3	0	—	—
Aeromonas hydrophilia	1(0.2)	0(0)	0.2	0	—	—
Bacteroides melanino-genicus	1(0.2)	1(0.3)	0.2	0.3	—	—
E. agglomerans	1(0.2)	1(0.3)	0.2	0.3	—	—
Proteus rettgeri	1(0.2)	1(0.3)	0.2	0.3	—	—
Citrobacter spp.	1(0.2)	0(0)	0.2	0	—	—
Clostridium spp.	1(0.2)	0(0)	0.2	0	—	0.8
Anaerobic streptococci	1(0.2)	0(0)	0.2	0	—	0.3
St. pneumoniae	1(0.2)	0(0)	0.2	0	0.1	0.1
Gaffkya sp.	1 (0.2)	0 (0)	0.2	0	—	—
Providencia alkalifa-ciens	1 (0.2)	0 (0)	0.2	0	—	—

E. hafnia	1 (0.2)	1 (0)	0.2	0	—	—
Pseudomonas maltophilia	—	1 (0.3)	—	0.3	—	—
Klebsiella/Enterobacter spp.	—	3 (0.9)	—	1	—	—
Nonhemolytic streptococcus	—	4 (1)	—	1	—	—
S. micrococcus	—	3 (0.9)	—	1	—	—
Acinetobacter lowffi	—	1 (0.3)	—	0.3	—	—
Yeast	—	5 (1.5)	—	2	—	0.06
Gram-negative rods (unidentified)	—	8 (2)	—	3	—	—
Gram-positive rods (unidentified)	—	1 (0.3)	—	0.3	—	—
Gram-positive cocci (unidentified)	—	3 (0.9)	—	1	—	—

Total isolates surveyed 1973—76 = 651; total isolates surveyed 1977—May 1978 = 348;

refers only to total number of organisms isolated at the University of Virginia Laboratory.

Sixty Hospitals in Virginia of varying sizes submitting data.

Based on 14 hospitals widely dispersed in the U.S., total discharges = 171,900.

Table 8A
POSTOPERATIVE WOUND INFECTION RATES
UNIVERSITY OF VIRGINIA, JANUARY 1973—JUNE 1978[a]

Service	Procedures	Number of infections/number of procedures = (%)
Neurosurgery	Laminectomy	23/761 = (3)
	CNS[a] Shunt	22/305 = (7.2)
	VP[b] — Wound infection	13/281 = (4.6)
	VP[b] — CSF infection	9/106 = (8.5)
	Non-VP[b] — wound infection	1/12 = (8.3)
	Non-VP[b] — CSF infection	1/9 = (11)
	Shunt revision	9/128 = (7)
Plastic surgery	Face lift	0/70 = (0)
	Craniofacial surgery	2/75 = (2.7)
	Blepharoplasty	0/62 = (0)
	Transfer rotation flap	36/307 = (11.7)
	Burn contraction release	6/63 = (9.5)
	STSG[c] (Nonburn service)	92/458 = (20)
Burn	STSG[c]	141/491 = (28.7)
Thoracic cardiovascular surgery	CABG[d]	18/495 = (3.6)
	Valve replacement	16/345 = (4.6)
	Bypass grafts	4/148 = (2.7)
	Femoral popliteal	8/121 = (6.6)
	Aorto-femoral	0/38 = (0)
	Other	2/60 = (3)
Urology	Nephrostomy	3/41 = (7.3)
	Cystostomy	0/88 = (0)
	Nephrectomy	7/144 = (4.9)
Otolaryngology	Radical neck dissection	17/104 = (16.3)
	With intra-oral surgery	6/28 = (21.4)
	No intra-oral surgery	1/29 = (3.4)
General surgery	Renal transplant	16/87 = (18)
	Appendectomy	40/688 = (5.8)
	Ruptured	16/72 = (22.3)
	Nonruptured	10/359 = (2.8)
	Cholecystectomy	31/722 = (4.3)
	Herniorraphy	17/924 = (1.8)
	Complicated	3/13 = (2.3)
	Uncomplicated	2/467 = (0.4)
	Colon resection	24/283 = (8.5)
	Below knee amputation	17/122 = (14)
Gynecology	TAH[e]	28/591 = (4.7)
	TVH[f]	28/580 = (4.8)
	Abortion (endometritis)	4/315 = (1.3)

Table 8A (continued)
POSTOPERATIVE WOUND INFECTION RATES
UNIVERSITY OF VIRGINIA, JANUARY 1973—JUNE 1978[a]

Service	Procedures	Number of infections/ number of procedures = (%)		
Orthopedics	THR[g]	10/422	=	(2.4)
	TKR[h]	5/163	=	(3.1)
	Menisectomy	6/982	=	(16.7)

[a]	CNS	= Cental nervous system shunt.
[b]	VP	= Ventriculo-peritoneal.
[c]	STSG	= Split thickness skin graft.
[d]	CABG	= Coronary artery bypass graft.
[e]	TAH	= Total abdominal hysterectomy.
[f]	TVH	= Total vaginal hysterectomy.
[g]	THR	= Total hip replacement.
[h]	TKR	= Total knee replacement.

there was a greater likelihood on the burn unit than on the wards that the organism in the bloodstream was resistant to commonly used aminoglycoside antibiotics. One of the uses of such data will be to help clinicians decide which antibiotic to initiate for suspected bloodstream infections until the antibiogram data are available 2 days later, by knowing where the patient is and where he has been located within the hospital.

THE WRITTEN REPORT

By definition, a report is a summary of collected data carefully organized for the purpose of informing others — it is a communication. The purpose of the infection control report, which is generally published monthly, is to educate, elicit interest, and change behavior of those in the health care field. Therefore, besides informing, the report may be an important instrument in effecting control of some infections. The basis for the requested behavior changes are the data gleaned from surveillance; in addition, there may be supportive information in the literature. The underlying assumptions important for effective reporting are as follows:

1. The reports must be relevant to the reader.
2. They should be easily understood.
3. They should be brief.
4. The major change in behavior requested, i.e., the "message", should be clearly indicated and underscored in the report.

Whenever possible, graphs and figures should be substituted for lengthy tables, and definitions and keys to various abbreviations and symbols should be clearly stated.

One of the problems with most infection reports is that the readers — nurses and physicians in medicine — do not know how to alter their practice based on data relating to overall rates or rates by site, service, and pathogen. It seems most obvious that ICPs must develop reports now that focus on specific operations and procedures and relate to specific hospital personnel. In the past, if the chief of general surgery were to read that the overall infection rate was 10% or that all clean-contaminated operations had an infection rate of 12.5%, there was very little that he or she could do with the infor-

Table 8 B
SUMMARY OF INFECTIONS FOLLOWING 100 OR MORE OPERATIONS (1968—1975)

	National Research Council			Foothills Hospital		
	Number of wounds	Infections Number	%	Number of wounds	Infections Number	%
General surgery						
Breast biopsy excision lesion	827	18	2.2	768	2	0.3
Radical mastectomy	227	43	18.9	—		
Modified radical mastectomy	—			446	19	4.3
Partial gastrectomy	288	29	10.1	194	26	13.4
Vagotomy and pyloroplasty	—			687	41	6.0
Partial colectomy with anastomosis	220	22	10.0	312	54	17.3
Abdominoperineal resection	190	22	11.6	101	25	24.8
Total colectomy	—			67	10	14.9
Appendectomy	551	63	11.4	1,821	180	9.9
Cholecystectomy	756	52	6.9	3,129	93	3.0
Cholecystectomy	—			1,466	28	1.9
Cholecystectomy with cholangiography	—			747	15	2.0
Cholecystectomy with appendectomy	—			399	18	4.5
Choledochostomy	111	19	17.1	470	40	8.5
"Negative" laparotomy	321	25	7.8	159	8	5.0
Inguinal hernia	1,312	25	1.9	2,360	11	0.5
Incisional hernia	314	12	3.8	239	10	4.2
Splenectomy	—			141	1	0.7
Stripping of varicose veins	204	12	5.9	1,374	8	0.6
Thyroidectomy	406	9	2.2	305	3	1.0
Nephrectomy	127	22	17.3	(Unilat.) 164	6	3.6
				(Bilat.) 79	5	6.3
Orthopedics						
Bone biopsy and excision of bone lesion	109	6	5.5	415	10	2.4
Open reduction and nailing of fractured femur	—			194	13	6.7
Open reduction of fractured tibia	144	6	4.2	83	7	8.8

Fractured hip	—			655	32	4.9
Excision of intervertebral disk	212	1.4	3	798	12	1.5
Excision of intervertebral disk with fusion	—	—	—	1,297	38	2.9
Site of donor bone	—	—	—	1,134	43	3.8
Hip arthroplasty	—	—	—	238	10	4.2
Meniscectomy	—	—	—	993	4	0.4
Keller's operation	—	—	—	853	7	0.8
Gynecology						
Abdominal hysterectomy with or without salpingo-oophorectomy	628	6.1	38	2,066	89	4.3
Cesarean section	—	—	—	1,113	72	6.5
Abdominal tubal ligation	—	—	—	3,497	18	0.5
Oophorectomy: unilateral or bilateral	136	3.7	5	104	4	3.8
Cardiovascular — thoracic						
Exploratory thoracotomy (with or without biopsy)	137	5.8	8	61	3	4.9
Lobectomy, segmental resection	131	6.9	9	155	6	3.9
Femoropopliteal bypass	—	—	—	369	25	6.8
Aortoiliac bypass	—	—	—	246	10	4.1
Neurosurgery						
Craniotomy — tumor	—	—	—	269	1	0.4
Craniotomy — aneurysm	—	—	—	104	3	2.9
Laminotomy	—	—	—	228	5	2.2
Plastic surgery						
Otoplasty	—	—	—	201	2	1.0
Augmentation mammaplasty	—	—	—	427	4	0.9
Reduction mammaplasty	—	—	—	196	6	3.1
Rhyodoplasty	—	—	—	254	1	0.4

Reprinted by permission from the *South. Med. J.*, 70(1), 6, 1977.

Table 9A
RISK OF URINARY TRACT INFECTION FOLLOWING INDWELLING FOLEY BLADDER CATHETERIZATION

Service	Cumulative risk — number of infections/number of procedures = (%)	Day of infection after catheterization[a] Mean	Median
General surgery	51/432 = (12)	24	8
Gynecology	14/302 = (5)	6	5
Medicine	212/1800 = (12)	15	10
Neurology	63/319 = (20)	12	11
Neurosurgery	52/207 = (25)	18	8
Obstetrics	5/487 = (1)	3	3
Ophthalmology	0/24 = (0)	—	—
Otolaryngology	0/42 = (0)	—	—
Orthopedics	375/615 = (60)	30	18
Pediatrics	11/115 = (9)	33	33
Plastic surgery	14/107 = (13)	46	23
Burn unit	28/68 = (41)	20	15
TCV surgery[b]	13/421 = (3)	13	10
Urology	35/290 = (13)	11	8
Total	873/5229 = (17)		

[a] Based on N = 209.
[b] TCV = Thoracic/cardiovascular.

Table 9B
RESPIRATOR-ASSOCIATED PNEUMONIA UNIVERSITY OF VIRGINIA HOSPITAL (1974—1977)

Service	Number pneumonia/ number on respirator[a] (%)	Mean day of infection after admission (n = 217)	Mean day of infection after placement on respirator (n = 146)
Burn	5/20 (25)	18	7
NICU[b]	13/83 (16)	—[c]	—[c]
General surgery	52/318 (16)	19	13
Urology	3/25 (12)	42	8
Neurosurgery	27/282 (10)	16	12
Gynecology	1/10 (10)	10	4
Medicine	52/859 (6)	20	12
TCV surgery[d]	48/893 (5)	21	14
Neurology	8/157 (5)	24	14
Orthopedics	3/86 (3)	20	12
Pediatrics	5/276 (2)	36	37
Otolaryngology	0/15 (0)	—	—
Obstetrics	0/3 (0)	—	—
Ophthalmology	0/1 (0)	—	—
Total	227/3096 (7)	21	14

[a] Of patients admitted, 4% are placed on a respirator.
[b] NICU = Newborn intensive care unit.
[c] Included in pediatrics.
[d] TCV = Thoracic/cardiovascular.

Table 10
RATES OF HOSPITAL ACQUIRED BSIª BY LOCATION WITHIN THE HOSPITAL: SPECIFIC REFERENCE TO INTENSIVE CARE AREAS — 1977

Location	Total admissions	Total patient days	Total number BSI	Total BSI caused by Gram-negative rods		Number BSI with isolates resistant			Isolates in blood resistant to aminoglycosides (%)		
				Infections	Isolates	Gentamicin	Tobramycin	Amikacin	Gentamicin	Tobramycin	Amikacin
Surgical ICU^b	1,735	5,351	58	37	43	15	13	2	41	35	5
Medical											
ACU^c	209	1,227	2	2	2	1	0	1	50	—	50
BU^d	121	1,349	32	26	34	13	13	5	50	50	19
CCU^e	1,013	2,510	4	1	1	0	1	1	—	100	100
NICU^f	406	8,042	27	19	24	2	2	2	11	11	11
General wards	17,024	173,968	153	92	102	9	10	2	10	11	2
Total	20,508	102,447	276	177	206	40	39	13	23	22	7

ª   BSI   = Bloodstream infection.
b   ICU   = Intensive care unit.
c   ACU   = Acute care unit.
d   BU   = Burn unit.
e   CCU   = Cardiac care unit.
f   NICU = Newborn intensive care unit.

mation. However, if one lists the specific procedure, stating that there was a 3 or 10% postoperative wound infection rate following a nonruptured primary appendectomy, then the chief surgeon has an idea if the rate is high, low, or average; and he knows who performed that type of operation. He can therefore have that physician specifically examine the techniques used and identify the types of patients associated with the operation in question. It seems reasonable to assume that most physicians and nurses in medicine are highly motivated and want the best for their patients, including a minimal risk of infection following a hospital procedure. No one wants to be identified with a procedure associated with a high infection rate. Therefore, the interpretation of the data, which are published widely within the hospital, should be scientific and cautious; and comments should reflect the sensitivity necessary to effect change without unnecessary embarrassment.

A second major focus for reports should be data related to hospital acquired bloodstream infections. This is important because bloodstream infections have a high mortality and because the organisms recovered are usually not contaminants since the bloodstream is a closed space area. Data related to both pathogens and antibiograms are important as well as data on patients' underlying diseases, in order to determine whether or not there is a new problem, i.e., an outbreak, perhaps related to a given procedure or secondary to infections at another site.

There are several types of infection reports possible based on the extent of the population surveyed:

1. A floor or ward report
2. A specific service report
3. A hospital-wide report
4. A regional or statewide report
5. A national report

A major question is how much information should be sent to whom. In its simplest fashion, the answer is that as much available information should be given as the readers are interested in absorbing. Caution, however, is necessary; although it is very easy to present a large report of great interest to the infection control team, such overwhelming epistles may have a negative effect on those interested only in the infections on a given ward or service. Generally, it is the experience of many epidemiologists that those nurses and physicians on one floor are not keenly interested in the infection rates for patients in other locations in the hospital. They are interested in their own patients and a fair assessment of the infection risks of their own procedures. Even a service report, such as pediatric or internal medicine report, does not have the same meaning for the floor if that service admits to several wards. Therefore, it seems reasonable to conclude that the ideal report for a ward or a service is one which limits the data to those areas specifically (or in some way highlights the specific ward or service report). On the other hand, it does seem important that certain people in the hospital receive the full hospital-wide report: administrators, chiefs of all the medical services, chiefs of all the support services, and the director of nursing services. In addition, complete reports should be available to anyone else who is interested. There is no question that the epidemiology service has a responsibility, within their capabilities and time constraints, to analyze the data critically, even though only portions of it are distributed to the rest of the hospital.

For purposes of continuing education in infection control and of changing behavior, it seems most important to review the data of the monthly report with the ward nurses and, if possible, with the physicians who work on any given ward. If only a single report is generated in the hospital, the practitioner who is assigned to surveillance on a given ward can circle in red all data related to the specific floor service being covered and briefly review the information with the head nurses and other nurses who are available. The information could then be passed on by the nurses at the time of the change of shift reports over the subsequent 24 hr. Any particular messages related to procedures, patients with bloodstream infections, and possible outbreaks are highlighted and covered in this brief 15-min summary between the ICP and the ward nurses.

There are no data to show that a particular type of illustration or report has influenced behavior in hospitals more than another type. It seems obvious that brief summaries, graphic illustrations, and comments are read more often than extensive tables. Examples of local reports from the University of Virginia Hospital showing the site, service, pathogen, procedure, and operation-related infection data are shown in the chapter entitled "Isolation Procedure and Infection Control Manual". In addition to monthly reports, reports illustrating secular trends have an important impact if the data relate to clinical cases. Examples might include infections on a given service for a specific procedure, results of antibiotic resistance in bloodstream pathogens, or rates for a procedure in which major changes have been instituted.

SPECIAL REPORTS

In general, there are three other reports which are generated by the infection control team. They include

1. The monthly Infection Control Committee report
2. Special announcements such as the institution of a new policy
3. A report identifying or summarizing work-up of an outbreak

The committee report should list all members and identify those present for the meeting. In addition it should acknowledge the review of the infection surveillance report and note if there were any unusually high infection rates and any explanations for the unusually high rates. In addition, the report should perform the following functions:

1. Briefly identify the question or problem presented to the committee (usually only one or two can be adequately handled in depth in the 1-hr meeting).
2. Present the background information and all options for decisions (usually provided by the infection control team or guest expert).
3. Summarize the subsequent discussion.
4. Record the final resolution by the committee.

If any subcommittees are formed, its membership should be listed, and duties of the group and report deadlines should be stated.

In the other two types of special reports, it is wise to give a full explanation to the chiefs of departments verbally and then follow with a personal letter outlining the substance of the report. It is this author's opinion that "To:/From:" letters should be avoided in dealing with heads of departments and hospital services. They carry a military and an impersonal connotation not helpful for the diplomacy needed to implement a new policy or describe a new outbreak. As in any report, the problem should be succinctly stated, background data briefly summarized, and simple charts and figures substituted for lengthy tables. The primary message should be clearly phrased and highlighted, and most importantly, specific requests of the chiefs of service be enumerated. If possible, some estimation of the duration of the investigation or problem should be included. If a new procedure is being instituted, then the expected (or known) benefits should be stated.

CENTRALIZED REPORTING

In 1970 the CDC organized the first system for generalized reporting of hospital acquired infections, NNIS. To initiate the program, the CDC originally supported the salaries of voluntary hospital ICPs. Currently there are over 80 hospitals from 30 states reporting monthly infection rates to Atlanta.[20] The purpose of this program and others is to standardize infection control at a high level of excellence, identify low frequency, common source outbreaks such as those associated with intrinsically contaminated I.V. products, and to be a central resource for new information.

The first statewide program in infection control was initiated at the University of Virginia Medical Center in 1974. Currently there are over 50 hospitals reporting nosocomial infection data monthly to Charlottesville. The program was originally funded totally by the CDC as a pilot project, with the goal that the state would eventually offer support necessary for maintaining it. In 1978, The State Health Department assumed full support of the program. All those contributing to the University of Virginia/State Health Department Program have been trained in Charlottesville in courses of eight to ten students each. Variations of the Kardex® systems of suveillance have been employed and standard definitions for infection are used throughout the state. The compliance to the program, i.e., the willingness of participating hospitals to send reports once they have sent their first report, has been estimated to be approximately 85%. Accuracy of surveillance was reassessed in comparative prospective reviews and was estimated to be approximately 70%.[23] The statewide surveillance system has been utilized to examine postoperative wound infection rates for specific procedures.[24]

FUTURE NEEDS

Currently there are no data to show that routine surveillance by itself in a hospital has led to a reduction in infection rates; nor are there data to show that surveillance has reduced morbidity or mortality in hospital acquired infections. However, there are many encouraging preliminary reports from the SENIC (Study of the Efficacy of Nosocomial Infection Control) that hospitals employing surveillance have lower infection rates than those not performing surveillance.[25] Moreover, since the alternative for surveillance, i.e., not knowing the infection rates for various hospital services and procedures, seems undesirable, the current emphasis favors performing some type of surveillance. Although the benefits of high visibility of the infection control team while performing surveillance and continual education seems obvious, the impact of education itself on long-term control of infection remains poorly documented. In the meantime, it seems worthwhile to develop more refined reporting in order to understand existing problems and perhaps begin to design studies to determine the effect of new infection control policies or behavioral changes.

Some practitioners begin to reach an impass or saturation point after several years of continual surveillance. They do not have time or help, including computer assistance, to become more sophisticated. At the same time, demands in other areas increase. It is the philosophy of the author that hospitals should spend at least 1 year performing in-depth continual surveillance of all wards. Thereafter if outside demands, e.g., teaching or working up new policies and procedures, exceed resources, it seems reasonable to focus surveillance on all the intensive care units (ICUs) and continue to relate infections to common hospital procedures.[26] Exactly how much time should be spent outside the ICU surveying postoperative wound infections following a selected number of procedures depends on the time available and data obtained. With more resources or surveillance efficiency, it seems wise to concentrate on the rate of infections in the urine and lung after Foley catheterizations and respiratory assistance, respectively.

Education using the surveillance system data should be an ongoing effort, and it is extremely important that the infection control team work closely with the in-service team, providing information to identify priority areas. It is the opinion of many that the ICP should not forfeit his/her identity as a clinical specialist and that more effort should be made to have that person collecting data not only skilled in the area of surveillance but also in the performance of many of the hospital procedures. Identification by other nurses working in the hospital that the ICP is also a skilled clinician lends important credibility to his or her skills as an epidemiologist. Perhaps a few days each month should be spent in an ICU actually performing the procedures important for infection control, e.g., bladder catheterizations, tracheostomy care, and others.

Certainly the literature is replete with articles that end with such statements that the hospital personnel were told to wash their hands more carefully and/or that intense teaching was instituted. Our success nevertheless in getting hospital personnel to wash hands between patient visits seems dismal more than 100 years after Semmelweis first illustrated the importance of this 15-sec procedure. In the future, it is possible that even if we develop effective alternatives to current handwashing procedures, we will also employ the expertise of psychologists, marketing professionals, and management experts.

There is no seminar in infection control which does not touch on the political issues associated with infection control, particularly those encountered in the workup of outbreaks. The data from surveillance should be carefully presented to those chiefs of services involved in various outbreaks in order to address the issues rather than the problems that may arise because of concern over "turf" or pride. The chiefs of services and chiefs of special care units in which outbreaks have been identified must be informed of the problem, the available data, and proposed workup before such information is more widely distributed.

Since the ICPs are among the few who operate throughout the hospital, their role is likely to expand to become a more general one of the patients' advocates.[27] In the future, surveillance of all procedures and equipment which could affect the safety of patients might come under the responsibility of the infection control team. With the development of local, statewide, and international programs and refinements of computer assistance, many policies and procedures affecting health care will be more carefully scrutinized. The problems of infection control certainly traverse national boundaries, and it is only a matter of time before the World Health Organization will extend its efforts and look at hospital acquired infections on an international scale.

REFERENCES

1. Rose, R., Hunting, K. J., Townsend, T. R., and Wenzel, R. P., Morbidity/mortality and economics of hospital-acquired blood stream infections: a controlled study, *South. Med. J.,* 70, 1267, 1977.
2. Townsend, T. R. and Wenzel, R. P., Nosocomial bloodstream infections among neonates in a newborn intensive care unit: a controlled study, Abstracts of the 18th Interscience Conf. Antimicrobial Agents and Chemotherapy, No. 376, 1978.

2a. **Freeman, J., Rosner, B., and McGowan, J. E.**, Adverse effects of nosocomial infection, *J. Infec. Dis.*, 140, 732, 1979.

2b. **Townsend, T. R. and Wenzel, R. P.**, Nosocomial bloodstream infections in a newborn intensive care unit: a case-matched control study of morbidity, mortality, and risk, *Am. J. Epidemiol.*, 113, 1981.

3. **Wenzel, R. P., Osterman, C. A. Hunting, K. J., and Gwaltney, J. M., Jr.**, Hospital-acquired infections. I. Surveillance in a university hospital, *Am. J. Epidemiol.* 103, 251, 1976.

4. **Kislak, J. W., Eickhoff, T. C., and Finland, M.**, Hospital-acquired infections and antibiotic usage in the Boston City Hospital 1964, *N. Engl. J. Med.*, 271, 834, 1964.

5. **Barrett, F. F., Casey, J. I., and Finland, M.**, Infections and antibiotic use among patients at Boston City Hospital, February 1967, *N. Engl. J. Med.*, 278, 5, 1968.

6. **McNamara, M. J., Hill, M. C., Balows, A., and Tucker E. G.**, A study of the bacteriologic patterns of hospital infections, *Ann. Intern. Med.*, 66, 480, 1967.

7. **Thoburn, R., Fekety, F. R., Cluff, L. E., and Melvin, V. B.**, Infections acquired by hospitalized patients, *Ann. Intern. Med.*, 121, 1, 1968.

8. **Oh, M. K., Matsen, J. M., Leonard, A. A., and Quie, P. G.**, Antibiotic therapy and hospital-acquired infections, *Minn. Med.*, 52, 1067, 1969.

9. **Adler, J. L. and Shulman, J. A.**, Nosocomial infection and antibiotic usage at Grady Memorial Hospital, a prevalence survey, *South. Med. J.*, 63, 102, 1970.

10. **Wenzel, R. P., Osterman, C. A., and Hunting, K. J.**, Hospital-acquired infections. II. Infection rates by site, service and common hospital procedures, *Am. J. Epidemiol.* 104, 645, 1976.

11. **Groschel, D. and Bradley, S. R.**, Surveillance of infection in a community teaching hospital, *Yale, J. Biol. Med.*, 44, 247, 1971.

12. **Mulholland, S. G., Greenhalgh, P. J., and Blakemore, W. S.**, Experience with detailed surveillance of nosocomial infection, *Surg. Gynecol. Obstet.*, 140, 941, 1975.

13. **Eickhoff, T. C., Brachman, P. S., Bennett, J. V., and Brown, J. F.**, Surveillance of nosocomial infections in community hospitals. I. Surveillance methods, effectiveness, and initial results, *J. Infect. Dis.*, 120, 305, 1969.

14. **Silberg, S. I., Paiker, D. E., Corrie, R. N., and Adess, M. L.**, Surveillance of nosocomial infections in two Oklahoma City area hospitals, *Okla. State Med. Assoc. J.*, 67, 134, 1974.

15. **Britt, J. R., Burke, J. P., Nordquist, A. G., Wilfert, J. N., and Smith, C. B.**, Infection control in small hospitals, prevalence surveys in 18 institutions, *JAMA*, 236, 1700, 1976.

16. **Shoji, J. T., Axnick, K., and Rytel, M. W.**, Infections and antibiotic use in a large municipal hospital, 1970—1972: a prospective analysis of the effectiveness of a continuous surveillance program, *Health Lab. Sci.*, 2, 283, 1974.

17. **Edwards, L. D.**, Infections and use of antimicrobials in an 800-bed hospital, *Public Health Rep.*, 84, 451, 1969.

18. **Stark, F. R. and Collins, T. C.**, Total surveillance program of infections: an analysis of two new programs in Army teaching hospitals, *Mil. Med.*, 141, 33, 1976.

19. **John, J. F.**, Nosocomial infection rates at a general Army hospital, *Am. J. Surg.*, 134, 381, 1977.

20. **Center for Disease Control**, National Nosocomial Infection Study Report, Annual Summary 1974, April 1977, 6.

21. **Post-operative wound infections:** the influence of ultraviolet irradiation of the operating room and of various other factors, report of an Ad Hoc Committee of the Committee on Trauma, Division of Medical Sciences, National Academy of Sciences, National Research Council, *Ann. Surg.*, 160 (Suppl.) 23, 1964.

22. **Moore, G. J.**, personal communication.

23. **Wenzel, R. P., Osterman, C. A., Townsend, T. R., Veazey, J. M., Jr., Servis, K. H., Miller, L. S., Craven, R. B., Miller, G. B., Jr., and Jackson, R. S.**, Development of a statewide program for surveillance and reporting of hospital-aquired infections, *J. Infect. Dis.*, 140, 741, 1979.

24. **Farber, B. F. and Wenzel, R. P.**, Postoperative wound infection rates: results of prospective statewide surveillance, *Am. J. Surg.*, 140, 343, 1980.

25. **Haley, R.**, The SENIC Report, Proc. 2nd Int. Symp. Nosocomial Infections, 1981.

26. **Wenzel, R. P., Osterman, C. A., Donowitz, L. G., Hoyt, J. W., Sande, M. A., Martone, W. J., Peacock, J. E., Jr., Levine, J. J., and Miller, G. B., Jr.**, Identifications of procedure-related nosocomial infections in high risk patients, *Rev. Infect. Dis.*, 1981.

27. **Hierholzer, W. J., Jr.**, Hospital epidemiology beyond infection control, *Infect. Control*, 1, 373, 1980.

COMPUTERS AND INFECTION SURVEILLANCE

Harvey A. Elder and Darrell A. Leonhardt

INTRODUCTION

Hosptal infection control is becoming a scientific discipline. It incorporates many principles from engineering, biology, and education. Infection control begins with a rational evaluation of accurate and pertinent data within the logic matrix of engineering, hygiene, microbiology, pathology, immunology, physiology, and pharmacology, using epidemiologic methods. When valid conclusions are derived, they need to be applied using the disciplines of education, psychology, communication, and administration. To miss any part—data collection, the logic matrix, epidemiologic methodology, or application of results—is to replace scientific hospital infection control with random responses to perceived catastrophies.

The computer assists in the collection of data and in the epidemiologic methodology. By its ability to present intelligible displays of significant data, the computer allows Infection Control Practitioners (ICPs) to develop hypotheses that can be tested statistically. Data manipulation is the computer's function. Logic, decision making, and decision implementation are human functions. In this chapter, the idea that the computer is merely a compiler of historic data for committees to ponder is not accepted by the authors. The computer frees ICPs from the tedium of what they do poorly (data manipulation), so that they can perform the logic, decision making, and implementation aspects of infection control. The problems and design constraints that these notions impose upon computer usage and the necessary decisions anteceding computer utilization are herein reviewed.

SURVEILLANCE

Infection surveillance utilizes various strategies of case finding, referred to as "case find", the identification of potentially infected patients. Patients (or their charts) are carefully examined to determine if they fulfill the criteria for infection, i.e., have verified infections. If case find is not followed by verification, surveillance is not selective, i.e., it includes noninfected patients along with the infected patients. If infection verification is done on only part of the infected population, then surveillance is not sensitive because some patients with infection are not identified and verified. It is too much useless work to examine every hospitalized patient; thus, some system of identifying potentially infected patients, case find, should be developed. This may include review of microbiology data, antimicrobial utilization, nursing reports, Kardex®,[1] etc. (see chapter entitled "Surveillance and Reporting of Hospital Acquired Infections").

Efficiency will be defined in terms of the utilization of the ICPs time and effort. The ICP must choose a proper balance between sensitivity, selectivity, and efficiency which is individualized for the needs, resources, and problems of the hospital. Important epidemiologic information may be stored and retrieved by the ICP and used to determine infection rates, the presence or absence of potential epidemics or epidemic agents, and the identification of services or wards with excessive infectious disease problems. Additionally, it may be possible to identify specific procedures (surgical, diagnostic, or therapeutic) associated with frequent infectious complications. From the epidemiologic study of endemic infections, a strategy for improved control may be designed to alter causitive factors, i.e., new procedures can be developed. Continued surveillance will show whether or not the instituted change (the new procedures) decreased the endemic infection rate.

THE ROLE OF THE COMPUTER

This section describes the demands for data entries and data displays. In the section on algorithmic diagnosis by computers, the approaches to computerized case find using the microbiologic laboratory data as case find are included. Such surveillance techniques may be of value in the absence of adequate ICP support. However, algorithmic diagnoses by computers are considered valuable only if they assist (not replace) the practitioner.

Data Entry

Data entry is any system that enters data into the data base. The data base is the stored data available for update, display, or retrieval. Some of the problems of data entry are data base specific (i.e., they depend on file structure, accessibility, or file content). Systems of data entry which are interactive ("on line") with the data base are subject to more problems with security than systems which are not interactive. Potentially the former method can accept more errors and therefore decrease the data base accuracy. However, an on line system is more convenient and available for use. In the rest of the chapter, it will be assumed that the data base is on line and available for interactive response with the user. As an alternative, the data base could require "batch" entry mode which is made by someone other than the user at a time and by a method chosen by the data processing center. Batch entry mode is not interactive with the user, although some computer centers have a very rapid "turn around" time, so that data entry and retrieval can be performed with only short delays.

Specific requirements for data entry are as follows:

1. Security
2. Error identifiction
3. Speed for interactive systems
4. Utilization of incomplete data
5. Simple means of updating data in the data base
6. Adequate codes and code translations
7. Simplicity, so that the system can be easily learned and run by clerks

Security

Security is the protection of data from unauthorized retrieval and/or use. People with varied levels of training and reponsibility may have access to the data base: the unskilled keypunch operator, who can enter data, but does not understand it; the hospital epidemiologist, who understands the data, but not the computer and may misuse the system; the ICP, who understands the data and computer; and the computer personnel, who are not entitled to see the data, but have access to it. One or more of these people may also wish to display data for illustrative purposes to students or visitors. Finally, others may share the computer system, and potentially they have access to the data base.

To help solve security problems at Loma Linda University, the authors have assigned an entry and retrieval security level to every field. Each individual with access to the data base has a security level assignment. Individuals can enter only those types of data allowed by their security level. Some individuals (clerks) cannot retrieve from data base, other can retrieve only certain types of data. For illustration, high levels of security are required to enter data base and to delete, edit, or update data. Some data require higher levels of security than others. If an individual attempts to enter or retrieve data requiring a level higher than the operator's security level, the system will give an error message. If the operator is persistent, the system will refuse further access to the computer.

To have a maximally functional system, one should be able to reassign security levels to clerks as skills and demonstrated reliability increase. In addition, one may want to alter the security level required for entry or retrieval of selected data.

Error Identification

It is the authors' policy to make all checks for error at the time of data entry. With an interactive system to identify the systematic and (most) nonsystematic errors, errors can be corrected before the data are entered into the data base. Error review and correction, which are carried on after data are in the data base, require relatively more time and the user is never certain of the data base's accuracy. Error identification can include patient identification, codes, spelling errors, incorrect data, or numerical sequences. The general steps are as follows:

1. The patient number is entered. The entry program gives the patient name and patient number, so that the clerk can be assured the data are assigned correctly.
2. The date is checked to be certain that the patient was hospitalized on the date indicated and that it is not a future time.
3. Coded information is used for most data entries. All codes are checked to be certain they exist and are legitimate entries for the specific field.
4. Selected fields must be completed for a particular segment to be accepted. For example, to enter an infection, the following must be entered: (a) the date of onset, (b) whether nosocomial or community acquired, and (c) the site of infection. Other data may or may not be entered.
5. When data for a segment are entered, the information is displayed for verification by the clerk. The display uses both codes and code translations, so that the clerk can confirm the correctness of the entry. (Note: the information is not yet in the data base.) If the clerk indicates that the data are accurate, they are placed into the data base, and the clerk can no longer make corrections.

Speed For Interactive Systems

An interactive system must check security levels and perform error reviews at speeds compatible with efficient employee work. When the data from a single source (i.e., microbiology laboratory) are entered, security and error checking should occur during the time the employee prepares the next slip for data entry (i.e., 2 to 10 sec). If multiple slips are entered before error checking, then the employee may have to retrieve a discarded slip to make the correction. This action wastes time. When timing computer interactions from entry until the computer has responded, one should include in the calculations not only the time for data entry, but also the expected time delay if there is time sharing and a heavy system load.

Ability to Utilize Incomplete Data

Surveillance data can describe ongoing problems very early. Ideally, infections must be identified within the first 24 to 48 hr of onset, so that epidemiologic evaluation by the ICP can occur while factors responsible for the infection are operative and discoverable. This would be easier with an interactive entry system. By contrast, batch entry data can be useful as historical review of what has happened prior to the current surveillance findings.

Data regarding ongoing problems are necessarily incomplete. At a minimum, microbiologic speciation and antimicrobial susceptibility are usually incomplete; and clinical diagnoses may not have been verified. Yet, even with incomplete data, the ICP is able to progress with case find and may discover ongoing practices or circumstances that perpetuate the problem. Thus, the epidemic may be interrupted. In contrast, historic review of complete data which are batch entered and returned at a later date is consistent with a more casual approach. The latter review, for example, often occurs after the epidemic is over or when crucial causitive factors are no longer apparent and discoverable.

While the practitioner should collect all requisite surveillance data at the first patient visit, some data may not be available or may be only preliminary. If the entry system is interactive, it can assist the practitioner by recognizing incomplete or preliminary data and identifying the need for followup. Data that require updating are usually microbiologic and can be obtained from the laboratory. For example, review of the bacteriology laboratory data for diagnosed infections may reveal that some have only Gram-stain reports and that final bacterial identification is still needed. For example, a purulent sputum from a patient with pneumonia with Gram-negative rods may be reported out as *Pseudomonas aeruginosa*.

Clinical data also require updating on occasion. Thus, early case find utilizes an accurate though incomplete data base, and patient files are updated later with previously unavailable data. Early surveillance speeds case find by including those with infection, but with preliminary data (i.e., a review of *Pseudomonas* pneumonias could include even those with Gram stains, the cultures of which are pending if the reports showed purulent sputum and Gram-negative rods on stain). This approach frees the ICP from compilation chores to do infection verification. Rapid infection verification may be of great importance if an epidemic is in progress.

Simple Means of Updating Data in the Data Base

The software should include programs that identify preliminary reports or initial impressions. All cases should be arranged in some appropriate sequence to speed completion. The programs should include routines for rapidly updating the data base, i.e., all incomplete bacteriology segments can be arranged in order by the microbiology laboratory sequence. Such updating will facilitate finding the date of culture. There must be a simple means of entering the data base and of correcting errors and/or deleting data (if for example it is decided that the patient was not infected).

Adequate Codes and Code Translation

It is important to have adequate infection and bacterial codes relative to the needs of the hospital. Some of the National Nosocomial Infection Study (NNIS) classifications of infections[2] are not differentiated at all hospitals. Thus, codes must be modified to fit the practices of the hospital. The bacterial codes must also be consistent with the microbiology laboratory's procedures. They must serve the hospital's needs, identify areas of importance, and be devoid of divisions into minutia which are of no interest to hospital personnel.

Codes work best under the following circumstances:

1.   If there is an internal logic
2.   If specific diagnoses are subsets of more general diagnoses
3.   If codes are not compact
4.   If antique code designations are not re-used

The last two items are probably self-explanatory; the first two will be expanded.

Table 1
MICROBIOLOGY CODES

A*	Gram pos. cocci	D*	Aerobic Gpr
A1*	Staph	D1	*Lactobacillus*
A11	Staph coag pos	D2	Diphtheroid
A12	Staph coag neg	D3*	*Corynebact* sp.
A2	*Micrococcus*	D31	*Corynebact diphtheriae*
A4*	Alpha growth	D39	*Corynebact* other
A41	Alpha strep	D4	*Listeria monocytogenes*
A42	*S. pneumoniae (Pneumococcus)*	D5*	*Bacillus* species
A5	Microaero strep	D51	*B. subtilis*
A9	Aer GPC N/ST oth	E*	Anaerobic GPR
B*	Anaerobic GPC	E1*	*Clostridium*
B1	*Peptococcus* sp.	E11	*C. tetani*
B11	*P. assacharolyticus*	E19	*Clostridium* other
B2	*Peptostrepto* sp.	E2	*Eubacterium*
B21	*P. anaerobious*	E3	*Proprionibacterium*
B22	*P. micros*	E4	Bifidobacterium
B23	*P. parvulus*	E9	Anaerobic GPR-other
B24	*P. productus*	F*	Gram neg rods
B3	*Sarcina*	G*	Enterobacteriaceae
B4	*Gaffkya*	G1*	*Escherichia coli* group
B9	Anaero GPC-other	G11	*E. coli enteropathogenic*
C*	*Streptococcus*	G12	*E. coli*
C1*	B hemo strep	G2*	K E S group
C11	B hemo strep A	G21	*Klebsiella*
C12	B hemo strep B	G212	*K. pneumoniae*
C18	B hem strp N/AB or D	G22	*Enterobacter*
C19	B hemo strp N/A	G221	*E. aerogenes*
C3	Strep viridans	G23*	*Serratia*
C5	N/hemo strp N/D	Etc.	
C6*	Group D		
C61	Enterococcus		
C69	Gr D N/Enterococci		

Internal Logic

At Loma Linda University, the various body systems are designated with letters B through L, and all infections have a first letter B through L. Specific surgery, procedures, specimen source, host susceptibility, X-ray, and radiation therapy have first letter codes B through L to designate the appropriate body system. Interpretation depends on the specific data segment in which the letter is placed; e.g., "D-Lower Respiratory" designates lung surgery in the surgery segment, pulmonary procedure in the procedure segment, sputum as specimen source in the bacteriology laboratory segment, pulmonary impairment in the host susceptibility, chest X-ray in the X-ray segment, and lung radiation in the radiation therapy segment.

Subsets

Each alphanumeric to the right indicates a subgroup of the more general group indicated by the alphanumeric to the left (see Table 1). There should be an attempt to follow a logical scheme of organization, so that subgroups are natural divisions. (Obviously logic can become a fetish and lose its usefulness.) However, natural divisions can make the system work smoothly.

The closer the logic of microbiology codes matches the (diagnostic) logic of the clinical microbiology laboratory, the easier it will be to utilize and update preliminary data. For example, an accurate Gram stain and 24-hr microbiology preliminary report obviate the need to wait for final reports. While such data are not adequate for epidemiologic work, they are effective for preliminary case find and investigation of concurrent problems. Thus, in the system at Loma Linda, the codes are initiated (first letter to the left) by type of organism shown on Gram stain. The 24-hr report will secure the first letter and probably the second alphanumeric (see Table 1). If the organism is one of the commoner pathogens, the clinical laboratory will finish the data by the second or third day, and the code can be completed. At any time, the computer can search for an organism or for a group of related organisms by using either the complete code for specific species name or by using the left-most alphanumerics to identify related species. In either case, simple allowances can be made for preliminary microbiologic identification.

Codes

If codes are not too compact, there is adequate "space" in the computer to change codes as taxonomy, nomenclature, or laboratory procedures are updated. Codes can therefore continue to reflect current practice.

Antique Codes

Codes that are no longer used (antique codes) are not reused, and thus the potential for ambiguity is avoided. It is important that whenever codes are used translations should be given, otherwise practitioners, though familiar with most codes, will require excessive time for handling uncommon and unfamiliar codes.

Simplicity

Data entry is not data specific if the data entry sequence is the same regardless of data (i.e., only the data differ not the method or sequences used for data entry). This practice reduces the number of sequences to be learned and decreases the possibility of error.

Identification of the specific code or appendix "lookup" should be possible without interrupting the sequence of data entry, further increasing efficiency in learning and data entry. If stroke-saving steps, such as one-key identification of the entry date and one-key recall and reentry of identification data are available, more time will be saved, and fewer errors will result.

The system should record the duration of each operator's work, number of items entered, and number of errors made. This allows management to evaluate work efficiency and to assess who is having trouble with accuracy and who may need more training. These data may also identify parts of the system that are slow and error prone—parts that need better programming. Not all infection control programs need so elaborate a data entry system. However, if a hospital opts for an interactive system, they are available and described.[3]

COMPUTER DIAGNOSIS WITH ALGORITHMS

There are several diagnostic decisions that must be made when performing surveillance of nosocomial infections. The following categories are important to consider:

1.   Significant organisms
2.   Infectious diagnosis

3. Date of onset of infection
4. Community vs. nosocomial acquisition
5. The role of antecedent procedure, surgey, or therapy

In general, significant decisions must be made regarding case find patients to determine if they are verified. The authors anticipate that the decisions will be made by the ICP utilizing the computer for assistance. However, the sections entitled "Significant Organisms" and "Nosocomial vs. Community-Acquired Infection" below were designed so that the computer could make diagnoses without the practitioner's participation.

Criteria must be developed for each diagnostic decision. If the criteria are met, the decision is yes; if they are not met, the decision is no. The criteria can be few and objective leading to nonambiguous decisions; however, decisions may be clinically inaccurate because the criteria do not cover all situations, (the situation is outside the domain of the criteria). Criteria can be subjective and judgmental covering all circumstances, but allowing variation in decision making. This leads to variable and inconsistent diagnoses.

Optimum diagnosis occurs if the computer assists the human. The computer can make a diagnosis when objective criteria are consistently used. The human evaluates the quality of the objective criteria used and limits the computer decisions to those domains where the objective criteria apply. Decisions external to the domain of the criteria cannot be made by the computer unless additional objective nonambiguous criteria are developed.

To illustrate, let the reader assume that the presence of bacteriuria is the definition of a urinary tract infection. Thus, if a urine culture shows bacteriuria, the computer can identify the fact and diagnose urinary tract infection. However, the computer cannot know if the specimen was collected properly, nor can the computer know whether there was asymptomatic bacteriuria or acute pyelonephritis with secondary bacteremia. In terms of morbidity, potential mortality, and hospital cost, the differences are not trivial. It would be difficult to develop objective, nonambiguous data which the computer could collect (without a diagnostician's input) for making the latter differentiations. On the other hand, to ignore all asymptomatic bacteriurias and to define urinary tract infections only in patients with significant symptoms would yield an ambiguous population of patients. If culture are then evaluated, infection would be defined as a subset of an ambiguous group determined by humans when making decisions using subjective biases. It is best to make objective criteria based upon microbiologic and/or X-ray data, physical findings (which the ICP can substantiate by examination), and evidence that the physician has initiated specific therapy. If other specific criteria are fulfilled, infection may be diagnosed whether or not the patient is treated. The only objective findings for many of the less common infections are the physician's physical examination and the histology and/or culture of biopsied specimens (culture may or may not have been ordered). One of these infections may be diagnosed if the physician encourages treatment in the absence of objective findings.

The following discussion of criteria is designed for computer identification of infection based solely on microbiologic data. It assumes a competent microbiology laboratory and laboratory requisitions which include at least the following: patient name, patient number, doctor (services), ward (room), specimen source, and date of specimen. Other assumptions are that the microbiology laboratory will do at least the following: Gram stain, organism identification, and quantification (if applicable) plus susceptibility (if applicable). In addition, the white blood count, percent polymorphonuclear cells (segmented plus bands), and urinalysis are assumed to be available to the data base from other laboratory sources. Finally it is assumed that certain census information is available, such as the day of admission and the number of discharges from each service and ward.

The authors have not examined the specificity and sensitivity for the ideas described; each would vary depending upon the indications for bacteriology culture and the appropriateness of culturing practices utilized by the various hospital services.

Significant Organisms

For discussion, the term "significant" organisms is defined as those microorganisms likely to be the etiologic agent for the infectious illness, as contrasted to noninvasive microbial colonization, i.e., the normal flora. Patients with significant organisms probably have a verifiable infection (the system is adequately predictive). Other patients not found to have significant organisms may or may not have infections. (The system may not be a sensitive or selective detector of some infections.)

In the next few paragraphs the "rules" which the computer "uses" to separate significant from nonsignificant organisms will be discussed. Specimen sources will be discussed under three groups, and rules will be discussed for each group.

Group 1 Specimen Sources

Group 1 specimen sources are those that normally are sterile. These include blood, spinal fluid, other body fluids, i.e., pleural, peritoneal, pericardial, synovial, tissues, or implanted foreign bodies. Organisms present in more than one specimen from Group 1 sources and in moderate numbers are probably significant. Significance increases with the number of specimens containing the same organism, increasing concentrations of organisms, and with isolation of a single microbial strain. *Staphylococcus epidermidis*, diphtheroids, *Bacillus subtilis*, and other common skin organisms when inconsistently present in low concentration or in mixed flora are not significant.[4]

Group 2 Specimen Sources

Group 2 specimen sources are those that have a normal flora, and a Gram stain can be used to assist interpretation if careful guidelines are used when examining the Gram stain. The primary example for this group is sputum. If a valid Gram stain is obtained without evidence of excess contamination (squamous epithelial cells),[5] and if significant pus and significant bacteria (among the pus) are noted, and if organisms grown on culture are morphologically consistent with the organisms seen on Gram's stain, then the species is considered significant. All other culture results are not significant and should be considered as contamination. If the specimen is contaminated, then a better specimen should be obtained.[6]

Group 3 Specimen Sources

Group 3 specimen sources have specific rules for each specimen source. (These are specific, not sensitive rules, because many epidemiologically important infections will be excluded.) Specific epidemic situations may necessitate modification of these rules:

1. Urine cultures — clean-voided urine cultures — Table 2 is a significance table that can be ued to evaluate voided urine specimens if consecutive cultures show one and the same species.
2. A specimen from a catheterized patient with a single species present in concentrations of 10^5 or greater is probably significant, even if a confirming urinalysis is not available. If two Gram-negative species are present in each of two consecutive cultures, each in concentrations greater than 10,[5] they probably represent significant organisms.[7]

Table 2
CLEAN-VOIDED URINE CULTURES—SIGNIFICANCE TABLE WHEN SUCCESSIVE SPECIMENS SHOW THE SAME ORGANISM

Quantitative culture ($>10^5$ organisms/ml urine) number of successive specimens	Number of white bloodcells/high dry field	
	0—5	>10
1	Not significant	Probably significant
2	Probably significant	Significant
3	Significant	Significant

3. Stool — If any Campylobacter *Salmonella* species or *Shigella* species are present in any number, these are significant. If *Staphylococcus aureus* or *Candida* species are present in moderate or high concentrations, these are considered significant organisms.[8]
4. Pharynx — If Group A *Streptococcus, Neisseria gonorrhoeae,* or *Corynebacterium diptheriae* are present, these are significant.[9]
5. Urethra — *Neisseria gonorrhoeae* is significant if present in the urethra.
6. Cervix — Beta hemolytic *Streptococcus* or *Neisseria gonorrhoeae* is significant if present.[9]
7. Wound/skin — Group A *Streptococcus* and or *Staphylococcus aureus* are significant if present.[9] (If the patient has burns *Pseudomonas* may be included, but the computer cannot identify significant pseudomonas infection without a quantitative culture.[9])
8. Abscess — Any positive type organism(s) aspirate from a closed abscess is significant.[9]
9. Organisms not meeting the about characteristics are considered contaminants.
10. It is possible to screen the data base for specific agents that are thought to be epidemic, realizing that the computer may have difficulty differentiating colonization from infections.

In addition to those above, several additional rules are helpful.

1. If there are multiple organisms, they should be arranged in sequence as follows:

    a. Beta hemolytic *Streptococus*
    b. *Straphylococcus aureus*
    c. *Neisseria gonorrhoeae*

    (If any of the three is present, it should be listed first.)

    d. All other organisms should be listed sequentially in order of decreasing concentration from the highest concentration to those present in lowest concentration.

2. Include significant infectious agents identified by nonculture methods (serology, antigen detection, tissue section, etc.).
3. Whenever epidemiologically indicated, organism identification should include antibiogram and other typing criteria.

Infectious Diagnosis

The illustration about urinary tract infections indicates that diagnostic criteria, if not objective, will lead to subjective inconsistency. The use of objective nonambiguous criteria will save the practitioner time. Instead of searching the data, the ICP can review the quality of the data input and the compatibility of the diganosis with the set criteria. Specific examples from common areas follow.

1. A positive blood culture may initiate a positive computer generated diagnosis of bacteremia. However, the ICP must evaluate the quality of each datum and also decide if the bacteremia is primary or secondary; if it is secondary, the primary source should identified. Whatever the diagnosis, the practitioner must evaluate the patient for contributing factors.
2. A positive urine culture may cause the computer to generate the diagnosis of urinary tract infection, but, as mentioned above, the practitioner must evaluate the quality of the data and determine the magnitude of the infection and the relationship to antecedent procedure, surgery, or host impairment.
3. A respiratory infection is diagnosed on the basis of purulent sputum and X-ray findings. In these patients, the ICP must know that the sputum specimen was valid for microbiologic evaluation and must note whether or not the true diagnosis is outside of the computer's diagnostic domain. (An infiltrate with purulent sputum is generally pneumonia, but could also be a lung abscess).
4. A wound infection is diagnosed by objective physical findings of infection and the presence of exudate. Again the practitioner must determine the quality of the specimen and its applicability. Wounds associated with some injuries (including burns) may have purulence with or without infection. The practitioner should evaluate skin and wound site for objective evidence of infection.[10]

Date of Onset

In general, the criterion for identifying date of onset of infection is based upon chart review. The computer may help by determining ward, service, and physician (if there have been recent changes).

If a computer is used to identify nosocomial infections from microbiologic data, then the date for onset of infection is the date of the first culture showing the nosocomial agent. (It is essential to recognize that this may be colonization which anteceded the infection.)

Nosocomial vs. Community Acquired Infection

In the following discussion, it is assumed that the microbiologic data are available to (or in) the data base. The authors' purpose is to suggest some algorithms that may be useful.

1. A positive specimen (a culture with a significant organism or purulent discharge) found at a site with (a) previous culture (this admission) that did not show a significant organism, (b) previous culture (current admission) that showed a significant organism of a different species, or (c) previous Gram stain without purulence is probably a nosocomial infection. It is necessary to know that the negative culture was valid and that the etiologic agent found on the positive culture was not present or incubating at the time of admission. These assessments are best made by the ICP.
2. A positive specimen with a significant organism in the first culture, but taken more than 48 hr after admission, is probably nosocomial. The practitioner needs

to be certain that there was no evidence of delay in culture and no evidence of an infection incubating at the time of admission. (A positive urine culture taken on the third hospital day in a patient without a urinalysis or history of previous urinary tract infection is by definition a nosocomial infection. If the patient had symptoms of previous urinary tract infection or pyuria at the time of admission and the culture did not follow urinary tract manipulation, then the urinary tract infection is considered community acquired.)

3. Culture of wound, operative sites, procedure sites, or of procedure equipment that lie within the host, such as catheters, monitors, etc., should be considered nosocomial until proven otherwise. Unfortunately, most of these cultures may not be specifically labeled. Thus, cutaneous, skin, wound, or tracheal cultures should be suspected and evaluated further. If the patient is a week postdischarge (and/or postprocedure), a cause-effect relationship between the procedure and infection may not be recognized as valid. It would be helpful if the computer could search for specimens from sites related to previous procedure or surgery. If such correlations are made by the computer, the practitioner should evaluate the final relationships. If the computer cannot make such a search, the practitioner may need to do this by hand.

The Role of Antecedent Procedures, Surgery, or Therapy

If the computer has only the microbiologic data and if the specimen source has been coded for site without any data on related hospital events, then no specific information regarding the relationship between infections and antecedent procedures will be available to the computer. If the computer knows the procedures, it can be programmed to look for specific specimen sources, i.e., in patients with total parenteral nutrition, the computer is programmed to search for bacteremia. In patients with endotracheal intubation, the computer will search for purulent respiratory secretions.

These schemes will not identify all nosocomial infections. However, they will give computer-generated data with relatively constant error. The sensitivity and selectivity may be knowable or may be variable. The practitioner may choose to limit surveillance to the infections found by computerized surveillance with further verification or to do additional surveillance on patients likely to be missed by these schemes.

DATA DISPLAY

The data base must be continuously available for data display and review by approved users. If there is a delay between data entry and correction of the data base, then data retrieval needs to be blocked during this time. It is necessary to differentiate clearly between preliminary data and erroneous data that must be corrected before it can be used.

Data display may utilize cathode ray tube (CRT) terminals and should be able to interface with printers, graphic plotters, and statistical (see chapter entitled "Choosing the Correct Statistical Tests") or other packages in other languages on other systems. The data base must not be output specific nor should the output be data base specific (i.e., output limited to the content or design of data base). It must be possible to present selected portions of data base to any one of the available output devices or systems.

DATA FORMAT

Output needs selective programs that present only the items of interest from the

	Community	This Hospital	Past Hospital	Other Hospitals	Nursing	Totals
Systemic	–	1	–	–	–	1
ENT	5	2	–	–	–	7
Respiratory	71	43	–	1	–	115
*Pneumonia	32	24	–	1	–	57*
*Br/trach	37	18	–	–	–	55*
Cardiovascular	2	1	–	1	–	4
GI	11	1	–	–	–	11
Genitourinary	51	39	–	–	2	91
Gynecologic	3	–	–	–	–	3
Musculoskeletal	1	–	–	–	–	1
CNS	2	–	–	–	–	2
Superficial	22	8	1	1	–	32
*Postoperative wound	–	6	–	1	–	7*
Bacteremia	7	7	–	1	–	14
*Primary Bacteremia	5	3	–	–	–	8*
Total	175	100	1	3	2	280

Note: Numbers are rates per 10,000 patient days based on 13,169 patient days.

FIGURE 1.   Infection surveillance output — all infections at Loma Linda University Medical Center; infection site vs. where acquired (11/1/1978 through 11/30/1978).

portion of data base under study. It is valuable to have routines that will isolate portions of the data base and display the desired data in an appropriate manner. Usually portions of the data base are selected by time (i.e., all infections with onset on a given date) ward, service (i.e., all *Pseudomonas* infections occurring on that ward or service), organism (i.e., all infections caused by *Klebsiella*), or infection site (i.e., all lower respiratory tract infections).

The display may be any item(s) that is (are) to be studied or compared. For example, the display may be a two-way table of two important characteristics in common (i.e., the number with enterococcal bacteriuria) in the selected population, the *rate* of the combined characteristics (i.e., rate of enterococcal bacteriuria), the *difference* in number or rate of the combined characteristics since the previous month (i.e., change in number or change in rate of enterococcal bacteriuria), or the *percent* of one characteristic with the second characteristic (i.e., percent of bacteriurics with enterococci, etc.).

Table displays should be fully labeled so they can be understood without translation (see Figure 1). The table should describe the population and dates included and identify its type (numbers, rates, etc.) and the day the table was run. The columns and rows should be clearly identified and all abbreviations explained in footnotes. If the table is a rate, the base population should be identified (if rate is number per 100 discharges, then number of discharges should be stated as a footnote). Similarly, graphs should stand alone. They should be fully described. If ranges are shown, a footnote should show they were derived.

Other outputs can include the following:

1.   Line listings with many items for each infection, such as name, patient number,

date of admission, date of onset of infection, name of infection, infecting agent, service, ward, etc. Such listings are useful for study and hypothesis testing.

2. Directories can arrange patients and/or infections for quick look-up. These might arrange patients by service, ward, infection, or by infecting organism in sequence determined by date of onset. These represent supportive data and are used to search for clusters and for referencing.

3. Special data arrangements may be needed to supply the specific needs of a ward, service, or situation. It may be valuable to tabulate bladder catheter-associated infections by date of onset for each ward, particularly when trying to motivate the wards to give better bladder catheter care.

DESIGN DECISIONS

Adequate and successful decisions regarding computer facilities in hospital infection control can be made if precise evaluations are carefully made. The following questions need to be answered.

1. Why are the data needed? The goals and objectives for infection control must be understood and clearly stated. Interactive data uilization is expensive with high demands for data manipulation to discover problems and how and why they occur. (This will require an "interactive" system.) In contrast, retrospective review is cheaper, requiring simple counting schemes to recognize and record problems of the past and those that continue to the present. (A "batch" system will suffice for such a review.)

   Who will review and understand the data? If management will read and respond to data, then output must include facts in formats which management understands. If output is interpreted for the decision makers, output demands are simpler. If the computer is to perform graphic, mapping, or statistical functions, additional demands on design will be made.

2. What is the estimated size of data base? Will the epidemiologist enter only infection data with etiologic agents for proven infections, or will he enter all of case find and supporting data? Will he enter data regarding surgery, procedures, and antibiotics? (Who will collect these data? Will they be collected on all patients or only on those with infections?)

   How will data be used? Which data must be collected from all patients? What will be done if data is not collected from all patients? Why collect them on any?

   How many pieces of data will be collected per patient in a file? Will any denominator data be entered? How much?

   How many of these data must be interactively available and how many can be in a format more slowly retrieved?

3. Who will have access to data? How many will have access? Is it possible that some people will have access to more data than the epidemiologist or practitioner want them to see?

4. What happens if the epidemiologist wants to update the input, output, definitions, criteria, or codes?

5. What interactions will the epidemiologist have with data? Will he only enter data and receive output or will the interactions with data base have the potential for inquiry?

6. Details regarding control of equipment and programmers are crucial. To whom is the computer assigned? Who hires the programmer? How responsive are these people to needs of infection control? Does infection control need priority to ob-

tain new formats or to change configuration? Who assigns priority? How supportive of the needs of infection control are the programmers, analysts, and technical people? Or is infection control to be satisfied with the available services? Will the programmers tailor programs to optimize utilization by infecton control? Must new programs be written for available machines in the available languages or can other surveillance programs be adopted?

7.   Response times and available times must be honestly described if one plans to use interactive programs. Turn-around times must be precisely understood for batch-oriented uses. The computer must serve infection control, not make demands and create bottlenecks.

8.   What are the personnel, fiscal, and space resources available? A batch-oriented system will save tabulation time, increase compiling time, and often force ICPs to perform added work. An interactive program will require additional clerical support, lure infection control personnel to take on additional tasks, and thus increase their work load. In addition, there will be the fiscal requirements for terminals, printed output, software, and the space required for storage and terminals.

DESIGN CRITERIA

Before deciding upon computer support for infection control, one must address critical design criteria.

Data Base Size

Data base size must be approximated so the system analysts can estimate storage and the time required for certain activities. The size estimates must separate "on line" storage from storage satisfied by delayed retrieval. One will need to include the following:

1.   Maximum number of patients to be in data base
2.   The number of data types (segments) per patient and the length of each data type (number of fields)
3.   The number of segments to be correlated (When will correlation occur, at the time of entry or later?)

Batch vs. Interactive Systems

Support for the authors' prejudices have been given above and will not be repeated here. Nonetheless, this is a basic decision that must be made early.

Security

The security needs must be defined precisely so the systems analyst can form proper design. Absolute protection of data makes for expensive hardware and software demands. Most people settle for reasonable security as described above.

Network

Can the computer access critical data from other sources so that the ICP need not reenter the data? Examples would include census data from "bed control", microbiologic data from clinical laboratory, or antibiotic data from the pharmacy.

Back-Up

Back-up is any method of saving the current system and data in the event of computer, disk, or system "crash". All systems should have both a duplicate copy of the data base and of all data entered since duplication. Infection control back-up should be updated daily. If update is infrequent, there is the danger of losing data during a "crash", and reconstruction of data base could be difficult.

Subsequent Changes

With time, infection control problems change; thus the data needs and the decision matrix must be updated to meet the new problems.

Once a computer system is developed, it will need frequent change to keep up with the needs of infection control. Fields and/or segments may need to be added or deleted. New codes may need to be defined, new responses may need to be developed, and new correlations may need to be tested. It is necessary that designs make possible simple implementation of change to optimize infection control.

CONCLUSION

The computer facilities for infection control at Loma Linda University Medical Center share a minicomputer, disk drive, communication gear, power control, air conditioning, and operating system with other patient care facilities. There are lines direct from the "mini" to terminals and printer in the work area. A dialect of Mumps called MIIS (Meditech) is used.[3] This system is an excellent information management system because of data base structure and interactive terminal communication processing. A table-driven data base management system called LUMPS has been developed that is described in a text by that name from the Mumps User's Group, 700 S. Euclid Avenue, St. Louis, Mo., 63110.

REFERENCES

1. Wenzel, R. P., Osterman, C. A., Hunting, K. J., and Gwaltney, J. M., Jr., Hospital-acquired infections. I. Surveillance in a university hospital, *Am. J. Epidemiol.,* 103, 251, 1976.
2. Center for Disease Control, NNIS Sites Definitions Manual (unpublished), 1975.
3. Munnecke, T. and Elder, H. A., *LUMPS: Loma Linda University LUMPS Programming System Design Manual,* Mumps User's Group, Loma Linda, Calif., 1977.
4. Bartlett, R. C., Ellner, P. D., and Washington, J. A., II, Blood cultures, in *Cumitech I.,* American Society for Microbiology, Washington, D.C., 1974.
5. Murray, P. R. and Washington, J. A., II, 1975 Microscopic and bacteriologic analysis of expectorated sputum, *Mayo Clin. Proc.* 50, 339, 1975.
6. Bartlet, J. G., Brewer, N. S., and Ryan K. J., Laboratory diagnosis of lower respiratory tract infections, in *Cumitech VII.,* American Society for Microbiology, Washington, D.C., 1978.
7. Kunin, C. M., *Detection, Prevention and Management of Urinary Tract Infections,* 2nd ed., Lea & Febiger, Philadelphia, 1974, 55.
8. Hornick, R. B., Gastroenterocolitis Syndromes, in *Infectious Diseases,* 2nd ed., Hoeprich, P. D., Ed., Harper & Row, New York, 1977, 543, 549, 562.
9. Isenberg, H. D., Washington, J. A., II, Ballows, A., and Sonnenwirth, A. C., Collection, handling and processing of specimens, in *Manual of Clinical Microbiology,* 2nd ed., American Society of Microbiology, Washington, D.C., 1974, 66, 69, 70.
10. Johnson, J. E., II and Cluff, L. E., Wound Infections, in *Clinical Concepts of Infectious Diseases,* Williams & Wilkins, Baltimore, 1972, 184.

Microbiologic Considerations

OPTIMAL USE OF THE LABORATORY FOR INFECTION CONTROL

Thomas F. Keys

INTRODUCTION

The microbiologist provides an etiology for hospital associated infectious diseases, an important responsibility in an era of frequent and sometimes unusual infection problems. The microbiology laboratory must have the expertise to accurately identify most microorganisms and the resources available to characterize unusual organsms.

It is crucial for the laboratory to maintain close communication with the infection control team. There is nothing more discouraging than finding out after the fact that a patient's sputum is laden with multiple acid-fast bacilli, or that a patient's serum is positive for hepatitis-B surface antigen, or that blood cultures from many patients in an intensive care unit are growing out *Serratia marcescens!*

The infection control team should check regularly (preferably daily) with the laboratory to obtain culture reports on hospitalized patients to see if any isolates of an alarming quality or quantity are being identified. Reports may be provided by a computer-assisted program or simply from copies of laboratory slips that will eventually be placed in the patient charts. Reports should at least provide the following information:

1. Patient name, patient identification number
2. Hospital service and hospital room number
3. Specimen type and source
4. Laboratory identification number
5. Microbiology identification and quantitation
6. Date received — date completed
7. Antibiotic sensitivities

Individual laboratory slips can be organized according to patient location or hospital service to ease the task of bedside surveillance. Isolates of potential epidemiologic significance should be preserved for future studies, if the need arises. Once a year they can be reviewed and discarded if they have no further usefulness.

COLLECTION OF CLINICAL SPECIMENS*

Blood Cultures

It is important that the skin site for venipuncture be adequately decontaminated of surface bacteria prior to collection of a blood culture. It is our practice to use an iodophor or 2% tincture of iodine for this purpose. Larger volumes of blood are more likely to yield organisms. Two bottles (total of 20 m*l* blood) are obtained from the same venipuncture site; 10 m*l* of whole blood is added to each enclosed bottle containing 90 to 100 m*l* of broth medium. Contamination can be avoided by not opening the bottles; however, one of the two bottles should be transiently vented, and it may be necessary to add penicillinase. Bacteria of unusual growth requirements may be detected by routinely subculturing within the first 12 hr after incubation onto appropriate solid medium. All blood culture bottles should be incubated for at least 7 days

---

* See Table 1.

Table 1
OPTIMAL COLLECTION OF CLINICAL MICROBIOLOGIC SPECIMENS

Material	Method	Remarks
Pus	Anaerobic transport tube or sterile syringe	Gram stain and culture for aerobes and anaerobes
Blood	Two-bottle kit	10% v/v blood to each bottle, do not vent
Urine	Midstream, catheter, or supra-pubic aspiration in sterile container	Process within 2 hr of collection
Sputum	Sterile container	Gram stain before setting up culture
Tissue	Sterile collection in sealed container	Process within 30 min of collection
Stool	Fresh stool preferred to rectal swab	Specify if enteric pathogens suspected
Nares	Swab anterior nares	Rarely indicated

before being discarded as negative. Occasionally, bottles may be held for 14 to 21 days if fastidious bacteria are suspected.[1]

Interpretation of blood culture results obviously depends on the individual clinical situation. Common skin contaminants are *Bacillus* species, diphtheroids, and *Staphylococcus epidermidis*. Rare contaminants are *Staphylococcus aureus*, Beta-hemolytic streptococci, members of Enterobacteriaceae and *Pseudomonas* species (including *Pseudomonas aeruginosa*).

Urine Cultures

Collection, transportation, and performance of a urine culture must be optimal to avoid a misrepresentation of the clinical problem. In general a clean, freshly voided, midstream collection is preferred. Prior to collection, the periurethral area should be decontaminated with an antiseptic solution. Optimally, all urine specimens should be processed by the laboratory within 2 hr of collection. If this is not possible, the collection should be refrigerated to prevent uncontrolled growth in the collection bottle.

As a general rule, a colony count of equal to or greater than 100,000 colonies per milliliter of urine indicates a significant urinary tract infection. When it is necessary to obtain a catheterized or suprapubic specimen, the area should be adequately cleansed and decontaminated with an iodophor solution. In this case, any number of orgnisms may indicate a significant urinary tract infection. For the patient who already has an indwelling urinary catheter in place, the specimen is collected by aspirating urine from the catheter with a small sterile needle and syringe.[2] The longer the catheter is in, the greater the likelihood of urinary tract infection.

Cultures must be assessed carefully for both their cinical and epidemiologic significance. Usually, hospital associated bacteriuria comes from endogenous intestinal flora. Common infecting organisms are *Escherichia coli*, *Proteus mirabilis*, Group D streptococci, and to a lesser extent *Klebsiella*, *Enterobacter*, and yeasts. Of greater concern, from the epidemiologic vantage point, are bacteria that may be introduced from the hospital evironment, such as *Pseudomonas*, *Serratia marcescens*, indole positive *Proteus*, *Providencia*, and *Acinetobacter* species.

Sputum Cultures

Pitfalls to the interpretation of bacterial growth in sputum cultures are well appreciated by the infectious diseases clinician. It is equally important for the infection control team to understand that results may not be representative of lower airways infection. For this reason, it is very important that the collection be of lower airway purulent bronchopulmonary secretions rather than saliva. A Gram stain should be carefully examined before setting up cultures. Sputum smears that contain an abundance of polymorphonuclear white blood cells are likely to contain important microbiologic information. Those with many epithelial cells are unlikely to be helpful and make it necessary to resort to other means to make a microbiologic diagnosis. Cultures of blood, pleural fluid, transtracheal aspiration, or lung biopsy may be required. Cultures of the nasopharynx, throat, and bronchoscopic washings are unlikely to yield important bacteriologic information.

Isolates from sputum may represent colonization or infection from either the patient's own endogenous flora or from exogenous sources. Common endogenous colonizers of the airway include viridans group of streptococci, *Neisseria* and *Haemophilus* species. Endogenous pneumonia is usually caused by *Streptococcus pneumoniae*, less often by *Staphylococcus aureus*, and rarely by *Haemophilus influenzae*. Exogenous hospital pneumonia is frequently due to *Pseudomonas aeruginosa*, *Serratia marcescens*, other antibiotic-resistant members of Enterobacteriaceae and, of course, *Staphylococcus aureus*.

Wound Cultures

A prompt, accurate identification of bacteria causing surgical wound infections is very important. The specimen must be truly representative of infection and not of colonized adjacent areas. Every attempt should be made to decontaminate the superficial area of a wound before collection. Specimens should be promptly forwarded to the laboratory, preferably within 30 min after collection. It is preferable to aspirate pus into a sterile syringe or anaerobic transport tube rather than using a dry cotton swab. This procedure allows the laboratory to culture the specimen for both anaerobic and aerobic organisms. Swabs of dry wounds including ischemic limbs, burn wounds, and sinus tracts are of little value.

For deep infections, it may be preferable to culture tissue directly.[3] This technique is recommended for burn wound infections and allows for quantitation of culture results. At least 1 g of clinically infected tissue should be obtained. After mincing or grinding into a suspension, serial dilutions are made in broth and subcultured onto solid media. Colony counts greater than 100,000 organisms per gram of tissue are associated with extensive infection. Of course, tissue should also be sent to pathology for special stains.

Autopsy Cultures

Any autopsied cases where infection was a major factor in death should be cultured from appropriate areas. This might include a vein from a case of suppurative thrombophlebitis, heart tissue from a case of infectious endocarditis, or material form a case of deep-seated surgical wound infection. As with any tissue specimen, all efforts should be made to decontaminate the overlying surface; it should be collected by aseptic means and promptly submitted to the laboratory.

COLLECTION OF ROUTINE ENVIRONMENTAL SPECIMENS

In the past, cultures from a variety of environmental sources were routinely collected

Table 2
OPTIMAL COLLECTION OF ROUTINE ENVIRONMENTAL MICROBIOLOGIC SPECIMENS

Material	Method	Frequency
Hospital-prepared infant formula	10 m*l* of liquid in sterile container	Monitor weekly
Steam sterilizer	Spore strip with *Bacillus stearothermophilus*	Monitor weekly
Ethylene oxide sterilizer	Spore strip with *Bacillus subtilis*	Monitor with every cycle
Reusable nonsterile inhalation therapy equipment	In-use sampling of effluent gas or culture of mainline nebulizers and reusable mainline tubing in enriched broth	Monitor monthly or more frequently if indicated

as part of a widely accepted hospital surveillance program. Within this decade, such culturing has been discouraged because it provided very little meaningful information.[4,5] At the present time, routine microbiologic surveillance is indicated only for hospital-prepared infant formula, sterilizers, and reusable nonsterile inhalation equipment (See Table 2).

Hospital-Prepared Infant Formula

Occasional outbreaks of food-related illnesses have been noted in hospitalized patients.[6,7] *Salmonella enteritidis* is the most common pathogen and can easily be introduced from contaminated cereals, eggs, and milk products. Fortunately, most hospitals now use commercial infant formula that is packaged as a single-use disposable item. Monitoring of these products on a routine basis is not necessary. However, if formula is prepared in the hospital kitchen, it should be monitored weekly. An aliquot of fluid (approximately 10 m*l*) is submitted to the laboratory in a sterile container for culture of aerobic and anaerobic bacteria. Counts above 25 colony-forming units per milliliter of formula are not acceptable and indicate significant contamination of the product.[8]

Pediatricians may elect to feed premature infants breast milk from nonmaternal donors. Breast milk for this purpose should be screened before donors are enrolled and thereafter on a weekly basis.[9] Persistent bacterial counts of equal to or greater than 100 colonies per milliliter of milk indicate significant contamination. In addition, because of the vertical transmission of hepatitis B from mothers to their offspring and a potential of contamination from breast milk, it would appear to be a good idea to screen nonmaternal mothers for HBsAg.

Sterilizers

To insure adequacy of sterilization, a biological spore challenge test is used. For steam sterilizers, spores of *Bacillus stearothermophilus* are incorporated into the indicator strip. The indicator is placed in the center of a test pack and run through a normal sterilization cycle. Afterward, the indicator and a control strip are placed in a small selfcontained incubator for 24 hr. Growth is detected by a color indicator. Growth in the control strip and no growth in the test strip indicate the sterilizer is functioning satisfactorily. Monitoring is recommended on a weekly basis.

For gas sterilizers (ethylene oxide), a similar indicator system is used, but with *Bacillus subtilis*. Monitoring for gas sterilizers is recommended with every cycle.

It is important to note that spore strips are not valid indicators for sterilizing liquids. In this case, ampules containing spores are used.[10]

Reusable Nonsterile Respiratory Inhalation Equipment

After the introduction of inhalation therapy to hospitals in the early 1960s, a serious problem with necrotizing Gram-negative pneumonia developed. Significant contamination of mainline nebulizers and tubing by Gram-negative bacteria was discovered.[11] Many hospitals now gas sterilize reusable equipment every 24 to 48 hr to control this problem. For hospitals that practice decontamination rather than sterilization, monthly monitoring of inhalation therapy equipment prior to usage is recommended.

One technique is to culture effluent gas from the machine during operation by directing an aerosol stream into broth culture medium.[12] A commercially available kit (Aerotest Sample®, Olympic Medical Corp., Seattle, Wash.) now provides for quantitating bacteria directly from agar plates. If more than 40 colonies of bacteria per plate are detected, this corresponds to an aerosol count of greater than 1000 colonies per 0.028 m³, consistent with high level contamination of equipment.[13]

A more conventional approach is to culture the nebulizers and tubing directly from the machines. They are irrigated with 50 ml of brain heart infusion broth enriched in 0.5% beef extract (enriched BHI). The irrigant fluid is collected by aseptic means into a 125-ml screw-capped flask and cultured. If desired, the machine exhalation valves may be cultured by swabbing with two sterile cotton applicators, each placed in screw-capped tubes containing 10 ml of enriched BHI. As a rule, growth of more than 100 colonies per milliliter broth from equipment indicates inadequate decontamination.

COLLECTION OF INVESTIGATIONAL SPECIMENS

When the probability exists of an outbreak of hospital associated infection, intensive microbiologic studies of the environment may be indicated. It is critical first to assess the problem objectively, analyzing variables common to the cases in question before proceeding with reckless abandon! Sources might include any items in intimate contact with patients. These range from catheters, vascular monitoring devices, surgical grafts, and foreign body prostheses to parenteral infusion fluids, as well as liquid soaps, lubricants, and lotions (See Table 3).

Although physicians often implicate hospital air (usually in operating rooms) as causing wound infections, in fact, air is rarely to blame if current ventilation standards are maintained. Air sampling is usually not indicated for investigation of hospital infections. Details for conducting such studies may be found by consulting other resources.[14]

Intravenous Catheters

I.V. catheters serve a useful purpose for administering fluids and drugs, but they are also a frequent source of hospital associated sepsis. After catheters are in longer than 48 hr, they become colonized and ultimately may cause a serious clinical infection. When this is suspected, the catheter should be removed immediately and a distal portion submitted to the laboratory for culture. A frequent practice is to decontaminate the skin entry with alcohol or an iodophor, aseptically remove the line, amputate the distal tip with a sterile scissors, and place it in a sterile screw-top tube containing 10 ml of trypticase soy broth (TSB).

Recently Maki et al. have reported a semiquantitative technique for identifying infection due to I.V. catheters.[15] A distal catheter segment 5 to 7 cm in length is rolled back and forth across the surface of a blood agar plate for quantitative culture. Counts of 15 colonies or more per plate invariably occur with catheter-associated sepsis.

Pressure Monitoring and Other Equipment

Vascular pressure transducers may be flushed with 10 to 20 ml of infusion fluid,

Table 3
OPTIMAL COLLECTION OF ENVIRONMENTAL SPECIMENS DURING INVESTIGATION

Material	Method(s)	Remarks
Intravascular catheters	Culture distal tip in broth or on agar	Indicated when catheter source suspected of sepsis
Pressure monitoring devices	Flush with 20 mℓ infusion fluid for culture or use premoistened swab to culture diaphragm or undersurface of dome	Process as for blood culture
Other equipment (small hardware, prostheses, etc.)	Swab area with premoistened swab or immerse object in broth	Neutralize residual disinfectants
Parenteral infusion fluids (blood, etc)	Draw 20 mℓ of fluid from I.V. line or bottle by aseptic means	Inoculate both agar plate and blood culture bottles
Other fluids	Pass 20 mℓ fluid through 0.22 μm Millipore® filter or culture directly	Culture filter or fluid in broth or on agar

exercising sterile precautions, for collection in a blood culture bottle. An alternative technique is to swab the transducer diaphragm or undersurface of the dome with sterile cotton applicators premoistened in enriched BHI broth.[16]

Portals from large equipment may also be swabbed with sterile cotton applicators premoistened with enriched BHI broth. Small hardware may be rinsed or totally immersed in enriched BHI broth. To prevent continued activity of residual disinfectant, the addition of 0.07% lecithin and 0.5% polysorbate-80 is recommended for neutralization. One aliquot should be cultured in broth for 4 hr, and another should be cultured for 24 hr, before transferring the specimen to solid medium.[17]

Parenteral Infusion and Other Fluids

Any infusion fluid, including blood, that is suspect of contamination should be promptly cultured. By aseptic means, 20 to 30 mℓ of fluid is drawn fom the infusion line or directly from the container; 1 mℓ is incorporated into an agar pour plate, and the remaining fluid is proportioned in two blood culture bottles. A much more sensitive method is to culture the entire volume of suspect fluid by adding an equal volume of enriched broth and incubating under standard conditions at 37°C.[18]

Other fluids, such as water and melted ice, can be most effectively cultured by passing 20 to 50 mℓ through a small (0.22 to 0.45 μm) Millipore® filter and culturing the filter either in enriched BHI broth or directly on agar.[17] Liquids, such as lotions and lubricants, that cannot be passed through a filter may be cultured directly in broth or on agar.

SIGNIFICANCE OF MICROBIAL ISOLATES

Most bacteria can be completely identified within 48 to 72 hr after a culture specimen has been submitted. Preliminary information may also be helpful to the infection control team, especially during an investigation. Bacteria have a characteristic appearance (size, shape, texture, and opacity) and odor when grown on solid media. In broth, bacteria may be distinguished by pellicle formation, turbidity, precipitates, and their ability to produce catalase and coagulase.

Table 4
MEMBERS OF THE FAMILY
ENTEROBACTERIACEAE[25]

Tribe	Genus
Escherichieae	Escherichia
	Shigella
Edwardsielleae	Edwardsiella
Salmonelleae	Salmonella
	Arizona
	Citrobacter
Klebsielleae	Klebsiella
	Enterobacter
	Serratia
Proteeae	Proteus
	Providencia
Yersinieae	Yersinia
Erwinieae	Erwinia
	Pectobacterium

Gram-Positive Cocci

In the preantibiotic era, beta-hemolytic streptococci were commonly recovered from life-threatening bacterial infections. Staphylococci were also a problem, later on becoming more difficult than streptococci when penicillin-resistance became widespread. Despite the availability of more effective chemotherapy, staphylococci remain the most serious Gram-positive infection in hospitalized patients, and recently methicillin-resistant strains have been isolated in several U. S. hospitals. *Staphylococcus aureus* is a virulent pathogen and can quickly be differentiated from other staphylococci by the coagulase test. The organism may be further classified by a phage typing system customarily used when investigating a suspected common source outbreak. Phage typing is not available in the usual hospital laboratory, but can be performed by a reference laboratory. In previous years, coagulase-negative staphylococci such as *S. epidermidis* were considered avirulent, nonpathogenic members of the normal skin flora. However, we know now that they may cause serious infections, especially after the insertion of prosthetic heart valves and total orthopedic joints.[19,20]

Despite the reduced frequency of beta-hemolytic streptococcal disease, sporadic outbreaks of wound and skin infections continue to occur; some have been traced to healthy carriers on the operating team.[21,22] Prompt identification of streptococci is required. Basic classification is according to the Lancefield grouping of cell wall antigens. The commercial availability of Group A, B, C, D, F, and G antiserums allows for the identification of over 99% of all beta-hemolytic streptococci.[23] Further grouping or typing procedures is not available to the hospital laboratory, but may be obtained by consulting the Directory of Rare Analyses (DORA).[24]

Enterobacteriaceae

Because of the increasing numbers of hospital acquired infections due to members of Enterobacteriaceae, their precise identification has become a necessity. Classification according to tribe and genus is based on that of Edwards and Ewing (See Table 4).[25] Further identification of species is made by testing for unique biochemical and serologic features. All ferment glucose, reduce nitrates, and are oxidase negative, a distinguishing feature from the nonfermentative group of Gram-negative bacteria. Fortunately, for the smaller laboratory, commercially available diagnostic kits have eased the identification of these organisms.

Table 5
NONFERMENTATIVE GRAM-NEGATIVE BACILLI[26]

Acinetobacter calcoaceticus
Alcaligenes sp.
Achromobacter
Bordetella
Cardiobacterium hominis
Commamonas terrigena
Eikenella corrodens
Flavobacterium
Moraxella
Pseudomonas

Nonfermentative Gram-Negative Bacilli

These organisms are being isolated from hospitalized patients in increasing frequency and are gaining in significance (See Table 5).[26] Nonfermenters are ubiquitous in the hospital environment. In the usual clinical setting, they often appear as innocent bystanders; however, they may cause serious life-threatening infections, especially in the immunologically compromised host. Of greatest concern to the clinician is *Pseudomonas aeruginosa*, but other organisms in this group may be implicated.

Fungi

Certain filamentous fungi are worrisome to the infection control team. An outbreak of aspergillus pneumonia in cancer patients traced to contamination of fire-proofing materials was reported recently.[27] We have described a series of skin and soft tissue infections due to *Rhizopus* species associated with contaminated adhesive occlusive dressings.[28] Filamentous fungi are distinguished by observing characteristic morphology on solid fungal medium.

Yeasts occur normally in small concentrations in the oral cavity and digestive tract. With encouragement from broad spectrum antibiotics, prolonged hospitalization, and serious underlying disease, they may proliferate and cause serious disseminated infection. Yeasts may be introduced into the blood stream during surgery or I.V. therapy, especially during total parenteral hyperalimentation.[29,30] Any yeasts found in normally sterile spaces, such as blood, synovial, and cerebrospinal fluid, should be identified completely. Of critical importance is the distinguishing of common yeast species from *Cryptococcus neoformans*, a known pathogen for healthy as well as compromised patients.

Mycobacteria

Mycobacterium tuberculosis is a well-recognized pathogen in man. The laboratory must have the resources to distinguish this organism from other *Mycobacterium* species, many of which are nonpathogenic. Sometimes health care workers and other patients are unknowingly exposed to a patient with far-advanced active pulmonary tuberculosis. Organisms seen on acid-fast or auramine-rhodamine smears may provide presumptive evidence of tuberculosis, but a definitive diagnosis can only be made by culture results.

Recently, the Runyon Group IV organisms (rapid growers) have been recovered in hospitalized patients. They commonly grow in water and rarely have caused clinical infections in the past. *Mycobacterium chelonei* has been reported to have caused an outbreak of postoperative thoracotomy wound infections.[31] These organisms have also been isolated from porcine heterografts implanted during cardiac surgery.[32] Rapid growing mycobacteria are optimally cultured by incubating specimens in thioglycolate broth at 28°C for up to 8 weeks.

Viruses

Viruses may cause infections in hospitalized patients. Becaue of its epidemiology, hepatitis B virus presents unique problems to the infection control team. A simple serologic test for detecting hepatitis B surface antigen is available (Ausria II ®, Abbott Laboratories, North Chicago, Ill). The test has had greatest usefulness in screening for hepatitis B infection in potential blood donors. It also has been used to screen individuals in high hepatitis risk areas, such as the dialysis center or clinical laboratory, where contamination from infected blood and blood products may occur.

Other viruses such as rubella, herpes and cytomegalovirus may play a role in hospital infection problems. Since most hospitals do not have culture facilities, reliance on serologic tests is necessary. If an outbreak of hospital associated viral infections is suspected, public health authorities should be consulted for assistance.

SAMPLING HEALTH CARE PROVIDERS

In addition to tuberculosis and hepatitis, hospital employees may also require assessment for other communicable diseases. Employees working in pediatrics and obstetrics may be at increased risk of acquiring rubella and cytomegalovirus. Women of childbearing age should be screened for rubella antibody and if none is detected, offered rubella vaccine. Screening for cytomegalovirus antibody may be also worthwhile, but a vaccine is presently not available.

Outbreaks of bacterial infections, especially those caused by penicillin resistant or methicillin-resistant *Staphylococcus aureus* and Group A streptococci, may be introduced by hospital staff. Open skin lesions should be cultured. Sometimes cultures of axillary skin, fingers, nose, and anus are required to detect an asymptomatic individual who is shedding large numbers of these organisms.

ANTIBIOTIC SENSITIVITY TESTING

All laboratories should be able to provide information on the susceptibility or sensitivity of clinically significant bacteria to antimicrobial agents. These tests are equally useful to the infection control team. Hospital associated bacteria are frequently antimicrobial resistant or have sensitivity patterns varying from those of community-acquired isolates. The "antibiotogram" may be a useful marker for tracing infections back to a common source. Antibiotic resistant patterns of hospital bacteria may be monitored on a monthly basis and used as an educative device to curtail inappropriate use of antibiotics.

The most widely used method presently is the Kirby Bauer single disk diffusion test. Agar and broth dilution techniques are not ordinarily done in the small hospital laboratory. For the Kirby Bauer test, filter paper discs with a specified content of antibiotic are placed on the surface of a Mueller-Hinton agar plate that has been streaked with a standard inoculum of the test organism.[33] After incubation for 16 to 18 hr at 35°C, the diameters of growth inhibition surrounding the disks are measured and translated to a "susceptible", "resistant", or "intermediate" category from a reference table. Quality control measures are necessary to minimize day-to-day and laboratory-to-laboratory variations in test results. These measures should include daily testing of established control strains: *S. aureus* (ATCC 25923), *Escherichia coli* (ATCC 25922), and *P. aeruginosa* (ATCC 27853). Common sources of error must be considered if zone diameters of the controls are outside of published tolerance limits.

It is customary to preselect sets of antibiotic tests depending on the general microbiologic category of the isolate. In our laboratory, staphylococci are routinely tested against penicillin, oxacillin, cephalothin, erythromycin, clindamycin, and chloramphenicol; streptococci are tested against penicillin, ampicillin, erythromycin, and chloramphenicol; and aerobic Gram-negative bacteria are tested against ampicillin, carbenicillin, cephalothin, tetracycline, chloramphenicol, gentamicin, tobramycin, and amikacin. Nitrofurantoin, nalidixic acid, and the combination of sulfamethoxazole-trimethoprim are tested against urinary isolates only.

These antibiotograms are satisfactory for routine surveillance of hospital bacteria. If necessary, other antibiotics may be added: vancomycin, tetracycline, sulfonamide, and aminoglycosides for staphylococci and polymyxin for Gram-negative bacteria.

ASSESSMENT OF MICROBIAL DATA

Microbiologic data must be readily available for review by the infection control team. Information should be transferred from laboratory report slips to separate epidemiology cards for individual patients with hospital infections. Data may be organized according to organism, source, and patient location, allowing for a regular survey of hospital infections and providing background information during investigation of an outbreak. This information can also be circulated to other members of the hospital infection committee for review at their regular meetings.

Some laboratories have a computer capacity that provides limited epidemiologic information to the infection control team.[34] Any computer system is only as good as the data input. Errors in collecting, labeling, processing, and identification may be compounded. It would be hazardous to rely solely on a laboratory-based computer system for data on hospital infections, since the system cannot distinguish between a community or hospital acquired infection, colonization or clinical infection, or identify infections that have not been cultured. It is essential for the infection control team to relate laboratory data to clinical events occurring at the bedside. No computer can substitute for the interest and support required of the microbiologist to maintain an effective infection control program.

REFERENCES

1. **Isenberg, H. D., Washington, J. A., II, Balows, A., and Sonnenwirth, A. C.,** Collection, handling and processing of specimens, in *Manual of Clinical Microbiology,* 2nd ed., Lennette, E. H., Spaulding, E. H., Truant, J. P., Eds., American Society for Microbiology, Washington, D.C., 1974, chap. 6.
2. **Kunin, C. M.,** *Detection, Prevention and Management of Urinary Tract Infections: A Manual for the Physician, Nurse and Allied Health Worker,* 2nd ed., Lea & Febiger, Philadelphia, 1974, 63.

3. Krizek, T. J. and Robson, M. C., Evolution of quantitative bacteriology in wound management, *Am. J. Surg.*, 130, 579, 1975.

4. American Publich Health Association, Committee on Microbial Contamination of Surfaces, Environmental Microbiologic Sampling in the Hospital, *Health Lab. Sci.* 12, 234, 1975.

5. American Hospital Association, Committee on Infections Within Hospitals, Statement on microbiologic sampling in the hospital, *Hospitals*, 48, 125, 1974.

6. Silverstolpe, L., Plazikowski, U., Kjellander, J., and Vahlne, G., An epidemic among infants caused by *Salmonella moenchen, J. Appl. Bacteriol.*, 24, 134, 1961.

7. Schroeder, S. A., Aserkoff, B., and Brachman, P. S., Epidemic salmonellosis in hospitals and institutions, *New Engl. J. Med.*, 279, 674, 1968.

8. American Academy of Pediatrics, Committee on Fetus and Newborn, *Standards and Recommendations for Hospital Care of Newborn Infants*, 5th ed., 1971.

9. Center for Disease Control, National Nosocomial Infections Study Report, Human Milk for Feeding Premature Infants, U.S. Department of Health, Education and Welfare, Annual Summary 1976 (issued February 1978), 16.

10. Bartlett, R. C., Groschel, D. H. M., Mackel, D. C., Mallison, G. F., and Spaulding, E. H., Control of hospital-associated infections, in *Manual of Clinical Microbiology*, 2nd ed., Lennette, E. H., Spaulding, E. H., and Truant, J. P., Eds., American Society for Microbiology, Washington, D.C., 1974, chap. 91.

11. Pierce, A. K., Sanford, J. P., Thomas, G. D., and Leonard, J. S., Longterm evaluation of decontamination of inhalation-therapy equipment and the occurrence of necrotizing pneumonia, *New Engl. J. Med.*, 282, 528, 1970.

12. Edmondson, E. B. and Sanford, J. P., Simple method of bacteriologic sampling of nebulization equipment, *Am. Rev. Respir. Dis.*, 94, 450, 1966.

13. Ryan, K. J. and Mihalyi, S. F., Evaluation of a simple device for bacteriological sampling of respirator-generated aerosols, *J. Clin. Microbiol.*, 5, 178, 1977.

14. Fincher, E. L. and Mallison, G. F., Intramural sampling of airborne microorganisms, in *Air Sampling Instruments Manual*, 4th ed., American Conference of Governmental Industrial Hygienists, Cincinnati, 1972.

15. Maki, D. G., Weise, C. E., and Sarafin, H. W., A semiquantitative culture method for identifying intravenous-catheter-related infection, *New Engl. J. Med.*, 296, 1305, 1977.

16. Center for Disease Control, National Nosocomial Infections Study Report, The Infection Hazards of Pressure Monitoring Devices, U.S. Department of Health, Education and Welfare Annual Summary 1974 (issued March 1977), 15.

17. Center for Disease Control, National Nosocomial Infections Study Report, Laboratory Aspects in the Control of Nosocomial Infections, U.S. Department of Health, Education and Welfare, Annual Summary 1974 (issued March 1977), 27.

18. Goldmann, D. A., Maki, D. G., Rhame, F. S., Kaiser, A. B., Tenney, J. H., and Bennett, J. V. Guidelines for infection control in intravenous therapy, *Ann. Intern. Med.*, 79, 848, 1973.

19. Keys, T. F. and Hewitt, W. L., Endocarditis due to Micrococci and *Staphylococcus epidermidis*, *Arch. Intern. Med.*, 132, 216, 1973.

20. Fitzgerald, R. H., Peterson, L. F. A., Washington, J. A. II, Van Scoy, R. E., and Coventry, M. B., Bacterial colonization of wounds and sepsis in total hip arthroplasty, *J. Bone Jt. Surg.*, 55, 1242, 1973.

21. Schaffner, W., Lefkowitz, L. B., Goodman, J. S., and Koenig, M. G., Hospital outbreak of infections with Group A streptococci traced to asymptomatic anal carrier, *New Engl. J. Med.*, 280, 1224, 1969.

22. Goldmann, D. A. and Breton, S. J., Group C streptococcal surgical wound infections transmitted by an anorectal and nasal carrier, *Pediatrics*, 61, 235, 1978.

23. Facklam, R. R. and Smith, P. B., The gram positive cocci, *Hum. Pathol.*, 7, 187, 1976.

24. Young, D. S., Hicks, J. M., and Pestaner, L. C., Directory of Rare Analyses, *Clin. Chem.*, 23, 323, 1977.

25. Washington, J. A., II, Laboratory approaches to the identification of Enterobacteriaceae, *Hum. Pathol.*, 7, 151, 1976.

26. Blazevic, D. J., Current taxonomy and identification of nonfermentative gram negative bacilli, *Hum. Pathol.*, 7, 265, 1976.

27. Aisner, J., Schimpff, S. C., and Bennett, J. E., *Aspergillus* infections in cancer patients, *JAMA*, 235, 411, 1976.

28. Keys, T. F., Haldorson, A. M., Rhodes, K. H., and Roberts, G. D., Nosocomial outbreak of Rhizopus infections associated with Elastoplast wound dressings — Minnesota, *Morbidity and Mortality Weekly Report (C.D.C)*, 27, 33, 1978.

29. **Plouffe, J. F., Brown, D. G., Silva, J., Eck, T., Stricof, R. L., and Fekety, R.,** Nosocomial outbreak of *Candida parapsilosis* fungemia related to intravenous infusions, *Arch. Intern. Med.,* 137, 1686, 1977.

30. **Montgomerie, J. Z. and Edwards, J. E., Jr.,** Association of infection due to *Candida albicans* with intravenous hyperalimentation, *J. Infect. Dis.,* 137, 197, 1978.

31. **Robicsek, F., Daugherty, H. K., Cook, J. W., Selle, J. G., Masters, T. N., O'Bar, P. R., Fernandez, C. R., Mauney, C. U., and Calhoun, D. M.,** *Mycobacterium fortuitum* epidemics after open heart surgery, *J. Thorac. Cardiovasc. Surg.,* 75, 91, 1978.

32. **Laskowski, L. F., Marr, J. J., Spernoga, J. F., Frank, N. J., Barner, H. B., Kaiser, G. and Tyras, D. H.,** Fatidious mycobacteria grown from porcine prosthetic heart valve cultures, *New Engl. J. Med.,* 297, 101, 1977.

33. **Matsen, J. M. and Barry, A. L.,** Susceptibility testing: diffusion test procedres, in *Manual of Clinical Microbiology,* 2nd ed., Lennette, E. H., Spaulding, E. H., and Traunt, J. P., Eds., American Society for Microbiology, Washington, D.C., 1974, chap. 46.

34. **Kuntz, L. J.,** Computerization in microbiology, *Hum. Pathol.,* 7, 1969, 1976.

IMPROVING USAGE OF ANTIMICROBIAL AGENTS

John E. McGowan, Jr.

INTRODUCTION

Antimicrobial agents have made a major impact on the practice of medicine, and because of their obvious virtues, they are among the most frequently prescribed of all chemotherapeutic agents. For many years, attention has been given to the problems of overuse and misuse of these drugs.[1,2] Recently, however, papers have focused on delineating specific problems of misuse[1,3-9] and upon suggestions for improving usage, including various forms of "peer review".[3,10,11] As a result, accreditation and regulatory agencies in the past few years have placed increasing emphasis on requirements for individual hospitals in the U.S. to conduct programs for improving the usage of these agents.[12,13]

Although conduct and implementation of these programs are stated to be requirements for the medical staff of the hospital,[12] infection control personnel are frequently asked to obtain information about usage or to carry out various other facets of such a review program.[14] It is probably helpful and appropriate for infection control workers to be involved in this effort. Surveillance has been defined as "the monitoring of hospital procedures and practices to detect and eliminate factors that may become determinants of infection".[15] How antibiotics are used may in part determine patterns of nosocomial infection and thus seems a reasonable focus for infection control efforts. Thus, programs for improving the usage of antimicrobial agents are an appropriate subject for consideration by workers in infection control.

Extent of Usage of Antimicrobial Agents[5]

Antimicrobial agents are among the most frequently prescribed of all chemotherapeutic agents and account for approximately 15% of all prescriptions. Moreover, in 1971 the number of antibiotic prescriptions presented to community pharmacies was equivalent to one prescription each for 89% of the total U.S. population. The production and use of antibiotics for both humans and animals increased over threefold in the decade between 1960 and 1970 (a period in which U.S. population increased 11%).

Usage in Hospitals

Within the hospital, antimicrobial agents are frequently prescribed. Castle and colleagues found that 34.2% of all patients at Duke University Hospital received antibiotics,[6] and other studies have indicated usage in 19 to 30% of hospitalized patients.[7,10,16,17] A study by the Commission on Professional and Hospital Activities ("PAS Study") estimated that about 27% of the 33 million patients discharged from general hospitals in 1972 received one or more antibiotics during their hospital stay.[5] During the period 1960 to 1970, the total cost of antibiotics to hospitals in the U.S. increased 320%.[10]

Usage for Prophylaxis

In the hospital setting, a large proportion of the antimicrobial agents used are apparently for prophylaxis. A study by Scheckler and Bennett in seven community hospitals found that 62% of treated patients had no evidence of active infection and therefore were presumed to be treated prophylactically.[18] Similar findings were reported from Latter Day Saints Hospital in Salt Lake City,[19] and prophylactic indications accounted for 30% of the courses of antibiotic therapy at the University of Wisconsin.[7] A study by the Intersociety Committee on Antimicrobial Drug Usage, convened by the American College of Physicians, showed that more than 25% of total antibiotic use in 20 randomly selected Pennsylvania hospitals was "apparently" for surgical prophylaxis.[20]

Potential Consequences of Misuse and Overuse

The volume of antibiotic usage is of concern because there is a measurable risk of adverse effect from any antimicrobial agent. Thus, indiscriminant prescribing of these agents is unwise. Many antimicrobial agents have the potential for producing serious toxic reactions in the patient.[9] Caldwell and Cluff have pointed out the magnitude of this problem in a hospital inpatient population and have described reactions to antimicrobial agents that ranged from extremely serious (e.g., shock, pancytopenia) to less severe, but yet a hindrance to patient care (e.g., drug-associated fever).[16]

These direct toxic effects to the patient are paralleled by adverse consequences to the population of the hospital and to the community as a whole.[21] For example, the widespread use of antimicrobial agents in the hospital setting can frequently lead to the selection of organisms resistant to these antimicrobial agents.[21-28] When patients acquire infection with these microorganisms from the hospital environment, the organisms often will be more difficult to eradicate.[29] In addition, the high cost of many of antimicrobial agents makes a compelling argument for giving an antibiotic only when necessary and for giving a particular agent only when equivalent, less costly alternatives are not available. Thus, use of antimicrobial agents is not without adverse consequences, and use of an antimicrobial agent without a definable benefit to outweigh the potential risk is inadvisable.[30]

MAJOR PROBLEMS IN USAGE OF ANTIMICROBIAL AGENTS

A number of reports have now reached the literature that describe some of the problems that have been encountered in both ambulatory[31-33] and hospital-based[1-8,10,34-36] clinical practice. It must be realized, however, that many of these reports have resulted from retrospective application of criteria drawn up by the authors of the studies and that the criteria may not have been agreed upon by (or even available to) the prescribers whose actions were reviewed. In such cases, decisions about "appropriateness" of usage may be somewhat subjective judgements and thus subject to dispute.[37] Therefore, exact frequencies of "appropriate" and "inappropriate" usage are probably somewhat misleading. However, a number of general areas have been found in which problems arise with the usage of antimicrobial agents. These can be divided into six general categories in which problems have arisen.

Use of an Antimicrobial Agent to Treat a Disease That is Unresponsive to Any Such Agent

There are a number of reasons why this situation might occur. Frequently, it may result from a simple lack of knowledge by the person who is giving the antimicrobial agent.[38] A study by Neu and Howrey[39] indicated deficiencies of knowledge about antimicrobial agent usage and reinforced the need for further postgraduate education in the use of antibiotics. A second factor involved here is that patients often come to the physician expecting to receive an antimicrobial agent. Thus, the physician is frequently under some pressure from the patient to prescribe one of these drugs, even if he or she is aware that the agent may not help much.[40-42] A review of medications given to patients with the common cold in physicians' offices in Pennsylvania during 1972 showed that 28% of these patients received a prescription for a broad- or medium-spectrum antibiotic, an additional 21% of the patients received penicillin, and 2% more received sulfa drugs.[5] Thus, about half of the patients received an antimicrobial agent for a syndrome in which antimicrobial agents will help only the very few patients with bacterial superinfection in association with viral respiratory illness.

Use as a Substitute for Diagnostic Procedures

On occasion, an antimicrobial agent will be employed as an empirical test for patients with fever or other signs of inflammation. If symptoms remit with therapy, it is presumed that infection was the cause. There are clinical circumstances in which this approach may not benefit the patient,[40] and so this course must be exercised with caution, In contrast, however, it has been suggested that "it has become common practice for antibiotic prescriptions to be given without examination of the patient, and expectant treatment with antibiotics in complicated and undiagnosed conditions is a widely accepted medical standard."[43]

Mistakes in the Mechanics of Usage

Errors in the way antibiotics are administered are a third area of concern. Use of the wrong route of administration, incorrect dosage of an agent, treatment for a too-long or too-short period, neglect of adjunctive procedures such as surgical drainage, or use of an ineffective agent for treatment of an infection that might be responsive to a different agent—all represent practices that are likely to lead to failure of therapy.[8]

Failure to Monitor the Patient's Course

Not watching closely for adverse effects during the period of administration is a fourth major problem. The failure to conduct the appropriate tests to minimize the possibility of toxic effects from the antimicrobial agent or to recognize toxicity at the earliest possible time is especially a problem when one is prescribing some of the newer antimicrobial agents such as aminoglycosides, for which toxicity is such a likely possibility.[16] The need to adjust the dosage of nephrotoxic agents in patients with altered renal function, the need to alter administration of potentially heptotoxic agents in patients with liver disease, and the need to look for known hematologic, auditory, vestibular, or other severe effects of administration are important issues that sometimes are not considered. For example, Gilbert and colleagues reviewed the use of gentamicin in a community hospital and found that only 50% of patients receiving this agent of known high potential for nephrotoxicity had their renal function assessed during the course of therapy.[44]

Misuse of Drugs for Prophylaxis

There are specific principles relating to the use of antimicrobial agents for preventing subsequent infection; most current recommendations based on these principles suggest use of prophylactic antimicrobial agents around the period of operation for 2 days or less.[45-48] In many cases, these principles are not being applied effectively. Kass surveyed antimicrobial agent usage in 20 randomly chosen hospitals in Pennsylvania and found that over 25% of total antibiotic use was apparently for surgical prophylaxis.[20] Only 22% of courses of therapy were given for less than 4 days, and 78% were given for longer periods. This survey suggested that using prophylactic antimicrobial agents according to current recommendations[45-48] would probably lower antimicrobial usage for an entire hospital by approximately 19%. This problem is particularly important because of the widespread use of antimicrobial agents for prophylaxis (see above).

Table 1

GUIDELINES FOR ANTIMICROBIAL AGENT REVIEW

1.   The review is a required function of the medical staff, coordinated with the Infection Control Program.
2.   It must be performed on a regular, frequent basis.
3.   It must review the use of the antimicrobial agents in all patients seen at the institution — inpatients, outpatients, emergency-care patients, long-term care patients, etc.
4.   The review must provide clinical, patient-specific data rather than an accumulation of statistical information unrelated to specific patients.
5.   The process must involve comparison of observed usage with defined criteria, includng those for prophylactic usage, approved by the medical staff.
6.   The review committee must provide written documentation of findings.
7.   The personnel concerned must provide evidence that corrective action has been taken if usage is found to vary from the standards that have been developed.
8.   Findings must serve as a subject for the continuing medical education of the medical staff and as a means of improving the quality of medical care.

STEPS TOWARD BETTER USAGE

Recognition that a Problem Exists

Recently there has been increasing recognition that in fact a problem exists with usage of antimicrobial agents. George G. Jackson, M.D., has noted that "hopefully, physicians have become aware of the need to protect the hospital environment, and to preserve the effectiveness of chemotherapy with the present drugs by some restrictions on the indiscriminant overusage of antibiotics."[43] In addition, a number of British[49,50] and U.S. journals[11,51,52] have recently published editorials that have focused attention on this problem. Thus, there is today a reasonable consensus that some attention must be given to improving usage. This is an essential step in attempting to establish "effective peer pressure" to overcome resistance to attempts at corrective action.[36]

Role of Regulatory Agencies

In part as a result of increasing recognition of this problem, a number of regulatory and accreditation agencies have begun to require efforts to improve antimicrobial agent usage in hospitals and extended-care facilities. The Joint Commission on Accreditation of Hospitals (JCAH) has been especially interested in this area and has directed hospitals to conduct such a review.[12] In adition, the JCAH has indicated a number of desirable attributes for a program of this type;[12,13] these are summarized in Table 1. Thus auditing usage of antimicrobial agents has been given a strong boost by regulation.

Usage Review Programs

It has been suggested that attempts to improve usage should be based on methods developed for auditing quality of care.[49,53-56] In these programs, people at a given institution attempt to delineate the problems present in their hospital so that corrective action then can be determined. My view of how this general process would apply to reviewing usage of antibiotics is in Figure 1.[57]

1.   In the first step of the process, one conducts surveillance to determine the ways in which antimicrobial agents are used in a given hospital or extended-care facility.
2.   One then develops an analysis of usage patterns that describes agents that are commonly used, situations in which they are employed, and methods used to

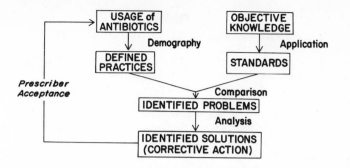

FIGURE 1. General process of review of antimicrobial agents. (Adapted from McGowan, J. E., Jr., *Q. Rev. Bull.*, 5, 32, 1979.)

ensure that the drug is administered in correct dosage and also to assure that the potential for toxicity is minimized.

3. People in the institution review knowledge of basic pathophysiology, pharmacology, and host-parasite-antimicrobial agent interactions to develop "usual" standards for optimal use of antimicrobial agents, paying particular attention to the agents and situations that are of special relevance to the institution. (For example, the antimicrobial agents to be used for the initial therapy of suspected septicemia would be of small interest to workers in a nursing home, but might be of great importance to those reviewing usage in a large general hospital).

4. Comparison of these standards with the analysis of actual usage within the institution should delineate specific problems. It then is the job of the committee to formulate reasonable solutions to these problems and to promulgate these findings so prescribers within the institution can speedily act on their recommendations.

PROBLEMS ENCOUNTERED IN USAGE REVIEW

The difficulty with usage review as an approach to improved prescribing is that optimal methods for conducting such a review and measuring its effects have not yet been established.[56,58-62] As noted by the *Lancet,* audit was "introduced on an axiomatic basis"; a directive to review usage was issued before sound and effective methods were derived for performing such an evaluation.[59]

Major Problem Areas

A number of authors recently have reported their experience in individual hospitals with programs of this type.[3,4,6-8,10,14,17,34-36,44,54,55,63-77] A wide range of results have been encountered; some programs showed marked improvement in usage patterns, some did not. Some of the problems with this approach fall into several fairly general categories.

Development of Therapy Standards

Standards for judging appropriateness of therapy should be based exclusively on objective data. Yet, unfortunately, there are still many areas of infectious disease diagnosis and therapy in which we act by empirical guidelines.[3,10,37,43,57,63,78,79] For these areas, the decision as to what is appropriate therapy (and therefore the definition of variation that is inappropriate) remains a subjective one.[60] The results of audits based on these subjective opinions often fail to generate the acceptance by the prescriber that

Table 2
APPROACHES TO CORRECTIVE ACTION

Education of prescriber
    Reports from infection control committee
    Reports from pharmacy
    Reports from clinical laboratory
    Added information in formularies
    Improved package inserts
    Teaching conferences, grand rounds, etc.
    Specific discussions of audit findings
Restriction of usage prior to administration
    Required consultation prior to release from pharmacy
    Removal of drug from formulary
    Required culture prior to therapy
    Not reporting susceptibility test results for selected agents
    Required justification in chart for ordering drug
Review interaction during administration
    Concurrent review
    Required written justification for continuing drugs
    Automatic stop orders
    "Counter-detailing" by clinical pharmacists
    Required consultation after specified period of therapy

is necessary for corrective action.[60,79,80] Thus, to produce effective audits, we must (1) clearly identify those areas in which we have sufficient knowledge to generate mandatory standards and (2) eliminate standards for those diseases about which we cannot agree.

Standards Are Not Universal

Even in situations where standards can be generated to deal with the "usual" case, most clinical situations are not yet sufficiently predictable to permit issuance of absolute standards. Thus, we are not currently confident enough about the validity of criteria to insist on compliance in every case. Failure to allow for the infinite variety of clinical situations that stretch our current "axioms" beyond the breaking point can produce programs in which rigorous application of the guidelines would not be to the patient's benefit.

Lack of Acceptance by Prescribers

Even when we do generate reasonable standards, we sometimes fail to improve usage of antibiotics because the prescriber still does not adhere to the recommended changes.[60] Thus, we need to identify the measures that will cause the prescriber to accept and implement corrective action. Some of the avenues employed in attempting to accomplish this are in Table 2.

1. The first of these, and the one most frequently employed, is education of the prescriber.[3,8,10,34,44,57] Certainly, if the reason for suboptimal therapy is simply a lack of knowledge, then making the prescriber more knowledgeable about the use of these agents should correct the situation. Some success has been reported with this technique.[10,34,44] Unfortunately, what little data we have about this approach suggest that often it does not produce fruitful results.[60,63] Jones and colleagues in Dallas, on attempting to implement an educational approach, found that "an educational program directed at specific prescribing errors produced little noticeable effect on the use of antibiotics in a university hospital. The study indicates that more direct measures, such as control of use of particular antibiot-

ics, may be required to produce a meaningful change in prescribing practices."[63] It also may be that we will need to increase our efforts to educate the patient.[40,81] So there are at least some situations in which we have not yet found the educational methods that will convince people to act, even when the standards that have been set are reasonable.

2. Control measures that have been employed for particular antibiotics have attempted to attack the problem from two directions—restriction of usage and interaction with the prescriber during the time in which the drug is being given (see Table 2). Some reports have shown that prescribing practices have been altered by control systems of this type.[3,4,17,34,65,67,72] However, these systems require much effort, and unfortunately none of these studies to date have provided objective information showing that the effort involved was justified by either cost savings on drug purchases or by improvement in patient care. For example, a system requiring justification for usage of certain antimicrobial agents did have a marked effect on prescribing patterns at Boston City Hospital,[4,17] but is not entirely clear whether these changes in usage patterns produced benefits to the patient that justified the work involved in providing consultations by infectious disease physicians 24 hr a day. Likewse, in reviewing a similar system,[67] Meyer questioned whether restriction merely resulted in a switch from one expensive agent to another.[68]

Thus, it appears that even in situations where the use of therapy standards has been moderately effective in identifying problems, these problems are not always corrected because we have yet to identify optimal methods for getting the prescriber to take corrective action.

Cost-Benefit Analysis

Even though programs have been mandated and found to be expensive,[78,82,83] there are still no objective data regarding the benefit in terms of the time and money involved in abstracting data, identifying variation, and attempting to implement corrective actions.

Errors of Omission

Most review programs select a case for review because an antimicrobial agent has been administered. Thus, cases in which drugs are given incorrectly can be examined. However, this mechanism cannot deal with cases in which the physician failed to treat with an agent that was needed.[9]

Problems Faced by Individual Hospitals in Attempting to Identify Optimal Review Methods

Determination of optimal methods will require careful assessment of the methods and techniques currently proposed. Experience reported to date suggests that it will be difficult for individual hospitals to derive these methods by themselves. Cases in which antimicrobial agents are misused represent a relatively small proportion of all cases in which these agents are employed. Thus, a large number of cases will have to be reviewed to determine whether differences exist between systems being studied.[62] Moreover, confounding variables are usually present in the hospital setting, e.g., other educational efforts besides those of the audit program. How much these factors confound measurement of the usefulness of the audit program can only be assessed by including a number of control groups in one's study.[56,62] However, the effort required to review a large number of cases and to include control groups would severely tax the resources of most hospitals, which have only limited resources for such review programs. Thus, it appears that controlled cooperative studies will be needed to determine optimal methods for review and that most individual hospitals will have to design their review programs on the basis of information generated by these larger research projects.

PRACTICAL CONSIDERATIONS FOR THE INDIVIDUAL PROGRAM

Audit has been placed in the "must do" category by the JCAH. Thus, for many hospitals and extended-care facilities, the question is now one of how best to go about his review. From the above considerations, it appears that there are certain elements that should be taken into consideration by those involved in conducting a review program.

Choice of Subjects for Review

1. Concentrate on achievable projects—those that can be completed successfully in the unique situation of an individual hospital. Attempts to review many areas at once may lead to failure in all. One might begin by reviewing a specific area of usage in which little disagreement is expected, to establish the principle of review and to familiarize all with the review process. Remember, as Komaroff says, "if we simplify what is required of mandated quality assurance activities, we may reduce the level of antagonism that such activities have generated."[62]

2. Concentrate on clinically significant problems instead of statistical surveys of overall use or "drug reaction". Just because a drug was used does not mean the drug was misused.[84] As Inglefinger points out, drug reaction is "part of the risk any doctor-patient combination must assume when the likely benefit from therapy is felt to outweigh the adverse effect of administering the drug".[85] In addition, statistical reviews are neither specific nor convincing enough to encourage change. By contrast, problems are more readily appreciated by those using the drugs when usage for specific patients and their circumstances are evaluated. Subjects for evaluation that fit well in this area include all patients receiving a particular antibiotic (to detect deviation from agreed-upon indications), dosage schedules, duration of therapy, monitoring for adverse effects of drug administration, indications for prophylaxis, and many other areas.[10]

3. Review all patients, regardless of location in the hospital. Not only is this a requirement of regulatory groups such as the JCAH, but also this prevents the feeling that a particular service or physician is being singled out.

Development of Standards[57]

Use only standards that can be agreed upon. Most physicians have been prescribing antibiotics throughout their careers and feel that they do a good job. Thus, the response when criteria run counter to physicians' opinions is that the criteria are in error. This attitude may be influenced by pharmaceutical company representatives.[40,75] As a result, there are as many disagreements in this area as in any area of medicine.[78] To avoid this, one might begin with the guidelines compiled by various groups—these are now beginning to appear in the literature.[45-48,86-87] These might be used as a basis for arriving at a policy for the individual hospital by taking into account specific local problems.[51] This process should be a combined activity of the various departments of the hospital.[10,12] After review and discussion, it should be possible to determine a "common ground" of guidelines that the staff being audited can agree to.[69] This consensus on usage practices (and only these commonly accepted guidelines) should then be the standard with which actual clinical cases should be compared.[51] This process also insures that the criteria are well understood by the group being audited. In particular, guidelines for prophylaxis must spell out duration of therapy to avoid situations like that reported by Kass.[20] In developing all of these guidelines, the key point is flexibility. The inclusion of controversial criteria will do nothing but encourage the ire of the staff, thus hampering one's ability to change things for the better.

Dealing with Variation

The review must be set up in such a way that variation from the criteria signal a need for further review, but do not necessarily imply error. As many of our standards are not perfect,[37] one must allow for cases in which variations from the criteria are to the patient's benefit.

Timing of Review Efforts

Recommendations from a single survey are more readily ignored than those repeatedly established by an ongoing program. Thus, evaluations should be performed repeatedly.

Achieving Prescriber Acceptance of Corrective Action

In attempting to achieve prescriber acceptance, remember that we do not yet know which approaches are the effective ones.[56-62] Until these are better defined, it may be necessary to employ a multifaceted approach in hopes that among the variety of methods employed, at least one will be effective. It also appears that the more successful efforts have been those in which corrective action involved implementing some group decision or manipulating objects or procedures (e.g., alteration of drug formulary) rather than actions aimed at changing habits of specific prescribers.

Attempts to achieve prescriber acceptance of corrective action will usually work best as a peer-review effort. Often, it is the prescriber that is most in need of education who rails against the idea of audit. This feeling may be heightened if it is felt that the review is being conducted by those the prescriber perceives as either superiors or inferiors.[10] In this case, it may be helpful to have the recommendations for corrective action come from the committee as a whole, or from the committee member whose background is most similar to the person's being reviewed. Incidentally, this is a major reason why review of antibiotic usage should not be viewed exclusively as the function of the infection control practitioner (ICP). While this person can be of inestimable value in obtaining and processing data for the review effort,[14] the above considerations explain why I feel that interpretation of, and action taken on, these data should remain (as required by the JCAH) a function of the medical staff.

The Role of Drug Restriction

Can we improve usage by restricting drugs? As noted above, some studies show that restriction leads to a marked change in usage pattern.[56] This is not an easy system to employ. It is difficult to start, as attempts to restrict physicians' usage patterns often meet with a great deal of resistance. Yet, as noted by the *British Medical Journal*, some review committee have "begun to challenge the freedom (so often claimed as fundamental!) of doctors to prescribe whatever they think best for their patient...".[80] Restriction requires a great deal of personnel time because a restriction system is useful only if the consultants are freely available to carry out the interaction.[4] Yet, this approach holds some promise for special situations, such as outbreaks due to specific resistant organisms where a decrease in usage of a given drug might reduce the selection pressure that permits survival of the organism. Another situation of this type would be the use of drugs that are so expensive that the cost and effort of restriction procedures are equalled or surpassed by savings from elimination of misuse.[83,88] To date, however, there are no studies showing clearly how cost and savings are related in a given hospital, although savings reported in some hospitals are most impressive.[3,66]

Complying with Regulatory Guidelines

The format for the review must comply with requirements of regulatory agencies.[12,13] Thus, one must have complete records showing that the review involved comparison with defined criteria, that findings and recommendations have been communicated to all concerned, that corrective action has been taken where necessary, and that follow-up review has been conducted to see that corrective action was effective in improving usage.

THE MOST IMPORTANT FACTOR

While attempting to develop a program to improve usage of antimicrobial agents, one may at times feel that this type of a program boils down to a contest between the reviewers and the prescribers. However, it is essential to keep in mind that physicians prescribe antimicrobial agents in a well-meaning attempt to improve the lot of their patients. Thus, information showing the prescriber how to provide even better care for patients will be welcomed by virtually all.[89] As Komaroff has noted, if we "expand research efforts designed to develop sound standards and effective quality assessment and assurance mechanisms, perhaps the insidious nihilism that undermines many of our efforts will be replaced by a spirit of cautious enthusiasm. It is easier and more enjoyable to 'do something' when you have learned what to do."[62]

Finally, it is worth reminding ourselves of the value of this activity. "Clinicians are naturally defensive about limitations on their rights to prescribe antibiotics, and about criticism about their less hygienic habits. But cross-infection and the abuse of antibiotics are socially unacceptable, and impose obligations on us all if we really do put the interests of patients, and potential patients, first."[50]

REFERENCES

1. **Reimann, H. A.,** The misuse of antimicrobics, *Med. Clin. North Am.* 45, 849, 1961.
2. **Myers, R. S., Slee, V. N., and Ament, R. P.,** Antibiotic study shows need for therapy audit in hospitals, *Bull. Am. Coll. Surg.,* 48, 61, 1963.
3. **Kunin, C. M., Tupasi, T., and Craig, W. A.,** Use of antibiotics — a brief exposition of the problem and some tentative solutions, *Ann. Intern. Med.,* 79, 555, 1973.
4. **McGowan, J. E., Jr. and Finland, M.,** Usage of antibiotics in a general hospital — effect of requiring justification, *J. Infect. Dis.,* 130, 165, 1974.
5. **Simmons, H. E. and Stolley, P. D.,** This is medical progress? — trends and consequences of antibiotic use in the United States, *JAMA,* 227, 1023, 1974.
6. **Castle, M., Wilfert, C. M., Cate, T. R., and Osterhout, S.,** Antibiotic use at Duke University Medical Center, *JAMA,* 237, 2819, 1977.
7. **Maki, D. G. and Schuna, A. A.,** A study of antimicrobial misuse in a university hospital, *Am. J. Sci.,* 275, 271, 1978.
8. **Smith, J. W. and Jones, S. R.,** An educational program for the rational use of antimicrobial agents, *South. Med. J.,* 70, 215, 1977.
9. **Bernard, H. R.,** Dangers of indiscriminate antibiotic therapy, *Surg. Clin. North Am.,* 55, 1303, 1975.

10. **Counts, G. W.,** Review and control of antimicrobial usage in hospitalized patients — a recommended collaborative approach, *JAMA,* 238, 2170, 1977.

11. **Aagard, G. N.,** Antibiotics under the drug spotlight, *Ann. Intern. Med.,* 79, 600, 1973.

12. Joint Commission on Accreditation of Hospitals, *Standards for Infection Control Adopted by the Board of Commissioners,* Joint Commission for Accreditation of Hospitals, Chicago, February, 1976.

13. **Porterfield, J. D., III,** Antibiotic prescribing patterns — a response from the JCAH, *Hospitals* 49, 14, 1975.

14. **Carruthers, M. M. and Grant, K.,** A practical method of antimicrobial surveillance, *Health Lab. Sci.* 15, 44, 1978.

15. **Moore, B.,** Surveillance of hospital infection, in *Proc. Int. Conf. Nosocomial Infections,* Center for Disease Control, August 3 to 6, 1970, Brachman, P. S. and Eickhoff, T. C., Eds., American Hospital Association, Chicago, 1971, 272.

16. **Caldwell, J. R. and Cluff, L.,** Adverse reactions to antimicrobial agents, *JAMA,* 230, 77, 1974.

17. **McGowan, J. E., Jr. and Finland, M.,** Effects of monitoring the usage of antibiotics — an interhospital comparison, *South. Med. J.,* 69, 193, 1976.

18. **Scheckler, W. E. and Bennett, J. V.,** Antibiotic usage in seven community hospitals, *JAMA,* 213, 264, 1970.

19. **Moody, M. L. and Burke, J. P.,** Infections and antibiotic usage in a large private hospital, *Arch. Intern. Med.,* 130, 261, 1972.

20. **Shapiro, M., Townsend, T. R., Rosner, B., and Kass, E. H.,** Use of antimicrobial drugs in general hospitals: patterns of prophylaxis, *N. Engl. J. Med.,* 301, 351, 1979.

21. **Eickhoff, T. C.,** Hospital infections, *Disease-a-Month,* September 1972.

22. **O'Callaghan, R. J., Rousset, K. M., Harkess, N. K., Murray, M. L., Lewis, A. C., and W. L. Williams,** Analysis of increasing antibiotic resistance of *Klebsiella pneumoniae* relative to changes in chemotherapy, *J. Infect. Dis.,* 138, 293, 1978.

23. **Shulman, J. A., Terry, P. M., and Hough, C. E.,** Colonization with gentamicin-resistant *Pseudomonas aeruginosa,* pyocine type 5, in a burn unit, *J. Infect. Dis.,* 124, S18, 1971.

24. **Søgaard, H., Zimmerman-Nelson, C., and Siboni, K.,** Antibiotic-resistant gram-negative bacilli in a urological ward for male patients during a nine-year period — relationship to antibiotic consumption, *J. Infect. Dis.,* 130, 646, 1974.

25. **Franco, J. A., Eitzman, D. V., and Baer, H.,** Antibiotic usage and microbial resistance in an intensive care nursery, *Am. J. Dis. Child.,* 126, 318, 1973.

26. **Roberts, N. J., Jr. and Douglas, R. G., Jr.,** Gentamicin use and *Pseudomonas* and *Serratia* resistance — effect of a surgical prophylaxis regimen. *Antimicrob. Agents Chemother.,* 13, 214, 1978.

27. **Isenberg, H. D. and Berkman, J. I.,** The role of drug-resistant and drug-selected bacteria in nosocomial disease, *Ann. N.Y. Acad. Sci.,* 182, 52, 1971.

28. **Finland, M.,** Changing ecology of bacterial infections as related to antibacterial therapy, *J. Infect. Dis.,* 122, 419, 1970.

29. **Gleckman, R. A. and Madoff, M. A.,** Environmental pollution with resistant microbes, *N. Engl. J. Med.,* 281, 677, 1969.

30. **Jonsen, A. R.,** Do no harm, *Ann. Intern. Med.,* 88, 827, 1978.

31. **Schaffner, W., Ray, W. A., and Federspiel, C. F.,** Surveillance of antibiotic prescribing in office practice, *Ann. Intern. Med.,* 89, 796, 1978.

32. **Ray, W. A.,** Federspiel, C. F., and Schaffner, W., Prescribing of tetracycline to children less than 8 years old, *JAMA,* 237, 2069, 1977.

33. **Benn, R. A. V.,** Antibiotics — use and abuse in office practice, *Drugs,* 13, 297, 1977.

34. **Achong, M. R., Theal, H. K., Wood, J., Goldberg, R., and Thompson, D. A.,** Changes in hospital antibiotic therapy after a quality of use study, *Lancet,* 2, 1118, 1977.

35. **Achong, M. R., Hauser, B. A., and Krusky, J. L.,** Rational and irrational use of antibiotics in a Canadian teaching hospital, *Can. Med. Assoc. J.,* 116, 256, 1977.

36. **Perry, T. L. and Guyatt, G. H.,** Antimicrobial drug use in three Canadian hospitals, *Can. Med. Assoc. J.,* 116, 253, 1977.

37. **Cluff, L. E.,** Antibiotic prescribing patterns—a new emphasis for the infection control practitioner, *A.P.I.C. (J. Assoc. Pract. Inf. Control),* 4, 11, 1976.

38. **Perry, T. L.,** Antibiotic abuse—the testimony of medical students, *Can. Med. Assoc. J.,* 112, 1428, 1975.

39. **Neu, H. C. and Howrey, S. P.,** Testing the physician's knowledge of antibiotic use — self-assessment and learning by videotape, *N. Engl. J. Med.,* 293, 1291, 1976.

40. **Kunin, C. M.,** Problems of antibiotic usage—definitions, causes, and proposed solutions, *Ann. Intern. Med.,* 89, 802, 1978.

41. **Chandler, D. and Dugdale, A. E.,** What do patients know about antibiotics? *Lancet,* 2, 422, 1976.

42. Editorial, Antibiotics for common colds?, *Lancet,* 1, 132, 1976.

43. **Jackson, G. G.,** Perspective from a quarter-century of antibiotic usage, *JAMA,* 227, 634, 1974.

44. **Gilbert, D. N., Eubanks, N. M., and Jackson, J. M.,** The effects of monitoring the use of gentamicin in a community hospital, *J. Med. Educ.,* 53, 129, 1978.

45. **Chodak, G. W. and Plaut, M. E.,** Use of systemic antibiotics for prophylaxis in surgery, *Arch. Surg.,* 112, 326, 1977.

46. Veterans Administration Ad Hoc Interdisciplinary Advisory Committee on Antimicrobial Drug Usage, Audits of antimicrobial usage—guidelines for peer review, *JAMA,* 237, 1001, 1977.

47. **Berger, S. A., Nagar, H., and Wertzman, S.,** Prophylactic antibiotics in surgical procedures, *Surg. Gynecol. Obstet.,* 146, 469, 1978.

48. **Chodak, G. W. and Plaut, M. E.,** Wound infections and systemic antibiotic prophylaxis in gynecologic surgery, *Obstet. Gynecol.,* 51, 123, 1978.

49. **Ruedy, J.,** Monitoring drug use, *Can. Med. Assoc. J.,* 118, 1483, 1978.

50. Editorial, Antibiotics for disease, *Lancet,* 2, 1055, 1974.

51. **Kunin, C. M.,** Guidelines and audits for use of antimicrobial agents in hospitals, *J. Infect. Dis.,* 135, 335, 1977.

52. Editorial, Antibiotics, *JAMA,* 226, 350, 1973.

53. **Gregory, J. M. and Knapp, D. E.,** State-of-the-art of drug usage review, *Am. J. Hosp. Pharm.,* 33, 925, 1978.

54. **Goldstone, J. and Way, L. W.,** The use of medical audits in surgical education, *Surgery,* 84, 25, 1978.

55. **Stolar, M. H.,** Model for a formal, prospective antibiotic use review program, *Am. J. Hosp. Pharm.,* 35, 809, 1978.

56. **Sieverts, S.,** The uses of utilization review, *N. Engl. J. Med.,* 295, 1505, 1978.

57. **McGowan, J. E., Jr.,** Continuing education — a critical component of attempts to improve usage of antimicrobial agents, *Q. Rev. Bull.,* 5, 32, 1979.

58. **Kessner, D. M.,** Quality assessment and assurance — early signs of cognitive dissonance, *N. Engl. J. Med.,* 298, 381, 1978.

59. Editorial, Audit of audit, *Lancet,* 2, 453, 1976.

60. **Nelson, A. R.,** Orphan data and the unclosed loop — a dilemma in P.S.R.O. and medical audit, *N. Engl. J. Med.,* 295, 617, 1976.

61. **McNerney, W. J.,** The quandary of quality assessment, *N. Engl. J. Med.,* 295, 1505, 1976.

62. **Komaroff, A. L.,** The P.S.R.O. quality assurance blues, *N. Engl. J. Med.,* 298, 1194, 1978.

63. **Jones, S. R., Barks, J., Bratton, T., McRee, E., Pannell, J., Yanchick, V. A., Browne, R., and Smith, J. W.,** The effect of an educational program upon hospital antibiotic use, *Am. J. Med. Sci.,* 273, 79, 1977.

64. **Zeman, B. T., Pike, M., and Samet, C.,** The antibiotic utilization committee — an effective tool in implementation of drug utilization review that monitors the medical justification and cost of antibiotics, *Hospitals,* 48, 73, 1973.

65. **Recco, R. A., Gladstone, J. L., Friedman, S. A., and Gerken, E. H.,** Antibiotic control in a municipal hospital, *Clin. Res.,* 26, 336A, 1978.

66. **Craig, W. A., Uman, S. J., Shaw, W. R., Ramgopal, V., Eagan, L. L., and Leopold, E. T.,** Hospital use of antimicrobial drugs — survey at 19 hospitals and results of antimicrobial control programs, *Ann. Intern. Med.,* 89, 793, 1978.

67. **Smolens, B., Gaylor, D. W., and Finegold, S. M.,** An antibiotics control program in a large teaching hospital, *Am. J. Hosp. Pharm.,* 20, 610, 1963.

68. **Meyer, R.,** Antibiotic prescribing patterns — a new emphasis for the infection control practitioner, *A.P.I.C. (J. Assoc. Pract. Infect. Control),* 4, 9, 1976.

69. **Freeman, J. and McGowan, J. E., Jr.,** Choice of potentially-toxic antibiotics — derivation of an internal standard of physician performance, *Clin. Res.,* 25, 327A, 1977.

70. **Edwards, L. D., Levin, S., and Lepper, M. H.,** A comprehensive surveillance system of infections and antimicrobials use at Presbyterian-St. Luke's Hospital, Chicago, *Am. J. Public Health,* 62, 1053, 1972.

71. **Madden, R. W.,** Monitoring the effectiveness of antimicrobial agents in a general hospital, *Am. J. Hosp. Pharm.,* 31, 262, 1974.

72. **Dillard, K. R., Yoshikawa, T. T., and Guze, L. B.,** Appropriate usage of antibiotics improved by surveillance program, *Hospitals,* 51, 81, 1977.

73. **Gibbs, C. W., Jr., Gibson, J. T., and Newton, D. S.,** Drug utilization review of actual versus preferred pediatric antibiotic therapy, *Am. J. Hosp. Pharm.,* 30, 892, 1973.

74. **Eliasson, C.,** Guidelines for clinical antibiotic usage review, *Hosp. Top.,* Jan-Feb 1977, 10.

75. **Simon, W. A., Thompson, L., Campbell, S., and Lantos, R. L.,** Drug usage review and inventory analysis in promoting rational parenteral cephalosporin therapy, *Am. J. Hosp. Pharm.,* 32, 1116, 1975.

76. **Greenlaw, C. W.,** Antimicrobial drug use monitoring by a hospital pharmacy, *Am. J. Hosp. Pharm.,* 34, 835, 1977.

77. **Shoji, K. T., Axnick, K., and Rytel, M. W.,** Infections and antibiotic use in a large municipl hospital 1970-1972 — a prospective analysis of the effectiveness of a continuous surveillance program, *Health Lab. Sci.,* 11, 283, 1974.

78. **Wagner, E. H., Greenberg, R. A., Imrey, P. B., Williams, C. A., Wolf, S. H., and Ibrahim, M. A.,** Influence of training and experience on selecting criteria to evaluate medical care, *N. Engl. J. Med.,* 294, 871, 1976.

79. **Finley, R.,** Antibiotic usage, *JAMA,* 239, 1280, 1978.

80. Editrial, Freedom to prescribe — in ignorance, *Br. Med. J.,* 2, 1573, 1978.

81. **Downs, G. E.,** What the patient needs to know about antibiotics, *Am. J. Pharm.,* 149, 169, 1977.

82. **McSherry, C. K.,** Quality assurance — the cost of utilization review and the educational value of medical audit in a university hospital, *Surgery,* 80, 122, 1976.

83. **Noel, M. W. and Paxinos, J.,** Cephalosporins — use review and cost analysis, *Am. J. Hosp. Pharm.,* 35, 933, 1978.

84. **Burnum, J. F.,** Preventability of adverse drug reactions, *Ann. Intern. Med.,* 85, 80, 1976.

85. **Inglefinger, F. J.,** Counting adverse drug reactions that count, *JAMA,* 294, 1003, 1976.

86. Veterans Administration Ad Hoc Interdisciplinary Advisory Committee on Antimicrobial Drug Usage, Audits of Antimicrobial usage, 16 — ordering antimicrobial agents for hospitalized patients, *JAMA,* 237, 1967, 1977.

87. **McCabe, W. R. and Finland, M. Eds.,** *Contemporary Standards for Antimicrobial Usage,* Vol. 13, Principles and Techniques of Human Research and Therapeutics, Futura, Mount Kisco, N.Y., 1977.

88. **Garrison, T. J. and Puckett, C. F.,** The automatic stop order — is it still needed?, *Am. J. Hosp. Pharm.,* 32, 994, 1975.

89. **Kunin, C. M.,** Impact of infections and antibiotic use on medical care, *Ann. Intern. Med.,* 89, 716, 1978.

CHOOSING THE BEST ANTISEPTIC, DISINFECTANT, STERILIZATION METHOD, AND WASTE DISPOSAL AND LAUNDRY SYSTEM

George F. Mallison

ANTISEPTICS

Definition

An antiseptic is a chemical used externally, on the skin or in and around wounds, in an attempt to control surface microbial contamination that could cause infection. The major use of antiseptics in health care facilities is for handwashing.

Handwashing

Handwashing is generally considered to be the most important single procedure in preventing the spread of nosocomial (hospital acquired) infections. Routine handwashing is required before and after any significant contact with patients and after any significant contact with a contaminated object.[1]

Acceptable soap for handwashing may come in the form of bars, liquids, granules, leaflets, or soap-impregnated tissues. If liquid products are used, dispensers may become contaminated with time; they should be dumped, cleaned, and dried, and refilled with fresh solution from time to time. If bars of soap are used, tiny "motel" bars should be used to help discourage expensive pilferage and to prevent individual bars from remaining for many days in pools of water that might support the growth of microorganisms; racks that permit bars of soap to dry between use are recommended.

Routine Handwashing

Handwashing with plain soap, warm water, and mechanical friction are sufficient to remove most transient microorganisms contaminating the hands. Under a moderate-sized stream of comfortably warm water, hands should be vigorously lathered and rubbed together for at least 15 sec. Then, the hands should be rinsed, dried with a paper towel, and the towel then should be used to turn off the faucet. Faucet aerators become contaminated, and should not be used in hospitals. Because rings and cracked nail polish make microorganisms on the hand difficult to remove, personnel who take care of patients should be discouraged from wearing rings or nail polish while on duty.[1]

Handwashing with Antiseptics

Antiseptic handwashing products should be used for handwashing before surgery and before other high-risk or invasive procedures (such as insertion of catheters), in the care of newborn infants, and in the care of isolated patients.[1]

The three major types of antiseptic handwashing products currently in use in the U.S. contain either an iodophor, hexachlorophene, or chlorhexidine. All three are effective in reducing transient flora of the hands. Iodophors are water-soluble complexes of iodine with organic compounds; iodophors release iodine during the handwashing process and for a short time thereafter, but in some people they cause excessive drying of skin if used many times a day. Hexachlorophene-containing preparations reduce populations of resident skin flora, particularly Gram-positive organisms, when used routinely, but they may result in an increase in the proportion of Gram-negative skin organisms, and the product is readily absorbed into the bloodstream when used frequently. Chlorhexidine-containing handwashing agents are essentially nonabsorbed into the bloodstream, are generally acceptable to patient-care personnel, and considerably reduce numbers of resident microorganisms on the skin for hours after a single use.

Preoperative Skin Preparation

Shaving of the operative site should be done immediately preoperatively, not the night before; skin areas with little hair need not be shaved. After being shaved (if done), the skin should be cleansed with a 2-min soap-and-water scrub. Then, just prior to the operative procedure, a 2- to 5-min scrub of the operative site should be carried out with an iodophor, 70 to 90% ethyl or isopropyl alcohol, tincture of chlorohexidine, or a sterile solution of cetylpysidinium chloride; this final skin preparation is done using sterile sponges by a person wearing sterile gloves.[2]

Use of Antiseptics in Wounds

For minor injuries with breaks in the skin for hospitalized patients, out-patients, or staff, the wound should be washed with unmedicated bar or liquid soap; if a soap solution is considered necessary, it should be made up only when needed to prevent microbial contamination that is likely to occur if the solution were to stand for more than a few hours. If the wound is large, after washing with soap and warm water and rinsing out all foreign material, an antiseptic such as ethyl or isopropyl alcohol (70 to 90%) or an iodophor should be used in and around the wound. Dressings should be applied to the wound only if necessary to keep it clean.

Dilute aqueous benzalkonium or benzethonium chloride products (e.g., Zephiran® and Roccal®) should never be used for any type of antisepsis in hospitals. This recommendation for non-use includes a policy change in the previous recommendation for use of such products for wounds exposed to rabies virus.[3] The current recommendation for treatment of wounds so exposed is for such wounds to "be thoroughly cleaned immediately with soap solutions."[4]

DISINFECTANTS

Definition and Levels of Disinfection Needed

A disinfectant is a product that is used to kill disease-causing organisms, except spores, on objects used in patient care and on environmental (inanimate) surfaces. Disinfectants in the U.S. are tested, registered, and regulated in interstate commerce by the U.S. Environmental Protection Agency (EPA).

Objects that contact skin or mucous membranes should receive at least a high level of disinfection. These objects include endoscopic instruments that do not enter tissue or the vascular system; oral and rectal thermometers; respiratory therapy and anesthesia equipment, including medication and humidification apparatus as well as masks and tubing; suction catheters; and similar equipment. The criterion for efficacy of high-level disinfection of such items should be the absence, after processing, of viruses and of all common vegetative microorganisms, including pathogens and opportunistic pathogens. Occasional (perhaps four times annually, but more if pathogenic contamination is found) culturing of disinfected items has been recommended.[5]

Many patient-care supplies not wet in use, not used by infected patients, and not used in direct skin contact generally need only thorough detergent cleaning and drying.

How to Disinfect

Thorough cleaning of surfaces is essential prior to disinfection of objects that will come into contact with skin or mucous membranes. Frictional ("elbow grease") scrubbing or detergent spray cleaning removes contaminants that may be poorly penetrated by disinfectants; such cleaning also greatly reduces the number of microorganisms to be subsequently destroyed by the disinfecting chemical or process.

After thorough cleaning, disinfection by the chemicals or processes listed under Disinfection in Table 1 should be carried out for at least 30 min. Then, items should be thoroughly rinsed either with sterile water or with tap water to which hypochlorite is added to produce at least 10 mg/ℓ (ppm) of chlorine to prevent recontamination from organisms that might be in tap water. A fresh 1:3000 dilution of 5% hypochlorite laundry bleach in tap water, prepared at least each work shift, will yield $\geqslant$10 mg/ℓ chlorine residual. After rinsing, items may be dried with filtered hot air which is preferable to open-air drying; drying may be done using sterile towels. After drying, the items should be packaged prior to reuse.

Alternate Processes to Disinfection

If sterilization is possible, particularly stream sterilization, it should be used instead of disinfection, because it is cheaper, as well as more effective than disinfection (see the section entitled "Sterilization", below). Reuseable tubing and other supplies that may be steam sterilized are available for use in anesthesia and respiratory therapy. Clean, disposable respiratory therapy or anesthesia tubing also may be used, but it is expensive, and it should be used only once. Dry thermometer-care systems, in which all thermometers are kept by the patients' bed and cleaned before and after each use under the faucet with soap and then dried (or washed and dried and then wiped with 70 to 90% alcohol), are a reasonable and safe alternative to wet disinfection for each patient.

STERILIZATION

Definition

Sterilization is a process that has as its objective the removal and/or destruction of all living microorganisms that may exist on the surface of an article or in a fluid. Instruments, catheters, or fluids that enter tissues or the vascular system, as well as extracorporeal equipment through which blood circulates, must be subjected to a procedure that produces sterilization.

Sterilization by Heat and Disposables

Some sterilization processes (particularly sterilization using heat-hot air or steam) may be less expensive, as well as more effective, than disinfecting processes. Thus, sterilization should be used whenever possible, even when it is not essential to prevent disease transmission. For instance, steam-sterilizable tubing for respiratory therapy and anesthesia is available.

Inexpensive sterile disposable items widely used in patient care, e.g., hypodermic syringes and needles, are customarily used in patient care because they are safe and convenient to use without any hospital processing. Items sold as disposable should never be re-used.

Steam Sterilization

Steam under pressure in an autoclave is used for most hospital sterilization. Both heat and moisture from steam are essential for effective steam sterilization; thus, each package placed in a steam autoclave must be free of air pockets (e.g., any item that could hold water must be placed on its side in the sterilizer or steam may not displace the air) or wrappers that would block ready steam penetration.[6]

Table 1

Object	(Will come in contact with skin or mucous membrane)		Sterilization (will enter tissue or vascular system)	
	Procedure[a]	Minutes	Procedure[a]	Hours
Smooth, hard-surfaced objects	A	≥30	C	18
	C	≥30	G	MR[g]
	D	≥30	H	12
	E	≥30	I	10
	F[b]	≥30	K	MR
	H	≥30		
	I	≥30		
	J	≥30		
Rubber tubing and catheters	D	≥30	G	MR
	E	≥30	K	MR
	I	≥30		
	J	≥30		
Polyethylene tubing and catheters[c,d,e]	A	≥30	C	18
	D	≥30	G	MR
	E	≥30	H	12
	I	≥30	I	10
	J	≥30	K	MR
Lensed instruments	H	≥30	G	MR
	I	≥30	H	12
			I	12
Thermometers (oral and rectal)[f]	B	≥30	C	18
	I	≥30	G	MR
			I	10
Hinged instruments			G	MR
			H	12
			I	10
			K	MR

[a]   A, ethyl or isopropyl alcohol (70 to 90%);
   B, ethyl alcohol (70 to 90%);
   C, formaldehyde (8%)-alcohol (70%) solution;
   D, iodophor (500 ppm iodine);
   E, phenolic solutions (3% aqueous solution of concentrate);
   F, sodium hypochlorite (1000 ppm available chlorine);
   G, ethylene oxide gas (for time, see manufacturer's recommendations);
   H, Aqueous formalin (40% formaldehyde).
   I, Glutaraldehyde (2% aqueous solution);
   J, Wet pasteurization at 75°C after detergent cleaning;
   K, Heat sterilization (see manufacturer's recommendations).

[b]   Not recommended for metal instruments.

[c]   Tubing must be completely filled for disinfection.

[d]   Instruments or catheters that enter tissue or the vascular system should be sterilized.

[e]   Thermostability should be investigated when indicated.

[f]   Thermometers must be thoroughly wiped, preferably with soap and water, before disinfection or sterilization. Alcohol-iodine solutions will remove markings on poor grade thermometers. Do not mix rectal and oral thermometers at any stage of handling or processing.

[g]   MR, manufacturer's recommendations.

Sterilization is produced by the high temperature of steam, not its pressure; pressurized steam is used in autoclaves only to obtain the high temperature necessary to kill microorganisms rapidly. Depending upon the size of a package placed into a conventional gravity-displacement sterilizer, once it reaches its operating temperature of at least 121°C (250°F), sterilization can be achieved in 15 to 45 min, depending on the size and type of item. Specific recommendations for time of sterilization necessary for various items are provided by manufacturers of sterilizers.[6]

High-vacuum, short-cycle steam sterilizers have been used more and more in hospitals in recent years because they permit a total sterilizing cycle time for fabric packs that is considerably shorter than that provided by a gravity-displacement sterilizer. High-vacuum sterilizers normally operate at 132 to 135°C (270 to 275°F). Both the conventional and the high-vacuum steam sterilizers require routine maintenance, as well as careful operation; the latter type, although faster, is more expensive than conventional sterilizers and requires more skill in operation and maintenance. With high-vacuum sterilizers only, a crossed-autoclaved-tape test (the so-called Bowie-Dick test) should be used in the center of the bottom front pack in the first load each day for quality control in addition to the tape and spore tests discussed below.

Linen packs to be sterilized should weigh no more than 5.5 kg (12 lb) and be no larger than 30 × 50 cm (12 × 12 × 20 in.). Double wrappers of cotton cloth, paper, and various synthetic materials all have been used successfully for linen and other packs that are sterilized by steam; no matter what type of wrappers used, however, only autoclave tape should be used to seal the packs prior to sterilization. Autoclave tape not only holds packs together dependably, but it will also show at a glance by color change that the pack has been through a cycle in a working steam sterilizer. It is neither necessary nor recommended that color-change indicators be placed inside packs sterilized by steam.

As soon as packs are removed from a steam sterilizer, they should be clearly marked with the date of sterilization and the date when they will no longer be considered to be sterile. Packs double wrapped with two wrappers each containing two layers of muslin (total of four layers of muslin) will remain sterile for 3 weeks when stored on open shelves. Recommendations for time of storage using this and other types of wrappers are in Table 2.

At least weekly testing of all steam sterilizers is recommended, using commercial preparations of spores of *Bacillus stearothemophilus*. Any positive spore tests should be followed immediately by another; if it also is positive, the sterilizer should be carefully checked immediately to correct any possible mechanical or operational problems. It is not necessary to recall any packs sterilized if only occasional nonconsecutive spore tests (1 to 2% of all tests) are positive because there is a considerable safety factor inherent in steam sterilization.

A pack that has been sterilized should no longer be considered sterile if it becomes wet, if it has been dropped onto the floor, or if any tape seal has been broken.[7]

Dry Heat Sterilization

Materials, such as petroleum products, powders, and complex instruments that cannot be disassembled or with edges that might be damaged by moist heat, and glassware may be sterilized in hospitals by using specially designed hot-air sterilizers. Muslin or foil are satisfactory wrappers for items sterilized by dry heat. These sterilizers should be monitored for efficiency using at least weekly tests with spores of *B. stearothermophilus*. Sterilization times in forced-convection hot-air sterilizers vary from 6 hr at 121°C (250°F) to 1 hr at 171°C (340°F).[6]

Table 2
STORAGE TIMES DURING WHICH
PACKS REMAINED STERILE[7]

	Duration of sterility[a]	
Wrapping	In closed cabinet	On open shelves
Single-wrapped muslin (two layers)	1 week	2 days
Double-wrapped muslin (each two layers)	7 weeks	3 weeks
Single-wrapped two-way crepe paper (single layer)	At least 8 weeks	3 weeks
Tightly woven pima cotton (single layer) over single-wrapped muslin (two layers)	—	8 weeks
Two-way crepe paper (single layer) over single-wrapped muslin (two layers)	—	10 weeks
Single-wrapped muslin (two layers) sealed in 3-mil polyethylene	—	At least 9 months

[a] Sterility was checked daily for the first week of storage and weekly thereafter.

Sterilization by Liquid Chemicals

Several EPA-registered liquid chemicals are capable of producing sterile surfaces on objects after periods of 10 to 18 hr of soaking (see Table 1). Sterilization using such chemicals is not recommended except for unusual, heat-labile items that cannot be successfully sterilized by ethylene oxide gas (see below) using a "cold" (less than 35°C [95°F] cycle.

Gas (Ethylene Oxide) Sterilization

Sterilization with gaseous ethylene oxide (EtO) is widely used today in hospitals for reuseable items that might be damaged by steam sterilization. Commercial "gas" sterilizers are available that process goods in about 3 to 8 hr at usual operating temperatures of 50 to 57°C (122 to 139°F). Items should be carefully cleaned just prior to sterilization. Any porous items, such as those made of rubber or plastic, accumulate residues of EtO during sterilization, and thus, they must be well aerated in a commercial aeration cabinet for 8 to 12 hr before they are safe to use. Items to be gas sterilized should be wrapped in muslin, paper, and films of commercial wrappers made of cellophane, polypropylene, polyvinylchloride, or low-density polyethylene.

Each package that is gas sterilized should be monitored by a color-change indicator on the outside of the package to show that that package has been through a cycle in a working sterilizer. At least weekly testing of gas sterilizers is recommended using spores of *Bacillus subtilis (globigii)* that are available from several commercial manufacturers. It is further recommended that any implantable items in any load sterilized by gas be held until the spore test be shown to be negative before these items are released for use in patients.[8]

Ethylene oxide is a moderately toxic and potentially mutagenic (causing birth defects) chemical. To avoid unnecessary exposure to EtO gas, a room with a gas sterilizing unit or an aerator should be well ventilated, and both types of units must be vented to the outside of the building where located. Additionally, it is recommended that staff members leave the room containing a gas sterilizer for 5 min immediately after the sterilizer door is opened after completion of a cycle of the unit.

SOLID WASTE DISPOSAL

Proper disposal of hospital solid waste is a responsibility generally delegated to the housekeeping department. Hospital solid wastes capable of producing injury or containing large numbers of infectious microorganisms should be handled in such a fashion that they will not cause any risk of disease. Waste from isolated patients and waste from microbiology laboratories must be steam sterilized or incinerated in the hospital. Pathology wastes should be incinerated or ground to the sanitary sewer. Materials capable of producing injury (such as hypodermic needles) should be placed into rigid containers immediately after use to prevent injury. Any liquid infectious waste should be carefully poured down a flushing hopper or toilet.[9]

Hospitals relying on municipal or commercial systems for ultimate disposal of solid wastes must assure that the method of terminal disposal is safe if a sanitary landfill or a municipal incinerator is not used.

LAUNDRY OPERATIONS

Laundry operations for health care facilities exist to process soiled linens into clean linens that are used to provide comfortable care for patients without the risk of disease transmission. Pathogen-contaminated soiled linens might cause infections, and improperly laundered linens can cause physical irritation of the skin of patients.

Soiled linens should be placed into carts or bagged at the location where they are used; they should never be thrown on the floor prior to collection or transfer for laundering. Hands should be washed after handling soiled linen. Soiled linen should not be sorted in patient care areas. Linens that are known to be highly contaminated, particularly linens from strict and respiratory isolation and from enteric and wound and skin precaution isolation, should be clearly labeled and handled with special care, preferably in impervious bags. Soiled linens should be sorted as little as possible in hospital wards or in the laundry. Soiled linens should never be prerinsed in the wards or steam or gas sterilized prior to laundering.

Laundering at water temperatures of 71°C (160°F) for 25 min kills or removes nearly all microorganisms other than resistant spores. Such temperatures have been conventionally used for hospital laundering for decades, and they are known to produce linens that are free from risk of microbial contamination sufficient to cause disease when used in patient rooms.[10] However, surgical gowns and surgical linens, delivery-room linens, and some nursery linens should be steam sterilized after laundering prior to use.

REFERENCES

1. Steere, A. C. and Mallison, G. F., Handwashing practices for the prevention of nosocomial infections, *Ann. Intern. Med.*, 83, 683, 1975.
2. American College of Surgeons, *Manual on Control of Infection in Surgical Patients*, American College of Surgeons, Philadelphia, 1976.

3. U.S. Department of Health, Education, and Welfare, Isolation Techniques for Use in Hospitals, 2nd ed), DHEW Publ. No. (CDC) 76-8314, U.S. Government Printing Office, Washington, D.C., 1975.
4. Center for Disease Control, Aqueous quarternary ammonium compounds and rabies treatment, *J. Infec. Dis.,* 139, 494, 1979.
5. Committee on Microbial Contamination of Surfaces, American Public Health Association, Proposed Microbiologic Guidelines for Respiratory Therapy Equipment and Materials, Health Laboratory Service 15, 177, 1978.
6. *Sterilization Aids,* American Sterilizer Company, Erie, Pa., 1968.
7. **Mallison, G. F. and Standard, P. G.,** Safe storage times for sterile packs. *Hospitals,* 48, 77, 1974.
8. Joint Commission on Accreditation of Hospitals, *Accreditation Manual for Hospitals,* Joint Commission on Accreditation of Hospitals, Chicago, 1979.
9. U.S. Department of Health, Education, and Welfare, Disposal of Solid Wastes from Hospitals, National Nosocomial Infections Study, Department of Health, Education and Welfare Publication No. (CDC) 74-8257, Center for Disease Control, Atlanta, 1974, revised 1980.
10. U.S. Department of Health, Education, and Welfare, The Hospital Laundry, Department of Health, Education and Welfare Publication No. 930-D-24, U.S. Government Printing Office, Washington, D.C., 1966.

Organization for Infection Control

UNIVERSITY OF VIRGINIA MEDICAL CENTER — ISOLATION PROCEDURE AND INFECTION CONTROL MANUAL*

Richard P. Wenzel, Charles A. Osterman, and Gerald L. Mandell

INTRODUCTION

Approximately 5 to 10% of hospitalized patients acquire an infection after admission, one which is not present or incubating at the time of admission. Such "nosocomial" or "hospital acquired" infections may significantly increase the duration of hospitalization and costs for many patients and may result in permanent disability or death. Furthermore, staff members working closely with patients with communicable diseases may be at increased risk of acquiring infections unless isolation techniques are instituted and strictly observed. In addition, those hospitals and staff members not adhering to a currently accepted infection control policy may be held legally liable for injury incurred by patients and can be sued. For many reasons (medical, economic, ethical, and legal) most hospitals have written guidelines for infections occurring within the hospital.

The risk of acquiring nosocomial (hospital associated) infections can be viewed in terms of a formula which lists the basic factors involved:

$$\text{Risk of infection} = \frac{\text{Dose} \times \text{virulence}}{\text{Host resistance}}$$

This means that if the total number of organisms in the environment is increased or if more virulent (invasive) strains of organisms are substituted for benign organisms, the risk of acquiring an infection increases. Similarly, if host resistance factors are lowered, e.g., by instituting immunosuppressive therapy, we are likely to see an increasing number of infections in such patients.

Proper handwashing influences the dose favorably by reducing the number of organisms which may inadvertently find their way into a patient's wound, bloodstream, urinary tract, or respiratory tract by contact with our hands. To carry this one step further, we may cover washed hands with sterile gloves to virtually eliminate dose from this particular source, providing that sterility is maintained.

Appropriate isolation affects virulence by confining the dangerous organisms to a small area within the hospital, protecting other patients, and the hospital's personnel. Host resistance is most influenced by the medical team's administering to the patient. For example, if indwelling catheter tubes can be discontinued or the dosage of steroid therapy can be reduced, then host resistance can be improved. A partial list of host resistance factors is shown in Table 1.

The components of infections shown above as a formula can be expressed as three circles (sets) of important factors (see Figure 1). Where the circles overlap, there is a greater risk of infection; e.g., when the dose of organisms is increasing while host resistance is decreasing (intersection of Sets I and III) or when the dose of organisms is increasing while virulence is increasing (intersection of Sets I and II). Obviously the worst possible circumstance would be the combination of increasing dose, increasing virulence, and least host resistance (intersection of Sets I, II, and III).

---

* Editor's note — The Isolation Procedure and Infection Control Manual is intended to be a frequently used reference. Thus, a copy is placed on every ward and clinic and in every medical, nursing, and administrator's office.

Table 1
HOST RESISTANCE FACTORS

Factors	Comment
Normal number of circulating white cells	Special risk if total neutrophils $\leqslant 500/mm^3$
Normal immunoglobulins (gamma globulins)	Patients with multiple myeloma may have added difficulty with infections
Normal functions of cellular immunity (lymphocytes and macrophages)	Often depressed with steroid therapy and immunosuppressive drugs
Intact skin and mucosa	Indwelling catheters disrupt intact skin and mucosa
Strong cough reflex	Anesthesia and sedatives may depress cough reflex

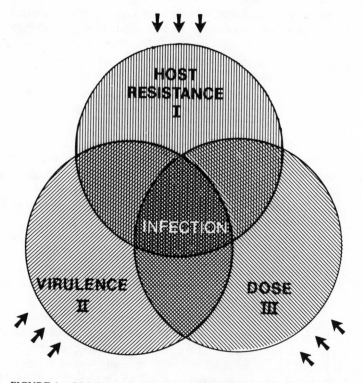

FIGURE 1.   Risk factors in infection. Intersecting areas indicate increased risk of infection. The greatest risk occurs in the center (small area where I, II, and III intersect), when all three factors combine, i.e., when both dose and virulence are increasing in a patient with decreasing resistance.

By its nature, the hospital is an area where ill people (some with infections) are concentrated. Therefore, there are more dangerous (virulent) organisms in this area than anywhere else in the community. Also, since clinicians have continued to use newer antibiotics, not only are there more virulent organisms in the hospital, but also there are more drug-resistant organisms. As physicians have become more proficient at treating malignancies, collagen vascular diseases, renal transplant rejections, etc. they have had to resort to drugs which lower host resistance (immunosuppression/ steroids). It is not surprising therefore that patients will develop hospital acquired nosocomial infections, for we expose the people with the least resistance to an increasing number of often virulent organisms. Moreover, once the patient enters a hospital, he is likely to have his skin and mucosa invaded (I.V. line and bladder catheter). He may have an operation which with the anesthesia may depress his cough reflex and increase the risk of pulmonary infections, in addition to a possible surgical wound infection. If he is seriously ill, he may receive immunosuppressive or steroid therapy and reduce his otherwise efficient function of lymphocytes and macrophages. Therefore, many hospital acquired infections are inevitable, and not all can be prevented.

Those interested in hospital acquired infections would do well to think of the basic factors: Dosage, Virulence and Host resistance, as we analyze the causes and look for solutions to these problems. Proper handwashing (15 sec minimum) between patient contact is the main way to decrease the dosage of organisms to which our patients are exposed. Other important factors are the limiting to the barest minimum the number of hours our patients have an indwelling I.V. or bladder catheter in place, as well as weighing the risk of all procedures against their presumed benefit prior to their institution.

Early institution of proper isolation procedures will limit the spread of virulent organisms from infected patients to the staff and in turn to other patients. The physicians and nurses have a large responsibility in monitoring host resistance factors and instituting measures to remedy deficiencies.

We wish to express our thanks to the following sources of reference material[1-4] on which we base much of this revision of our "Isolation Procedure and Infection Control Manual." *Isolation Techniques for Use in Hospitals, Control of Communicable Diseases in Man, The Infection Control Manual, University of Virginia Medical Center Isolation Procedure and Infection Control Manual.*

INFECTION CONTROL COMMITTEE

Every hospital seeking accreditation is required by the Joint Commission on Accreditation of Hospitals (JCAH) to have an infection control committee. The purpose of the committee (see current listing of members) is to utilize the expertise of members from various departments of the hospital, so that the existing policies of infection control can be continually reviewed and nosocomial infection problems can be identified and resolved. The qualifications for membership should include interest, expertise, and, if possible, influence within the hospital. It is also likely that administrative changes can more easily be effected if the representatives possess the desired qualities of tact and charisma. The administrator on the Infection Control Committee is also a member of the hospital's Policy Committee, therefore, all issues resolved at the former are routinely presented for necessary approval and action by the latter committee.

In acute situations, the Infection Control Committee does have executive power to institute all necessary changes to control infection within the hospital. In addition, the Infection Control Committee, the hospital epidemiologist, or Infection Control Practitioners, (ICPs) do have authority to place a patient on isolation until a diagnosis is resolved. Any differences of opinion must be referred to the hospital epidemiologist or chairman of the committee for resolution.

Current Listing of Members of the University of Virginia Medical Center Infection Control Committee

		Extension
1.	Dr. Gerald Mandell, Internal Medicine, Chairman	5241
2.	Dr. Richard P. Wenzel, Hospital Epidemiologist	2777

3.	Mr. Charles A. Osterman, R.N., Epidemiology Nursing Supervisor	2143
4.	Dr. Nuzhet Atuk, Employee Health Service	2013
5.	Dr. Ivan Crosby, TCV Surgery	5052
6.	Dr. Richard F. Edlich, Plastic Surgery	2085
7.	Dr. Jack M. Gwaltney, Jr., Internal Medicine	2093
8.	Dr. J. Owen Hendley, Pediatrics	2218
9.	Ms. Sandra M. Landry, R.N., Infection Control Practitioner	2143
10.	Mrs. Emma Hunt, R.N., Employee Health Service	2013
11.	Dr. Dieter Groschel, Bacteriology	2796
12.	Ms. Sherry Y. Thompson, R.N., Infection Control Practitioner	2143
13.	Dr. John Hoyt, Anesthesiology	5241
14.	Miss Jewell Reeves, R.N., Central Sterile Supply Supervisor	5461
15.	Mr. Edward Smith, Administrator	2257
16.	Dr. Edward Rose, Internal Medicine	5210
17.	Mrs. Anna Sutphin, R.N., Supervisor, Surgical Specialties, Recording Secretary	2482
18.	Dr. Matthew Lambert, General Surgery	2028
19.	Miss Jackie A. Young, Director, Hospital Pharmacy	2013
20.	Ms. Brenda S. Russell, R.N., Infection Control Practitioner	2143

JOB DESCRIPTION PHYSICIAN-EPIDEMIOLOGIST[4a]

The primary function of the physician—epidemiologist is to direct a program of infection control within the hospital. The program includes surveillance of nosocomial infections, continuing education, control of infectious disease outbreaks, protection of the employee staff, and advice on new products and procedures. The infection control program is enforced by way of the Infection Control Committee, of which the physician-epidemiologist is a member and to which he is responsible. He must have delegated authority from the hospital administration and the Infection Control Committee to institute emergency measures and studies when indicated for infection control.

Broadly speaking, the physician-epidemiologist should be a consultant in infectious diseases and be familiar with nosocomial problems. He should have a working understanding of statistics and envision himself as an advisor and as a member of a large interdisciplinary health team.

Surveillance — He should be able, together with the ICP(s), to establish a form of routine surveillance, with the goal of identifying background endemic rates as well as new outbreaks. The surveillance, once established, can be maintained by the ICP(s). The physician, however, has the responsibility of maintaining quality control, directing and advising the nurse or technician in all of his/her responsibilities, and assisting in the analysis and distribution of data.

Continuing education — He should be prepared to teach and/or lead others in the teaching of proper isolation techniques, good wound care, tracheostomy care, etc. to medical and paramedical staff.

Control of infectious disease outbreaks — If new problems become apparent, such as recognition of contaminated I.V. fluids, the physician-eidemiologist should implement necessary changes to protect patients and/or personnel. He should be prepared to institute emergency and urgent measures to control any outbreak of infection in either patients or staff within the hospital. Such control measures may involve special surveillance bacteriologic studies, isolation procedures, or changes of procedures from the routine.

Protection of employee staff — Routine surveillance of PPD (Tuberculin) skin testing of employees should be carried out at all hospitals, and the physician-epidemiologist should assist in this surveillance. In addition, he should assist and/or direct the student and employee health services in proper updating of necessary immunizations, use of immune serum globulin, etc. He should be able to advise the paramedical staff (dietary, housekeeping, etc.) of the risks within a hospital and ways of avoiding or limiting these infectious risks.

Advice on new products and procedures — He should be prepared to advise on the infection control risks and benefits prior to acceptance of a new procedure or product within the hospital.

JOB DESCRIPTION FOR NURSING SUPERVISOR IN HOSPITAL EPIDEMIOLOGY

Distinguishing Features

The epidemiology nursing supervisor helps coordinate the activities of the Division of Hospital Epidemiology, provides technical supervision on hospital infection control, coordinates and assumes direct responsibility for nosocomial infection surveillance and reporting, communicable diseases follow-up and reporting, investigation of outbreaks in the hospital, and continuing education of the staff on infection control matters, and assists the Hospital (physician) epidemiologist. This position is unique in that the supervising nurse epidemiologist functions primarily as a specialist trained in hospital epidemiology rather than as a nurse or technician. However, the position involves regular contact with physicians, nurses, and administrators at all levels within the hospital and state health departments.

The work is directed and evaluated by the hospital epidemiologist and/or the Medical Center Infection Control Committee. During investigations of outbreaks in the hospital, the epidemiology nursing supervisor reports directly to the hospital epidemiologist, with whom he/she assesses the nature and extent of the problem, determines the proper course of the investigation, and assigns priorities to the rest of the infection control program. The supervising nurse epidemiologist delegates the various aspects of the overall infection control program to the other ICPs according to the priorities established. Effective performance depends upon sound comprehension of the principles of epidemiology, management, organization, and the ability to stimulate medical, nursing, bacteriology, and other staff in the hospital to improve the infection control program.

Examples of duties characteristic of the epidemiology nursing supervisor include:

1. Review and compilation of weekly/monthly nosocomial infection surveillance data, completion of special forms, and the preparation of regular (written as well as verbal) epidemiologic status reports for the Infection Control Committee, the State Bureau of Epidemiology, and for appropriate persons throughout the Medical Center.
2. Contacting of department heads in the Medical Center (physicians, microbiologists, nurses, administrators, etc.) for additional information on incomplete reports or whenever there is reason to believe an epidemic or infection hazard situation exists.
3. Initiation, coordination, and completion of investigations of infectious disease outbreaks in the hospital, including supervision of the investigative staff and implementation of control measures directed by the physician-epidemiologist.
4. Participation in special hospital epidemiological studies or projects in a consultative, coordinating, liaison role.

5. Consultation on infection control problems to all departments in the hospital, particularly in the absence of the hospital (physician) epidemiologist.
6. Assigning priorities to various activities of the division together with the hospital epidemiologist, scheduling and delegating responsibilities for various aspects of surveillance, investigation, teaching, follow-up and reporting of infection control problems, and assuming final responsibility for completeness of all of the assigned tasks.
7. Planning and participation in-service training and other teaching programs on hospital epidemiology and infection control for new employees, periodic programs for nurses and nursing students, medical technologist students, housekeeping personnel, etc.
8. Attendance at epidemiologically or infection control-oriented workshops, in-service and training conferences, and otherwise actively participating in the development and maintenance of hospital-wide and state-wide standards of infection surveillance, investigation, control and reporting.
9. Assessment, evaluation, recommendation, and clinical trials of new or improved products or procedures and their relationship to infection control in the hospital, requiring thorough knowledge of products and procedures in use, the ability to prepare comparative cost analyses, and a comprehensive understanding of the purchasing procedures of the hospital.

Qualification Standards

Qualification standards include registration or eligibility for registration in Virginia as a graduate professional nurse either from a baccalaureate degree program or diploma program approved by the National League for Nursing, with additional preparation in the specialized field of infection control.

One must also have 2 years of hospital epidemiology nursing experience at the Nurse Epidemiologist B level. Additional college-level education in nursing or nursing experience in infection control may be substituted for the required hospital epidemiology nursing experience. No substitution may be made for at least 1 year of hospital epidemiology nursing experience at the Nurse Epidemiologist B level (see chapter on "The Infection Control Practitioner").

JOB DESCRIPTION—INFECTION CONTROL PRACTITIONER/ NURSE-EPIDEMIOLOGIST*

Definition

The ICP has traditionally been a registered nurse serving on the Infection Control Committee and responsible to the physician epidemiologist. This position may also be filled by a microbiologist, epidemiologist, pharmacist, or a trained sanitarian. The position involves professional responsibilities in the following areas, as assigned by the supervisor of the Epidemiology Division.

1. Surveillance, analysis, and reporting
2. Case finding
3. Investigation, consultation, and education
4. Liaison with all hospital departments

*   See chapter entitled the "Infection Control Practitioner," for proposed guidelines to enter infection control from various disciplines within and outside of nursing.

5.   Prevention of infections occurring in hospitals and evaluation and implementation of recommendations
6.   Working with and comprehension of statistics

Qualifications

The individual should be interested and knowledgeable in the areas of infection, be familiar with the facilities of the hospital, and be well-known by the hospital's personnel. He/she should have considerable knowledge of nursing theory and practice, as well as functional knowledge of microbiology and epidemiology. The person should have the ability to instruct and supervise medical, nursing, and ancillary personnel within the hospital and should be skillful in public relations.

Functions

1.   Perform routine surveillance on hospital acquired infections and investigate common source outbreaks. He/she should be able to compile the data into a monthly report for presentation to the Infection Control Committee for action.
2.   Conduct studies or special investigations with the physician epidemiologist or head of the Infection Control Committee when appropriate. The findings of these investigations should be reported to the supervisor and physician epidemiologist.
3.   Serve as consultant and instructor on proper isolation techniques and other aspects of control and prevention of infections.
4.   Serve as a liaison between the hospital Infection Control Committee and hospital personnel, particularly nursing and ancillary staff, in implementing programs with procedural changes, as outlined by the physician epidemiologist or recommended by the Infection Control Committee, or as assigned by the division supervisor.
5.   Establish and maintain close contact with the Public Health Department, both in the local community and when necessary the National Center for Disease Control (CDC) in Atlanta, Ga.
6.   Compile "contact lists" of personnel exposed to unisolated patients with communicable diseases for the purpose of referrals to Employee Health Service for appropriate follow-up.
7.   As time permits, meet with product representatives for the purpose of evaluating products which may have infection control importance. Attend periodic educational meetings within the hospital necessary to maintain expertise in the area of infection control.

SURVEILLANCE OF HOSPITAL ACQUIRED INFECTIONS[5,6]

In the second week of every month, a report of the previous month's hospital acquired infections is released. All infections are listed by infection site and by individual medical or surgical services (see Table 2). At the top of the report, the overall monthly rates are shown on the line graph. Particular attention to increasing infections should be made, and any questions regarding the report should be referred to the physician epidemiologist or ICP.

We urge the staff to document clearly in the patient's progress notes any new infections. *Ideally, the dates of insertion and discontinuation of all indwelling catheters should be noted in the nursing care plan (KARDEX®) as well as in the patient's progress notes.*

An accurate system of surveillance for hospital acquired infections is essential for

Table 2

U VA. HOSPITAL

MONTHLY NOSOCOMIAL INFECTION SURVEILLANCE REPORT
FOR THE MONTH OF JAN 80
OVERALL NOSOCOMIAL INFECTION RATE

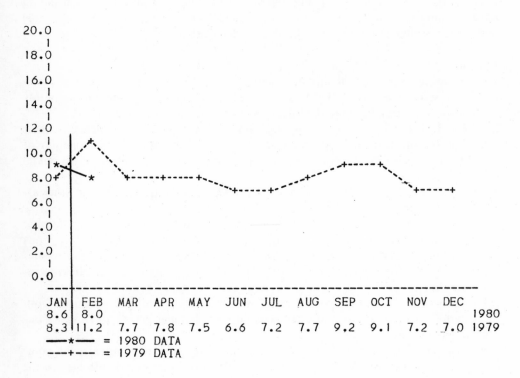

	JAN	FEB	MAR	APR	MAY	JUN	JUL	AUG	SEP	OCT	NOV	DEC	
	8.6	8.0											1980
	8.3	11.2	7.7	7.8	7.5	6.6	7.2	7.7	9.2	9.1	7.2	7.0	1979

—*— = 1980 DATA
---+--- = 1979 DATA

U. Va. Hospital Monthly
Nosocomial Surveillance Report (continued)

```
                            U VA. HOSPITAL
                  JAN NOSOCOMIAL    UNIT REPORT              3/14/80
```

UNIT	TOTAL POPULATION	TOTAL # OF INFECT NUMBER	%	BLD	PUL	UTI	POW	OTH
N-5	★ 74	15	20	2	3	10	0	0
S-5	★ 57	3	5	1	0	1	1	0
SDU	★ 00	1	0	0	0	1	0	0
W-5	★ 68	14	21	1	2	11	0	0
N-4	★ 64	13	20	3	1	7	0	2
ACU	★ 5	3	60	1	0	0	0	2
W-4	★ 85	5	6	2	1	1	0	1
CCU	★ 66	0	0	0	0	0	0	0
N-3	★ 83	9	11	1	1	4	2	1
S-3	★ 73	3	4	0	0	1	1	1
BU	★ 10	2	20	0	0	0	1	1
W-3	★ 00	4	0	1	1	2	0	0
N-2	★ 98	3	3	0	2	0	1	0
S-2	★ 111	4	4	1	0	0	0	3
W-2	★ 78	6	8	2	1	1	0	2
N-1	★ 85	3	4	0	1	2	0	0
S-1	★ 144	3	2	0	0	0	3	0
NICU	★ 29	9	31	5	0	0	0	4
B-I	★ 70	4	6	0	1	3	0	0
B-II	★ 42	4	10	1	2	0	0	1
B-III	★ 83	7	8	0	2	0	0	5
B-G	★ 68	4	6	0	1	1	1	1
ICU	★ 103	23	22	5	7	7	0	4
D-3	★ 54	1	2	0	1	0	0	0
T-N-2	★ 56	6	11	1	0	5	0	0
T-S-2	★ 52	6	12	4	0	1	0	1
T-N-5	★ 23	0	0	0	0	0	0	0
T-S-5	★ 26	0	0	0	0	0	0	0
BR5-WEST	★ 18	0	0	0	0	0	0	0
BR2-WEST	★ 19	2	11	1	0	0	0	1
BR1-WEST	★ 14	0	0	0	0	0	0	0
CRC	★ 39	0	0	0	0	0	0	0
BR2-EAST	★ 9	0	0	0	0	0	0	0
BR3-WEST	★ 3	0	0	0	0	0	0	0
TOTAL	1809	157	9	32	27	58	10	30
PERCENT OF TOTAL				20.4	17.2	36.9	6.4	19.1

U. Va. Hospital Monthly
Nosocomial Surveillance Report (continued)

SERVICE	MEAN RATE 72-78	#INF'S/#ADM'S=(%) JAN 1979	JAN 1980	SERVICE	MEAN RATE 72-78	#INF'S/#ADM'S=(%) JAN 1979	JAN 1980
G-SGY	12%	23/168 (14%)	16/162 (10%)	TCV-SGY	9%	13/97 (13%)	7/74 (9%)
GYN	4%	9/86 (10%)	5/89 (6%)	UROL	8%	0/67 (0%)	4/61 (7%)
MED	6%	29/438 (7%)	38/363 (10%)	PSYCH	0%	0/67 (0%)	0/0
NEURO	4%	2/75 (3%)	4/81 (5%)	DIALYSI		0/0	0/0
N-SGY	9%	18/158 (11%)	23/119 (19%)	DERM	0%	0/12 (0%)	1/10 (10%)
OB	2%	9/143 (6%)	3/140 (2%)	DENT/OR		0/0	0/0
OPHTHAL	0%	1/37 (3%)	0/35 (0%)	FAM PRA	14%	1/6 (17%)	1/7 (14%)
OTOL	1%	0/85 (0%)	3/104 (3%)	RADIOL		0/1 (0%)	0/1 (0%)
ORTH	7%	11/120 (9%)	26/118 (22%)	ANETH		0/1 (0%)	0/0
SP CD I	43%	6/23 (26%)	3/58 (5%)	CRC		0/0	0/62 (0%)
PED	4%	2/89 (2%)	6/142 (4%)	B.R.-TB		0/0	2/25 (8%)
NICU	31%	13/28 (46%)	10/29 (34%)	B.R.-NE		0/0	0/16 (0%)
MED ICU		0/0	0/0	B.R.-DI		0/0	0/6 (0%)
P-SGY	10%	6/100 (6%)	5/96 (5%)	B.R.-NU		0/0	0/0
BURN SE	95%	8/10 (80%)	0/10 (0%)	BR-AMB		0/0	0/9 (0%)
				TOTAL	7%	151/1811 (8%)	157/1817 (9%)
				TOTAL UVA	7%	151/1811 (8%)	155/1699 (9%)
				TOTAL CRC		0/0	0/62 (0%)
				TOTAL BR		0/0	2/56 (4%)

157 INFECTIONS OCCURRED IN # 115 PATIENTS

U. Va. Hospital Monthly
Nosocomial Surveillance Report (continued)

```
                          SERVICE GRAPH


SERVICE          RATE

OPHTHAL    ( 0/ 35= 0%)  |
MED ICU                  |
BURN SERV  ( 0/ 10= 0%)  |
PSYCH                    |
DIALYSIS                 |
DENT/ORAL  ( 0/  0= 0%)  |
RADIOL     ( 0/  1= 0%)  |
ANETH      ( 0/  0= 0%)  |
CRC        ( 0/ 62= 0%)  |
B.R.-NE(EP( 0/ 16= 0%)   |
B.R.-DIABE( 0/  6= 0%)   |
B.R.-NUTRI               |
BR-AMB TB  ( 0/  9= 0%)  |
OB         ( 3/140= 2%)  |==
OTOL       ( 3/104= 3%)  |===
PED        ( 6/142= 4%)  |====
NEURO      ( 4/ 81= 5%)  |=====
SP CD INJ  ( 3/ 58= 5%)  |=====
P-SGY      ( 5/ 96= 5%)  |=====
GYN        ( 5/ 89= 6%)  |======
UROL       ( 4/ 61= 7%)  |= ===== ==
B.R.-TB    ( 2/ 25= 8%)  |=========
TCV-SGY    ( 7/ 74= 9%)  |==========
G-SGY      (16/162=10%)  |======= ===
MED        (38/363=10%)  |=== == == ===
DERM       ( 1/ 10=10%)  |=========
FAM PRAC   ( 1/  7=14%)  |===============
N-SGY      (23/119=19%)  |======= ==========
ORTH       (26/118=22%)  |========== ===========
NICU       (10/ 29=34%)  |====== === =================== ========== ====
                         +---+---+---+---+---+---+---+---+---+---+
                  %         5   10   15   20   25   30   35   40   45   50
```

U. Va. Hospital Monthly
Nosocomial Surveillance Report (continued)

BLOODSTREAM   3/14/80
PATHOGENS ISOLATED FROM BLOOD
JAN 80

33   INFECTIONS IN 26 PATIENTS WITH 34 ISOLATES

5/34	(# 1) S AUREUS	4->10 IV'S	
		2-H.A.-C	
		3-MBT	
			2/5 R-N
5/34	(# 2) S EPIDERMIDIS	2->10 IV'S	
		1-H.A.-C	
		1-H.A.-P	
		3-MBT	
5/34	(# 22) S. PN (PNEUMOC)	4->10 IV'S	
		1-H.A.-C	
		3-MBT	
3/34	(# 72) E. COLI	1->10 IV'S	
		1-MBT	
2/34	(# 87) S. MARCESCENS	2->10 IV'S	
2/34	(#157) BACTEROIDES SPP.	1->10 IV'S	
		1-H.A.-C	
		1-MBT	
2/34	(#249) ENTEROCOCCUS	1->10 IV'S	
			2/2 R-N
1/34	(# 29) LI. MONOCYTOGENES	1-H.A.-C	
		1-MBT	
			1/1 R-N
1/34	(# 73) K. PNEUMONIAE		1/1 R-G
			1/1 R-T
1/34	(# 86) SERRATIA SPP	1->10 IV'S	
		1-MBT	
1/34	(#122) PS AERUGINOSA	1->10 IV'S	
1/34	(#130) PS MULTIVORANS (CEPACIA)	1->10 IV'S	
		1-MBT	
			1/1 R-G
			1/1 R-T
			1/1 R-A

U. Va. Hospital Monthly
Nosocomial Surveillance Report (continued)

BLOODSTREAM   3/14/80
PATHOGENS ISOLATED FROM BLOOD
JAN 80

1/34	(#188) C. ALBICANS	1-MBT		
1/34	(#194) TOR. GLABRATA	1-H.A.-C		
		1-MBT		
1/34	(#333) PS CEPACIA		1/1	R-G
			1/1	R-I
			1/1	R-A
1/34	(#403) GM - RODS			
1/34	(#446) PROVIDENCIA SPP			

33 INFECTIONS
34 ISOLATES   18->10 IV'S
                                        7-H.A.-C
                                        1-H.A.-P
                                       16-MBT

KEY: > 10 IV'S=MORE THAN 10 INTRAVENOUS INFUSIONS PRIOR TO POSITIVE CULTURE
     H.A.-C=HYPERALIMENTATION--CENTRAL
     H.A.-P HYPERALIMENTATION--PERIPHERAL
     MBT=MULTIPLE BLOOD TRANSFUSIONS

U. Va. Hospital Monthly Nosocomial Surveillance Report (continued)

EXAMPLE OF

U VA. HOSPITAL
LINE LISTING
FROM JAN 01 TO JAN 31
SITE: BLD

3/14/80

NAME-AGE / STORY #	WARD	ADM DT / SERV	DIAGNOSIS / SURGERY	RISK	DT / ORG/INF	DT-PV NG / DT/TYP-C&S	SITE/INF / COMMENTS/RX
KINNEY,DONNA-20Y 6676	N-5	122479 ORTH	AVULSION OF DORSUM MULT. METACARPAL FX'S FX L CLAVICLE PEN ALLERGY 122679 DEBRID RT HAND 011080 DEBRID RT HAND	12/24 >10 IV' 12/24 ANTIBIO 12/26 SGY 12/26 3-4 TU 01/09 SGY 01/09 1-2 TU 01/09 1-2 TU	01/12 PS AERUGINOSA	122479 NORM. P.E. 01/12 BLOOD	1' 01/12 ANCEF RX-II 01/15 MANDO RX-TI
RD,GEORGE-70Y 2248	N-5	122879 ORTH	GANGRENE R FOOT VENTRICULAR ECTOPY ABN CXR (PROB. CA) P.V.D.	01/04 >10 IV'	01/09 ENTEROCOCCUS	010380 NEG PR C&S 01/09 BLOOD	1' 01/13 PEN RX-TI 01/17 AMP RX-TI
NES,MELVIN-54Y 6685	S-5	112280 ORTH	FX. OF RT FEMUR CHRONIC OSTEOMYELITIS 112380 SEQUESTRECTOMY 112380 SAUCERIZATION	12/17 CVP/ART 12/25 >10 IV'	12/30 S. MARCESCENS S. MARCESCENS	NO DATA 12/30 BLOOD 12/31 CATH	2' CVP LN 11/23 GENTA RX-PI 11/23 NAF RX-PI
RBELL,RODGER-23Y 2718	W-5	110479 ORTH	C.H.I. T4 PARAPLEGIC HYPOTHERMIA LIVER LACERATION OBTUNDATION	11/04 >10 IV' 11/06 H.A.-C 11/06 CVP CAT 11/15 MBI 11/26 CVP CAT	01/02 S AUREUS R-NAF	121580 NEG PR C&S 01/02 BLOOD	1' 01/17 FANC RX-TI
X,ASHTON-54Y 8201	N-4	122879 MED	LIVER FAILURE ASCVD E.T.O.H. ABUSE H/O HYPERTENSION STAPH EPI SEPSIS	01/01 MBI	01/07 S AUREUS	010680 NEG PR C&S 01/07 BLOOD	1' 01/12 NAF RX-TI

LLIS,LEE-53Y   N-4   010480   01/12 OTH INF   01/12   NO DATA   2' PERITO
            MED   E.T.O.H. ABUSE   S. PN (PNEUMOC)   01/12   BLOOD   01/12 GENTA   RX-TI
3586   HEPATIC FAILURE   01/12 AMP   RX-TI
                  ASCITES   01/15 PEN   RX-TI
                  ANEMIA
                  HEPATIC ENCEPHALOPATHY

FORD,SHERMAN-53Y N-4   101279   123180 NEG PR C&S   22' ENDOCA
            MED   AORTIC REGURG.   12/11 ANTIBIO   01/04   01/04 BLOOD   01/07 AMP   RX-TI
2402   AORTIC STENOSIS   12/07 ANTIBIO   C. ALBICANS
                  ANEMIA   12/29 ANTIBIO
                  HX SUBDURAL HEMORRHAGE 10/26 >20 TU
                  102680 AORTIC VALVE REP 10/26 SGY
                                         10/26 MBT
                                         10/26 MBT

*PATIENTS' NAMES AND HISTORY
NUMBER HAVE BEEN OBLITERATED TO
PREVENT IDENTIFICATION

U. Va. Hospital Monthly
Nosocomial Surveillance Report (continued)

GENERAL COMMENTS

THE CURRENT OVERALL INFECTION RATE IS 9%, WHICH IS UP 2 PERCENTAGE POINTS FROM LAST MONTH, AND IS UP 1 PERCENTAGE POINT FROM JAN 1979 (8%).

THIS MONTH 157 INFECTIONS OCCURED IN 115 PATIENTS FOR A 6% 'PATIENTS-INFECTED RATE', WHICH WAS 6% LAST MONTH.

THE DISTRIBUTION OF INFECTIONS WAS AS FOLLOWS:

```
   3 PATIENTS HAD   4 INFECTIONS EACH      ( 12)
   8 PATIENTS HAD   3 INFECTIONS EACH      ( 24)
  17 PATIENTS HAD   2 INFECTIONS EACH      ( 34)
  ---                                      ------
  28                                       ( 70)
```

87 PATIENTS HAD 1 INFECTION EACH, ACCOUNTING FOR 55% OF ALL INFECTIONS.

28 PATIENTS WITH MULTIPLE INFECTIONS ACCOUNTED FOR 70 INFECTIONS, OR 45% ALL INFECTIONS.

115 PATIENTS HAD 157 INFECTIONS.

```
LATE ENTRIES:
 1 BLD
      HX #: 341558 = 1
 1 POW
      HX #: 593066 = 1
 1 OTH
      HX #: 349184 = 1
```

defining "problem" areas, for detecting microepidemics early, and for maintaining an infection awareness in the hospital. Our ICPs examine the nursing Kardex® seeking clues to high-risk patients (see Table 3). The charts of all patients with the procedures or diagnoses listed below are examined weekly. We define a hospital acquired infection as one that is not present or incubating on admission (usually not present within the first 3 days of admission). The criteria (see Table 4) we employ are simple and objective, and we therefore feel this should make them generally acceptable to all disciplines.

The ICPs make daily rounds, and the entire hospital is surveyed in a week's time. Therefore, there are four or five surveys contributing to the monthly nosocomial infection report. During their rounds, the ICPs talk with the physicians and nurses on each floor and are often alerted to other problems related to infection control, such as patients on isolation or employees exposed to patients with infections.

Many hospitals advocate use of the microbiology laboratory as a "starting point" in case finding. We have not found this as helpful as the Kardex® system for our hospital, since the laboratory method depends on the infected sites being cultured.

Obviously clinial judgment must be exercised in defining an infection; ICPs must be able to dismiss an obvious contaminant found, e.g., a *Staphylococcus epidermiditis* in one of six blood cultures or list as an infection a patient with 50,000 colonies per milliliter in the urine who obviously has new symptoms referable to the urinary tract. He/she must accept the clinician's judgment concerning the differentiation of pulmonary infarction and infection. Occasionally a viral syndrome may appear with diarrhea (intestinal infection), but one must rule out noninfectious diarrhea, e.g., that secondary to tube feeding.

The ICPs list the hospital acquired infections on line-listing sheets. The line listing includes the patient's name, ward, admitting diagnosis, date of admission, and infec-

Table 3
NOSOCOMIAL INFECTION SURVEILLANCE SYSTEM

Diagnoses of condition
    Leukemia, lymphoma, carcinoma, granulocytopenia, collagen vascular diseases, sarcoid, widespread dermatoses (diagnoses often requiring steroid therapy)
    Burns
    Organ transplantation
    Hepatitis (check of earlier transfusions)

Operations or procedures
    All surgery requiring general anesthesia
    Tracheostomies
    CNS shunts
    Bladder catherization (any entry into the urinary tract)
    Hyperalimentation
    Respiratory assistance therapy
    Special wound or decubitus care
    Arteriograms
    Myelograms
    All invasive diagnostic procedures

All patients hospitalized for 3 weeks or more

Table 4
HOSPITAL ACQUIRED INFECTION

Infection site	Criteria for infection
Wounds/tracheostomy site	Presence of pus
Blood	Positive culture
Pulmonary	Infiltrate on chest X-ray not present on admission associated with new purulent sputum production
Urine	$\geqslant$100,000 colonies of bacteria per milliliter
Intestinal	Positive cultures for pathogen or unexplained diarrhea for $\geqslant$2 days
Burns	New inflammation or new pus not present on admission
Miscellaneous (hepatitis, upper respiratory infections, peritonitis, etc.)	Alternatively $\geqslant$10^6 organisms per gram of biopsied tissue Clinical diagnosis

tion date, type, and evidence of hospital acquired infection. These data are kept on file and summarized monthly. Only patients with infections are listed on the line-listing forms. An example of our monthly report is shown in Table 2 which lists the complete hospital-wide report figures for 1 month.

TUBERCULOSIS CONTROL IN THE HOSPITAL[7-9]

During the year, several patients with active tuberculosis will be admitted to the hospital before a diagnosis is suspected, and proper respiratory isolation is instituted. In order to protect all employees, students, and other patients, an ICP will compile contact lists (see Table 5) of those individuals who have had contact with the undiagnosed patient. Copies of these lists are forwarded to both Student Health and Employee Health Services, where plans will be made to call in contacts for serial PPD skin testing or chest X-ray, and subsequent follow-up. Other patients, who may have

Table 5

FORMAT OF THE TUBERCULOSIS CONTACT LIST USED AT THE UNIVESITY OF VIRGINIA HOSPITAL

University of Virginia
Infectious Disease Contact List

Patient	History (#)	Location	TB status	Date
			Patient suspect Acid fast bacillus growth/smear TB diagnosed	Admitted: Isolated: Discharged:

*** Please print ***

Students
(Medical, nursing, university)

Last name	First	Middle Initial	Title	Department

Employees
(Medical Center)

Last name	First	MI	Title	Department

been roommates of the patient in question, are also at risk of contracting the disease. Therefore whenever roomates are involved, their attending physician is notified of this, so that he may take the necessary steps to protect his patient.

All regular employees, whether they are aware of a recent contact with a tuberculosis patient or not, are nonetheless re-skin tested by Employee Health Service periodically to assure their protection. Since yearly tuberculin skin testing is required, any new convertors are easily recognized. Annual chest X-rays are taken of those with a known positive skin test. For the health of all of us, your cooperation in all phases of tuberculosis control is needed. Therefore, we urge you to notify us when you know or suspect that you have had contact with a patient in whom tuberculosis was suspected and proper isolation had not yet been instituted. Call the ICP responsible for tuberculosis control, or the Epidemiology Nursing Supervisor at Ext. 2143.

Since there is active surveillance of all infections and a close working relationship with Student/Employee Health Services and the Hospital Epidemiology Division, we can readily institute rapid control with this same reporting mechanism for other communicable diseases occurring in the hospital. These may include viral hepatitis, salmonella gastroenteritis, meningococcal meningitis, and others.

REPORTING OF COMMUNICABLE DISEASES

Title 32-48 and 32-49 as amended in Chapter 16 of the Code of Virginia, entitled "Virginia Hospital Licensing and Inspection Law," require that every physician (or: other person if no physician is in attendance) report any case of communicable disease known to his local health department. The following is a list of diseases and methods for reporting them to the Virginia Health Department.

A. Nosocomial outbreaks

   An outbreak will be considered to be present when there is an increase in incidence of any infectious disease or infection above the usual incidence. Please complete form CD-24.2 to report outbreaks.

B. Reportable diseases

   Report Influenza by number of cases only.

   Venereal disease cases should be reported on a special health department form (VD35C) available through the state venereal disease program or the local health department. Cases of venereal disease will be investigated by health department personnel after consultation with the patient's physician. Enter minimal identifying data on all other diseases listed below.

Report diseases preceded by an asterisk (*) immediately by telephone to the local Health Director or State Epidemiologist as well as by completing the reporting form.

Amebiasis	*Foodborne diseases	Meningococcal infections	Reye's Syndrome
*Anthrax	Gonorrhea	Mumps	Rocky Mountain spotted fever
Arboviral infections	Granuloma Inguinale	*Nosocomial outbreaks	Rubella
Aseptic Meningitis	Hepatitis A (Infectious)	Occupational illnesses	Salmonellosis
Bacterial Meningitis	B (Serum)	Opthalmia Neonatorum	Shigellosis
(specify etiology)	Unspecified	Pertussis	*Smallpox
*Botulism	Histoplasmosis	Phenylketonuria (PKU)	*Syphilis
Brucellosis	Influenza	*Plague	Tetanus
Campylobacter infections	Kawasaki's Disease	*Poliomyelitis	Trichinosis
Chancroid	Legionellosis	*Psittacosis	Tularemia
Chickenpox	Leprosy	Q Fever	*Tuberculosis[a]
*Cholera	Leptospirosis	*Rabies in man	Typhoid Fever
Congenital Rubella Syndrome	Lymphogranuloma Venereum	Post exposure Rabies treatment	Typhus, Flea-Borne
*Diphtheria	Malaria	in man	Vibrio infections
Encephalitis	*Measles (Rubeola)	Rabies in animals	Waterborne outbreaks
primary (specify etiology)			*Yellow Fever
post infectious			

Any other disease or outbreak of public health importance

[a] An additional report will be filed with the Bureau of Tuberculosis Control by the local health department.

Retain Copy (3) for your records. Mail Copies (1) and (2) to your local health department.

DIVISION OF EPIDEMIOLOGY　　　　　FORM CD-24.1 1980

Listing of Health Officers Within the State

> Richard Prindle, M.D., Director, Thomas Jefferson Health District
> Grayson B. Miller Jr., M.D., State Epidemiologist
> James B. Kenley, M.D., State Commissioner of Health

HANDWASHING[10]

Handwashing is the single most important factor in reducing the spread of micro-organisms.

Special Instructions

1. Wash hands before and after contact with each and every patient. Special attention should be paid to this with those patients who are immunosuppressed.
2. Handwashing must be done before and after each procedure in patient care and after handling contaminated material and equipment.
3. Minimum length of time required for removal of most transient bacteria is 15 sec.
4. Since faucets are considered contaminated, turn faucets off with the paper towel used for drying hands.
5. Apply hand lotion frequently to assure good skin care. Individual new containers of hand lotion should replace old ones, and there should not be large stock containers of lotion used to refill smaller containers.

Procedure

1. Moisten hands and apply good lather with soap tissues, covering well beyond the area of contamination.
2. Use friction, one hand upon the other, with fingers interlaced.
3. Rinse throughly under running water, holding elbows higher than hands to allow water to flow from fingertips.

Additional Information

1. Liquid or cake soap may be used, but since these are prone to becoming contaminated themselves, single-use, dry, soap-impregnated tissues are preferred. If cake soap is used, rinse it thoroughly before returning to a drained dish.
2. Areas between fingers and under nails require special attention.

UNIVERSITY OF VIRGINIA MEDICAL CENTER PROCEDURES FOR ISOLATION OF PATIENTS

Purpose

The purpose is to provide a simple, workable guide to the hospital staff for the care of patients with potentially communicable diseases and to protect patients with diminished resistance to infection from unnecessary exposure to a potentially contaminated environment.

The recommendations for various types of isolation are based on available information on the mode of transmission of infecting agents. They are not based on critical studies proving their efficacy, but are intended to be reasonable precautions subject to changes as new information develops.

Of particular note is that we have abandoned the full recommendation by the CDC to don gown, gloves, and mask for visiting patients in protective isolation. Because of the lack of data to support such procedures in routine hospital rooms and because of the disadvantage of psychological isolation that may result, we suggest only private room and insist on rigorous handwashing before and after visiting patients. No one with any infection — even a minor skin infection — should enter the room. If any essential medical personnel must visit the patient and he/she has a "cold", then a mask should be worn.

It should be noted that in institutions where laminar airflow (LAF) systems are available and oral nonabsorbable antibiotics are administered, then protective isolation with gowns, gloves, and masks is appropriate. Since the University of Virginia Hospital has no such LAF system, we choose a more simplified version for protective isolations.

Responsibility

Everyone, including the physicians, medical students, nursing personnel, housekeeping staff, and technicians, is responsible for complying with isolation procedures and for tactfully calling observed infractions to the attention of offenders. The responsibilities of the hospital staff cannot be effectively dictated, but must arise from a personal sense of responsibility. Every member has an important role to play. There must be careful attention to details, continuous education, and awareness of the problems of infection control.

The physician directly responsible for the care of the patient is expected to order isolation or precaution procedures according to the outline provided below. He/she may add certain special procedures which may be deemed worthwhile in special situations. The nursing staff is responsible for insuring that all procedures are carried out according to policies determined by the Hospital Epidemiology Division and the Infection Control Committee. Physicians, medical students, and all others are expected to comply with the procedures as posted on the patient's door and listed within this manual. Everyone on the hospital staff is encouraged to consult the Epidemiology Division, Extension 2143 or 2777, or the Hospital Infection Control Committee when special problems are encountered. (See section entitled "Current Listing of Members of the University of Virginia Medical Center Infection Control Committee".)

Isolation or Precaution Classification

In the past, five major isolation or precaution categories have been developed to guide the staff. In 1980, in response to the problem with Methicillin-resistant *Staphylococcus aureus,* a new type of isolation was instituted: "Cohort Isolation". Essentially, this is a "wound and skin" type of isolation, except that in a two-bed room only patients harboring the same organism may be roommates. This type of isolation should be instituted whether the patient is infected or only colonized. These are specifically marked within the section entitled "Alphabetical Listing of Diseases with Type and Duration of Isolation or Precaution Required," and listed below. Space is provided on the Protective Isolation card for additional instructions which the physician may wish to add.

Note: Any patient infected or colonized with Amikacin-resistant Gram-negative rods, should be placed on the isolation/precaution appropriate for infection at that site, i.e., positive sputum cultures, place patient on respiratory isolation, etc.

	Instruction cards	Color code	Stock number
1.	SI—strict isolation	Yellow instruction card	HS-555
2.	RI—respiratory isolation	Blue instruction card	H -642

3.	WSP—wound and skin precaution	Pink instruction card	HS-554
4.	EnP—enteric precaution	Tan instruction card	HS-553
5.	PI—protective isolation	Green instruction card	H -552
6.	BDP—body discharge precautions	White instruction card	HS-845
7.	BP—blood precautions	No instruction card	
8.	CI—cohort isolation	Orange instruction card	HS-884

Facilities

Private rooms should be used when available. Placing more than one patient (even with the same disease) in a room is discouraged, but may be necessary in special situations. Isolation carts are assigned to Nursing Units and supplies are replaced by nursing staff as needed. (See the section entitled "Detailed Procedures for Setting Up and Carrying Out Isolation Techniques.")

Geographic Isolation

In view of the difficulty of adhering to strict isolation procedures in children with certain common childhood diseases (pertussis, measles, chickenpox, and mumps) geographical isolation may be necessary. This means that such children should be located in a section of the Pediatric Wards, where they will not be in contact with immune-suppressed patients.

Duration of Isolation

To prevent unnecessary exposure of other patients as well as the staff, isolation should be instituted as soon as there is strong suspicion that the patient has a transmittable disease (e.g., with tuberculosis), rather than to wait until bacteriological data confirm the diagnosis. Conversely, isolation of patients should be discontinued as soon as there is reasonable evidence that the hazard from infection is minimal. These procedures are costly, tend to interfere with close observation of the patient, and may interrupt otherwise good morale. The exact isolation or precaution category for the diagnosed illness can be determined from information given in the section entitled "Alphabetical Listing of Diseases with Type and Duration of Isolation or Precaution" as well as on the reverse side of the "Door Cards". Samples are in the section entitled "Instruction (Door) Cards."

SPECIAL INSTRUCTIONS

1. A physician's written order must be obtained when a patient is placed on or removed from Isolation or Precaution. However, the charge nurse may place a patient on Isolation or Precaution to protect the patient or to prevent the spread of infection to other patients. The ICP does have authorization to request a patient be placed on Isolation by the ward nurse.

2. If the physician is unavailable or does not wish to place the patient on Isolation or Precaution, then the head/charge nurse should request a decision on this matter from the hospital epidemiologist or the epidemiology nursing supervisor at extension 2777 or 2143.

3. The physician must at all times observe the proper procedures associated with the type of Isolation or Precaution stipulated for the patient. *The actions of the physician must teach by example.*

4. It is the responsibility of the nurse to display conspicuously the appropriate "instruction card" in the places indicated (outside the door and on the foot of the bed for Wound and Skin or Enteric Precautions). The type of "Isolation" must also be indicated on front of patient's chart by affixing one of the specially pro-

vided labels to the front of the chart jacket and on the admission sheet in the front of the chart. (See the section entitled "Isolation/Precaution Labeling of Patient's Charts".)

5. The clothes of a patient on strict isolation are to be wrapped in a clean, uncontaminated paper bag and sent home with the family, giving them instructions to wash, dry clean, or disinfect them. If the family is not present, keep clothes in a bag in the room with the patient.

6. Patient's requisitions (consultation requests) sent to other departments, such as X-Ray, Laboratory, etc., are also to be labeled with the specially provided labels, indicating the type of isolation or precaution. When patients are posted for surgery in the O.R., it should be indicated if he/she is on Isolation or Precaution in the same manner as in (4) above. (See the section entitled "Isolation/Precaution Labeling of Patient's Charts.")

7. If the patient has been found not to have an infectious disease and is removed from Isolation, it is not necessary to terminally disinfect the room.

DEFINITIONS (AS USED IN THIS MANUAL)

1. Concurrent disinfection refers to routine practices that are observed daily in the care of the patient's room and equipment which aid in limiting or destroying nosopoietic organisms.

2. Terminal disinfection refers to additional measures which must be taken in caring for the patient's room and belongings after he has ceased to be a source of infection.

3. Direct contact refers to any physical contact with the patient, his discharges (secretions and excretions), and articles, including bed linen, contaminated therewith.

4. Dressings ("No-Touch" Technique) from infected wounds should not be touched with bare hands. Wear clean gloves when removing soiled dressings. Don sterile gloves to apply fresh dressing. (Wash hands between glove changes.) (See the section entitled "Handwashing.")

5. "CMC" (Contaminated material container) is for the disposal of all needles, syringes, masks, etc. Masks are disposed of in this manner when the CMC is stationed outside an Isolation Room. For needle and syrine disposal, see the section entitled "Care of Contaminated Equipment (Concurrent or Terminal) — Articles which can be Autoclaved."

ALPHABETICAL LISTING OF DISEASES WITH TYPE AND DURATION OF ISOLATION OR PRECAUTION*

Disease	Type of Isolation or Precaution**	Duration***
Actinomycosis		
Draining lesions	BDP	DI
Other	None	
Agranulocytosis	PI	DI
Amebiasis (amebic dysentery)	EnP	DI
Amikacin-resistant		
Gram negative rods	Depends on site	DI
Anthrax		
Cutaneous	BDP	CN
Inhalation	SI	DI

* Keys to abbreviations and numbers appear at the end of this section.

Arthropod-borne viral encephalitis (eastern equine and western equine encephalomyelitis, St. Louis and Venezuelan equine encephalitides)	N	
Arthropod-borne viral fevers (dengue, Colorado tick fever)	BP(1)†	DH
Ascariasis	None	
Aspergillosis	None	
Blastomycosis, North American	None	
Brucellosis (undulant fever, Malta fever, Mediterranean fever)		
Draining lesions	BDP	DI
Other	None	
Burn wound	SI,WSP, or BDP (2)†	
Candidiasis		
Mucocutaneous	None	
Other	None	
Cat-scratch fever	None	
Chancroid (ulcus molle, soft chancre)	None	
Chickenpox (varicella)	SI	(3)
Cholera	EnP	DI
Clostridium difficile	EnP	DI
Clostridium perfringens	BDP	DI
Food poisoning	BDP	DI
Wound infection		
Gas gangrene	WSP	DI
Other	BDP	DI
Coccidioidomycosis		
Pneumonia	None	
Draining lesions	BDP	DI
Congenital rubella syndrome	SI	DH
Conjunctivitis, acute bacterial (sore eye, pink eye)	BDP	U
Conjunctivitis, viral (neonatal inclusion blennorrhea, paratrachoma, swimming pool conjunctivitis)	BDP	DI
Creutzfeldt-Jakob disease	N/WSP	(36)
Cryptococcosis (torulosis, European blastomycosis)	None	
Cysticercosis	None	
Cytomegalovirus	BDP	
Diarrhea, acute-suspected infectious etiology	EnP	DI
Diphtheria (pharyngeal or cutaneous)	SI	(4)
Ebola virus	SI	DI
Echinococcosis (hydatidosis)	None	
Eczema Vaccinatum	SI	DI
Encephalitis or encephalomyelitis, arthropod-borne (See Arthropod-borne viral encephalitides)	None	
Enterobiasis (pinworm disease, oxyuriasis)	EnP	DI
Enterocolitis, staphylococcal	EnP	CN
Escherichia coli gastroenteritis		
Enteropathogenic	EnP	(5)
Enterotoxic	EnP	DI
Fever of unknown origin		
Associated with foreign travel	SI	DI
Other depends on diseases under consideration		
Food poisoning		
Botulism	None	
C. perfringens (*C. welchii* food poisoning)	BDP	DI
Salmonellosis (*Salmonella* food poisoning)	EnP	DI
Staphylococcal food poisoning	BDP	DI
Furuncolosis-staphylococcal	WSP	DI
Gas gangrene (due to *C. perfringens*)	WSP	DI
Gastroenteritis		
Campylobacter	EnP	DI
Enteropathogenic *E. coli*	EnP	(5)

Enterotoxic *E. coli*	EnP	DI
Nonspecified	EnP	DI
Salmonella sp. (except *S. typhi*)	EnP	DI
Salmonella typhi	EnP	(7)
Shigella sp.	EnP	(7)
Viral	EnP	DI
Yersinia enterocolitica	EnP	DI
German measles (rubella) (see also congenital rubella syndrome)	RI	(8)
Giardiasis	EnP	DI
Gonococcal Ophthalmia Neonatorum (gonorrheal opthalmia, acute conjunctivitis of the newborn)	BDP	U
Gonorrhea	BDP	U
Granuloma inguinale (donovaniasis, granuloma venereum)	BDP	DI
Hand, foot, and mouth disease	BDP	DH
Hepatitis, viral hepatitis		
Type A (infectious, epidemic hepatitis)	EnP/BP	DH(9)
Type B (Serum hepatitis, homologous serum hepatitis)	EnP/BP	(11)
Non-A, non-B hepatitis	EnP/BP	DH
Hepatitis B antigen carrier	BP	DH
Herpangina	BDP	DH
Herpesvirus hominis (herpes simplex)		
Disseminated neonatal (neonatal vesicular disease)	SI	DI
Mucocutaneous	BDP(12)†	DI
Herpes zoster		
Disseminated	SI	DI
Localized (to within two dermatomes)	WSP	DI
Histoplasmosis	None	
Hookworm disease (ancylostomiasis, uncinariasis)	None	
Infectious mononucleosis	BDP	DI
Influenza	RI(13)†	(5)
Jakob-Creutzfeldt disease	N/WSP	(36)
Keratoconjunctivitis, infectious (epidemic keratoconjunctivitis, infectious punctate keratitis)	BDP	DI
Lassa fever	SI	DI
Legionnaire's disease (*L. pneumophila*)	RI	DI
Legionella micdadei (Pittsburgh pneumonia agent)	BDP	DI
Leprosy (Hansen's disease)	None	
Leptospirosis (Weil's disease, canicola fever, hemorrhagic jaundice, Fort Bragg fever)	BDP(14)†	DH
Listeriosis	BDP	DI
Lymphogranuloma venereum (lymphogranuloma inguinale, climactic bubo)	BDP	DI
Malaria	BDP(15)†	DH
Marburg virus disease	SI	DI
Measles (rubeola), including encephalitis	RI	(16)
Melioidosis		
Pulmonary	SI	DI
Extrapulmonary, with draining sinuses	SI	DI
Extrapulmonary, without draining sinuses	None	
Meningitis		
Aseptic (nonbacterial, viral, or serous meningitis)	BDP	DH
Listeria monocytogenes	BDP	DI
Neisseria meningitidis (meningococcal)	RI	U
Other bacterial	None	
Meningococcemia	RI	U
Methicillin-resistant *S. aureus*	CI	DH
Mononucleosis, infectious (glandular fever, monocytic angina)	BDP	DI
Mumps (infectious parotitis)	RI	(17)
Mycobacteria, atypical	None	

Mycoplasma pneumoniae	RI	DI
Neonatal vesicular disease (herpes simplex, *Herpesvirus hominis*)	SI	DI
Nocardiosis		
Draining lesions	BDP	DI
Other	None	
Orf	BDP	DI
Pediculosis	None	(18)
Pertussis (whooping cough)	RI	(19)
Plague		
Bubonic	WSP	CN
Pneumonic	SI	CN
Pleurodynia (Bornholm disease, epidemic myalgia)	RI	DI
Pneumocystis carinii pneumonia	None	
Pneumonia		
Bacterial—not listed elsewhere	BDP	DI
Mycoplasma (primary atypical pneumonia, Eaton agent pneumonia)	RI	DI
Pneumocystis carinii	None	
Staphylococcus aureus	SI	DI
Streptococcus, group A	SI	U
Viral	RI	DI
Poliomyelitis (infantile paralysis)	EnP	DH (20)
Psittacosis (ornithosis)	None	
Puerperal sepsis, Group A *Streptococcus* (vaginal discharge)	WSP	DI (21)
Q-fever	None	
Rabies (hydrophobia)	SI	DI
Rat-bite fever		
(*Streptobaccillus moniliformis* disease, Haverhill fever)	None	
Spirullum minus disease (sodoku)	None	
Relapsing Fever (Borrelia recurrensis)	None	
Respiratory infectious disease, acute (if not covered elsewhere)		
Acute febrile respiratory disease	BDP	DI
Common cold	BDP	DI
Rheumatic fever (acute articular rheumatism)	None	
Rickettsial fevers, tick-borne (Rocky Mountain spotted fever), New World spotted fever, tick-borne typhus fever	None	
Rickettsialpox (vesicular rickettsiosis)	None	
Ringworm (dermatophytosis, dermatomycosis, tinea)	None	
Roseola infantum (exanthem subitum)	None	
Rubella (German measles)	RI	(22)
Rubella, congenital syndrome	SI	DH
Rubeola (measles), including encephalitis	RI	(23)
Salmonellosis (for *Salmonella typhi* see Typhoid fever)	EnP	DI
Scabies	None (24)	
Schistosomiasis (bilharziasis)	None	
Shigellosis, including bacillary dysentery	EnP	(25)
Skin infections	SI,WSP, or BDP	(26)
Smallpox (variola)	SI	(27)
Sporotrichosis	None	
Staphylococcal disease (*Staphylococcus*)		
Burns	SI	DI
Dermatitis	WSP	DI
Enterocolitis	SI	DI
Methicillin-resistant	CI or RI	DH
Pneumonia and draining lung abscess	SI	DI
Wound infection	WSP	DI
Streptococcal disease (Group A *Streptococcus*)		
Burns	SI, WSP, or BDP (26)†	DI

Endometritis (puerperal sepsis)	WSP	U
Erysipelas	None	
Impetigo	WSP	
Pharyngitis	RI	U
Pneumonia	SI	U
Scarlet fever	RI	U
Skin infection	SI, WSP, or BDP (26)†	DI
Wound infection	SI, WSP, or BDP (26)†	DI
Streptococcal disease (not Group A) unless covered elsewhere	None	
Syphilis, mucocutaneous	BDP	U
Tapeworm disease		
Hymenolepsis nana	EnP	DI
Taenia solium (pork)	EnP	DI
Other	None	
Tetanus	None	
Toxoplasmosis	None	
Trachoma, acute	BDP	DI
Trichinosis (trichinellosis, trichiniasis)	None	
Trichomoniasis	None	
Trichuriasis (trichocephaliasis, whipworm disease)	None	
Tuberculosis		
Pulmonary, sputum-positive or suspected	RI	(28)
Extrapulmonary, draining lesion	RI	DI
Tularemia		
Pulmonary	None	
Draining lesion	BDP	DI
Typhoid fever (entereic fever, typhus abdominalis)	EnP	(29)
Typhus fever, (endemic flea-borne {murine typhus}, endemic louse-borne {typhus exanthematicus, classical typhus fever}	None	
Urinary tract infection (including pyelonephritis)	None (30)	
Vaccinia		
At vaccination site	None	(31)
Generalized and progressive, eczema vaccinatum	SI	DI
Varicella (chickenpox)	SI	(32)
Variola (smallpox)	SI	(33)
Venezuelan equine encephalomyelitis	RI	
Vincent's angina	None	
Viral diseases		
ECHO, or Coxsackie, gastroenteritis, pericarditis, myocarditis, or meningitis	BDP	DH
Respiratory (if not covered elsewhere)	BDP	DI
Whooping cough (pertussis)	RI	(34)
Wound infections	SI, WSP, or BDP	(35)
Yersinia enterocolitica gastroenteritis	EnP	DI

** Type of isolation or precaution: SI, strict isolation; RI, respiratory isolation; WSP, wound and skin precautions; EnP, enteric precautions; PI, protective isolation; BDP, body discharge precautions; BP, blood precautions; CI, Cohort Isolation; and None, no isolation or precautions. (See the section entitled "Instruction {Door} Cards".)

***Duration of isolation or precautions: CN, until off antibiotics and culture negative; DH, duration of hospitalization; DI, duration of illness (with wounds or lesions, DI means until they stop draining, and/or culture or Gram stain reveals that the offending organism has been eradicated); and U, until 24 hr after initiation of effective therapy.

† Key to numbers in parenthesis:

1.   Screened room where mosquito vector is prevalent
2.   Depending on the extent of infection and on the organism
3.   For 7 days after eruption first appears in normal host; in immunosuppressed hosts, DI; in asymptomatic susceptible patient exposed to varicella, for 3 weeks after exposure
4.   Until two cultures from both nose and throat and from skin lesions, if present, taken at least 24 hr apart after cessation of antimicrobial therapy are negative for *Corynebacterium diphtheriae*
5.   Until three consecutive cultures or fluorescent antibody tests of feces, taken after cessation of antimicrobial therapy, are negative for infecting strain
6.   Patients with fever of unknown origin usually need not be isolated; however, if a patient has signs and symptoms compatible with a disease that calls for isolation, it is appropriate to isolate that patient pending confirmation or exclusion of that diagnosis
7.   Until three consecutive cultures of feces taken after cessation of antimicrobial therapy are negative for infecting strain
8.   For 5 days after onset of rash
9.   Need for isolation may be reconsidered 2 weeks after onset of jaundice
10.   Need for isolation may be reconsidered when blood becomes consistently negative for hepatitis B surface antigen (HBsAg)
11.   Until infectious etiology is excluded, otherwise same as required for the responsible agent
12.   Persons with eczema should avoid contact with oral secretions of patients with herpetic lesions
13.   There may be instances when respiratory isolation of patients with influenza cannot be instituted especially during a widespread outbreak
14.   Urine only
15.   Screened room where mosquito vector is prevalent
16.   For 4 days after onset of rash
17.   For 9 days after onset of swelling
18.   Close contact with patient or his personal effects could result in transmission; initiation of effective treatment rapidly reduces this hazard
19.   For 7 days after onset of therapy with either erythromycin or ampicillin
20.   Need for isolation may be reconsidered 6 weeks after onset of disease, since carriage of virus has not been documented after that time
21.   For 24 hr after onset of chemotherapy
22.   For 5 days after onset of rash
23.   For 4 days after rash appears
24.   Close contact with patient or his personal effects could result in transmission; initiation of effective treatment rapidly reduces this hazard
25.   Until three consecutive cultures of feces (taken 24 hr apart after cessation of antimicrobial therapy) are negative for infecting strain
26.   Depending on extent of infection
27.   Until all crusts are shed
28.   Until effective therapy begins and there is clinical improvement; for a minimum of 10 days of effective therapy (two drugs)
29.   Until three consecutive negative cultures of feces taken after cessation of antimicrobials are negative for *Salmonella typhi*
30.   Bacteriuric catheterized patients may serve as a source of microorganisms transmitted by direct contact to others, especially others with urinary catheters; adequate handwashing must be performed; spatial dispersal of catheterized patients should also be considered
31.   Should be isolated if there are patients on floor with conditions that make them unusually susceptible to vaccinia virus, such as an unvaccinated infants or patients with eczema, burns, varicella, and leukemia
32.   For 7 days after onset of eruption in normal host; in immunosuppressed hosts, DI; in asymptomatic susceptible patients exposed to varicella, for 3 weeks after exposure
33.   Until all crusts are shed
34.   For 7 days after onset of therapy with either erythromycin or ampicillin; if no therapy is given, for 3 weeks after onset of paroxysms
35.   Depending on the extent of infection
36.   No isolation required until after surgery or brain biopsy; then wound and skin precaution until lesions are healed and no exudate is present; contact with blood or secretions must be avoided by wearing gloves to handle these and all other body fluids; items contaminated with body fluids or secretions must be disinfected with sodium hypochlorite (Clorox®), or preferably *autoclaved for 60 min.*[26]

INSTRUCTION (DOOR) CARDS

Strict Isolation Card
(Front-Yellow)
Strict Isolation

Visitors—Report to Nurses'
Station Before Entering Room!
1. *Private Room—necessary;* door must be kept closed; specially ventilated room is essential.
2. *Gowns*—must be worn by all persons entering the room.
3. *Masks*—must be worn by all persons entering the room.
4. *Hands*—must be washed after contact with patient or dressing.
5. *Gloves*—must be worn by all persons having contact with patient or dressing.
6. *Articles*—special precautions necessary for instruments, dressings, linen and dishes.

HS-555

(Back)
Diseases Requiring Strict Isolation*

1. Anthrax, inhalation
2. Burns, extensive, infected with *Staphylococcus aureus* or Group A *Streptococcus*
3. Diphtheria
4. Eczema vaccinatum
5. Melioidosis, pulmonary, or extrapulmonary with draining sinus(es)
6. Neonatal vesicular disease (herpes simplex)
7. Plague (pneumonic)
8. Rabies
9. Congenital rubella syndrome
10. Smallpox
11. Staphylococcal enterocolitis
12. Staphylococcal pneumonia
13. Streptococcal pneumonia
14. Vaccinia, generalized and progressive
15. Herpes zoster (disseminated)
16. Varicella (chickenpox)
17. Ebola virus
18. Lassa fever

* A room with negative-pressure ventilation is essential.

Additional Information Regarding Strict Isolation

1. Mode of spread—highly communicable diseases which are spread both by contact and airborne routes of transmission.
2. The patient should be placed in a specially ventilated room (negative pressure). The door must be kept closed since leaving the door open defeats the ventilating system. All entry into patients' room must be via the adjoining anteroom, not the main door.
3. Specially ventilated rooms are located on the south side of the third and fourth floors of the main hospital and are numbered 35 and 36. (These rooms have "negative pressure" ventilation and should be used for all highly communicable airborne diseases). In other areas of the hospital, where no special rooms are available, negative pressure ventilation may be created by the temporary installation of an exhaust fan in the window of the room. Such fans are obtained by contacting the Maintenance Department or Epidemiology Division at Ext. 2267 or 2143, respectively. The Medical Center Maintenance Department should be asked periodically (once a month) to check these rooms for negative pressure. There are no specially ventilated rooms located in the Barringer Wing of the hospital, nor the Towers Nursing Facility. (No patient requiring strict isolation may be housed in the Towers Nursing Facility. Such patients must be isolated in the main hospital.)
4. Masks—these must be worn covering the mouth and nose in order to be effective and must be changed when the mask becomes moist (or after 45 min of continued wear) and should be capable of filtering out particles in the 0.5 + μm size range.

It is considered contaminated once it is removed and must be discarded. Masks must be worn by personnel, during stripping of linen and cubicle curtains and drapes (which are done prior to starting the 1-hr recommended airing period), following Strict and Respiratory Isolation. After the 1-hr airing period, housekeeping personnel need not wear masks while performing terminal cleaning of the room.

5. Articles—use only disposable articles whenever possible. Nondisposable articles and examining instruments must be cleaned with disinfectant or cleansed, wrapped, and autoclaved. No unnecessary equipment should be taken into an Isolation Unit to avoid possible contamination.

6. Linen—linen should be double-bagged and placed in yellow striped linen bag to be removed from contaminated area.

7. Dressings—these should be placed in waxed bag and placed in a covered trash can within patient's room.

8. Dishes—disposable dishes should be used.

9. Leaving the Isolation Unit—after hands have been washed, a paper towel should be used as a "barrier" to open the door; the paper towel may then be discarded into the contaminated material container (CMC) outside the door, along with the mask.

Respiratory Isolation Card
(Front—Blue)
Respiratory Isolation

(Droplet nuclei)
Visitors—Report to Nurses' Station
Before Entering Room

1. *Private Room*—necessary; door must be kept closed, specially ventilated room is essential.
2. *Masks*—must be worn by all persons entering room and by patient if possible.

H-642

(Back)
Disease Requiring Respiratory Isolation*

1. Measles (rubeola)
2. Meningococcal meningitis
3. Meningococcemia
4. Mumps
5. Pertussis (whooping cough)

6. Rubella (German measles)
7. Tuberculosis, pulmonary—sputum-positive (or suspect)
8. Venezuelan equine encephalomyelitis
9. Legionnaire's disease

* A room with negative-pressure ventilation is essential.

Additional Information Regarding Respiratory Isolation

1. Mode of spread—droplet and droplet nuclei coughed, sneezed, or breathed into the environment.

2. The patient should be placed in a specially ventilated room (negative pressure). The door must be kept closed, since leaving the door open defeats the ventilating system. All entry into patients' room must be via the adjoining anteroom, not the main door.

3. Specially ventilated (negative pressure) rooms are located on the south side of the third and fourth floors of the main hospital and are numbered 35 and 36.

(These rooms have "negative-pressure" ventilation and should be used for highly communicable airborne diseases). In other areas of the hospital, where no special rooms are available, negative pressure ventilation may be created by the temporary installation of an exhaust fan in the window of the room. Such fans are obtained by contacting the Maintenance Department or Epidemiology Division at Ext. 2267 or 2143, respectively. The Medical Center Maintenance Department should be asked periodically (once per month) to check these rooms for negative pressure. There are no specially ventilated rooms located in the Barringer Wing of the hospital, nor in the Towers Nursing Facility.

4. Masks—these must be worn covering the mouth and nose in order to be effective and must be changed when the mask becomes moist (or after 45 min of continued wear) and should be capable of filtering out particles in the 0.5μm size range. It is considered contaminated once it is removed and must be discarded. The patient must wear a fresh mask (if physically able) when anyone enters the room or when being transported to another area. Masks must be worn by personnel during stripping of linen and cubicle curtains and drapes (done prior to starting the 1-hr recommended airing period) following strict and respiratory isolation. After the 1-hr airing period, housekeeping personnel need not wear masks while performing terminal cleaning of the room.

5. The patient on respiratory isolation must be instructed by the nursing staff to cover his mouth with disposable tissues when coughing, and notation should be made on the Kardex® when this has been done. The patient must also be taught how to properly wear, remove, and dispose of the mask, as well as where to dispose of soiled tissues.

6. No unnecessary equipment should be carried into an isolation unit to avoid possible contamination. Some of the organisms responsible for illness listed in this category can be spread by freshly contaminated articles.

7. Leaving the isolation unit—after hands have been washed, a paper towel should be used as a "barrier" to open the door; the paper towel may then be discarded into the CMC outside the door, along with the mask.

8. Linen—yellow linen should be used. It should be double-bagged and placed in a yellow-striped linen bag to be removed from the contaminated area.

9. Avoid carrying any unnecessary articles into an isolation unit to avoid the possibility of accidental contamination. Equipment or articles having been left in the room, and not used, must be resterilized or disinfected and discarded if this is not practical. Disposable items, which theoretically are not resterilizable, should therefore be discarded if there continued sterility is in question, resulting in unnecessary waste.

Wound and Skin Precautions
(Front-Pink)
Wound and Skin Precautions

Visitors—Report to Nurses' Station
Before Entering Room

1. *Private Room*—desirable (two-bed room permissible).
2. *Gowns*—must be worn by all persons having direct contact with patient or dressings.
3. *Masks*—not necessary except during dressing changes.
4. *Hands*—must be washed before and after contact with patient or dressing.
5. *Gloves*—must be worn by all persons having direct contact with patient or dressings.
6. *Articles*—special precautions necessary for instruments, dressings, and linen.

(Back)

Diseases Requiring Wound and Skin Precautions

1. Burns (infected)—$\geq 10^6$ colonies per gram tissue biopsied
2. Gas gangrene
3. Impetigo
4. Staphyloccccal skin and wound infections
5. Streptococcal skin infection and wound infection
6. Wound infection, extensive (with purulence draining)
7. Plague, Bubonic
8. Herpes zoster, localized

Additional Information Regarding Wound and Skin Precautions

1. Mode of spread—transmissible by direct contact (most commonly from infected patient via personnel, to previously uninfected patient via hands) with wounds and heavily contaminated articles.
2. It is desirable to place a patient on Wound and Skin Precautions in a private room if one is available. However, when no private room is available, the patient may be placed in a two-bed room and the following precautions adhered to: a. patient placed on Wound and Skin Precautions should be placed in bed nearest the sink (the "A" bed); b. care must be taken that the uninfected patient in the room does not come in contact with or share any of his roommmate's articles, which might possibly be contaminaed with secretions or discharges from the infected patient's wound; c. both patients should be advised of the precautions necessary, but tact should be used to avoid arousing undue alarm in either patient. Keep in mind that the organisms and not the patients are being isolated; and d. The door card indicating that a patient in that room is on wound and skin precaution should be affixed to the outside of door (directly under the name plate) of the patient who is placed on precaution, as well as on the foot of his bed.
3. Masks—these must be worn during dressing changes (covering the mouth and nose) and must be changed when the mask becomes moist. It is considered contaminated once it is removed and must be discarded. If there is another patient in the room, he should leave the room or wear a mask at the time of the dressing change, if possible. Dispose of mask into the CMC outside the door.
4. Instruments—use only disposable instruments whenever possible. Nondisposable articles must be cleansed with disinfectant or cleaned, wrapped, and autoclaved.
5. Dressings—these should be placed in a waxed bag and then placed in covered trash cans within the patient's room. No-touch dressing technique should be used when changing any dressings. (See the section entitled "Dressings—No-Touch Technique.")
6. When giving direct nursing care to extensively burned patient receiving sulfamyalon or silver sulfadiazine treatment, mask, unsterile gown, and gloves may be worn to protect your clothing.

Enteric Precautions Card

(Front-Tan)

Enteric Precautions

Visitors—Report to Nurses' Station

Before Entering Room

1. *Private Room*—necessary for children. Private room desirable for infants and adults. Two-bed room permissible.

2. *Gowns*—must be worn by all persons having direct contact with patient.
3. *Hands*—must be washed after contact with patient.
4. *Gloves*—must be worn by all persons having direct contact with patient or with articles contaminated with fecal material, blood, or urine.
5. *Articles*—special precautions necessary for linen, dishes, and articles contaminated with urine and/or feces.

HS-553

(Back)
Diseases Requiring Enteric Precautions

1. Cholera
2. Enteropathogenic *Escherichia coli* gastroenteritis—diarrhea
3. Hepatitis, type A, type B, type Non-A or Non-B
4. Salmonellosis (including typhoid fever)
5. Shigellosis
6. Viral gastroenteritis
7. Acute diarrhea, suspected infectious etiology
8. Staphylococcal enterocolitis
9. *Yersinia enterocolitica*, gastroenterocolitis
10. Campylobacter
11. Poliomyelitis

Additional Information Regarding Enteric Precaution

1. Mode of spread—transmission of infection depends on ingestion of pathogens or by direct inoculation.
2. Private room—necessary for pediatric patients, among whom fecal-oral cross-infection is difficult to prevent. Adults requiring precaution may be effectively cared for in a two-bed room if the patient on precautions is adequately instructed in the measures necessary to prevent the spread of his disease to others. The patient in question should be placed in the bed nearest the sink ("A" bed). Door cards should be affixed to the outside of the door under the name plate of the patient on precaution, as well as on the foot of his bed. The uninfected patient is instructed not to come in contact with a roommate's bedlinen, food, or personal articles, nor should both patients share the same bathroom facilities.
3. The importance of handwashing to prevent transmission of enteric diseases must be stressed, not only for hospital personnel, but also for the patient as well as his roommate, who should be instructed to wash his hands carefully, especially after defecating and before eating.
4. In a two-bed room, the patient on precautions should use the toilet, and his roommate should use a portable commode. It is safer for the staff to handle the uninfected stool. If the patient is not ambulatory and therefore unable to use the toilet, both patients must be issued separate bedpans and/ or urinals and brushes. The only situation where the uninfected rommate may use the toilet is when the infected patient is limited to bed and is using only his own bedpans and/ or urinals and brushes. The precaution patient's brush should be labeled with the patient's name and disposed of during terminal cleaning of his room.
5. Articles—use only disposable articles whenever possible. Nondisposable articles must be cleansed with disinfectant or cleansed, wrapped, and autoclaved.
6. Linen—yellow linen should be used and double-bag technique employed in handling the linen to be removed from a contaminated area.
7. Dishes—disposable dishes should be used.
8. No unnecessary equipment should be taken into an isolation unit in order to avoid the possibility of accidental contamination. Unused equipment or articles

left in the room must be resterilized or discarded if continued sterility is in question, resulting in unnecessary waste.

9.   When caring for a patient with hepatitis particular care should be taken by the employee to avoid accidental blood or stool contact with the patient. In the event of a blood or stool contact, the employee is advised to report the incident to the Employee Health Service immediately for evaluation and possible prophylactic measures on his behalf.

Protective Isolation Card
(Front-Green)
Protective Isolation
Visitors—Report to Nurses' Station
Before Entering Room

1. *Private Room*—preferred.
2. *Hands*—must be washed *before* direct contact with patient.
Note: *No one with any infection—even mild—should enter the room.*

H-552

(Back)
Conditions That May Require Protective Isolation
1. Agranulocytosis or severe neutropenia
2. Severe and extensive, noninfected vesicular bullous, or eczematous dermatitis
3. Certain patients receiving immunosuppressive therapy
4. Certain patients with lymphomas and leukemia

Additional Information Regarding Protective Isolation

1.   Purpose—to protect uninfected persons who have seriously impaired resistance from potentially pathogenic organisms. There is limited evidence that protective isolation is effective; however, some physicians feel that it may reduce infections in some patients.

2.   All equipment and articles not specifically needed for the care of the patient should be kept outside the unit.

3.   In some instances it may be necessary to provide linen sterilized prior to use, and this may be noted in the space provided on the card along with other measures which the physician may deem necessary.

Body Discharge Precautions Card
Body Discharge Precautions
Sputum—urine—blood—spinal fluid—
feces—wound drainage
Physical segregation of patient from others may be indicated.

1. Purpose:
To prevent transmission of causative organisms and antibiotic-resistant organisms from any of the above sites.
2. Comments:
Strict handwashing before and after any contact with patient and/or secretion-contaminated articles,
i.e., suctioning/respiratory assistance equipment, dressings, urine/stool, etc.
        Emptying Foley bag every shift
    * Suctioning patients
       Assisting with any diagnostic procedure
       Caring for incontinent patients
    * Any dressing changes/wound care/burn care

a. No-touch technique
b. Dispose of soiled dressings and equipment in a waxed paper bag into contaminated trash to be incinterated

* Please Use Gloves

Note: These precautions apply until it is culture proven that the patient is free of infecting organisms.

HS-845

Additional Information Regarding Body Discharge Precautions

1. Purpose—to prevent cross infection of personnel and patients by direct contact with bloody wounds, secretions, or contaminated articles.
2. General comments:

   a. Basically, a barrier to transmission is interposed by use of the "no-touch" technique when changing dressings on these lesions and by use of proper handwashing procedures.
   b. Patients with diseases in this category need not be in private rooms or handled differently from patients without infections, except that precautions detailed in dressing techniques should be taken. These precautions should be maintained as long as the lesion is considered infective, which usually will be as long as there is a discharge from the lesion or until it has been proven by Gram stain and/or culture to be free of the infectious organism.
   c. Dressing techniques consist of handwashing before and after patient contact, use of sterile equipment when changing dressings, double-bagging the soiled dressings and equipment, and the "no-touch" technique when changing the dressings.
   d. These precautions apply only with lesions, from which there is a discharge.
   e. In some of these diseases, such as enteric infection with poliomyelitis or ECHO viruses, the virus may be isolated from the oral secretions for up to 14 days after the first clinical signs of disease. However, it has not been demonstrated that these secretions can be the natural source of infection for susceptibles.
   f. Only hospital personnel who have been immunized with poliomyelitis vaccine should have direct contact with patients with known or suspected active poliomyelitis.
   g. At the direction of the infection control team and/or committee, certain lesions with antibiotic-resistant organisms may require Body Discharge Precautions. Institution of such precautions are to be instituted whenever multiply-resistant organisms are isolated from any site on a patient, in an attempt to minimize spread of such organisms, which are difficult to treat. Beginning in 1978, all amikacin-resistant organisms fell into that category. See sample card entitled "Body Discharge Precautions". (Consult Hospital Epidemiology Division for additional recommendations, Extension 2777 or 2143.)

3. Conditions warranting body discharge precautions
   Actinomycosis
   Anthrax (cutaneous)
   Brucellosis (draining lesions)
   Burns, minor (infected)

Coccidiodomycosis (draining lesions)
Conjunctivitis, (acute bacterial)
Conjunctivitis, (gonococcal)
Cryptococcosis (blastomycosis)
Cryptococcosis (torulosis, European blastomycosis)
Food poisoning
  Clostridium perfringens (C. welchii)
  Staphylococcal
Gonorrhea
Granuloma inguinale (donovaniasis, granuloma venereum)
Hand, foot, and mouth disease
Herpangina
Herpes simplex
Keratoconjunctivitis, infectious
Legionnella micdadei (Pittsburgh pneumonia agent)
Leptospirosis (Weil's disease, Canicola fever, hemorrhagic jaundice, Fort Bragg fever)
Listeriosis (other than meningitis)
Lymphogranuloma venerum
Meningitis, aseptic (nonbacterial or abacterial meningitis, viral meningitis)
Nocardiosis (draining lesions)
Orf
Pleurodynia (Bornholm disease, epidemic myalgia)
Pneumonia (other bacterial, unless listed differently under specific pathogens)
Pneumonia, mycoplasmal, (primary atypical, eaton agent)
Pneumonia (viral)
Poliomyelitis (infantile paralysis)
Psittacosis (ornithosis)
Q-fever
Respiratory disease, acute viral, acute febile respiratory disease, common cold
Streptococcal disease (pharyngitis, scarlet fever)
Syphilis, mucocutaneous
Taeniasis (tape worm)—pork
Trachoma, acute
Tuberculosis (extrapulmonary open)
Tularemia (draining wounds)
Viral diseases, ECHO, coxsackie, pericarditis, myocarditis, meningitis (or if not covered elsewhere)

4.   The following diagnoses if not previously covered:

Closed cavity infection (draining)
Colostomy, draining
Empyema (draining)
Lung abscess, nontuberculosis, nonstaphyloccal (draining)
Peritonitis (draining)
Wound (draining)
Wound infections (not extensive)

Information Regarding Blood Precautions*

1. Purpose—to prevent cross-infection of patient and personnel from infection transmissable by contact with blood or items contaminated with blood. All blood must be considered as potentially contaminated with hepatitis virus. High-risk patients are those with chronic hemodialysis, drug addicts, and some with GI bleeding.

2. General comments—The following precautions must be observed for all patients:

    a. Disposable equipment should be used whenever possible. For high-risk patients, it is advisable to wear gloves when handling blood or blood products.

    b. Used disposable needles and syringes should be discarded directly into a specially designated container (CMC) with minimum manipulation, in order to avoid accidental injury. (See the section entitled "Contaminated Material Container".)

    c. These specially designated containers when filled are to be sealed and removed by housekeeping to be incinerated.

    d. Personnel should be careful not to prick themselves with any used needles. When caring for a patient with hepatitis, particular care should be taken by the employee to avoid accidental blood or stool contact with the patient. In the event of a blood or stool contact, the employee is advised to report the incident to the Employee Health Service for evaluation and possible prophylactic measures on his behalf.

    e. High visibility labels for hepatitis—high-visibility labeling of blood or blood products from patients with viral hepatitis (A, B, or non-A, non-B) should be employed (see below). The labels are yellow with black lettering which bear the word "Hepatitis". They are on every ward and additional supplies are available from the nursing office. The same label should be placed on all specimens from the nursing office. The same label should be placed on all specimens from patients with known serum carriage of hepatitis B surface antigen (HBsAg), as well as on specimens of patients suspected of carriage. In addition these patients' charts should also be so labeled, by affixing a label to the outside of the metal jacket and on the inside to the admitting sheet.

HEPATITIS

Cohort Isolation Card
(Front-Orange)
Cohort Isolation
Visitors—Report to Nurses' Station
Before Entering Room

1. *Room*—limited to patients infected or colonized with same organism.
2. *Gowns*—must be worn by all persons having direct contact with patient or dressings.
3. *Masks*—not necessary except during dressing changes.
4. *Hands*—must be washed *before* and *after* any direct contact with patient or dressings.
5. *Gloves*—must be worn by all persons having direct contact with patient or dressings.
6. *Articles*—special precautions necessary for instruments, dressings, and linen.

HS-884

(Back)
Blank

---

* Blood Precautions should always be in effect in this institution. Therefore, there is no card for Blood Precautions.

DETAILED PROCEDURES FOR SETTING UP AND CARRYING OUT ISOLATION TECHNIQUES

The Isolation Cart

Purpose

The purpose of the isolation cart is to provide a clean working surface and to maintain a compact central storage unit for the special articles necessary to carry out isolation technique properly (see Figure 2).

Equipment

Equipment kept in cart	Where stocked
Gowns	Linen room
Linen bags	Linen room
Gloves (sterile if indicated)	Central supply
Masks	Storeroom
Paper towels	Storeroom
Autoclave tape	Storeroom
Unwaxed paper bags (10 and 20 lb)	Storeroom
Waxed paper bags (#3 size)	Storeroom
Several "Information for Patients Placed on Isolation" pamphlets	Storeroom (Order #Hs-681)

Special Instructions for Nursing Staff

1.   Call the Linen room (Extension 2049) each morning to notify them of the number of patients on isolation, so that an adequate amount of yellow linen may be sent to the unit.
2.   Call Central Supply Room CSR (Extension 5461) daily if patient requires sterile linen.

Steps

1.   Stock the cart properly. Refer to illustration on the following page.
2.   Place the cart in the corridor beside patient's door. Some fire codes may necessitate putting carts in rooms.
3.   Check and replenish supplies every 4 hr (at least once each shift). Wash the cart top daily, more often if necessary. The patient's chart and other equipment which may not be carried in the unit may temporarily be left on top of the cart.
4.   Give the patient and his visitors a copy of the pamphlet entitled "Information for Patients Placed on Isolation" (order #Hs-681).
5.   Proceed to set up isolation room (refer to following page).

Setting Up an Isolation Room

Purpose

The purpose of an isolation room (see Figure 3) is

1.   To separate an infected person from others during the period of communicability
2.   To prevent direct and indirect transmission of the infectious agent
3.   To prevent secondary infection in the isolated patient

General Information

1.   Single rooms should be used for Isolation/Precaution if at all possible. Placing more than one patient (even with the same disease) in a room is discouraged.

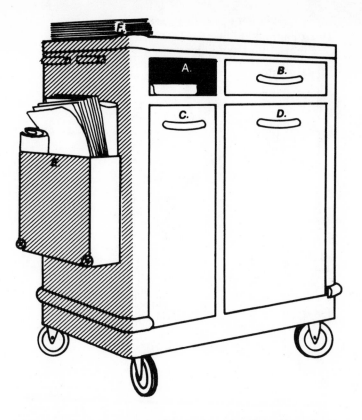

FIGURE 2. Isolation cart. This cart is stationed outside patient's door and should be well stocked at all times. The top of the cart should be washed daily with a germicide. A — gloves and autoclave tapes; B — masks; C — isolation linen bags; D — isolation gowns; E — bags (unwaxed paper bags, size 10 lb and 20 lb, and waxed size #3).

2. When no single room is available, the patient may be placed in a two-bed room for Wound and Skin or Enteric Precautions.

3. Whenever possible, place isolation patients in rooms on the same corridor, adjacent to each other, so that one cart may serve two patients.

4. Items which cannot be disinfected, autoclaved, or are not disposable should remain outside the room whenever possible. Disposable items are to be used whenever available. The emergency cart must be left in the corridor if required for the patient.

5. Help the patient and his family to understand their responsibility in carrying out correct isolation techniques! Give patient and visitors the pamphlet "Information for Patients Placed in Isolation" (Hs-681).

6. The surfaces within a patient's room are considered contaminated, including walls, floors, windows, door knobs, sink and faucets, and bathroom.

7. Remove linen and pillow from second bed in semiprivate room and replace with one single yellow sheet over mattress. Save linen, if not contaminated. Remove wool blanket in room, replacing with a cotton one.

8. Do not write patient's disease or diagnosis on instruction (door) card.

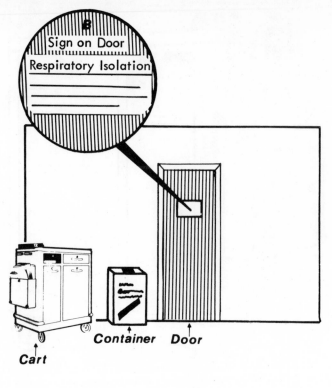

A

FIGURE 3.   This outline is used at the University of Virginia to con-
vert a hospital room to an isolation room. The second bed may be
removed from the room, depending upon the type of isolation. A =
isolation cart; B = sign on door; C = closed trash can; D = dirty
linen hamper; E = sink with soap paper dispenser; F = paper towel
dispenser; G = trash can; H = container (CMC) for used masks,
needles, and syringes. X = place where white "discard cards" should
be attached to wall. The cards clearly indicate where contaminated
articles should be discarded. These white cards are identified by the
following code numbers and may be ordered from storeroom by these
numbers: (a) contaminated gowns and linen, H-669; (b) masks,
needes, and syringes, H-670, and (c) gloves, dressings, food, and disposable dishes, H-671.

Equipment Kept in Patient's Room (in Addition to Standard Bedside Equipment)

Equipment	Additional information
1. Isolation "Instruction Cards."	Obtained from Ward Supplies, order from store room.
2. Linen hamper and stand.	
3. Large (20 gal) yellow, plastic-lined trash can with cover.	Obtained from Housekeeping.
4. Tall (21 in.) yellow trash can with plastic liner.	For discarded paper towels obtained from Housekeeping.
5. Box of masks and tissues for patient on Respiratory Isolation (i.e., tuberculosis).	In addition to those stored on the cart.

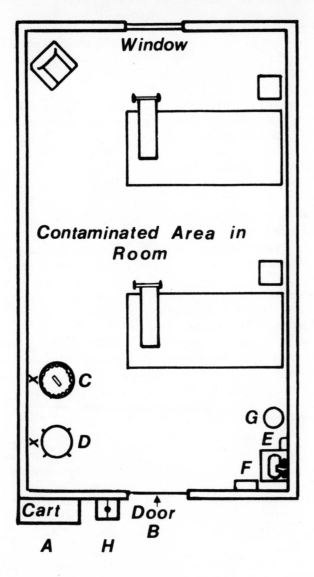

FIGURE 3B

6. Special tuberculosis instruction card for tuberculosis patient (cartoon card).

Reads: "Please cover mouth when coughing" (blue, H-643).

7. Tourniquet, vacutainer holder, and "red box" for disposable needles and syringes.

Red box when filled is disposed of into CMC (see section entitled "Contaminated Material Container").

8. Metal-topped, waxed disposable container for drinking water.

The metal top is reusable, the waxed container discarded.

9. White signs, indicating where to dispose of contaminated articles (see Figure 3).

Obtained from Ward Supplies, attach to wall above appropriate receptacles in patient's room.

10. Dry thermometer kit and ample cover sheaths; lubricant, if rectal temperature is indicated.

Obtained from Ward Supplies.

11. New bedpan brush (for patient on Enteric Precautions).

Obtained from Housekeeping, label with patient's name, discard when precaution is discontinued.

Steps (see Figure 3)

1. Attach appropriate "Instruction Card" to outside of door and to foot of bed for Wound and Skin or Enteric Precaution.

Special instructions may be added to bottom of Protective Isolation card.(e.g., "Patient must have sterile linen.")

2. Place linen hamper stand in room near door (outside room for Protective Isolation).

Bag with yellow marking for soiled linen and gowns.

3. Place yellow trash can (21 in.) near sink in room for paper towels.

4. Place covered yellow trash can (20 gal) in room near linen hamper.

Refer to Figure 3 for disposal of food, plastic utensils, soiled dressings, etc.

5. For patients on respiratory isolation, place a box of disposable masks and a box of tissues on the bedside table.

Obtained from Central Supply Room.

6. Place special "Tuberculosis Instruction Card" in room where it can be easily read by patient.

Blue card reads: "Please cover mouth with tissue when coughing" (Order from storeroom, #H-643)

7. Using autoclave tape, attach small-sized (#3) waxed paper bag to bedside table for patient on Respiratory Isolation.

For patient's soiled masks and tissues.

8. Place dry thermometer kit and cover sheaths on shelf over sink.

Also lubricant if rectal temperature is indicated (thermometer kit may also be placed in bedside stand drawer).

9. Tourniquet, vacutainer holder, and "red box" for disposable needles and syringes are also kept on the shelf above the sink in patient's room.

Red box when filled is discarded by placing in CMC.(See section entitled "Contaminated Materials Container.")

10. Use metal-top and disposable waxed container for the patient's drinking water.

Fill and place on bedside table.

11. Check supply of paper towels and soap tissues in dispensers near sink.

Supply replenished by Housekeeping maid.

Equipment

1. Isolation cart (see section entitled "The Isolation Cart").

Kept just outside the room, near the door (fire regulations permitting).

2. "CMC" contaminated material container for disposal of masks.

Should be kept immediately outside patient's room for all categories except Enteric Precaution (masks are not necessary for enteric precaution).

Donning Gown, Mask, and Gloves
General Information
1. Gowns, masks, and gloves can be obtained from the isolation cart.
2. Doctors' and medical students' coats are to be removed and hung on hooks on the end of the cart or on the coat rack before donning the gown.
3. Nurses need not remove their caps before entering an Isolation Room.

Steps	Additional information
1. Put on gown, overlapping well in back to cover clothing. Tie waist strings securely.	Neck band, tapes, and inside of gown are considered clean unless contaminated prior to donning. Gown must not be worn out of room.
2. Apply mask over mouth and nose, pinching soft metal band above nose to make mask conform to contour of nose after slipping elastic "tie" over head.	Change when moist and at least every 45 min. Front of mask should not be touched after it is applied. Only the "ties" are considered clean.
3. Put on gloves, pulling up over cuff of gown to protect wrist.	Use when indicated on "Instruction Card".
4. Enter room, leaving all unnecessary articles on cart outside room.	Patient's chart is not to be carried into room; instead it may be left on top of cart outside the door.

Removing Gloves, Gown, and Mask

1. Remove gloves. (If gloves are not worn, wash hands at this point.)	Gloves are "peeled off", turning them inside-out, and then they are discarded in the covered trash can in the room.
2. Unfasten waist ties of gown if tied in back.	If tied in front, this is the first step before removing gloves.
3. Unfasten neck ties and remove gown, turning inside out. Roll gown so that contaminated side is inside.	Discard in linen hamper.
4. Wash hands!	See the section entitled "Handwashing."
5. Exit from room.	Use paper towel "barrier" to protect hands when opening door to exit Isolation Room.
6. Remove mask, handling only elastic tie of mask and discard in CMC.	If front of mask is accidentally touched, wash hands again at nearest sink, not in isolation room.
7. For patients on Protective Isolation, mask, gown, and gloves should all be removed outside of room.	

To Take Temperature, Pulse, and Respirations

1. Leave pencil and pad outside room on cart.	
2. Take temperature, pulse, and respirations.	Record results on note pad on isolation cart outside door.

3.   Wash hands!

Care of the thermometer with the "Dry-Temp" system requires only sheathing with polyethylene cover which is discarded after use. Cleansing between uses is necessary only if sheath is ruptured, and in ER and Outpatient Department because thermometers are reused . . . ! Alternatively, thermometers may be cleansed with soap tissue and cold water, rinsed and soaked in 95% isopropyl alcohol and 0.2% iodine solution for 10 min. Rinse and dry before reuse.

Administration of Medication
1.   Leave medication cart and Kardex® in the corridor outside of the patient's room.

Follow procedure for administration of medications as listed in Nursing Procedure Manual. When possible leave medication for isolation patients until last. When one administers i.m. medications, a gown should be worn for all types of isolation except Respiratory Isolation.

2.   Wash hands!

See the section entitled "Handwashing."

Food Service and Disposal
1.   A tray should be placed on the cart in the corridor by a dietary aide.

The dishes on the tray are all disposable.

2.   Roll the overbed table to the doorway.
3.   Unit personnel will transfer food and utensils to overbed table in patient's room.

Cut meat before transferring patient's tray. Pour contents of thermos into cup and leave thermos outside unit.

4.   Discard liquid wastes into toilet.
5.   Place disposable dishes, utensils, and leftover food in waxed bag and discard in covered trash can.
6.   Wash hands!

See the section entitled "Handwashing."

To Fill Water Pitcher
1.   Fill disposable water container with ice and take to the unit.
2.   Remove metal top, pour water into sink, and discard water container into covered trash can.
3.   Replace metal top.
4.   Wash hands!

Care of Contaminated Linen (Double-Bag Method)

1. Place soiled linen and gown in yellow marked laundry bag.

   Laundry bag and hamper should be placed in the patient's room.

2. To remove soiled linen from room, close the top of the laundry bag and carry it to the doorway.

3. Person outside room holds clean isolation bag to receive contaminated bag.

   Form cuff with top of clean isolation bag to protect hands. Outside of isolation bag must be kept clean.

4. Person outside room closes isolation bag and places in laundry chute.

   No unbagged linen may be placed in laundry chute!

5. Replace laundry bag on hamper stand inside room.

   Soiled linen should be removed after a.m. care at the end of each tour of duty or whenever two thirds full.

6. Wash hands!

To Take Blood Pressure

1. Leave sphygmomanometer and stethoscope in room and clean terminally. Disposable cuff is preferable.

   To clean: wash off cuff, gauge, bulb, and stethoscope using cloth well moistened with germicide.

2. Wash hands!

To Fill Ice Cap

1. Fill paper bag with ice and take into unit.

   Use disposable cold pack if available.

2. Fill ice bag at sink. Cover bag and apply.

3. Wash those hands!

   See the section entitled "Handwashing."

To Collect Specimens

1. Open clean paper bag on chair in corridor (or leave on top of isolation cart).

   Leave all unnecessary equipment on cart outside door.

2. Take labeled specimen container into room and place on clean paper towel.

   Use disposable container, when possible. When collecting specimens from patients suspected of hepatitis, special yellow label should additionally be affixed to the specimen container.

3. Collect specimens as indicated; avoid unnecessary contact with the outside of the container. Cover container.

   Measure specimen, as necessary, within unit.

4. Place container in clean (nonwaxed) paper bag outside room.

   Do not contaminate top edge or outside of bag.

5. Wash hands!

6. Fold over top edge of bag twice and secure with autoclave tape.

   Stamp with addressograph patient's name and history number on pressure-sensitive label and affix to outside of bag. Additionally affix

7.   Place specimen and requisition in the messenger pick-up basket.

label indicating type of Isolation/ Precaution to outside of bag. (Labels-kept at nurses' station). Get specimen to laboratory with the lease possible delay. Label indicating type of Isolation/ Precaution should also be placed on requisition slip.

Disposal of Body Discharges (Stool, Urine, Vomitus)

1.   Pour discharge into toilet and flush.

Avoid soiling outer edges of commode.

2.   Wash hands!

Disposal of Body Discharge—Sputum

1.   Instruct patient to expectorate into a cup.

2.   Cover and place in 10-lb bag and discard in covered trash can.
3.   Wash hands!
4.   A patient with sputum positive for tuberculosis must have the bag and sputum cup burned in the incinerator, along with other trash material from the patient's room.

When one third filled, have the patient place a tissue over sputum. Change sputum cup twice a day and more often as necessary.

This is done by housekeeping. Place in red plastic trash bag. Keep I.V. bottles or any other closed bottles or cans out of trash to be incinerated.

Disposal of Soiled Tissues

1.   Place in unwaxed paper bag attached to bedside stand.
2.   Discard paper bags into yellow covered trash can once daily and more often if necessary.

Replace paper bag (unwaxed).

3.   Wash hands!

See the section entitled "Handwashing."

Dressings—"No-Touch" Technique

1.   Wash hands!
2.   Don mask.
3.   Don clean gloves.
4.   Loosen dressing all around.
5.   Place one gloved hand on top of dressing and then with the other hand (size permitting), peel the glove down over the hand holding the dressing. This permits the glove to act as a disposal bag.
6.   Place in waxed paper bag and discard in yellow covered trash can.
7.   Wash hands again!

See the section entitled "Handwashing."

8.   Don sterile gloves and proceed to apply the new dressing, using aseptic technique.

To Secure Signatures (For Strict Isolation Only)

Steps	Additional information
1. Place two unfolded paper towels on the overbed table.	
2. Place document to be signed on top of towels.	Allow patient to read document or read it to him.
3. Cover top and bottom portions of document leaving signature area exposed, so that patient's hands will not rest on the document.	
4. Have patient sign, remove covering paper towels, and discard.	
5. Wash hands!	See the section entitled "Handwashing."
6. Pick up document without contaminating hands.	Discard paper towels from table, touching only the clean side.

Outgoing Mail

1. Provide the patient with some water for moistening the stamp and sealing the envelope, instead of letting him lick the stamp or envelope.

Skin Clean-Up Basket

1. Set up individual tray to be used in the room, using disposable containers when available.
2. If unit clean-up basket is taken into room, it must be cleaned with a germicidal detergent applied with a pistol grip sprayer and articles replaced with sterile and clean towels.

To Draw Blood for Laboratory

1. Leave laboratory tray on top of isolation cart in corridor.	Place tray on extreme corner of cart next to patient's door.
2. Put on mask and gown before entering room; put on gloves when indicated.	Check information on instruction card on door.
3. Take only necessary equipment into room from tray. (Tourniquet is kept in room.)	Two paper towels from cart are to be opened and placed on overbed table for equipment. Equipment is to be placed nowhere else in room except on towels or sink.
4. Draw blood; take tubes and equipment and place in the sink.	
5. Discard needles and syringes in "red box" within the unit.	Preferably into CMC.
6. Untie waist ties of gown.	
7. Wash equipment and hands.	Use soap tissues and friction under running water. Rinse and dry with

paper towels. If the patient has hepatitis, discard the needle holder and tourniquet when discharged. Affix yellow "Hepatitis" label to specimen tubes and requisition slips (see the section entitled "Information Regarding Blood Precautions" and "Hepatitis Precaution: Labeling of Specimens").

8. Standing in doorway, place tubes and tray in corridor.

9. Remove gloves if worn.

10. Untie neck ties and remove gown turning it inside out. Roll gown with contaminated part inside.

Discard in linen hamper.

11. Wash hands!

See the section entitled "Handwashing."

12. Remove mask, handling only the ties.

Discard it in the CMC outside of the room.

To Keep EKG Paper Clean

1. Attach clean pillow case to the side of the EKG machine and allow EKG paper to loop into it.

With clean hands fold paper and secure with a paper clip.

Visitors

1. Visitors must follow the instructions on the door card indicating type of isolation.

Give visitors each a brochure (HS-681) explaining isolation and their responsibility, and use it for teaching visitors. Visitors are to be limited to one person to a patient at any one time.

2. Hats and coats of visitors should be placed on a chair outside unit.

3. Only articles that can be discarded, washed, disinfected, or autoclaved may be taken into the room.

Instruct visitor to leave purse with a relative outside of the room. If the visitor wants to carry a handbag or other articles into the room, place the articles in a clean paper bag. Dispose of paper bag into CMC when visitor leaves.

4. If card indicates, assist or instruct the visitor on donning a mask.

5. If the card indicates, assist visitor in putting on a clean gown.

Gown and mask are to be put on outside the room and should be removed before leaving the anteroom.

6. Instruct visitors not to sit on the patient's bed and to avoid handling any articles used by the patient.

Leaving Room

1. Instruct visitor to remove gown by turning it inside out, rolling it, and placing it in a laundry hamper.

   Gowns must be removed and discarded in the room.

2. Instruct visitor to wash hands and not to touch anything before leaving the room.

3. Remove mask.

   Masks must be removed and discarded outside the patient's room, into CMC.

Transportation of Patient to Other Areas

1. Drape yellow sheet over stretcher or wheelchair.

   Entire area which would touch bed or patient should be covered.

2. Put on a gown, mask, or gloves if instruction card indicates. For a helpless patient, have attendant don a gown, mask, and gloves also.

   Mask patient and have him carry tissues and a paper bag for disposal of respiratory secretions. Explain reason to the patient.

3. Patients on Respiratory Isolation should wear masks when being taken from their room to some other department or area.

   Patients on Strict Isolation may not be transported to other parts of the hospital until the danger of comminicability is over. Tranport of patients on Respiratory Isolation is discouraged.

4. Assist patient to stretcher or wheelchair and cover patient with a yellow sheet.

   Avoid touching the uncovered portion of the vehicle.

5. Wash hands and grasp the clean underside of the sheet folding over the patient. Use a second sheet if necessary.

   The patient's hands should be kept under the sheet. Fasten stretcher straps over the clean sheet. Avoid touching clean sheet with gown.

6. Remove gown and mask!

7. Wash hands!

   See the section entitled "Handwashing."

8. Specially designed labels have been provided and should be affixed to the front of the patient's chart and on the admitting sheet in order to alert persons in other departments to take necessary precautions.

   See quote from memo on page 176.

9. Report to personnel receiving patient that the patient is isolated and make sure they know the precautions that are necessary.

   Transportation aid should apprise the department receiving patient of his Isolation/Precaution status. This is performed by Housekeeping Department.

10. If a child needs to be transported, use an extra crib if at all possible. When finished using, wash the crip with a germicidal detergent, applied with a pistol grip sprayer.

11. If the patient must be transported in a bed, wipe exposed areas of the bed with a germicidal detergent (applied with pistol grip sprayer) and cover the patient with a clean sheet.

    When finished transporting patient, scrub the transportation vehicle with germicidal detergent.

Isolation/Precaution Labeling of Patient's Charts

On several occasions in the past, problems have been encountered regarding patients on some type of isolation, who were transported within the hospital for surgical or diagnostic procedures. The isolation status was not always clear to the receiving department. On at least one occasion recently, a patient on Enteric Precautions for confirmed hepatitis-B was taken to the OR and operated on, without the OR staff's knowledge of his precaution status.

A policy regarding identification of isolated patient's charts has existed and is stated in the "Isolation Procedure and Infection Control Manual", 1973. On January 1, 1976 this policy and the need for such identification was distributed in the form of a memo, which stated more emphatically:

> "It is essential that <u>everyone</u> coming in contact with patients on isolation or preautions be aware of the medical hazards and necessary precautions. Nonadherence to hospital policies could seriously jeopardize the health of your colleagues and co-workers as well as your hospital's ability to protect you from medico-legal action, in the event the disaese for which a patient is being isolated is transmitted to someone else due to ignorance (by that individual) that the patient was "Isolated".
>
> Every effort must be made to <u>label the chart</u> and the <u>consult sheet</u> and to <u>inform the transportation aide</u> that the patient is on a particular isolation or precaution. The aide, in turn, should then so inform the person receiving the patient in the other department.
>
> Any questions regarding infection control policies should be directed to the offices of the Hospital Epidemiology Division."

In view of the above experiences and the obvious ineffectiveness of previous efforts to avoid such episodes in the future, we are now instituting a system of Isolation/ Precaution identification labels to resolve this on-going problem. The specially provided labels have been designed to coincide with color-keyed door cards presently in use throughout the Medical Center. These labels, bearing only the type of Isoation/ Precaution, are to be affixed to the exterior metal jacket, of any patient's chart when he/she is placed on any of the isolation or precaution categories. Additionally, the label is to be affixed to any consult sheets on these patients.

Labeling should be done at the time when an order for Isolation/Precaution has been written by the physician and remain in the chart permanently thereafter. Responsibility for placing the labels on the chart rests with the Unit Assistant or anyone else who is "taking" orders from the chart. However, assuring that the labeling is carried out is the responsibility of the Head/Charge Nurse of the unit and will also be monitored by the Epidemiology Staff. Additionally, the date of the order should be written in the lower left corner of the labels themselves when they are placed in the chart. When isolation is terminated, the date should be written in the lower right corner of the labels, rather than removing the labels! This constitutes an easily noted, permanent part of the patient record. Only the label on the outside metal jacket may be removed when isolation is terminated!

The initial supply of labels and dispensers will be distributed by the Epidemiology Staff. Resupply will be from the hospital storeroom.

Hepatitis Precaution: Labeling of Specimens

All clinical specimens from patients with suspected or confirmed viral hepatitis (A or B or NANB) are to be labeled upon collection with a bright yellow "Hepatitis" label (see below). These will include specimens from any known HB antigen-positive patient, anyone diagnosed as or suspected of having hepatitis (A or B or NANB), and all hemodialysis patients.

The reason for such labeling is to advise special precaution to those handling the specimens, since these patients/specimens represent a high risk in the transmission of hepatitis to others.

A label should also be affixed by whoever collects the specimen to the patient's chart (on the face of the metal chart holder and admitting sheet). This will alert the staff to the potential danger of hepatitis.

HEPATITIS

(Yellow, black print)

Care of Patient After Death

Steps	Additional information
1. Put on gown, mask, and gloves if indicated on door card.	
2. Prepare patient. Cover any draining area with dressing.	See procedure on "Care of Deceased" (Nursing Manual).
3. Drape stretcher with a yellow sheet.	This is done to protect stretcher from contamination.
4. Place patient on stretcher and cover patient with second yellow sheet.	Fasten stretcher straps over clean sheet. Avoid touching clean sheet with gown.
5. Wash hands!	
6. Remove gown, masks, and gloves and wash hands.	
7. See that the ankle identification tag has an Isolation/Precaution label affixed to it. (See quote from memo on page 176.	If patient had hepatitis, yellow "Hepatitis" labels should be affixed to all identification of the body. (Both types of labels are available at nurses' station.
8. Transport patient to Morgue Number 2 and leave on stretcher.	
9. Wash hands again.	See the section entitled "Handwashing".
10. Give patient's clothing to family; if relatives are not present, take to Nursing Office in a paper bag labeled with patient's name and "Isolation/ Precaution" label.	Discard comb, toothbrush, and powder puff, etc. if expendable and if not requested by family.

Daily Cleaning of Room (Concurrent Cleaning)

1. Wash sink basin and faucets, bathroom doorknobs, radiator, window sills, chairs, lockers, overbed table, and bedside table with germicidal detergent applied with a pistol grip sprayer.	Done by Housekeeping aide.
2. Replenish paper towels and soap tissues.	Done by Housekeeping aide.
3. Empty trash can.	Done by unit janitor.
4. Damp-mop floor with general detergent.	Done by unit janitor.

Care of Contaminated Equipment (Concurrent or Terminal) — Articles Which Can Be Autoclaved

Steps	Additional information
1. Open clean unwaxed paper bag outside room on chair (or have someone outside hold bag open).	Use 20-lb paper bag or smaller from the cart. Do not use waxed bags; only equipment that will withstand autoclaving is to be placed in the bag.
2. Wash contaminated articles in room with germicidal detergent and dry with a paper towel.	Separate equipment with multiple parts. Small articles and sharp equipment should be placed in a small basin before placing in a paper bag.
3. Place articles in bag.	Avoid touching outside or top edge of bag. If outside of bag becomes moist or contaminated, a second bag must be used.
4. Wash hands!	See the section entitled "Handwashing."
5. Fold over top edge of bag twice and secure with autoclave tape.	Label bag with type of isolation and name of unit.
6. See section entitled "Primary Disinfectants and Antiseptics Used at the University of Virginia Medical Center" for care of other contaminated equipment.	

Care of Contaminated Equipment (Masks, Needles, and Syringes)
1. Discard masks, needles, and syringes into the CMC after using them.

Care of Patient After Removal from Isolation

1. If possible transfer patient to a clean room.	A bath is recommended before transferring (see the section entitled "Special Instructions").
2. Place patient's clothing and personal things in a clean paper bag and move with him.	

Terminal Disinfection of Room
Terminal disinfection is required following all types of isolation or precaution except Protective Isolation.

Steps	Additional information
1. a. Following Strict and Respiratory Isolation, there must be a 1-hour airing period of all rooms. In the "main hospital", windows and doors must	Windows must be closed before patient is admitted to room.

remain closed. In the Barringer Wing, the windows must be left open and the doors closed, and room is aired for 2 hr.

b. Before starting airing period, all linen, cubicle curtains, drapes, etc. should be stripped and placed in the linen hamper. When this is completed, inform the ward clerk to call housekeeping in 1 hr to begin terminal cleaning of the room.

Bed linen, including woolen blankets and uncovered pillows, should removed by unit housekeeping. Call the Housekeeping Department to remove cubicle curtains and drapes. During this procedure personnel must wear masks, following Strict and Respiratory Isolation.

c. Following the 1-hr airing period, personnel need no longer wear masks to complete terminal cleaning of the room.

Room is then cleaned in the same way as for any other patient discharge.

2. Respiratory Assistance Therapy and suction equipment should be cleaned by unit personnel, following these steps:

a. Empty water from drainage jar, nebulizer, or humidifier if used.

b. Double-bag and label with this information: "type of isolation, Respiratory Assistance Therapy Equipment".

For example, if patient is on Respiratory Isolation, label with the words "Respiratory Isolation—Respiratory Assistance Therapy Equipment".

3. The "red needle box" kept in the unit during the isolation period for the disposal of needles and syringes should be placed in CMC outside of the unit. It should then be removed by Housekeeping for incineration.

This task done by unit personnel. Thermometers may be discarded in the trash can within the room.

4. See section entitled "Primary Disinfectants used at the University of Virginia Medical Center", for care of other contaminated equipment.

a. Bedside utensils are washed with germicidal detergent, dried, and placed in a large paper bag which is left outside the room in the corridor, for pick-up.

Any questions regarding items not listed there should be referred to the offices of the Hospital Epidemiology Division.

This is done by the housekeeping maid. Avoid touching the outside of the bag. If the outside of the bag becomes contaminated, a second bag must be used.

b. Fold over top of bag, secure top with autoclave tape, and label: 1. type of Isolation/Precaution label; and 2. name of unit.

This task done by personnel.

c. Autoclave for 30 min in Isolation Utility Room.

6. Wipe with germicidal detergent all beds, mattresses, pillows, furniture, sink,

The Housekeeping supervisor, or in his/her absence, the charge nurse bathroom, windowsills, and door knobs (walls, doors, and windows).

7.   Bedpan brush used for Enteric Precaution patient must be discarded.

8.   Damp mop the floor with a germicidal detergent.

9.   Housekeeping personnel should notify unit personnel when the room is ready for occupancy. This should also be noted on the door of the room.

should inspect the walls, doors, and windows and give instruction for cleaning if needed.

Discard in contaminated trash.

This is done by unit janitor.

CONTAMINATED MATERIAL CONTAINER

Proper disposal of needles and syringes is essential to minimize personal injury to the hospital staff and to avoid possible transmission of hepatitis from this source. The CMCs (see Figure 4) distributed throughout the hospital were designed specifically for the disposal of syringes and needles (and masks in the case of isolation units) to reduce the injuries sustained by the staff. These containers are to replace the small red containers that were used in the past. In instances where the red container cannot be replaced with the CMC due to size limitations (e.g., on the medication cart), they should be placed inside the CMC when filled.

The correct usage of these disposal cartons is essential if they are to fulfill the objectives intended! When needle destruction equipment is used, all remaining parts are also to be discarded into the CMC. It is urged that the practice of "resheathing" of needles after use, as well as the disassembling of the needle from the syring, be discontinued. Instead, needle and syringe should be discarded into the CMC as a single unit in order to minimize manipulation of this accident-prone instrument.

It is further urged that all needles and syringes be disposed of in this manner, as this insured proper and final disposal of these items through incineration of the entire carton and contents.

The CMC is not intended to be a "disposable trash can", and we urge therefore that no I.V. bottles, soft drink bottles, or cans, etc. be disposed of in these containers. (Particularly dangerous are I.V. bottles or ether cans which upon incineration will explode!). I.V. tubing with the needle attached, but without the bottle, are to be disposed of in the CMC. No attempt should be made to retrieve any item once it has been deposited into the CMC, as this may result in personal injury.

The CMC, when filled, will be removed by Hospital Housekeeping personnel and replaced with a new container. No container should remain unchanged longer than 1 week, regardless of whether it is filled or not. The cooperation of everyone is necessary and will be greatly appreciated. The advantages of this container over others are

1.   Construction of heavy-weight paper board.
2.   A triple-thick inner bottom, plus 2-in. false outer bottom, to prevent penetration.
3.   A large, 6-in. diameter opening on top, eliminates the need to "stuff" items into the container.
4.   The fact that the container is not emptied, but instead is incinerated with its contents.
5.   A polyethylene liner to contain all liquid effluent within the CMC.

All of the advantages noted above are expected to contribute significantly to an

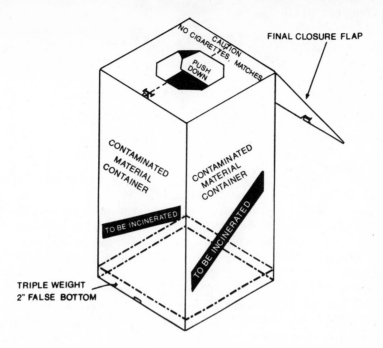

FIGURE 4. The CMC is a container 24 in. high by 12 in. square. It is used at the University of Virginia Medical Center for the disposal of masks, needles, and syringes.

overall reduction in puncture wounds sustained by the staff of this hospital (see Table 6) and thereby reduce the potential risk of hepatitis to the staff.

In laboratories, blood bank, etc., this container is also used to dispose of burnable contaminated waste (agar plates, culture tubes, etc.) to be incinerated. Since moderate amounts of liquid (blood) may be disposed as part of the contaminated waste, the CMC is lined with a 2 to 4mℓ polyethylene bag before placing the container in use (to prevent escape of any liquid). This is done by Housekeeping personnel.

All contaminated solid waste is to be disposed of in the CMC which is collected by the Housekeeping Department and transported to the incinerator for final disposition. No contaminated solid waste may be depositied in the hospital's trash chute!

Any questions regarding this policy may be directed to the Director of the House-keeping Department, (Extension 4-5186) or the Epidemiology Division (Extensions 4-2777 or 4-2143).

HOSPITAL GUIDELINES

Antiseptics, Disinfectants, and "Cold Sterilization" — General Information

Chemical disinfectants are important tools in the control of the spread of infections (see section entitled "Definitions" among patients and staff. As with any tool, maximum benefit is derived when the tool is employed to do the job for which it was intended. An antiseptic will be ineffective if used as a disinfectant. The following information is provided to help in selecting the proper "tool" for a particular job.

One need not have extensive knowledge of chemistry in order to make an intelligent selection from the myriad of trade-name formulations available. Being familiar with a relatively small group of compounds is usually all that is necessary. Important agents are those which are usually the active ingredients in most preparations — usually noted

Table 6

NEEDLE-STICK INJURY RATE[23]

Year	Total injury rate/1000	Total # injuries	Needle-Stick Rate/1000	Distribution of needle sticks (Rate/1000)			
				Nursing	Sub-nursing	Housekeeping	Others
1971	137	384	35	15.7	2.9	11.1	5.4
1972	127	380	45	19.0	4.5	12.1	9.7
1973	94	395	31	14.8	3.3	8.1	4.5

on manufacturer's labels, e.g., phenolics, hexachloraphenes, iodines, alcohols, chlorines, and quaternary ammonium products (see Table 7).

Unfortunately, there is no universal "best" chemical agent for use in hospitals for all applications. Some agents are very good as antiseptics, but are utterly useless as disinfectants, while others may be good disinfectants, but are too toxic for use as antiseptics. Some, however, may be used as antiseptics or disinfectants depending on the use-diluting (see Table 8).

The reference table (Table 9) will help you identify the group to which a given antimicrobial agent belongs. It lists some of the advantages and disadvantages of various agents, as well as recommendations (as listed in the CDC isolation manual) and methods for disinfection of various objects.

The only method that will provide sterilization almost instantly is incineration. All other methods require varying amounts of time to take effect.

The amount of time required for a specific preparation to yield a desired effect depends upon numerous factors. Generally, the longer the active agent is left in contact with a surface, the greater the number of microorganisms that will be inactivated or killed. For example, alkalinized gluteraldehyde (Cidex®) is generally considered a disinfectant when objects are immersed in the preparation for only brief periods (10 to 30 min). However, when sterility (death of all microscopic life, including all spores) of objects is required, it becomes necessary to immerse them in the same preparation (Cidex®) for much longer periods. Emersion for 10 hr or more is sometimes adequate to sterilize an object; but it is possible, in the case of viral hepatitis, for instance, that 10 hr of immersion of Cidex® may not provide sterilization.

Because no single preparation will fulfill all requirements, the hospital Infection Control Committee cannot make a brand recommendation in favor of one specific preparation which should be used exclusively throughout the hospital. The committee recommends against the use of a specific preparation, particularly if that preparation presents a potential hazard, e.g., the committee's recommendation for the elimination of aqueous benzalkonium chloride (Zephiran®) or similar products stems from the finding that such products are generally ineffective against Gram-negative organisms and only marginally effective against Gram-positive organisms. In addition, there are numerous published reports that these preparations are easily and frequently contaminated with organisms to such a degree that they have actually caused outbreaks of clinical illness.

The following specific recommendations are made by the committee for the specific applications listed. It should be understood that the alternatives to the use of benzalkonium chloride (Zephiran®) are preferred over other means currently available. While tincture of Zephiran® is still stocked (in limited quantity) in the hospital pharmacy in 8-oz (1:750) bottles, it is important that medical personnel adhere to the following practices:

Table 7

ADVANTAGES AND DISADVANTAGES OF SOME ANTIMICROBIALS

	Chemical group	Advantages	Disadvantages
Effective as antiseptics and disinfectants	Alcohol	Inexpensive; rapidly effective against vegetative bacteria; effective against tubercle bacillus; evaporates without leaving residual chemical	Volatile, with no residual activity; on prolonged contact, damaging to rubber and plastic
	Chlorine preparations	Economical	Inhibited by extraneous organic matter; in high concentration, corrosive to metal
Effective as antiseptics only	Iodine preparations, iodophors	Highly active; compatible with soaps and detergents	In high concentration may toxic; leaves temporary stains
	Hexachloraphene compounds	Generally nonirritating to tissue; compatible with soaps	Bacteriostatic only; slow acting, with repeated and frequent application required; insoluble in water; inactivated by extraneous organic matter
Effective as disinfectants only (theoretically Cidex® will sterilize if given enough time to act)	Glutaraldehyde: 1. Alkaline (Cidex®) 2. Acid (Sonacide®)	Broad-spectrum activity	Relatively expensive; unstable, toxic; on prolonged contact corrosive to metal; weakly sporicidal; in high concentration, irritating to human tissue
	Phenolic compounds	Rapidly effective; compatible with soaps and detergents; not reaidly inactivated by extraneous organic matter	Phenolics are not recommended in newborn nurseries
Partially effective as antiseptics and disinfectants	Cationic quaternary ammonium compounds (quats); benzalkonium chloride	Relatively nontoxic to tissue; nearly odorless, no staining properties	Against some organisms bacteriolostatic only; not effective against tubercle bacillus; neutralized by soap and anionic detergents; absorbed by gauze and fabrics; inhibited by extraneous organic matter, use in aqueus

Table 7 (continued)
ADVANTAGES AND DISADVANTAGES OF SOME ANTIMICROBIALS

Chemical group	Advantages	Disadvantages
		form, both 1:750 and 1:500 concentration
Chlorhexidine gluconate	Generally nonirritating to tissues; nonstaining, broad spectrum activity; rapid acting, some residual activity for some time after application	Avoid contact with eyes and ears; relatively expensive; limited to handwashing preparation at present

Effective as antiseptic only

Table 8
TYPICAL ANTISEPTICS AND DISINFECTANTS WITH
RECOMMENDED USE-DILUTIONS

Phenolic compounds	Cen-O-Phen®	Disinfectant	0.6% (1:175)
	Lysol®	Disinfectant	1% (1:100)
	Phenol	Disinfectant	5% (1:20)
	Staphene®	Disinfectant	0.5% (1:200)
Hexachloraphene compound	pHisoHex®	External antiseptic	Undiluted (3%)
Iodine preparations (iodophors)	Betadine®	External antiseptic	Undiluted (1%)
	Iodine tincture	External antiseptic	2% (1*50)
Chlorine preparation	Clorox®	Disinfectant	5% (1:20)
Quaternary ammonium compounds ("quats")	Zephiran®[b]	External antiseptic	Undiluted (1:750)
Alcohol	Usually tincture	External antiseptic	Undiluted (70%)
		Disinfectant	Undiluted (95%)
Aldehydes (gluteraldehyde)	Cidex®	Sterilant/ disinfectant	Undiluted (2%)
	Sonacide®	Sterilant/ disinfectant	Undiluted (2%)
Chlorhexidine	Hibiclens®	Antiseptic	Undiluted (4%)

[a]   Disinfectant.
[b]   Aqueous solution is not recommended, since it will support growth of Gram-negative rods.

Table 9
HOW TO IDENTIFY SOME COMMON ANTIMICROBIALS

Chemical group	Trade product	Identifying phrase	Active antimicrobial(s)
Phenolic compounds	Lysol®	-sol	Orthophenyl phenolics
	Pheno Cen®	pheno- -phene	(and other substituted phenolics)
Hexachloraphene compounds	pHisoHex®	-hex	Hexachlorophene
	Gamophen®	-phen	
Iodine preparations (Iodophors)	Betadine®	-dine	Povidone-iodine complex
	Prepodyne®	-dyne	
	Wescodyne®	-dyne	Polaxamer-iodine complex
			Iodine complex
Chlorine preparation	Clorox®	cl-	Sodium hypochlorite
Quaternary ammonium compounds ("quats")	Zephiran®	None for trade name	Benzalkonium chloride
	Roccal®		Benzalkonium chloride
	A-33[a]		
Alcohol	Usually tincture	None	Ethyl alcohol
			Isopropyl alcohol
Gluteraldehydes	Cidex®	Cid-	Aldehyde
	Sonacide®	-cide	
Chlorhexidine preparations	Hibiclens®	None	Chlorhexidine gluconate

Note: The trade name of an antiseptic or a disinfectant often reveals the antimicrobial(s) it contains through use of a prefix, infix, or suffix derived from the chemical name.

1. Use of the solution should be limited only to situations where more effective antiseptics are contraindicated.
2. It should only be used directly from a small, pharmacy-issued, single-use bottle which will be emptied and discarded by the end of a 24-hr period.
3. No small bottles or containers should be refilled from larger stock bottles.
4. No large stock bottles will be dispensed from the pharmacy, in order to minimize the chance for common source outbreak of infection.
5. Care must be taken to avoid contaminating any bottles in use during the 24-hr usage period.

General Recommendations*

1. Whenever possible the use of transfer forceps should be avoided in favor of alternative methods. However, in the few instances when transfer forceps are necessary, they should be individually wrapped and sterilized in Central Supply. If they must be kept ready for continuous use, they should be stored in 95% isopropyl alcohol with "antirust" (0.2% sodium nitrite) added. That solution can be obtained from the pharmacy. The forceps should be dated and used no longer than 1 week, and then they should be autoclaved again.
2. ENT mirrors may be disinfected by soaking in 95% isopropyl alcohol with antirust for a minimum of 15 min , after a soap and water wash and a thorough rinse.
3. Mercury thermometers are best stored dry when not in use. The system currently in use in this hospital employs polyethylene cover slips to provide a "barrier" between the thermometer and the patient's mucous membranes. With this system it is essential that new cover slips be used each time a temperature is taken to avoid contamination of the thermometer (even if it is the patient's own thermometer). If contamination of the thermometer has occurred, or is suspected, the thermometer should be scrubbed with soap and cold water before resheathing for reuse.
4. Telethermometer probes may be ethylene oxide gas sterilized (in Central Supply) or soaked in 95% isopropyl alcohol with 0.2% iodine, for a minimum of 15 min. The latter solution will not kill spore-forming organisms or hepatitis viruses, while ethylene oxide (ETO) gas sterilization is thought to do so.
5. Eye instruments may be disinfected by soaking in 95% isopropyl alcohol with antirust for a minimum of 15 min after a soap and water wash and a thorough rinse.
6. Forceps lubricant—Delivery Room—sterile normal saline may be used, as a lubricant only.
7. Perineal preparation—Delivery Room—povidone or polaxamer iodine solution may be used to cleanse external genitalia. Caution should be exercised to avoid contact with mucous membranes and open wounds.
8. Douching should be avoided if possible. However, when indicated, povidone or polaxamer iodine preparation may be used for this purpose, as well as for gynecologic preparation.
9. Clean-catch urines—babies, including prematures—mild, neutral soap and water may be used.

---

*   Additional requests or recommendations regarding specific preparations and applications will be considered by the Infection Control Committee upon request or may be referred directly to the Division of Epidemiology, Extensions 4-2777 or 4-2143.

10. Commercially packaged catheterization trays are available containing either sterile acqueous benzalkonium chloride or povidone-iodine preparations. The latter are now being stocked in Central Supply at this hospital and are preferred over the former for this application.

Definitions[11-16]

Antiseptic — arrests or prevents growth of microorganisms by inhibiting their activity, but does not necessarily destroy them; the term is used to designate chemical agents applied to living tissue.

Cold sterilization — prolonged treatment in a sporicidal germicidal solution, particularly on sharp-edged metal instruments and other equipment that could be damaged by heat; this treatment theoretically renders object free of all life.

Detergent — agent which reduces surface tension, used with water to aid in cleaning and removing organic matter.

Disinfectant — frees from infection. Destroys microorganisms, but not ordinarily bacterial spores. The term is used especially to designate chemical agents applied to inanimate objects.

Germicidal detergent — germicidal detergent is a cleaning and disinfecting agent (see Tables 8-10) which is registered by the Environmental Protection Agency (EPA). It is often used synonymously with the term disinfectant, but implies an additional capability. The most frequently used germicidal detergent at University of Virginia for general cleaning is a phenolic compound.

Sterilization — process used to destroy all microscopic life, including spores, e.g., steam under pressure (autoclave), hot-air oven, or gaseous ethylene oxide.

Use-dilution — recommended or actual dilution of an antimicrobial preparation for maximum effectiveness and safety.

Primary Disinfectants and Antiseptics Used at the University of Virginia Medical Center

The primary disinfectant compounds used at University of Virginia are

1. Phenolics on hard surfaces (such as walls, on some floors — O.R. and Isolation Room floors)
2. Quaternary ammonium detergent disinfectants (in newborn area)
3. Soap and water on floors (all-purpose detergent)
4. Sodium hypochlorite (1%) and formalin (2%) on spills of hepatitis-contaminated blood, followed by routine clean-up with phenolic disinfectant

The primary antiseptics used at the University of Virginia are

1. Alcohol and iodine (in O.R.)
2. Chlorhexidine (for handwashing)
3. Hexachloraphene (for handwashing)
4. Povidone/Polaxamer iodine (handwashing and skin preparation)

Hospital Guidelines for the Care of Respiratory Therapy Equipment[17]

All equipment, especially moist equipment, can serve as a reservoir for infection. Infection from these reservoirs can occur if:

1. The patient's own organisms grow in the equipment and then reinfect him.
2. Equipment is stored wet or allowed to collect dust for long periods of time.

Table 10
RECOMMENDATIONS FOR CHEMICAL DISINFECTION AND STERILIZATION

Objects	Low level (vegetative bacteria, fungi, and influenza viruses are killed)		Intermediate level (low-level organisms plus the tubercle bacillus and enteroviruses are killed)		High level (low- and intermediate-level organisms plus bacterial and highly resistant fungal spores and probably hepatitis viruses are killed)	
	Agent[a]	Duration (min)	Agent[a]	Duration (min)	Agent[a]	Duration (hr)
Smooth, hard-surfaced objects	A[b] for	10	B for	15	D[b] for	1—2
	D[c] for	5	D for	10	L for	3—12
	E[c] for	10	G[b] for	20	M for	12
	F[c] for	10	I[b] for	20	N for	10
	H[c] for	10	M for	15	—	—
	M for	5	N for	15	—	—
	N for	5	—	—	—	—
Rubber tubing and catheters[c]	E[b] for	10	G[c] for	20	L for	3—12
	F[b] for	10	I[c] for	20	—	—
	H[b] for	5	—	—	—	—
Polyethylene tubing and catheters[c]	A[b] for	10	B for	15	D[b] for	12
	E[b] for	10	G[b] for	20	L for	3—12
	F[b] for	10	I[b] for	20	M for	12
	F[b] for	10	N for	15	N for	10
Lensed instruments	E[b] for	10	M for	15	L for	3—12
	F[b] for	10	N for	15	M for	12
	H[b] for	10	—	—	N for	10
Thermometers (glass)[d]	C for	10	C for	15	D[b] for	12
					L for	3—12 (cold cycle only)
					M for	12
					N for	10
Hinged instruments[e]	A[b] for	15	B for	20	L for	3—12[f]
	D[b] for	10	D[b] for	15	M for	12
	E[b] for	20	G[b] for	30	N for	10
	F[b] for	20	I[b] for	30	—	—
	H[b] for	15	M for	20	—	—
	M for	10	N for	20	—	—
	N for	10	—	—	—	—
Inhalation and anesthesia equipment	A[b] for	15	B for	20	L for	3—12[f]
	E[b] for	20	N for	20	N for	10
	N for	5	—	—	—	—

Table 10 (continued)
RECOMMENDATIONS FOR CHEMICAL DISINFECTION AND STERILIZATION

Objects	Low level (vegetative bacteria, fungi, and influenza viruses are killed)		Intermediate level (low-level organisms plus the tubercle bacillus and enteroviruses are killed)		High level (low- and intermediate-level organisms plus bacterial and highly resistant fungal spores and probably hepatitis viruses are killed)	
	Agent[a]	Duration (min)	Agent[a]	Duration (min)	Agent[a]	Duration (hr)
Floors, furniture, walls, etc.						
	E[b]	—	G[b]	—	None	—
	F[b]	—	I[b]	—	—	—
	H[b]	—	K	—	—	—
	J	—	—	—	—	—

[a] A, ethyl or isopropyl alcohol (70 to 90%);
B, ethyl alcohol (70 to 90%);
C, A plus 0.2% iodine;
D, formaldehyde (8%) plus alcohol (70%) solution
E, quaternary ammonium solutions (1:500 aqueous);
F, Iodophor — 100 ppm available iodine;
G, Iodophor—500 ppm available iodine;
H, phenolic solutions (1% aqueous);
I, phenolic solutions (2% aqueous);
J, sodium hypochlorite (2000 ppm);
K, sodium hypochlorite (1%);
L, ethylene oxide gas
M, aqueous formalin (20%);
N, activated glutaraldehyde (2% aqueous) Cidex®; and
O, Sonacide®.

[b] Sodium nitrite (0.2%) should be present in alcohols, formalin, formaldehyde-alcohol, quaternary ammonium, and iodophor solutions to prevent corrosion; sodium bicarbonate (0.5%) should be present in phenolic solutions to prevent corrosion.

[c] Be certain tubing is completely filled.

[d] Thermometers must be thoroughly wiped, preferably with soap and water, before disinfection or sterilization. Alcohol-iodine solutions will remove markings on poor-grade thermemeters.

[e] Must first be cleansed, grossly free of organic soil.

[f] Depending upon procedure used; more rapidly cidal for microorganisms killed with low-level and intermediate-level disinfection.

3. Equipment is shared between patients.
4. Terminal sterilization is incomplete or ineffective.

Autoinfections

All patients harbor potentially pathogenic bacteria which when exhaled into the unit can multiply. Then each succeeding treatment provides an opportunity to force bacteria back into the patient's airway. Careful attention to nebulizer chambers and the use of disposable tubes and mouthpieces or frequent replacement of this equipment with sterile units can cut down on this self-infection.

Cross-contamination can occur when two or more patients are utilizing a single

IPPB machine. This can be prevented if each patient has a separate circuit (mouthpiece nebulizer, exhalation valve, and tubing).

Equipment Storage
1. Equipment, including humidifiers and nebulizers, should be kept dry to prevent growth of pseudomonas and other bacteria. Once in service, these should be exchanged for clean units every 24 hr. They should be filled with sterile distilled water only. Tap water is often contaminated, especially when there are aeraters on faucets.
2. Equipment should be packaged, kept closed, and/or kept in dust free cupboards to maintain cleanliness. IPPB units and respirators should have the tubes and manifolds protected from settling dust. "Baggies" can be very useful.

Terminal Sterilization
1. All equipment must be well washed with mechanical scrubbing to remove gross dirt.
2. Autoclaving (steam sterilization) is the preferred method for most inhalation therapy equipment. "Spore strips" should be used to verify the effectiveness of this method.
3. Both ethylene oxide (ETO) sterilization and the use of disposable equipment are less economical than steam sterilization. If ETO is used, the clean and slightly moistened equipment should be placed in ETO-sterilizable plastic bags and sterilized according to the manufacturer's recommendations. Care must be taken to insure adequate aeration of all equipment that is gas sterilized. "Spore strips" should be used with each load to verify the effectiveness of this method.
4. Chemical disinfection is probably best done by an alkalinized glutaraldehyde solution (Cidex®).
5. Bacteriological monitoring of equipment is carried out routinely every month depending on usage of equipment by the Respiratory Therapy Department. Specimens collectd are sent to the Clinical Laboratory for processing.

Some General Comments
 Nebulized droplets provide transportation for organisms from the nebulizer to areas deep within the patient's lungs. If a humidifier is used, there will be no particles on which the organisms can ride into the patient's tracheo-bronchial tree. Thus, humidifiers are safer than nebulizers.

1. Chemical disinfection is not considered complete unless the air-lock in each capillary tube of the nebulizer is broken and these little tubes are filled with the disinfectant or the disinfectant is actually nebulized through the equipment.
2. Copper wool sponges (Chore Girls®) in humidifier units have been shown to have a bacteriostatic effect and are employed here to provide a simple, inexpensive means of preventing bacterial growth in respiratory therapy equipment.[17]

Specific Information for Inhalation Therapy Equipment with Isolated Patients
1. When inhalation therapy or suction equipment is delivered to a room where any form of isolation/precaution is posted:
    a. Read and follow all instructions posted on the instruction card on the door.
    b. Do not take any unnecessary equipment into the isolation unit.
    c. Insofar as possible, use disposable equipment (disposable IPPB set-ups, humidifiers for trial use, etc.).

2.   Patients on Protective Isolation are being protected from organisms which we or our equipment may carry; such patients lack the ability to fight infections. With isolated patients requiring IPPB equipment, leave equipment in the room for the duration of isolation, if possible.

3.   Recommended procedures for disinfection of equipment removed from isolation areas:

    a.   From Protective Isolation (Cidexed) — No additional precautions or disinfection needed. Treat as equipment from any other patient room.

    b.   From Enteric Precaution or Wound and Skin Precaution (Cidexed):

        1.   Discard any disposable equipment in the room.
        2.   Scrub all outside surfaces of equipment (which may be contaminated from handling) with germicidal disinfectant (Cleanaseptic Germicidal Surface Cleaner® — 14% isopropyl alcohol, 0.25% ammonium chloride). Rinse with water to remove disinfectant.
        3.   After it is washed with germicidal detergent disinfectant, the equipment is no longer considered infectious and may be handled as any other patient equipment.
        4.   Exception — suction equipment which has been used for wound drainage is to be treated as if it is from Strict Isolation.

    c.   From Respiratory Isolation or Strict Isolation (ETO sterilized):

        1.   Discard all disposable equipment in the room.
        2.   Place all permanent tygon tubing, masks, tubes, nebulizers, empty cascades, and metal and plastic connectors in separate or appropriate bags — using approved isolation techniques.
        3.   Scrub all external surfaces of equipment with phenolic solution. Rinse with water.
        4.   Move equipment to departments.
        5.   With Bennett or Bird IPPB pressure ventilation machine:

            a.   Using gloves, carefully remove valve.
            b.   Completely submerge valve cover and valve in 70% isopropyl alcohol for 30 min.
            c.   Pack empty valve casing in unit with alcohol-saturated sponges for a full 30 min.
            d.   Soak all parts from Bennett in alkalized glutaraldehyde for 30 min (all surfaces must be in contact with alkalized glutaraldehyde — no air bubbles blocking tubes). Rinse three times with sterile water.

        6.   For all other respiratory therapy equipment (Flowmeters®, Birds®, Emersons®, M.A.-1's®, etc.):

            a.   Remove all customarily disassembled parts: soak all plastic and rubber parts in glutraldehyde (alkaline) for a full 30 min.; autoclave metal parts from Emerson®, filters from M.A.-1 and similar items (Circuit on M.A.-1® is gas sterilized).

b.   Scrub external surfaces of flowmeters, ventilators, etc., with phenolic disinfectant solution. Rinse with water.
c.   Reassemble equipment for use.
d.   Oral/nasal secretion precautions — all equipment believed to have been in contact with these secretions should be treated as if from Strict or Respiratory Isolation.

Guidelines: Endoscopic Sterilization Procedures

Current CDC recommendations for disinfection/sterilization of all endoscopes (proctoscopes, sigmoidoscopes, colonoscopes, aparoscopes, esophagoscopes, and bronchoscopes) are the following:

1.   Steam sterilize all possible instruments or parts thereof.
2.   Gas sterilize all scopes which cannot be subjected to steam sterilization.
3.   Cidex® (alkalinized glutaraldehyde) sterilize those instruments that cannot be gas sterilized — because of the high cost and great turnover requirements in gas sterilization (aeration time is long in the gas sterilization process). The Cidex® procedure requires 30 min soaking after a thorough soap and water cleansing. Following the Cidex® soaking, all instruments must be rinsed three times with sterile water (or tap water with 10 ppm chlorine).

Rubber gloves and gowns should be worn by those performing the endoscopic procedure. There are no official CDC recommendations for those hospital workers who clean such instruments.

Current University of Virginia procedures for disinfection/sterilization of endoscopes include the following:

1.   Proctoscopes, sigmoidoscopes, and anoscopes — obturator and tubes should be autoclaved. The light source, cord and transformer should be wiped with 70% alcohol.
2.   Bronchoscopes — these instruments are washed with a brush and placed in a sterile solution (Betadine®, alcohol, and water). Then they are rinsed with water and wiped dry. The ocular lens is cleaned with 70% alcohol. The instrument is then allowed to dry.
3.   Gastroscopes and esophagoscopes — these instruments should be cleansed initially with septisol (a hexachloraphene compound). The insertion tube should be wiped with povidone iodine solution and rinsed with distilled water. The control section, light guide tube/plug, and camera are wiped with 70% alcohol. Biopsy forceps and brush are cleaned with septisol solution. Fiberscopes and biopsy forceps should be stored in a dry area.
4.   Colonoscope — the suction channels are cleaned with soapy water, clear tap water, then alcohol, and are air dried. The outside of the colonoscope should be cleansed with a germicide soap and water and allowed to air dry.

Additional Notes

1.   All physicians (and students) who perform endoscopy should wear gowns and gloves (masks also during bronchoscopy). Surely all who handle the instruments during sterilization procedures should protect themselves by wearing a gown and protective gloves. Personnel should wear new sterile gloves when handling sterilized instruments.
2.   The Scientific Director at Olympus Corporation of America (Medical Instrument

Division) warns that if the endoscope lining has a small tear in it, and the instrument is placed in glutaraldehyde, the metal parts holding the fibers may become oxidized. Then the instrument will rapidly become dysfunctional. Recently, the manufacturer of Olympus fiberscopes has stated that iodophor (Wescodyne®) or glutaraldehyde (Cidex®) disinfectants have been found not to damage Olympus fiberscopes when they are used according to the manufacturers recommendations. The same manufacturer has also stated that ethylene oxide gas sterilization can be performed without damage, provided that the fiberscope is clean and that the following conditions are met:

- Temperature: less than 135°F (57°C)
- Pressure: less than 20 psi
- Aeration time: 7 days at room temperature, 12 hr at 122°F (50°C) in an aeration chamber

3. It makes good sense, if we must care for so many patients with a limited number of scopes, to follow the manufacturer's recommendations (which insist on thorough washing before disinfection). As an additional precaution, it is recommended that all instruments be gas sterilized as frequently as possible.

Hospital Guidelines for Prevention of Infection in the Administration of I.V. Fluids[18]

I.V. therapy is a potential source of bacteremia and septicemia in patients receiving such therapy. Even with I.V. solutions which are sterile to begin with, the risk of contamination (of the I.V. set-up) is directly proportional to how long the bottle and/or the line has hung unchanged and the number of additives. Consequently, the hospital's Infection Control Committee has adopted the policy of requiring a once daily change of each patient's I.V. system (bottle plus all tubing) down to, but not including, the needle. Needles or I.V. catheters should, with rare exceptions, be changed at least every 48 hr. The routine use of three-way stopcocks is equally discouraged. We recommend use of 250-cc bottles of fluid — if available — for "keeping vein open" lines.

Intracath Warning

Risk of thrombophlebitis and infections is too high for routine use. Limit this to patients who require rapid volume replacement or other urgent need. Remove or change within 48 hr and justify continued use by note in chart by physician.

General Statements

Use new bottle only if clear and vacuum is present. No bottle, set, or tubing should hang longer than a 24-hr period.

Changing I.V. Tubing

1. All I.V. tubing should be changed daily. It is the responsibility of the charge nurse and/or team leader to see that this is done. We recommend that this be done on the 7 to 3 shift.
2. Needle sites should be inspected at the time tubing is changed.
3. Vein needles should be changed by the I.V. team every 48 hr.

Changing Needles and/or Intracaths

1. Every 48 hr notify the I.V. team to change vein needle or intracath.
2. In critical care areas such as the Intensive Care Unit, nurses who have been supervised in the procedure may start or change I.V. needles and intracaths.

3.   Needles and intracaths must be inserted under aseptic conditions. A povidone iodine preparation should be used on the skin prior to insertion.
4.   Individual packets of an iodophor ointment may be used on the insertion site. The site must be covered with a sterile dressing.

Changing Bottles
1.   Any time a setup is changed on a closed rubber stopper-type bottle, the top of the stopper should be cleansed with an alcohol sponge.
2.   Primary bottles with medications added may be allowed to continue until finished.
3.   A "keep open" bottle should be dated, timed, and changed every 24 hr between 7 and 12 noon, along with the tubing.
4.   A bottle attached to a "soluset" for the purpose of diluting medications should not hang longer than 24 hr. It should also be changed daily.
5.   When an I.V. infiltrates, this is usually a good opportunity to change the entire set-up (bottle, tubing, and needle). If this is not feasible because (a) the bottle was just started, (b) calculation of received fluids is difficult, or (c) large amount of medication remains in the bottle or soluset, then immediately connect new tubing and/or soluset to the existing bottle. Do not attach the new needle or intracath at this time and do not clear tubing or hang bottle until ready to restart I.V.

Charting
1.   Every bottle must be clearly labeled with the patient's name, room number, added medications, time started, and signature of the person hanging the bottle. When the solution has infused, the peel-back label should be removed from the bottle and put in the chart on an "I.V. administrative record sheet".
2.   Nurses should record in progress notes any time tubing, needles, intracaths, bottles, etc. are changed.
3.   When an I.V. is started, changed, infiltrated, discontinued, or medication is added, time, solution, amount, and condition of the site should be charted on I.V. label and in the Kardex.®
4.   I.V. labels are a permanent part of the patient's chart.

Management of Suspected Bloodstream Infection in Patients Receiving I.V. Therapy
   If septicemia of obscure origin (no obvious source such as infection at catheter site) develops in a patient receiving I.V. therapy:

1.   Obtain blood cultures from at least two independent venipunctures, and immediately discontinue the system (bottle, administration set, and cannula).
2.   Remove cannula aseptically and clip off the tip with sterile scissors into blood culture or other appropriate media. Discontinued unit (bottle) should be sent to lab for culture.
3.   Lot numbers and type of solution should be recorded on all suspected solutions. If contamination during manufacture is suspected, all other solutions bearing the same lot number should be saved for testing by the Food and Drug Administration (FDA).

   One consideration in patients who develop signs and symptoms of sepsis (shock or sudden fever and chills) while receiving I.V. therapy is a bloodstream infection related to contaminated I.V. solutions or catheters.

Although contamination at the manufacturing plant is very uncommon (intrinsic contamination), several national outbeaks have occurred. More likely, contamination occurs within the hospital setting related to handling I.V.s and administration of additives. This is called extrinsic contamination. The extent of the latter is unknown, but may be an important contribution to bloodstream infection and is potentially preventable.

Therefore, if a patient receiving I.V.s suddenly develops signs and symptoms suggesting bloodstream infection, the following four steps are recommended in addition to the history, physical examination, and obtaining of blood cultures:

1. Discontinue the I.V. immediately.
2. After iodine prep of the latex injection port at the distal end of the I.V. tubing (allow iodine to remain at least 2 min and then remove with 70% isopropyl alcohol), aspirate 10 cc of the I.V. contents. Place 5 cc into each of the two blood culture bottles (one set). Complete bacteriology requisition slip indicating I.V. solution and immediately send slip and blood culture bottle to Microbiology Laboratory.
3. Remove the I.V. and if an indwelling catheter is present (as opposed to needle), remove it and hold the external portion directly upwards. Have assistant cut the distal portion of the catheter with sterile screw-top beginning several millimeters inside the former skin surface/catheter interface and place into a sterile screw-capped container (see Figure 5A-5B). If the catheter is longer, cut 5-cm segments and place each into a sterile screw-top container. Complete bacteriology requisition slip indicating indwelling catheter and immediately send slips and container to the Microbiology Laboratory.
4. Record the steps in the progress notes. Record lot number of all I.V. products which the patient was receiving.

In the clinical Microbiology Laboratory, the technician will do the following:

1. Treat the blood culture bottles containing I.V. solution in the same manner as blood culture.
2. Roll the catheter piece(s) back and forth across the surface of a blood agar plate four times for quantitation of bacteria.
3. Report any growth immediately to the clinician and infection control group (Extensions 4-2777 or 4-2143).

Guidelines: Total Parenteral Nutrition (Hyperalimentation)

In the guidelines set forth regarding hyperalimentation, we have modified and adopted many of the policies of the Walter Reed Hospital and Massachusetts General Hospital. These institutions have great interest and experience in the procedue and have enjoyed relatively few complications.

Written hospital policy now exists outlining the procedure for insertion of the subclavian line. This is to be treated as a surgical procedure requiring strict aseptic technique.

Procedure for Care of the I.V. Hyperalimentation Fluid, Filter, Tubing, and Site of Entry

The solution bottle, I.V. tubing, and final filter are changed every 24 hr in the afternoon, when fresh solution arrives from the pharmacy. The solution should be kept refrigerated until 1 hr before use and should never be used after the expiration date on the bottle! Steps:

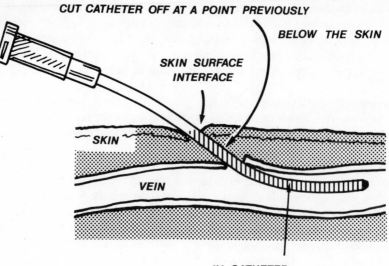

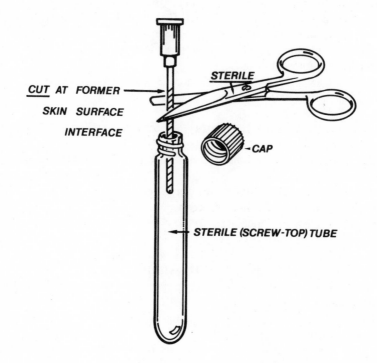

FIGURE 5A,B.   Management of suspected bloodstream infection in patients receiving I.V. therapy.

1. Place the patient absolutely flat in bed (without a pillow). This maneuver de-creases the chance of air entering the vena cava by causing the pressure in the vena cava to become less negative.

2. Remove tapes securing tubing and filter to dressing and tapes securing the catheter hub to the tubing.

3. Wash hands before handling a new filter.

4. Prime the I.V. with fluid and carefully handle the filter during its attachment to avoid contamination. Aim filter toward the ceiling, flush with fluid, tapping filter gently to dispel air. (The entire surface of the filter must be completely wet in order to obtain adequate flow of fluid).

5. Have the patient perform valsalva (tell him to "bear down') and quickly rotate old filter out, grasping catheter hub with a kelly clamp. Replace with new filter and I.V. setup. Tell the patient to breathe normally and adjust the flow rate to the prescribed order.

6. Place a strip of 1-in. adhesive tape lengthwise over the catheter hub and tubing to prevent their separation.

7. Anchor final filter and tubing above it to elastoplast dressing with 1-in. paper tape to prevent their separation. The paper tape allows delineation of basic dressing from filter/tubing anchors.

8. Mark tape on tubing with initials, date, and time changed, and record in progress notes.

9. Label the bottle with time-tape to check the infusion rate compared to its intended schedule.

10. Never allow I.V. bottle to run dry. If bottle empties and no more hyperalimentation solution is readily available, hang a bottle of dextrose 10% and water ($D_{10}W$).

Procedure for Changing Superior Vena Cava "Lifeline" Dressings When Hyperalimentation is Used

Equipment

1. Sterile tray (from Central Supply) containing:
   - 4 kelly clamps with gauze attached
   - 3 medicine glasses
   - 6 4 × 4 in. gauze
   - 6 2 × 2 in. gauze
   - 2 Q-tips®

2. Solutions (from floor/Pharmacy)
   - A tape remover
   - 30-cc plastic disposable container of iodophor solution
   - 70% isopropyl alcohol
   - Packet of iodophor ointment
   - Spray benzoin
   - One swab iodophor solution

3. Dressing cart
   - 1 sterile gown
   - 2 pairs sterile gloves
   - 1 sterile kelly calmp
   - 1 unsterile kelly clamp
   - Special hyperalimentation tubing with filter
   - 2-in. porous transpore water-repellant tape (clear)
   - Culture media

- Q-tips®
- 2 packages sterile 4 × 4 in. gauze pads

Procedure
1. Tubing change (wash hands!) (see section on ''Handwashing'')
    a. Explain procedure to patient.
    b. Don sterile gown and mask.
    c. Position patient flat in bed with head rotated to the opposite side of the catheter. Place a mask on patient.
    d. Clamp off old tubing at the hub, using an unsterile kelly clamp. Disconnect old tubing and bottle.
    e. After prepping top of new bottle with iodophor solution, pierce top of bottle with new hyperalimentation tubing with filter attached.
    f. Hang bottle and clear tubing of all air. Connect to hub of catheter, and check for blood return by lowering bottle.
    g. Regulate flow rate.

2. Removal of old dressing (wash hands!) (see section on ''Handwashing'')

    a. Pour tape remover onto sterile 4 × 4 in. gauze.
    b. Don sterile gloves.
    c. Remove old dressing by using gauze with tape remover, being careful not to touch the insertion area.
    d. Discard soiled dressing in wastebasket.
    e. Remove gloves.
    f. Inspect catheter site thoroughly for any day-to-day changes (e.g., purulence, redness, extravasation, crust, skin rash, blood, or any other significant findings).
    g. Culture site with Q-tip® and place in holding media. Transport to lab as soon as possible.
    h. Wash hands (see section entitled ''Handwashing'').

3. Cleansing the site
    a. Set up sterile tray. Pour iodophor solution and alcohol into medicine glasses (the third glass may be used where liquid benzoin must be used rather than aerosol, i.e., NICU). Drop iodophor ointment onto tray.
    b. Don sterile gloves.
    c. Using 2 kellys clamped with gauze, one at a time, cleanse the insertion area, working from the center to the periphery. Do not retrace steps. One hand is used to do the cleansing, while the other hand manipulates the catheter hub.
    d. Wait 2 min for the iodophor to have optimum effect. Then repeat the above steps using 70% isopropyl alcohol. Alcohol is used to reduce any allergic reaction to the iodophor.
    e. Using another sterile kelly clamped with 4 × 4 in. gauze, pat the site dry.
    f. Apply iodophor ointment to the site using a sterile Q-tip®.

4. Apply sterile dressing
    a. Using 2 × 2 in. gauze, cover the site and needle guard. Keep dressing small and neat, covering the entire site.
    b. Spray area around dressing with benzoin.
    c. Apply 2-in. water repellant tape securely around all edges of dressing.

d. Loop tubing so that it is directed upward over the shoulder to prevent pulling and tension on the catheter and tape.

e. Label with initials and the date.

5. Charting and surveillance

a. Record date and time of dressing change in the progress notes. Also note the appearance of the site and whether a culture was taken.

b. Record the same information, as well as diagnosis, any blood cultures taken, patient's temperature, fluid and electrolyte status, weight gain or loss, antibiotic therapy, and any significant findings in special hyperalimentation log book (kept by the Hyperalimentation Nurse).

General principles

a. Bandages should be changed every Monday, Wednesday, and Friday.

b. Strict aseptic technique with gloves, gown, and masks must be employed.

c. Preferably the same physician or nurse should perform the procedure for a given patient, so that day-to-day changes are readily noticed and so that standardization of the procedure becomes more likely.

Hospital Guidelines for Prophylaxis Against Viral Hepatitis[19]

On Injuries Caused by Articles Possibly Contaminated with Human Blood

Blood from all human beings must be considered as a potential source of one of the hepatitis viruses. Thus, any injury caused by needles, scalpels, scissors, etc. that have been in contact with blood from another individual must be considered as a "hepatitis-prone wound". Because of the efficacy of immune serum globulin (ISG) in preventing hepatitis A ("infectious hepatitis" or short-incubation disease) and the possible efficacy of hyperimmune globulin for hepatitis B (HBIG), we recommend that employees inform their supervisors of injuries sustained on the job and present themselves to Employee Health Service where a decision as to the appropriate prophylaxis will be made.

Following is the algorithm used as a guideline by the employee health team and recommended by the Infection Control Committee.

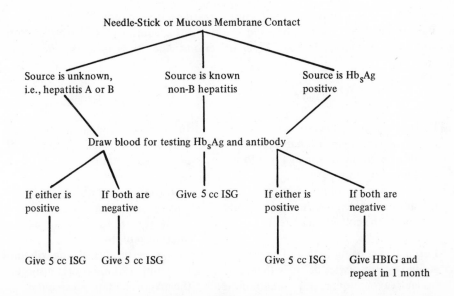

Proposal for Medical Management of Personnel Who require Viral Hepatitis Gamma-Globulin Prophylaxis

Cost of standard immune serum globulin: $4.00/cc. Cost of hyperimmune anti-B globulin: approximately $300.00 per course of two injections.

Follow-up:

All involved personnel have liver function enzyme studies and blood tests for Hb Ag$_s$ and antibody to Hb$_s$Ag initially, at 3 months, and at 9 months. Similar studies should be drawn if any illness suggestive of viral hepatitis occurs at any time.

Recent guidelines on control of viral hepatitis B have been elaborated by the Joint Committee on Viral Hepatitis and the Public Health Service Advisory Committee on Immunization Practices. These recommendations include the following for hospital workers:

1. Careful handwashing is the single most important practice in the protection against hepatitis B.
2. Boiling (10 min at 100°C), autoclaving (15 min at 15 lb/in.²) or dry heat (2 hr at 160°C) is thought to be effective in killing the virus.
3. During procedures that could result in splattering or splashing infective material, a surgical-type mask or facial covering to protect the eyes, nose, and mouth has value.
4. Hemodialysis workers should use gloves during procedures where there is contact with blood, such as in handling shunts, drawing blood, or cleaning or dismantling dialysis machines.
5. Abrasions, lacerations, and other breaks in the skin should be bandaged to protect hemodialysis and laboratory workers from infectious material.
6. Seronegative pregnant women working in high-risk environments (hemodialysis, cancer wards and clinical laboratories) should be transferred to work areas where the risk is lower, since hepatitis B infections during pregnancy can be transmitted to infants.

Hospital Guidelines for Urinary Catheter Care[20,21]

Purpose

The purpose is to minimize the infection hazard related to indwelling urinary catheters. We support the principles of good bladder care as outlined in *Detection, Prevention and Management of Urinary Tract Infections.* The major principles are outlined below:

Principles	Rationale
1. Personnel providing catheter maintenance must wash hands before handling equipment and again before caring for another patient.	Infection causing microorganisms may be transmitted from hands of personnel to patient.
2. Strict aseptic technique must be maintained while inserting catheter and setting up the collection system.	The urinary tract is a sterile system. Any invasive procedure provides a mode of entry for infection causing microorganisms.
3. Perineal care using soap and water should be done twice daily, with care taken to avoid unnecessary manipulation of the catheter tubing.	Proper perineal cleansing will limit the number of microorganisms at the meatus and may lessen the occurrence of infection. Too

4. A closed drainage system must be maintain at all times. The junction of the catheter and the drainage tube should never be "broken" without a physician's order.

5. The Foley catheter should never be clamped and disconnected for the purpose of ambulating the patient. The use of leg bags is discouraged. The patient should be transported or ambulated with the entire system intact. The tubing should be kept free of kinks to allow free flow of urine. Small coiled loops may be pinned to mattress surface to prevent kinking of tubing. The portion of the tubing lower than the bed must be straight to allow free flow of urine into the bag.

6. Bags must at all times be placed below the level of the patient's bladder.

7. Bags should be emptied at least every 8 hr or when necessary, with care taken to avoid contamination of mouth of the spigot. The bag should be emptied by means of the bottom of the drainage port, in an upright position, and never inverted. The bag should not be allowed to touch the floor.

8. Catheters should not be irrigated without physician's order; when necessary, sterile technique must be maintained. A fresh, sterile, large-volume syrine must be used with each irrigation employing sterile solution. Irrigating solutions should be prepared in the pharmacy in quantities to be used within a 24-hr period. Any remaining quantities must be discarded.

9. Urine specimens should be aspirated with a sterile syrine from the proximal lumen of the catheter or specimen port (not the drainage bag). The catheter should be cleaned with an alcohol sponge prior to the specimen collection. Specimens must be sent to the lab soon after collection or refrigerated until delivery is possible.

virgorous manipulation of tubing will cause urethral irritation. Any opening into the collection system provides entry for microorganisms into the patient's urinary tract.

Any obstruction to the free flow of urine would cause a backup of fluid into bladder and predispose the patient to infection. Large loops of coil below the bed level will not allow gravitational flow of urine into collection bag.

Gravitational pull will cause urine to flow downward into the collection system if the bag is placed below the level of the patient's bladder. Microorganisms are known to migrate from the collection bag up the lumen or the outside of the tubing. Microorganisms in the collection bag double in number every 30 min. This contaminated urine should never be forced up the tubing and into the patient's bladder. Any disconnecting of catheter and tubing allows entry of microorganisms into the system. Introducing fluids into the urinary system increases the risk of contamination. Microorganisms introduced into a container of standing irrigating solution will multiply within 24 hr to a number significant to contaminate the fluid. Only fresh bladder urine will provide an accurate bacterial colony count necessary for proper analysis.

10. A sterilely obtained urine specimen for culture should be sent to the Bacteriology Laboratory when the catheter is inserted, once each week (if long term) and when the catheter is removed.

Baseline data (admission urine culture and sensitivity) are necessary in order to clearly identify hospital acquired urinary tract infections.

11. By order of the physician, the catheter and/or the drainage system may be changed if the tubing becomes clogged or the system is otherwise disfunctional.

Infection risks increase with the number of catheterizations performed. With proper care, a functioning drainage system may remain in place for as long as 30 days.

12. When feasible, patients with Foley catheters should not share the same room. A UTI patient with a Foley should not have a roommate with a Foley catheter.

As microorganisms are transmitted primarily on the hands of personnel, the risk is great that a UTI infection will spread to other catheterized patients.

Pediculosis and Scabies[22]

Pediculus humanus capitis (Head Lice)

These are small (0.5 to 2 mm), blood-sucking insects which live on the scalp and hair. Transmission from person to person occurs by close contact or by sharing infested garments, combs and brushes, or bedding materials. Head lice will not survive more than 55 hr on fomites. Therapy is with A-200 Pyrinate®, Cuprex®, and Kwell® which are all shampoos. An initial shampoo should be followed by a second one in 7 to 10 days. It is thought that there is no risk of transmission after initial shampoo therapy. Disinfection of combs and brushes and laundry will be effective if they are placed in water of ⩾60°C for ⩾10 min.

Pediculus humanis humanis (Body Lice)

These survive longer (4 to 10 days) off the host than head lice. Pediculicides are not indicated, since good personal hygiene is sufficient. Machine washing of bedding and combs and brushes will be sufficient to remove the risk of transmission.

Phthirus pubis (Crab Lice)

These will die in less than 24 hr away from the host. Transmission via toilet seats and the sharing of underwear or bedding has been reported. Therapy with 1% Lindane (Kwell®) is recommended.

Scabies (mites)

These are 0.3 to 0.4 mm in diameter, and infestation may lead to severe itching and rash. Transmission is thought to be possible by sharing a bed, sponge-bathing a patient, or applying body lotions. Therapy with 1% Lindane (Kwell) is recommended as a cream or lotion applied to the entire body. A second application seven days later is recommended. Bedding and brushes should be cleaned with hot water (>60° for >10 min.) soaking or cleaning.

Myiasis (Fly Larvae)

A rare nosocomial problem is hospital acquired myiasis or infestation of a wound or mucous membrane with larvae of flies *(Phaenicia serricala)*. Management consists of physical removal of the larvae and debidement of necrotic tissue.

Arterial and Other Pressure-Monitoring Lines[25]

Investigation of an outbreak of *Serratia marcescens* nosocomial bloodstream infections in patients located in the Intensive Care Unit led to the recognition of the risk associated with pressure-monitoring devices. A summary of the investigation and conclusion that the transducer head was the reservoir for the bloodstream infections are listed below. In addition, the specific recommendations for routine disinfection of the transducer head are included.

Seventeen patients in an intensive care unit developed *S. marscescens* bacteremia between January 1 and July 31, 1978 (rate 2.4 vs. 0.3% for previous 6-month period, p <0.005). Infection in all cases occurred after a minimum of 12 hr of exposure to an arterial, Swan-Ganz®, or intracranial pressure-monitoring device. New pressure transducers with disposable domes had been introduced just prior to the outbreak. No increase occurred in *S. marcescens* urinary tract, pulmonary, or postoperative wound infections during the same period. Cultures of in-use I.V. fluid (n = 51) revealed a 0% rate of contamination. On the other hand, fluid from arterial lines (n = 110) was contaminated with *S. marcescens* at weekly rates of 10 to 40%. Investigation directed at defining the reservoir revealed: (1) no contamination of the pressure calibration apparatus, (2) no intrinsic contamination of the prepackaged arterial line components or fluid (n = 70) and, (3) 100% contamination of the permanent transducer heads with *S. marcescens*. Institution of routine glutaraldehyde disinfection of the transducer heads before use resulted in immediate sterilization of all in-use pressure monitoring lines and complete absence of additional cases of *S. marcescens* bacteremia. The fortuitous combination of a reservoir of *S. marcescens* on the permanent transducer plus a yet unexplained mechanism for transfer of these organisms to the disposable fluid-filled dome permitted this serious outbreak to occur. In conclusion, the control of the outbreak involved a simple disinfection procedure heretofore not considered essential for infection control in patients requiring pressure monitoring.

Recommendations for the care of pressure monitoring equipment at the University of Virginia Hospital:

1. The reusable transducer head should be disinfected (method as shown below) between patients requiring pressure monitoring
2. The transducer head should be disinfected (below) with each 48-hr line change if one patient requires monitoring for greater than 48 hr.
3. The method for disinfection of transducer head is as follows:
   a. Dip transducer head in Cidex® (activated glutaraldehyde) for 20 min.
   b. Rinse transducer with 100 cc of sterile water.
   c. Cover the disinfected transducer with a sterile red plastic transducer head cap.

Appendix 1
TERMINAL STERILIZATION AND DISINFECTION CHART

Article to be cleaned	Clean with friction-germicidal detergent, and rinse	Autoclave on unit	Bag, label, send to CSR (label: "Isolation Sterilization")	Discard	Remarks
Airways			X		Soak in hydrogen peroxide and rinse, first
Alternating pressure mattress	X				
Armboards	X			X	If disposable type
Bedboards	X				
Bedpan brush				X	Follow enteric precautions
Bedside equipment	X	X		X	If disposable type
Bedside scales	X				
Catheters					
French				X	
Foley				X	
Plastic				X	
Oxygen				X	
Chair commode	X				
Circulating bed	X				
Deoderizer	X				
Dressings (unused)			X		
Drug box (emergency)					Double bag Label "Isolation" and return to pharmacy
EKG machine	X				
Endotracheal tubes				X	
Enema tubes (red tubber)				X	
Fans	X				

Equipment				Instructions
Heating lamp	X			
Hemovac®	X		X	
Hot plate	X		X	
Hot water bottle	X		X	
Ice cap or collar	X		X	If disposable
Ice mattress	X			
Instruments		X	X	Wash with soap and water and rinse (if reusable)
Isolation cart	X		X	
I.V. bottles			X	Place in paper bag, then in white trash can in utility room
I.V. tubing	X			
"K"-pads	X			
Laryngoscope	X		X	In CMC
Nebulizers	X		X	Bag, label, and return to Respiratory Therapy Department
Ophthalmoscope	X			
Orthopedic (traction) equipment	X			
Oxygen cylinder and flow meter	X		X	
Oxygen mask			X	Wipe off only
Oxygen tubing			X	If disposable type
Oxygen, wall set-up		X		Place flow meter, empty humidifier bottle, delivery tube, etc. in paper bag, send to CSR
Perineal lamp	X		X	
Pleur-Evac (also see suction)			X	

Appendix 1 (continued)
TERMINAL STERILIZATION AND DISINFECTION CHART

Article to be cleaned	Clean with friction-germicidal detergent, and rinse	Autoclave on unit	Bag, label, send to CSR (label: "Isolation Sterilization")	Discard	Remarks
Respirators, IPPB machines, etc.	X				Wipe off only, then notify Respiratory Therapy Department to pick up
Sand bags	X				
Scales, stand-up	X				
Shock blocks	X				
Sitz-bath chair	X				
Sphygmomanometer	X				
Stethoscope	X				
Stryker® floatation pad	X			X	Cuff
Stryker® frame	X				Wipe off only
Stryker® foam leveling pad				X	
Tourniquet				X	
Toys	X			X	Depending upon type
Tracheostomy tubes		X			Rinse and then soak in hydrogen peroxide
Tracheotomy tube ("Briggs") adaptors					Bag, label, and return to Respiratory Therapy Department
Trash cans	X				

	Rinse and then wash with soap and water	In CMC	Rinse and then wash with soap and water	Wipe off only
Treatment rays	X			
Tubing, plastic		X		
Vacuetainer holder and needle		X		
Ventilating trays			X	
Water bed			X	
Water thermometer			X	

Appendix 2
RESPIRATORY THERAPY EQUIPMENT AND DISINFECTION IN ROUTINE PROCEDURES[a]

Equipment	Frequency of cleaning or replacement	Method	Location of disinfection
Anesthesia bag	Daily	Cidex®	Respiratory department of Central Supply
Blow bottles	Every 3 days	Disposables	N/A
Bourns	Daily	Cidex® and ethyl alcohol	Respiratory Department
Bennett® IPPB circuits	Daily	Disposables	N/A
Bird® circuits	Daily	Disposables	Respiratory Department
Emerson® circuit	Daily	Cidex®	Respiratory Department
Engstrom® circuit	Daily	Cidx®	Respiratory Department
MA-1® circuits	Daily	Gas sterilization	Central supply
Continuous positive-pressure breathing	Daily	Cidex®	Respiratory Department
Croupette tents	When D/C	Soap or ethyl alcohol	Respiratory Department or on location
Flowmeters — air and oxygen	When D/C	Soap or ethyl alcohol	Respiratory Department or on location
High-pressure hose (air and oxygen)	When D/C	Cidex®	Respiratory Department or on location
Humidity pots	Daily	Cidex®	Respiratory Department
Intermittent mandatory ventilation (IMV)	Daily	Cidex®	Respiratory Department
Incentive spirometer	After D/C	Gas Sterilization	Central Supply
Manual resuscitators	When D/C	Soap or ethyl alcohol	Respiratory Department or on location
Nasal cannula	Daily	Disposables	N/A
Nebulizers (Blount®)	Daily	Disposables	N/A
Nebulizers (Venturi®)	Daily	Cidex®	Respiratory Department
Needle valve, air, and oxygen adapters	When D/C	Soap or ethyl alcohol	Respiratory Department or on location
Oxygen analyzer	When D/C	Soap	Respiratory Department
Oxygen and air "T" hook-ups	When D/C	Soap or ethyl alcohol	Respiratory Dpartment or on location
All regulators and gauges	When D/C	Soap or ethyl alcohol	Respiratory Department or on location
Respirometers	Daily	Cidex®	On location
Servo	Daily	Cidex® and ethyl alcohol	Respiratory Department
All suction equipment	When D/C	Soap	Respiratory Department
Ventimasks	Daily	Disposables	N/A

Note: For patients on isolation refer to "Isolation Procedure and Infection Control Manual" or "Isolation Procedures in the Respiratory Therapy Procedure Manual."

[a]   D/C, discontinued; N/A, not applicable; and Cidex®, trade name for activated alkaline gluteraldehyde.

REFERENCES

1. Isolation Techniques for Use in Hospitals, National Center for Disease Control publication, 2nd ed., 1975.
2. Control of Communicable Diseases in Man, 12th ed., The American Public Health Association Publ, 1975 (adopted as the official rules and regulations for the control of communicable diseases in Virginia by the State Board of Health).
3. The Infection Control Manual, New York Hospital, Cornell Medical Center, 1970 (revised).
4. *University of Virginia Medical Center Isolation Procedure and Infection Control Manual*, Reynolds Printing, Charlottesville, Va., 1973 (revised).
4a. Haley, R. W., The "hospital epidemiologist" in U.S. hospitals, 1976—1977: a description of the head of the infection surveillance and control program. Report from the SENIC project, *J. Infec. Control*, 1, 21, 1980.
5. Wenzel, R. P., Osterman, C. A., Hunting, K. J., and Gwaltney, J. M., Jr., Hospital acquired infections. I. Surveillance in a university hospital, *Am. J. Epidemiol.*, 103, 251, 1975.
6. Wenzel, R. P., Osterman, C. A., and Hunting, K. J., Hospital acquired Infections. II. Infection rates by site, service and common procedures in a university hospital, *Am. J. Epidemiol.*, 104, 645, 1976.
7. Craven, R. B., Wenzel, R. P., and Atuk, N. O., Minimizing tuberculosis risk to hospital personnel and students exposed to unsuspected disease, *Ann. Intern. Med.*, 82, 628, 1975.
8. Atuk, N. O. and Hunt, E. H., Serial tuberculin testing and Isoniazid therapy in general hospital employees, *JAMA*, 218, 1795, 1971.
9. Atuk, N. O. and Hunt, E. H., Close monitoring is essential during Isoniazid prophylaxis, *South. Med. J.*, 70, 156, 1977.
10. Steere, A. C. and Mallison, G. F., handwashing practices for the prevention of nosocomial infections, *Ann. Intern. Med.*, 83, 683, 1975.
11. Kretzer, M. P. and Engley, F. B., Jr., Effective use of antiseptics and disinfectants, *R.N. Magazine*, May 1969.
12. Reddish, G. F., *Antiseptics, Disinfectants, Fungicides and Sterilization*, Lee & Febiger, Philadelphia, 1961.
13. Spaulding, E. H. and Mallison, G. F., Recommendations for chemical disinfectant and sterilization, *Hospital Tribune*, February 1971.
14. Mallison, G. F., "A.P.I.C. Newsletter," Vol. 2 (No. 2), 1974.
15. Isolation Techniques for Use in Hospital, 2nd ed., Center for Disease Control, Education and Welfare, 1975.
16. Wenzel, R. P., Hospital-acquired infections: sterilization, disinfection, and hospital waste, in *Principles and Practice of Infectious Disease*, Mandell, G. L., Douglas, R. G., and Bennett, J. E., Eds., John Wiley & Sons, 1979.
17. Deane, R. S., Mills, E. L., and Hamel, A. J., Antibacterial action of copper in respiratory therapy apparatus, *Chest*, 58, 373, 1970.
18. Maki, D. G., Weise, C. E., and Sarafin, H. W., A semiquantitative culture method for identifying i.v. catheter-related infections, *N. Engl. J. Med.*, 296, 1305, 1977.
19. Perspectives on the Control of Viral Hepatitis, Type B, Center for Disease Control Morbidity and Mortality Weekly Report (Suppl.), May 7, 1976, 25: #17, U.S. Dept. of Health, Education and Welfare.
20. Maki, D. G., Hennekens, C. H., and Bennett, J. V., Prevention of catheter-associated urinary tract infection, *JAMA*, 221 (11), 1270, 1972.
21. Maki, D. G., Bennett, J. V., Nosocomial urinary tract infection with *Serratia marcescens*: an epidemiologic study, *J. Infect. Dis.*, 128, (5), 579, 1973.
22. Juranek, D. D., APIC Newsletter 4:(i), Feb. 1976. Center for Disease Control Morbidity and Mortality Weekly Report, Vol. 24, No. 13, March 29, 1975, pp. 118-123.
22a. Jacobson, J. A., Kolts, R. L., Conti, M., and Burke, J. P., Hospital acquired myiasis, *Infec. Control*, 1, 319, 1980.
23. Osterman, C. A., Infection control-relation of new disposal unit to risk of needle puncture injuries, *Hosp. Top.*, Mar./April, 1975.
24. Kunin, C. N., *Detection, Prevention and Management of Urinary Tract Infections*, 2nd edition, Lea & Febiger, Philadelphia, 1974.
25. Donowitz, L. G., Marsik, F. J., Hoyt, J. W., Wenzel, R. P., *Serratia Marcescens* bacterema from contaminated pressure transducers, *JAMA*, 242(16), 1749, 1979.
26. Gajdusek, D. C., Gibbs, C. J., Jr., Asher, D. M., Brown, P., Diwan, A., Hoffman, P., Nemo, G., Rohwer, R., and White, L., Precautions in medical care of, and in handling materials from, patients with transmissible virus dementia (Creutzfeldt-Jakob Disease), *N. Engl. J. Med.*, 297, 23, 1977.

AN EMPLOYEE HEALTH SERVICE FOR INFECTION CONTROL

Nuzhet O. Atuk, Timothy R. Townsend, Ella H. Hunt, and Richard P. Wenzel

ORGANIZATION AND NECESSARY PERSONNEL

The goals of a newly organized employee health service should be practical and feasible. They should emphasize relatively simple means of keeping employees in the hospital setting healthy. The problems faced could be categorized as those:

1. Serving to maintain employees' health.
2. Increasing employees' efficiency through decrease in absenteeism because of sickness.
3. Providing greater efficiency by rendering care to those employees who become sick while on duty.

The need for conscientious and comprehensive surveillance of diseases and occupational hazards will increase as the necessary level of efficiency and the time value of employees is increased.

As the employee-patient load increases (see Figure 1), the Department of Employee Health will need to develop a multifaceted role in the hospital. Surveillance and control of infectious diseases is of top priority. Caring for the ill and injured employees, referring employees to other specialty areas when necessary, and counseling, all involve medical and administrative actions on diverse levels. Programs resulting from these activities must provide for the efficient recall of employees for testing purposes at the appropriate time, maintenance of individual health records, and documentation of procedures for statistical reports. Administrative responsibilities include enforcement of comprehensive infection screening for the benefit of employees and patients; maintaining lines of communication between departments to facilitate exchange of information regarding employees' health and fitness for work; and responsible reporting to appropriate personnel, with regard to the presence of infections, health hazard, or educational information developed through department activities that is of value to the medical field.

In order to assure the effectiveness of the department programs, it is of prime importance to have the support of the administration. The administration works with the department director and head nurse in establishing policies, screening new employees, and modifying programs when necessary to meet the needs of the Medical Center.

The Department of Employee Health (see Figure 2) is usually under the directorship of the medical director, a faculty member of the Department of Internal Medicine, who is available at all times for administrative consultation. The director is administratively responsible to the hospital administrator and professionally responsible to the physician-in-chief. He maintains close communication with the hospital (physician) epidemiologist.

At the University of Virginia Hospital, the department consists of a head nurse, a general-duty registered nurse, attendant specialist, two full-time secretaries, and one full-time receptionist. Medical assistant residents who cover the morning visiting hours also take calls for the afternoons for on-the-job illnesses and accidents. The Department of Employee Health provides health services for a pool of slightly over 6000 employees; of these 1200 (20%) represent newly employed personnel each year. Specific activities are outlined in Figure 3.

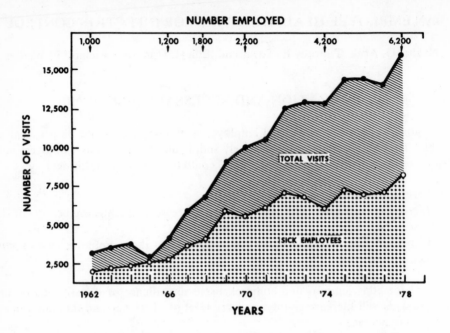

FIGURE 1.   The relationships are shown for increased total visits and increased visits by ill employees with time (from the University of Virginia Hospital Employee Health Department). The nonsick employees represent those screened for antibody to rubella, for PPD-S skin test reactions, etc. These figures do not include routine chest X-ray requests, PPD-S readings, assistance to employees in referrals, or health assistance by phone.

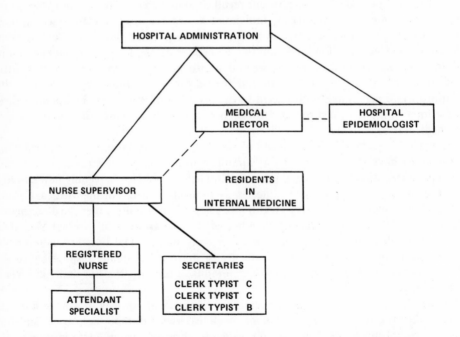

FIGURE 2.   Organization for Employee Health at the University of Virginia Hospital. A single medical resident is on duty from 10:00 to 12:00 a.m., Monday through Friday, and is on call for patients in the afternoons. In the evenings and weekends/holidays, the Emergency Room staff covers all employee heath needs, including referrals to the Department of Employee Health the following day.

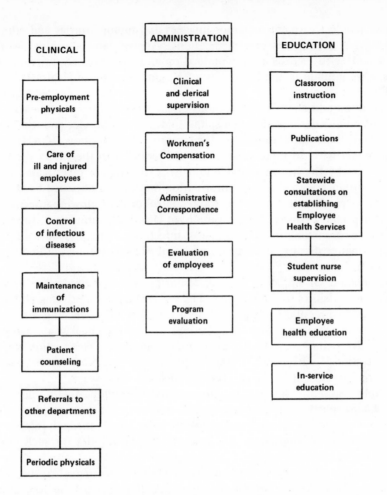

FIGURE 3.   Outline of the activities of an effective Employee Heatlh Service.

Outline of Activities

The following clinical administrative and education activities are those used at the University of Virginia. They are published only as guidelines for other hospitals to develop specific activities pertinent to their own institutions.

Clinical

1. The object of a placement examination is to determine whether an applicant is medically qualified to perform the work which he is to be assigned. He must be able to do such work without danger to himself or others for the protection of other employees, patients, and visitors. Screening medical examinations are given to all new, temporary, and permanent employees (approximately 1200 annually). This examination includes appropriate clinical laboratory tests in accordance with the employee's medical history and area of work. Complete physical examinations are given when deemed necessary according to the guidelines set forth by the medical director.
2. Injured and ill employees are screened by the head nurse or general-duty registered nurse to determine appropriate treatment. When necessary, arrangements are made for the employee to be seen by a physician. Activities related to patient

care include treatment of minor illnesses and minor injuries and administering emergency treatments and medications. Appropriate laboratory work is collected. Health records are maintained on all procedures. Approximately 16,820 visits were made to the University of Virginia Employee Health Department in 1978.

3. Prevention and control of infectious diseases are maintained in accordance with the recommendations of the Hospital Epidemiology Service and with the requirements of the Joint Commission for Hospital Accreditation (JCAH). Employees in contact with an infectious disease are reported to the Employee Health Department by the hospital epidemiologist. Contacts are investigated and treated in accordance with the latest information that can be obtained by the Employee Health Department. Surveillance and control of the following infectious diseases are of primary concern to the Employee Health Depatment: a. tuberculosis, b. hepatitis, c. meningitis, d. herpesvirus infections, e. staphylococcal infections, f. Legionnaires disease, influenza, and g. rubella (see section entitled "Immunizations").

4. Maintenance of employee immunizations protects the employees, as well as patients and visitors to the hospital. The service includes notifying all hospital employees on a regular basis of their need for tuberculin screening. Employees who have been in contact with an infectious disease are checked on a regular basis for a designated period after exposure to the disease (see section entitled "Immunizations"). Isoniazid (INH) drug therapy is provided for employees whose tuberculin skin tests indicate recent contact with the disease.

5. Simple counseling and guidance are offered to employees with minor emotional problems. Further support and specific treatment for those employees who have serious physical and emotional problems are available through referral to appropriate clinics or physicians. The financial responsibilities for such referrals rest with the employee.

6. Referrals of personnel to other departments are processed when specialized medical care is necessary. This entails communication between the designated department and the employee's department. Referrals are contingent upon the rules set forth by the administration.

7. Periodic physicals for those employees over 45 years of age are recommended every 2 years. These physicals include an electrocardiogram, blood work, chest X-ray, blood pressure checks, etc. These physicals maintain up-to-date baseline vital data which facilitate detection of abnormalities in middle-aged and older employees who desire to use this service When long-range health care is necessary, the Employee Health Department makes every effort to keep lines of communication open with the employee's primary care physician.

Administrative

1. Supervision of all clinical and clerical activities entails documentation of all procedures of the clinic. Appropriate records must be maintained to facilitate responsible care for employees over extended periods of time in which they may be examined by different physicians. In order to maintain effective disease control programs, patient records must be orderly and accessible. This is a continuous operation which occupies much of the secretaries' time. Final documentation must meet the approval of the medical director and/or head nurse. Approximately 6200 employee charts are maintained, with a turnover rate of 20% per year. Employee turnover varies and is dependent on the national economy and job availability.

2. Workmen's Compensation communication channels must be established for all job-related illnesses and accidents as set forth by law. Incident sheets must be recorded daily, and employees' departments informed of workers' conditions. Communication between the Personnel Department, head nurse, director, and employee's department regarding time lost, job restrictions, etc. is essential. Records and statistics for all cases must be maintained and submitted to appropriate safety committees as requested. Compensation bills coming to this department must be reached for approval or denial. Currently, the department handles approximately 840 cases a year, of which approximately 50 are major compensation cases requiring follow-up care for an extended period of time.

3. Administrative correspondence is necessary to maintain lines of communication with hospital department regarding immunization programs, employee status, and appropriate utilization of the Department of Employee Health benefits. This includes letters and directives from the director and head nurse, notices to employees regarding disease screening at regular intervals (approximately 12,500 notices a year), and Workmen's Compensation associated letters. Communication with the Health Department is necessary upon detection of certain infectious diseases, such as hepatitis, tuberculosis, shigella, salmonella, meningitis, and others.

4. Employee examinations are to determine an employee's fitness to begin work activities, or in the case of a period of disability, to return to his or her work activities. The decision as to whether an employee is fit to work is an administrative decision, contingent upon appropriate physical fitness.

5. All departmental programs are analyzed regularly for their effectiveness. Such analysis allows the director to determine the need for modification or discontinuation of existing programs, or the adoption of new programs. In addition, a benefit/cost evaluation of all programs is utilized in order to reduce the overall cost of health programs.

Education

1. The medical director and head nurse coordinate activities to teach part of the University of Virginia Hospital Epidemiology course. This activity is done on a regular basis in cooperation with the hospital epidemiology service.

2. Significant information obtained from various health programs of the hospital is organized and sponsored by the department director and head nurse in cooperation with colleagues.[1-3]

3. Upon request, organizational information is supplied to institutions inquiring of this department's rules and regulations. Requests frequently focus on this department's emphasis on immunizations, disease screening, and conscientious follow-up.

4. Rotating student nurses are assigned to this department for a short period of time during their schooling. While in this department, they have the opportunity to observe the physician and work with the nurses. They are encouraged by the nurses to participate as fully as is possible at their stage of schooling.

5. Employees are instructed in appropriate procedures for handling patients and patients' biological fluids and substances. These preventative measures are important in protecting employees from contracting patients' diseases and in preventing muscle strains. Alerting employees to likely modes of infection transmission also serves to protect patients from potential pathogens carried by employees.

6. The Employee Health Department nurses attend courses and meetings concen-

trating on current developments in their field of nursing and employee health services. These meetings may be held in the University of Virginia Hospital or out of town under the auspices of the State Health Department, Division of Occupational Health. In addition to the nurses attending various in-service programs, the clerical staff and attendant specialist attend various in-service programs; the clerical staff and attendant specialist attend programs which expose them to facets of the hospital they would not otherwise contact, but which broaden their understanding of the hospital.

CURRENT METHODS FOR TUBERCULOSIS SURVEILLANCE AND CONTROL IN THE MEDICAL CENTER OF THE UNIVERSITY OF VIRGINIA

Routine Tuberculosis Surveillance for all Medical Center Employees
Routine tuberculosis surveillance for all Medical Center employees includes:

1. An intermediate-strength protein precipated derivative of Siebert (PPD-S) is used for initial routine tuberculin tests, except for those employees with a family or personal history of tuberculosis, prior tuberculin sensitivity, or BCG administration, in which case testing is begun with first-strength PPD-S.
2. A chest X-ray film is obtained in addition to initial PPD-S skin test.
3. The tuberculin skin test is repeated annually in all previous nonreactors without any additional chest X-ray film.
4. Positive reactors to tuberculin receive chest X-rays annually.
5. Employees of certain services (i.e., Acute Care Unit Pulmonary Medicine, Dietary, Emergency Room, Intensive Care Unit, Thoracic Surgery Wards, Acute Internal Medicine Wards, and Radiology, Department) are given a tuberculin skin test or chest X-ray every 6 months.
6. All contacts of initially unrecognized and unisolated tuberculosis cases are advised on the symptoms of incipient tuberculosis.

Conversion of Tuberculin Test Within 1 Year
Chest X-ray examinations are obtained at the time a conversion occurs. If the X-rays are normal, the following schedule is used:

1. An appointment is made with the medical director.
2. INH prophylaxis for 1 year is recommended, with close monitoring under the direction of the medical director.
3. Chest X-ray examinations at 2, 6, and 12 months are recommended.
4. Tuberculin skin tests are given at the completion of the INH therapy. If a positive tuberculin reaction has reverted to negative, then the tuberculin test is repeated annually. If the tuberculin reaction remains positive, employees are followed by yearly chest X-ray examinations.
5. Employees with abnormal chest X-ray films are referred to the Pulmonary Disease Department for further evaluation and treatment.
6. All tuberculosis convertors are reported to the local Health Department.

AN EXAMPLE OF COST ANALYSIS AND SAVINGS IN AN EFFECTIVE EMPLOYEE HEALTH SERVICE

After the initial employee chest X-ray and tuberculin skin test, all negative reactors receive periodic skin tests without accompanying chest X-ray films. Employee compliance over a period of 8 years at the University of Virginia has been excellent. As a result, there has been a significant reduction of the radiation exposure to employees who have negative skin tests and a marked reduction of the annual expenditures for disease surveillance. For example, the total annual cost of X-rays for the 6200 employees of the Medical Center would be $204,707.00. Under the existing program, only the positive PPD-S reactors (17%) receive X-rays. This program results in an estimated savings of $152,454.50 (see Table 1).

A further reduction in costs has resulted from limiting the numbers of employees tested after contact with suspected disease. From 7/1/77 to 6/30/78, the Employee Health Service detected 27 PPD-S converters at the University Hospital through the tuberculosis surveillance program. Of the 27, only 3 (11%) were detected among 800 employees tested because of reported contact with active disease. The remaining 24 (89%) were detected during routine (annual or biannual) tuberculin testing. It appears that routine PPD testing efficiently detects newly converted employees. Therefore, unless an employee has close and direct contact with tuberculosis secretion, such as involvement with resuscitation, bronchoscopy, etc., tuberculin testing of employees is now limited to the annual routine programs.

Recently, the Center for Disease Control has suggested that a repeat tuberculin skin test may demonstrate a significantly larger reaction than the initial test in the absence of a new infection.[3a] In their opinion the so called "booster effect" may identify up to 6% with initially false negative PPD-S skin tests. They suggest that new employees who initially skin test negative receive a second skin test between 8 and 21 days after the first.[3b] The issues of the booster phenomenon and CDC recommendations have been carefully addressed[3c] and it is the opinion of the authors of this chapter that repeat skin tests should not be routinely instituted in hospitals until further studies, demonstrating benefits, are published. In part, our caution on this point stems from our own data on the booster phenomenon. Our recent studies of 407 employees have shown 15 (3.7%) initially were positive, 4 (1%) initially were negative and received the second skin test (5 tu) 8 days later and became positive, and the remaining 388 (95.3%) were negative in both tests.

IMMUNIZATIONS

A major question that the employee health program director must ask is how much medical service should be available to employees. Most hospitals have available a program to vaccinate women of childbearing age against rubella, a preventable disease with serious consequences for the unborn fetus. The program for such vaccinations is in Table 2.

In addition to rubella vaccine, employees may receive diptheria-tetanus vaccines at 10 year intervals at many hospitals. Influenza vaccine and vaccine to protect against pneumococcal infections are offered to high-risk employees, according to the Center for Disease Control (CDC) recommendations. It should be emphasized that vaccines are generally offered to employees, and the latter are not compelled to take them. It is important that some discussion of potential risks and benefits should be available on an individual basis to the employee.

MANAGING EMPLOYEE EXPOSURES TO INFECTION

Exposure to Viral Hepatitis

Viral hepatitis is an acute inflammation of the liver caused by at least three viruses,

Table 1

COST ANALYSIS OF TUBERCULOSIS SURVEILLANCE PROGRAMS EMPLOYING SKIN
TESTS RATHER THAN CHEST X-RAY FILMS TO SCREEN PPD-S NEGATIVE
EMPLOYEES

Number of employees screened	Cost of annual X-rays for all employees ($)	Cost of PPD screening and limited annual X-rays ($)
5,753 (negative PPD-S)	PA[a] (28.00) — 161,084.00	PPD-S (1.50) — 8,629.50
1,179 (positive PPD-S)	PA[a] and lateral (37.00) — 43,623.00	PA[a] and lateral (37.00) — 43,623.00
Totals 6,932[b*]	204,707.00	52,252.50

Note: Cost reduction of $152,454.50.

[a] PA = posterior — anterior.
[b*] The total number of employees screened is larger than the number of hospital employees because of the biannual screening of personnel in certain high risk areas of the hospital.

Table 2
RUBELLA VACCINE PROGRAM

A.   Rubella titers are drawn on female employees under 35 years of age in the following units:

    1. Emergency Room
    2. Newborn Nursery
    3. Newborn Intensive Care Unit
    4. Obstetrics
    5. Delivery Room
    6. Pediatrics
    7. Pediatric Clinic — Outpatient Department and Private
    8. Children's Rehabilitation Center

B.   Each employee is notified of the result of her titer:

    1. A positive titer is a titer $\geqslant$1:16.
    2. A negative titer is a titer <1:16.
    3. The rubella vaccine is recommended by letter, along with a form regarding birth control for the employee's personal physician to sign.

C.   Procedure for giving the vaccine:

    1. The employee reports to the department during her menstrual period with the signed form from her doctor.
    2. A consent form for the vaccine is signed by the employee.
    3. There is a review of the contraindications to the vaccine with the employee.
    4. Vaccine is administered according to the manufacturer's direction.

D.   Follow-up procedure:

    1. Recheck rubella titer in 6 weeks, then every 2 years.
    2. If titer is still negative, repeat the procedure for giving the vaccine.

type A, type B, and type non-A-non-B. In general, type A disease is a childhood infection, is highly communicable, has a brief (2 to 8 weeks) incubation period, and carries less morbidity than type B. Prophylaxis of contacts with immune serum globulin (ISG) is highly efficacious in preventing illness. In contrast to type A infection, type B is generally a disease of adults, less easily transmitted from person to person, has a long (2 to 8 months) incubation period, and has greater morbidity than type A. Prophylaxis of contacts of patients with ISG does not appear as good as with high-titered antibody to hepatitis B (HBIG) (see below).

Type A and type B viral hepatitis infections can be transmitted by either the fecal-oral or the parenteral route; for this reason, patients suspected of either illness are placed on enteric precautions, and all laboratory specimens are marked with the "hepatitis" label. (See "University of Virginia Medical Center — Isolation Procedure and Infection Control Manual", section entitled "Hepatitis Precaution: Labeling of Specimens".) Within the hospital, frequent handwashing and general attention to good technique in handling specimens are the mainstays of preventing acquisition by the fecal-oral route. Major problems arise primarily in two situations: (1) when hospital workers manage a patient with active GI bleeding, who has viral hepatitis, and (2) when an employee accidentally gets a finger-stick injury with a needle containing blood from an infectious patient, especially if the blood contains markers for hepatitis B.

Much work has been performed in the last 15 years to identify various serologic markers to hepatitis B. As a result, information has been obtained regarding the infectious nature of blood for patients with existing or past viral hepatitis B. The hepatitis B antigen HBAg is a complex of particles: 20-nm spheres and tubules, 100-nm tubules,

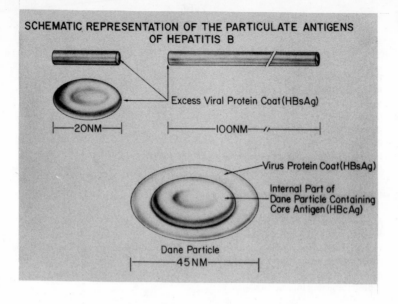

FIGURE 4.   Schematic representation of the particles forming the hepatitis B antigens as seen in the electron microscope.

and a 45-nm Dane particle (see Figure 4). It now appears that the first three are likely to be excess viral protein coat, whereas the Dane particle contains the virus plus its external protein coat. With detergents, one can separate the external coat of the Dane particle from the internal virus-like structure. The outer coat of the Dane particle and the 20- and 100-nm particles are collectively known as the hepatitis B surface antigen (HBsAg). It is the HBsAg which is currently measured in blood banks and clinical laboratories to screen for the serum carrier state of hepatitis B. The internal part of the Dane particle contains what is referred to as the hepatitis B core antigen (HBcAg).

If one could see the structure of the internal aspect of the Dane particle, one would note a circular double strand of DNA surrounded by core antigen HBcAg (see Figure 5). Closely associated with HBcAg is the enzyme, DNA polymerase, necessary for viral replication. A soluble antigen known as e antigen (eAg) is frequently found wherever one finds DNA polymerase and may be located within the virus; new data suggest that the eAg may arise from host cells, however.

In general, it appears that carriers of HBsAg who are also carriers of eAg are likely to have active liver disease and frequently can transmit their disease to susceptible needle-stick contacts.[4,5] In contrast, carriers of HBsAg who are eAg negative (and thus usually negative also for DNA polymerase) are not likely to transmit viral hepatitis B to contacts. The presence of antibody to surface antigen in the recipient is also an important determinant for infection. For, although the functions of HBcAg and the antibody core antigen (anti-HBc) are unknown, it does appear that antibody to surface antigen (anti-HBs) is the protecting antibody (or marker of protection). Persons with anti-HBs are usually immune to hepatitis B. Thus, needle-stick injuries in which the blood contains HBsAg usually does not result in hepatitis B in the recipient if they (recipients) have serum containing anti-HBs.

Since the dialysis unit is a high risk area, special surveillance efforts are often performed there. The current surveillance (1979-1980) of the hepatitis B exposure in the dialysis unit at the University of Virginia includes the following:

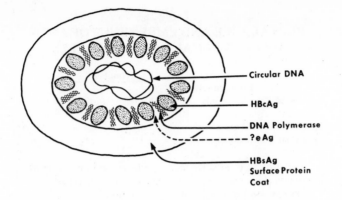

FIGURE 5. Schematic view of the internal structure of the 45nm Dane particle and relationship of the circular DNA, core antigen, and surface antigen.

All dialysis patients with negative serology are tested for hepatitis B (antigen or antibody) on a monthly basis, whereas the nurses at risk in the unit similarly are surveyed on a 3 month basis. Thirty-two of the previously negative Anti-HB,Ag employees were followed prospectively for 12 months after the original testing (Table 2a). The prevalence rate of anti-HB, was 9% in April 1979, and in 1 year, the development of anti-HB,Ag occurred in three (9.3%) employees who were known to have negative antibodies previously. Epidemiologic survey in these three convertors revealed that two were actually exposed to an undiagnosed and unsuspected hepatitis B antigen positive patient. The other was an attendant who could not be traced to any known exposure.

Duty schedules for the two convertors and other nurses in the dialysis unit have also been studied. It appears that there was no relationship between the frequency of contact with the known antigen positive patients and the development of hepatitis or antibodies for hepatitis B (Table 2b). There were many nurses who had a greater number of contacts with the antigen positive patients; however, one had a skin abrasion which allowed blood contact with a patient's blood.

PREVALENCE AND EMERGENCE OF ANTI-HB, IN HOSPITAL EMPLOYEES—UNIVERSITY OF VIRGINIA

Table 2c depicts the prevalence and emergence of anti-HB, in 62 employees (nursing, laboratory, and housekeeping personnel) following accidental needle-sticks. The prevalence rate was 8% in 1979. Forty of the previously negative anti-HB, employees were followed for 9 to 12 months after the original testing. The conversion rate of negative reactors during this period was 5%. Of these two persons, one, following the initial needle-stick, remained antibody negative for 9 months. In the 10th month he had another needle-stick. In the ensuing 2 months he became antibody positive. This may suggest the second accident was due to a contaminated needle which was in the trash.

The second person, following a needle-stick, has shown antibodies against HB,Ag at the third month testing period and this development was confirmed by further testing 6 months afterwards. One employee who was given HBIG immediately following the needle-stick maintained positive antibodies for a period of 12 months which was suggestive of passive and active immunization. However, in the 13th month his antibodies became negative. None of these patients had history or laboratory information indicative of clinical hepatitis.

Furthermore, the presence of anti-HB, among hospital employees did not correlate

Table 2a
PREVALENCE AND EMERGENCE OF ANTI-HB,AG IN RENAL UNIT EMPLOYEES

Year tested	Prior anti-HB,Ag status	Number		
		Tested	Positive	Percent
April 1979	Unknown	45	4	9%
April 1980	Previously negative	32[a]	3[b]	9.3%

[a] A total of 10 (9 negative and 1 positive) were lost to follow-up because of termination of employment or failure to report.
[b] A new case of hepatitis B still antigen positive for 6 weeks.

Table 2b
INCIDENCE OF THE DEVELOPMENT OF HB,AG, ANTI-HB, AND ANTI-HB$_c$ RELATION TO THE NUMBER OF CONTACTS MADE BY RENAL UNIT PERSONNEL WITH HEPATITIS PATIENTS

Number of contacts	Number of employees	Development		
		HB,Ag	Anti-HB,Ag	Anti-HB$_c$
1	1	—	—	—
2	2	—	—	—
3	1	—	+	+
3	1	—	—	+
4	1	—	—	+
5	1	+	—	+
5	1	—	—	—
7	1	—	—	—
8	1	—	—	—
9	1	—	—	—
10	1	—	—	—
12	1	—	—	—

Table 2c
PREVALENCE AND EMERGENCE OF ANTI-HB,AG IN HOSPITAL EMPLOYEE NEEDLE-STICKS

Year tested	Prior anti-HB,Ag status	Number		
		Tested	Positive	Percent
1979	Unknown	62	5	8%
1980	Previously negative	40[a]	2[b]	5%

[a] A total of 17 employees (1 positive and 16 negative) were lost to follow-up because of termination.
[b] Both of these 2 conversions occurred following needle-sticks.

well by duration of employment of the personnel (Figure 5a) however, when the presence of anti-HB, was examined by age of the employees there seemed to be a positive correlation between the age of the employee and the presence of antibodies (Figure 5b) although the possibility of out-of-hospital contact has not been ruled out.

A study was made of 301 accidental needle-sticks occurring during a 13 month period in an effort to determine what factors play a role in these accidents. Both age group and duration of employment were examined.

1. Age — the accident group was divided into 5 year age brackets and then compared to a sample of the entire population which was divided into 5 year age brackets. As can be seen in Figure 5c, 55% of the accidents were sustained by the 21- to 25-year-olds whereas 29% of the sample population fell into this age bracket. This suggests that the younger age group is prone to sustain a higher incidence of needle-sticks.

The frequency of needle-stick accidents may well relate to the frequency of needle usage, however there was no relationship between frequency of the needle-stick accident and work location in the hospital.

2. Duration of employment did not seem to influence the rate of needle-stick accidents.

The cost analysis of 1 year of hepatitis surveillance and control program was rather high and is demonstrated in Table 2d.

For employees who are exposed to needle-stick injuries or who have mucous membrane contact with blood from hepatitis patients, the following steps are recommended (Table 3):

1. Establish the degree of exposure, the identity of the donor (if known), and record the event.

2. Draw blood on both employee (recipient) and patient (donor) for tests of HBsAg and anti-HBs, serum glutamic oxaloacetic transaminase, (SGOT), and serum glutamic pyruvate transaminase (SGPT). Administer either ISG or high-titered hepatitis B immune globulin (HBIG).
   a. If the employee is negative for HBsAg and anti-HBs and the donor is known to be a non-B hepatitis case, then 5 mℓ of ISG are administered i.m. for hepatitis A prophylaxis.
   b. If the employee is negative for HBs Ag and anti-HBs and the source of exposure is unknown, administer 5 mℓ of standard ISG. A similar dose is administered in 30 days. The dosage has been suggested in earlier reports.[7,8]
   c. If the employee is negative for HBsAg and anti-HBs and the source of exposure is known to be HBsAg positive (hepatitis B), the HBIG is administered i.m. according to body weight (0.05 to 0.07 mℓ/kg). A similar dose is administered i.m. in 30 days.
   d. If the employee is positive for either HBsAg or anti-HBs, then 5 mℓ of ISG are administered.

3. Repeat liver function tests whenever the patient becomes ill with symptoms suggestive of viral hepatitis and routinely at 3 months. Repeat tests for HBsAg and anti-HBs at 3 and 9 months.

4. Record all findings in the employee's health records and in a separate report of the exposure.

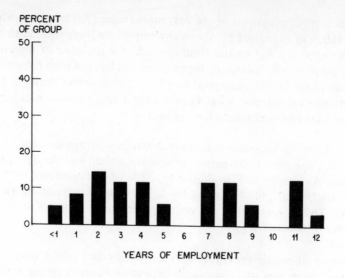

FIGURE 5a. Breakdown by length of employment of 34 anti-HB,Ag positive employees.

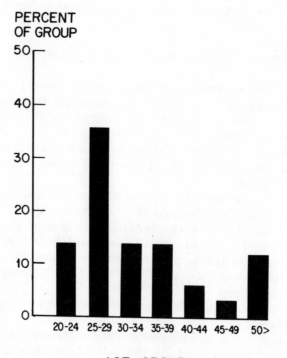

FIGURE 5b. Breakdown by age group of 34 anti-HB,Ag positive employees.

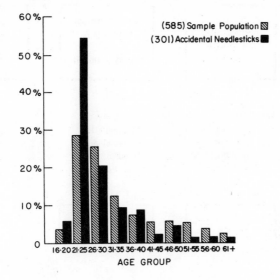

COMPARISON OF SAMPLE POPULATION TO NEEDLESTICK POPULATION
BY 5 YEAR AGE GROUP AS A PERCENTAGE OF IT'S GROUP

FIGURE 5c. Comparison of sample population by 5 year age group as a percentage of its group.

Table 2d
COST ANALYSIS FOR NEEDLE-
STICK PROTOCOL

Liver enzymes	38,892
Serology hepatitis panel	55,560
H-Big gamma globulin	8,928
Immune gamma globulin	1,313
Totals	$104,693

Note: This report is confined to that portion of the hepatitis expense relating to needle-sticks and not to actual treatment of work related cases of hepatitis diagnosed among the employees.

Note: Since routine laboratory testing for eAg is not generally available, no prophylactic guidelines are included regarding the presence or absence of this antigen in donor's blood.

More than 90% of lots of ISG manufactured after 1972 have detectable anti-HBs.[7] It is unclear whether this material costing approximately $5/ml will definitely protect against viral hepatitis type B. Lots of ISG prepared prior to 1972 are less likely to possess anti-HBs, and those which do have detectable anti-HBs have lower titers than the more recently manufactured lots. Recent evidence strongly suggests that HBIG does have a beneficial effect in prophylaxis of hepatitis B (see Table 3a) when compared to ISG containing no anti-HBs.[4] It is also possible that lots of ISG containing lower titers of anti-HBs may also prevent or modify hepatitis B in recipients, but current data are unclear.

Since a large hospital may have several hundred needle-stick injuries each year, and in many the sources of exposure is unknown, it is financially impractical to give all

Table 3

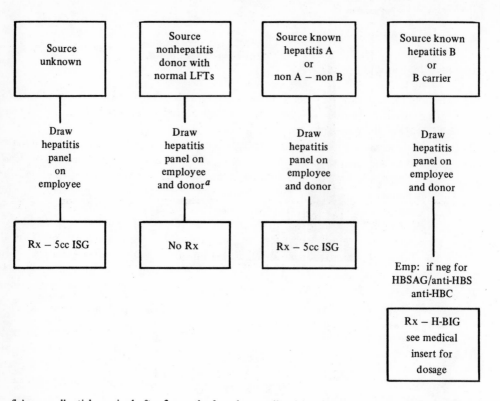

a Any needle-stick received after 2 months from last needle-stick — boost with 2cc gamma globulin, get % of inhibition on all positive anti-HB$_c$ tests, notify physician in charge, and secure Rx order.

Table 3a
DATA SHOWING THE EFFICACY OF HBIG FOLLOWING NEEDLE-STICK EXPOSURE TO HBsAg POSITIVE DONORS

Outcome after needle-stick injury in recipients with no prior anti-Hbs or HBsAg	Type of globulin administered	
	HBIG (N = 216) (%)	ISG + [a] (N = 203) (%)
Hepatitis B	1.4	5.9
HBsAg only	1.9	0
Anti-HBs	5.6	20.7

[a]   +, number of anti-HBs.

Adapted from Seeff, L. B., Wright, E. C., Zimmerman, H. J., *Ann. Intern. Med.*, 88, 285, 1978.

employees HBIG (cost of $300 per series of two injections). HBIG is generally reserved for susceptible employees (who have neither HBsAg nor anti-HBs) whose needle-stick or mucous membrane exposure to HBsAg is clearly recognized.

It should be noted that pregnancy is not a contraindication to using ISG and HBIG, that hypersensitivity reactions have been reported, and that approximately 3% of recipients of HBIG or ISG may develope fever, nausea, itching, rash, dizziness, or joint pains.[4]

Exposure to Tuberculosis

Surveillance of all employee contacts of patients with suspected active tuberculosis includes the following:

1. Suspected contact list — Upon discovery of a suspected active case, the Hospital Epidemiology Service develops a list of all personnel and roommates who were exposed to the patient.
2. Activated contact list — If tuberculosis is bacteriologically or pathologically confirmed in the suspected patient, the contact list is activated and sent to: a. Hospital Employee Health and Student Health Departments; b. physicians of the roommates; c. the patient's local health department, for tracing the family and community contacts; and d. other concerned personnel departments. All those employees called in routinely for 6-month tuberculin tests will not be recalled.
3. Detection of new converters — a. Tuberculin skin tests are performed on all previously negative reactors immediately and at 3 months after exposure. New converters are treated with INH therapy as described previously. b. Previously known reactors with normal chest X-rays are promptly X-rayed again at 3- and 12-month intervals and annually thereafter.

A random sample population of 2384 employees was tested in 1977 to demonstrate the age distribution of tuberculin reactivity among the hospital personnel (see Table 4). This study indicated that older people (50 years and above) have the highest percent of positive skin tests, although the conversion rate is highest among the younger employees (20 to 30 years).

Monitoring of INH Prophylaxis

Procedure used to detect INH toxicity is illustrated below.

1. Prior to the institution of INH therapy, the following blood control tests are obtained: liver function studies, including Alk Phophatase, SGOT, and bilirubin.
2. The above tests are repeated on the following schedule: the second month, sixth month, and twelfth month.
3. Caution employee to report to the Employee Health Department if any of the following symptoms are noted:* loss of appetite, fatigue, weakness, nausea, dizziness, and/or anthralgia.
4. Routine physicians visits are scheduled for: second month, sixth month, and twelfth month.

From 1/5/75 to 8/1/78, 25 University of Virginia Hospital employees were treated with INH. Of these 25, 10 did not complete a year of therapy. The status of the 15 employees who did complete a year of therapy is outlined in Table 5. It is significant that of the 10 employees whose conversions were detected within 1 year, the reversion rate was 80%. The cost of a year on INH is outlined in Table 6. The total is not what an employee would be charged elsewhere, as the amount does not include private physicians' fees.

---

* If any of the above symptoms occur for more than 3 days, have physician see patient.

Table 4

AGE DISTRIBUTION OF TUBERCULIN REACTIVITY AMONG THE HOSPITAL PERSONNEL

Age		Prevalence of employess with positive tuberculin (PPD) test[a]		Tuberculin conversions detected during employment compared to prevalence of PPD positive employees		Estimated risk of converting PPD while employed[b]
Distribution	Percent	Number	Percent	Number	Percent	(%)
Under 20	3.1	1	1	1	100	1
20—30	54.6	103	8	35	35	3
30—40	19	87	19	14	16	3
40—50	11.8	89	32	13	15	5
50—60	7.5	92	52	7	8	4
Over 60	3.3	36	46	11	31	14

Note: These statistics suggest:

1. Older people (50 to 60) have the highest positive tuberculin skin test rate.
2. The tuberculin conversion rate is highest among the young (20 to 30 years) and those over 60.
3. Most of the older people had positive tuberculin tests at the time of their employment.

[a] Representative sample of 2384 employess (1977).
[b] No attempt made to correct for length of employment.

Table 5

THE RESULTS OF INH THERAPY ON TUBERCULIN CONVERTERS

	Recent converters after therapy		Converters by history
Treated — 25	<3 months	3—12 months	(>1 year)
Tuberculin reaction			
Reverted	2[a]	5	—
Decreased	—	3	1
Unchanged	—	—	4

Note: Ten employees were lost to follow-up; eight moved away or terminated employment at the hospital; and two discontinued because of medical reasons.

[a] One patient had a negative reaction to her PPD of 8/3/76. Later (2 months, 10/18/76), she had a positive reaction, with an induration of 18 × 20 mm. She received a prescription for Isoniazid in February 1977. She left the hospital and discontinued her INH therapy. She did not receive a prescription from this department for her 6-month supply of Isoniazid. In July 1978, on her return to the hospital as an employee, she had a negative reaction to her routine employee examination PPD. She evidently reverted on a 200-day, or less than 7-month, supply of INH.

Table 6
COST OF INH THERAPY

	Initial visit ($)	2-month follow-up ($)	6-month follow-up ($)	12-month follow-up ($)
Skin test	0.09 (1.50)[a]	—	—	0.09 (1.50)[a]
X-ray	37.00	37.00[b]	37.00	37.00
Blood work	38.00	38.00	38.00	38.00
Medicine	5.00	5.00	10.00	—
Total	80.09	80.00	85.00	75.09

Note: Total cost of 1 year on INH therapy is $320.18.

[a] A patient skin tested at his expense would be charged $1.50. The total cost of therapy would be increased by $2.82.

[b] A converter by history is not X-rayed as part of the 2-month check-up. This would reduce the total cost of therapy for a nondocumented conversion by $37.00, making the cost $283.18.

Exposure to Meningococcal *(Neisseria Meningitidis)* Infections

Infections caused by the miningococcus (*Neisseria meningitidis*) are usually acute life-threatening illnesses characterized by meningitis and/or bloodstream involvement. A petechial rash or purpura may accompany the infections. The responsible organism is a Gram-negative diplococcus which is sensitive to I.V. penicillin; the treatment of choice in such cases. Patients acquire the disease after pharyngeal acquisition of a virulent strain of one of the serogroups (A,Y,B,C, etc.) of *N. meningitidis*.

It is important to emphasize that within any one serogroup, there are a number of types of *N. meningitidis*, only one of which is unusually virulent. The other serotypes are usually found in asymptomatic individuals, who are carrying the organism. Thus, contacts of a case of meningococcal infection who are carriers of the meningococcus, even those with the same serogroup, are not necessarily about to develop illness; they may have been long-term carriers of a different (nonvirulent) serotype.

It is unclear whether the organism enters the bloodstream directly from the pharynx or via the lung after aspiration. The most likely mode of spread from an infected person or carrier to a susceptible person involves large droplet secretions. Airborne (droplet nuclei) spread seems less likely, but possible, perhaps more so with pneumonia caused by *N. meningitidis*.

Certainly the risk of meningococcal infection in hospital employees is very low, and reports are limited. In Feldman's experience, it is most likely to happen after mouth-to-mouth resuscitation.[9] He has also reported a patient who acquired group C meningococcal infection following the transplantation of a kidney inadvertantly obtained from a donor who had died of (unrecognized overwhelming) meningococcal infection.

Recently the CDC reported the case of a 39-year-old nurse who developed group B meningococcal septicemia 3 days after exposure to a patient with group B meningococcal meningitis.[10] The patient had not been placed on respiratory isolation nor had the nurse received prophylactic antibiotics. The patient had been vomiting and did require intubation, and the nurse on careful questioning recalled that she had had exposure to nasopharyngeal secretions from the index patient.

Two other patients (both with cancer) were reported to develop nosocomial transmission of group Y *N. meningitidis* infection while in a clinical research center.[11] The patients were housed in adjacent rooms and became ill within 4 days of each other. Group Y organisms especially seem to be associated with respiratory symptoms, and the suggestion was made that airborne transmission seemed likely in this outbreak.

Furthermore, the recommendation was made that respiratory isolation may be particularly important for patients with meningococcal pneumonia.

The CDC estimates that there is up to 1000-fold risk of acquiring meningococcal illness in family members with a sporadic case compared to the risk in the general population.[12] During an epidemic, the risk to family members exposed to an index case may be 15,000 times the risk in the general population. Those family members of greatest risk seem to be young children, perhaps because they have not yet been exposed to the nonvirulent meningococcal organisms which appear to elicit protective antibody responses. Furthermore, up to one third of secondary cases in households occur within 4 days of hospitalization of the index patient.[13] Thus, by extrapolation of these data, it would appear that the risk to hospital employees is very low in general; that the greatest risk would be after mouth-to-mouth resuscitation or after obvious secretion contact; that pediatric roommates of unisolated cases would be at especially high risk; and that prophylactic antibiotics should be administered to those at risk as early as possible.

The general approach recommended in the medical management of contacts of meningococcal disease includes the following:

1.   Development of a contact list of those who had (or probably had) secretion contact
2.   Reassurance of employees of the low risk of subsequent illness
3.   Administration of prophylactic antibiotics (rifampin in the U.S.) to personnel who may have had exposure to respiratory secretions of the patient
4.   Close monitoring of contacts and immediate evaluation if new symptoms occur which are compatible with meningococcal infection (Note: No attempt is made to culture contacts to identify carriers of the same serogroups since serotyping is not performed.)

The contact list is generated by the nurse epidemiologist as soon as a case is suspected or confirmed, and the ward is visited to be sure that the patient is on Respiratory Isolation. The contact list includes those people who have written in the chart or who are otherwise identified to have close contact with the patient. The list is carried to the employee health nurse, who conducts brief interviews to determine which personnel may have had secretion contact. The latter are instructed about the disease, its low risk to employees, and the need to observe symptoms compatible with other meningococcal infection or side effects of rifampin.

In the U.S., rifampin is the drug choice, since virtually all new isolates of *N. meningitidis* are sensitive and because the drug enters the oral secretions in concentrations effective in erradicating the pharyngeal carrier state.[14] Penicillin, the drug of choice in treating illness, does not reach the oral secretions in sufficient concentration to eradicate the carrier site and therefore is not effective as a prophylactic agent. Other prophylactic agents which can get into oral secretions include sulfonamides and minocycline. The problem with sulfonamides is that a significant percentage of isolates in the U.S. are resistant,[15,16] and thus it may not be effective against many strains of *N. meningitidis*. Minocycline, an effective prophylactic agent, has associated vertigo in such high frequency to make it a second choice only.[17,18]

The dosage of rifampin[4] is as follows:

Adults	600 mg po	q 12 h for 4 doses
Children > 12 months	10 mg/kg po	q 12 h for 4 doses
<12 months	5 mg/kg po	q 12 h for 4 doses

Serious side effects of rifampin are not common, but patients may manifest red discoloration of secretions (tears, stool, and urine), allergy, and elevation of liver enzymes. Its half-life is increased in hepatic dysfunction. Since resistance has developed rapidly in patients treated with rifampin alone, infection control practitioners (ICP) should do their best to minimize unnecessary prescription of rifampin for meningococcal prophylaxis.

The TORCH Diseases and Female Employees of Childbearing Age: The Role of an Employee Health Program

The infection control team working in conjunction with employee health personnel can play a significant role in educating and counseling female employees who may be pregnant or contemplating pregnancy, regarding the possible risk to their unborn child that may be related to their type of employment. In addition to their role in counseling and educating employees, they should work with the administrators of the hospital to formulate hospital policy which will facilitate an understanding of the risks and responsibilities of employee and employer alike. Although there are a wide variety of elements in the hospital setting that are potentially harmful to the unborn children of pregnant personnel, such as ionizing radiation and accidents, this discussion will be limited to a group of infectious diseases known as the TORCH diseases. TORCH is an acronym for *t*oxoplasmosis, "*o*ther", *r*ubella, *c*ytomegalovirus, and *h*erpes simplex infections. The term "other" in the acronym has been used to describe a variety of perinatal infections, such as syphilis, mumps, varicella, variola and vaccinia, hepatitis, the enteroviruses, and various bacteria and protozoan diseases. These "other" infections, although important, will also be excluded from discussion.

The TORCH diseases in the past have been considered a syndrome. The reason for grouping these separate diseases into a single syndrome is that on clinical grounds alone, it is often impossible to distinguish one disease from the other. Table 7 demonstrates the similarities in clinical findings that one may find among infants born with these diseases. The diagnosis often cannot be made without serological confirmation or isolation of the responsible agent or both. Laboratory diagnosis often takes weeks or occasionally months, so it usually is impossible to diagnose precisely the infant's illness during the first few days of life. The inability to make a rapid diagnosis prevents one from precisely defining the risk of spread to susceptible hospital personnel who are caring for the infant. Hospital policy must therefore address the question of the management of these infants prior to a definitive diagnosis, making allowances for all possible etiologic agents.

Toxoplasmosis

Toxoplasma gondii, a protozoan parasite, is the etiologic agent for toxoplasmosis. This organism is found world-wide and is usually associated with animals. Humans are only incidentally infected, usually through contact with cat excreta or eating improperly prepared meat such as raw hamburger. Approximately 70% of infants born with toxoplasmosis are asymptomatic. Although *T. gondii* has been found in saliva and sputum and the organisms are able to survive in cow's milk, saliva, urine, and tears, human-to-human transmission is not thought to occur.[19] The infant with toxoplasmosis presents essentially no risk in terms of infecting nursery personnel.

Rubella

Rubella virus is a small RNA virus. It normally produces a mild febrile illness in young children. If, however, a susceptible pregnant woman comes in contact with the virus during the first or early second trimester of pregnancy, fetal infection may occur.

Table 7

COMPARISON OF SOME OF THE CLINICAL MANIFESTATIONS OF TORCH DISEASES

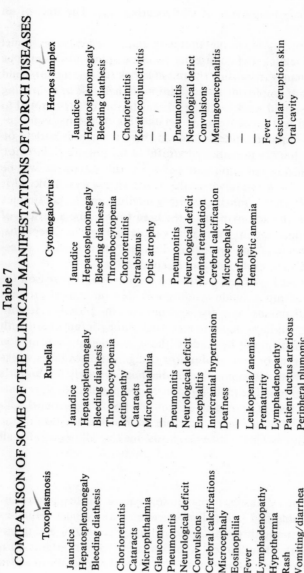

Toxoplasmosis	Rubella	Cytomegalovirus	Herpes simplex
Jaundice	Jaundice	Jaundice	Jaundice
Hepatosplenomegaly	Hepatosplenomegaly	Hepatosplenomegaly	Hepatosplenomegaly
Bleeding diathesis	Bleeding diathesis	Bleeding diathesis	Bleeding diathesis
	Thrombocytopenia	Thrombocytopenia	
Chorioretinitis	Retinopathy	Chorioretinitis	Chorioretinitis
Cataracts	Cataracts	Strabismus	Keratoconjunctivitis
Microphthalmia	Microphthalmia	Optic atrophy	
Glaucoma			
Pneumonitis	Pneumonitis	Pneumonitis	Pneumonitis
Neurological deficit	Neurological deficit	Neurological deficit	Neurological deficit
Convulsions	Encephalitis	Mental retardation	Convulsions
Cerebral calcifications	Intercranial hypertension	Cerebral calcification	Meningoencephalitis
Microcephaly	Deafness	Microcephaly	
Eosinophilia		Deafness	
Fever	Leukopenia/anemia	Hemolytic anemia	Fever
Lymphadenopathy	Prematurity		Vesicular eruption skin
Hypothermia	Lymphadenopathy		Oral cavity
Rash	Patient ductus arteriosus		
Vomiting/diarrhea	Peripheral plumonic stenosis		
	Coarctation of aorta		
	Growth retardation		
	Bony changes		
	Micrognathia		
	Undecended testicles		
	Myocardial necrosis		

Once a fetus becomes infected in utero, abortion or stillbirth may occur, or the fetus may be born with many, few, or no symptoms or signs. Congenital rubella is a chronic infection in that the virus persists in the fetus throughout gestation and can be recovered for up to 24 months following delivery from multiple sites, such as urine, feces, pharynx, conjunctiva, and CSF. Approximately 70% of infants infected with rubella virus are asymptomatic.

Close contact appears to be necessary for the efficient transmission of rubella virus. Since the virus can be easily recovered from the upper respiratory tract, transmission through the air is possible, but it is unclear whether infectious particles can travel great distances and infect susceptible individuals. Direct contact with infective secretions appears to be an efficient mode of transmission. Virus has been recovered from fomites that have been in contact with the excretions and secretions of affected infants, so transmission is theoretically possible via these inanimate objects. Of particular interest is the report by Schiff and Dine[20] that virus was recovered from the nipple of a bottle used by an infant with congenital rubella. Seeff[4] and Harty et al.[21] have reported studies in which hospital personnel apparently have acquired rubella from congenitally infected infants. Seventy-five percent of susceptible student nurses studied by Schiff and colleagues,[20,22] acquired rubella while caring for affected infants. A susceptible student nurse developed rubella 12 days following a deliberate exposure for 1½ hr to a congenitaly infected infant during which time she fed, held, changed the diaper, and generally played with the infant. Susceptibility to rubella correlates well with a hemagglutination inhibition antibody titer ≤1:8. Commercially available tests seem to be reasonably accurate, as long as nonspecific inhibitors are removed from test sera according to manufacturer's directions.

Cytomegalovirus

The cytomegalovirus (CMV) is a DNA virus of the herpesvirus family. This virus is found world-wide and nearly everyone at some time or another during his life is infected with this virus. Despite considerable research, the pathogenesis of CMV is poorly understood; and, like others of the herpesvirus family, latency and reactivation or reinfection often make it difficult to distinguish a primary infection from reinfection or reactivation of a latent viral infection. CMV infection is the most common of the TORCH diseases. Some 1 to 5% of all newborns are infected, and many more neonates acquire the virus shortly after birth. Approximately 95% of infants born with CMV infections are asymptomatic. There appear to be several different strains of CMV that are genetically unique. The AD 169 strain is the most commonly used antigen for serological testing, but since it does not cross react with all other known strains, serologic testing may be an unreliable indicator of all infections. The complement fixation antibody test is the most widely used antigen-antibody test system and titers ≥1:8 probably indicate prior contact with the virus. Since complement fixing antibody does not persist for more than several years, low titers may mean nothing more than infection in the more distant past.

The potential routes of transmission are numerous, since CMV has been recovered from urine, pharynx, feces, milk, semen, tears, and cervical secretions, as well as from a variety of organs, such as liver, lung, kidney, brain, etc. The precise mechanism of transmission is essentially unknown. Yeager performed complement fixation and indirect hemagglutination antibody tests on three groups of hospital personnel over a period of approximately 1½ to 2½ years.[23] No seroconversions occurred among personnel who had no patient contact, whereas two seroconversions occurred among a group of nursery nurses and three seroconversions occurred among ward nurses. These differences were not statistically significant, and other sources of infection outside of the hospital setting were not considered. Cox and Hughes studied two groups of children with acute lymphoblastic leukemia to determine if isolation procedures during outpatient visits and hospitalizations influenced their acquisition of CMV.[24] He was not able to demonstrate any difference between the two groups.

Herpes Simplex

The herpes simplex viruses (HSV) are DNA viruses of the herpesvirus family and can be divided into two antigenically distinct strains — type 1 and type 2. The majority of infections among neonates have been associated with type 2 virus. As with the CMV, the HSV can produce a latent infection, so it is often difficult to distinguish primary infection from reinfection or reactivation of a latent viral infection. In addition, it is difficult serologically to distinguish primary from recurrent infection. Furthermore, in spite of circulating neutralizing antibodies, the virus can be shed from various body sites. Close intimate contact probably is necessary for transmission of the virus, and there is no well-documented evidence that HSV can be spread via the airborne route. Outbreaks of herpetic whitlow among medical personnel who have handled patient's oral secretions demonstrate that transmission can occur via infective oral secretions, even in the absence of obvious oral lesions. Francis et al.[26] described an infant 6 weeks of age who acquired fatal herpes simplex type 2 disseminated disease shortly after three other infants in an intensive care unit died of maternally acquired herpes simplex disease. Transmission of the virus was thought to have occurred via the hands of nursery personnel. Linneman et al.[27] reported an outbreak involving two infants due to HSV type 1, and by DNA "fingerprinting" the isolates were shown to be identical.[9] The source of virus was thought to have been either the herpes labialis lesion of the father of one of the infants or hospital personnel. Serological testing is not widely available. Neonates infected with HSV are usually symptomatic — fewer than 5% will be asymptomatic.

Conclusions

The suggested guidelines found in Table 8 may be useful in establishing hospital policy regarding occupational exposure to the TORCH diseases. It is reasonable to screen and vaccinate susceptible female employees who may be at risk of developing rubella. Rubella's high communicability, its demonstrated ability to produce infection among susceptibles when exposed to affected infants, and the availability of good serological testing procedures support the rationale for such a program. The situation with CMV is somewhat different. Since there is no vaccine available, there is no convincing evidence that patient contact is associated with increased risk of infection, and since there is no widely available serologic test that is easily interpretable, there seems at present to be no need for a formalized screening program. Hospital personnel, however, should become knowledgeable regarding the mode of transmission of CMV and be aware that many infants that appear normal may be excreting the virus. Good handwashing practices and avoiding direct contact (nuzzling and kissing newborns or putting their fingers in the newborn's mouth) are common sense precautions that should be incorporated into hospital policy. A formalized screening procedure to determine susceptibility to HSV is not warranted because of the general unavailability of serological testing methods and the inability to interpret the results rationally. Unlike rubella and CMV, the asymptomatic infant infected with HSV is infrequently encountered, but common sense precautions such as good handwashing or the use of gloves during suctioning procedures or other manipulations in which the hands are in contact with body secretions/excretions, should be part of a hospital's policy and educational effort. A formalized policy for determining susceptibility to toxoplasmosis is unneces-

Table 8
SUGGESTED GUIDELINES FOR ESTABLISHING HOSPITAL POLICY REGARDING OCCUPATIONAL EXPOSURE TO TORCH DISEASES

1. Refer to accepted guidelines for isolation procedures for specific disease entities when a diagnosis of toxoplasmosis, rubella, CMV, or HSV infection is established (e.g., *Isolation Techniques for Use in Hospitals*[58]).
2. Since TORCH diseases are difficult to distinguish clinically one from another and various modes of transmission (or nontransmission in the case of toxoplasmosis) to hospital personnel might be involved, it is suggested that until the diagnosis of a specific TORCH disease is confirmed that all infants suspected of having TORCH syndrome should be placed in strict isolation. Once a specific diagnosis is established, appropriate isolation techniques can be utilized.
3. Screen all female hospital employees with patient contact for susceptibility to rubella using the hemagglutination inhibition (HAI) method. Vaccinate all susceptibles (titer ≤1:8) who can remain nonpregnant for 3 months following vaccination. Retest all vaccinees 6 weeks following vaccination to confirm response (see Note below). Susceptibles should refrain from patient contact, particularly high-risk patient populations, such as newborn nurseries and pediatric wards, until protective antibody status is assured.
4. Develop common sense policies and procedures for managing all infants and children that take into account known modes of transmission of the TORCH diseases, since a high percentage of infected patients are asymptomatic. Educate personnel as to the "state of the art" of knowledge about TORCH diseases, so they can make informed decisions about personal risks relating to their employment.

Note: The numbers of female employees who have antibody titers <1:8 will vary among hospitals, but generally the numbers should be small. Each hospital should examine its experience in this regard to determine if it is cost benefcial to retest vaccinated employees. Some 90 to 95% of vaccinees seroconvert, so it may be worthwhile retesting only those employees in contact with high-risk populations.

sary because of the lack of evidence of human-to-human transmission. Sound policies constantly updated as new data are available and education and counseling provided by members of the infection control team and employee health personnel should go a long way to minimizing risks.

MANAGEMENT OF EMPLOYEES WHO ARE CARRIERS OF COMMON PATHOGENIC ORGANISMS

Staphylococcus aureus Carriers

Humans are the reservoir and in most instances the direct transmitters of staphylococci. Nahmias and Eickhoff outlined the sources and modes of nosocomial transmission of staphylococci (see Figure 6) and indicated there are only two sources: a person with a lesion and the asymptomatic carrier.[28] Although the two sources are closely linked epidemiologically and clinically (e.g., the person with a lesion may be a patient or a hospital employee, and one may have transmitted the organism to the other), the following discussion will be limited only to the asymptomatic carrier of *Staphylococcus aureus.*

Why a particular individual, when he or she comes in contact with *S. aureus*, develops clinical disease, becomes a carrier, or does neither is incompletely understood in spite of considerable study by many investigators for nearly 100 years. There are several clinical situations that favor carriage of this organism, including increasing length of hospitalization[29] and treatment with antimicrobial drugs.[30] Shinefield et al. demonstrated that the "take" rate of *S. aureus* 502A was lower among carriers treated with placebo prior to challenge with 502A than those treated with oxacillin.[30] In contrast, in noncarriers the use of oxacillin or placebo made no difference in the "take" rates. The number and phage type of organisms existing at any particular body site seem to influence the ability of that site to become colonized with *S. aureus*.[30] The role of local and systemic immune factors in the development of the carrier state are poorly understood.

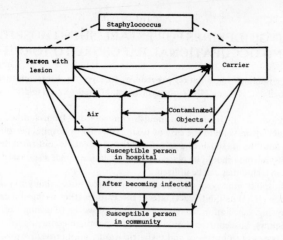

FIGURE 6. Epidemiologic cycle of staphylococci in the hospital and community. (From Nahmias, A. J. and Eickhoff, T. C., *N. Engl. J. Med.*, 265, 74, 1961. With permission.)

Table 9
SKIN CARRIAGE OF *STAPHYLOCOCCUS AUREUS*

Body part	Williams (1946) (%)	Ridley (1959) (%)	Noble (1969) (%)
Nose	88	84	9
Chest	24	—	1
Abdomen	32	32	1
Groin	—[a]	44	1
Thigh	32	30	1
Shin	32	—	1
Axilla	16	16	<1
Forearm	40	—	1
Back	24	—	<1
Total respondents	50 males	50 males	378 males and females

[a] Site not sampled.

Adapted from Nobel, W. C., *Contrib. Microbiol. Immunol.*, 1, 537, 1973.

Classification of Carriers: Body Site

S. aureus may be carried asymptomatically on almost any skin or mucous membrane surface of the body; Table 9 summarizes the experience of three investigators regarding the relative frequency of recovering this organism according to body site.[31] Since the anterior nares are a convenient body site to sample and seem to be one of the most commonly colonized sites, most reports in the literature and most epidemiological surveys focus on nasal carriage. However, when attempting to solve a particular outbreak, one should keep in mind the other body sites. Hill et al.[32] and Mitchell and Gamble[33] have demonstrated that males are often heavy dispersers of this organism from their perineal/groin areas, so these sites should not be overlooked when seeking the source of an outbreak.

Most staphylococci carried in the nose are carried in the anterior portion (vestibule) of the nasal cavity.[34] It is thought that the skin of the nasal vestibule (mucosal-skin interface) is the site of multiplication of the bacteria. This has practical implications for culturing techniques. Often nasopharyngeal (N-P) swabs are requested by clinicians seeking to determine nasal carrier status. N-P cultures are uncomfortable for the patient, and if improperly done can traumatize the nasal cavity. Persons being cultured, particularly those involved in epidemiological work-up of a problem, are often defensive and feel that the mere fact that they are being cultured is an indictment of their guilt in causing disease. An unnecessarily painful culturing technique adds nothing to dispel these feelings or encourage cooperation in the investigation. A simple swabbing of the skin just inside the nose is painless and an adequate sample when staphylococcal nasal carriage status is one's objective.

Classification of Carriers: Duration of Carriage

Depending on the length of time that a particular individual carries *S. aureus*, it is possible to classify carriers into the following groups: persistent carriers (15 to 35% of persons), intermittent carriers (15 to 65%), and noncarriers (15 to 25%). Persistent carriers harbor the same or different strains of *S. aureus* for long periods of time, whereas noncarriers rarely if ever are found to be colonized with the organism. Intermittent carriers alternate periods of carriage with periods of free from colonization. Among persistent and intermittent carriers, some are disseminators or dispersers of the organism (see Figure 7). These persons seem to be particularly effective in transmitting their organisms from their sites of carriage to other persons or inanimate objects and are epidemiologically important particularly if the strains are "virulent". Unfortunately, simply by culturing the noses of a group of people, one cannot determine which ones are persistent carriers who are good dispersers of virulent organisms.

Therapy

When indicated clinically and epidemiologically, therapy designed to eradicate or suppress the carrier state should be chosen according to the body site involved and the particular drug allergy history of the carrier. For body sites other than the nose or mucous membranes, hexachlorophene (3%) bathing on a regular daily basis will reduce the number of organisms transiently. It has been noted, moreover, that showering without an antibacterial soap may increase the numbers of resident bacteria on the skin surfaces, presumably by allowing organisms which normally reside in skin appendages (hair follicles, sebaceous glands, etc.) to spread over the skin surface after the transient flora has been removed.[31] It must be remembered that the use of antibacterial soaps are suppressive and do not eradicate the carrier state. During hospital epidemics of *S. aureus*, the Hospital Infections Branch, Bureau of Epidemiology, CDC has recommended (personal communication) the use of creams containing bacitracin or gentamicin for treating epidemiologically implicated nasal carriers. Nahmias and Eickhoff, however, point out that these topical agents should be used with caution because of their potential for selecting antibiotic-resistant staphylococci.[35] Again such forms of treatment are often only suppressive; thus, adequate follow-up is necessary. Recently a regimen of orally administered cloxacillin and rifampin has been used to treat occasional individuals (epidemiologically linked to a problem) from whom the organism could not be eradicated using topical nasal antibiotics.[36] In patients who have a history of allergy to the usual topical antibacterial agents, erythromycin has been shown to be effective in temporarily suppressing nasal colonization.[37] Efficacy of topical ointments remain unproven, and a recent pilot study suggested no benefit of either bacitracin ointment (500 units/g) or vancomycin ointment (5 mg/g) four times a day for 14 days compared to the untreated control group.[37a]

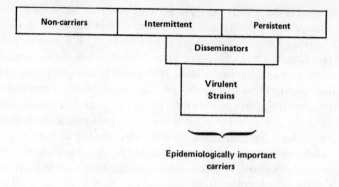

FIGURE 7.   *Staphylococcus aureus* carriage — a schematic representation.

An Approach to Problems Involving Carriers

Those with responsibility for the health of the hospital's employees should work
closely with the infection control team in establishing an approach to staphylococcal
disease and the carrier state. Routine culture surveys of personnel a. are not cost effective, b. generate data that are difficult to interpret, and c. generate data that may be
impossible to act on in terms of treating those found to be positive (imagine 50% of
hospital personnel on nasal gentamicin!). A more reasonable approach would be to
monitor the occurrence of staphylococcal disease such that, for example, when two
cases of disease among personnel or patients occur on the same ward during the same
week, an epidemiologic investigation would be initiated. If there were epidemiologic
evidence that the two cases were linked, then the epidemiologiclly implicated persons
would be cultured. Remember that the mere presence of *S. aureus* in the nose of a
hospital employee does not imply that that person was the "source" — he or she could
just as easily be the "victim" of a patient with a lesion. Once the epidemiologically
involved persons have been cultured, one must realize that the culture results will not
be known for 24 to 48 hr, and antibiograms and phage typing will take even longer.
What should one do with the individuals that have been cultured? Depending on the
severity of the problem and the numbers of personnel involved the following options
are open: a. remove all involved personnel from duty until culture results indicate they
are not harboring the organism, and b. allow all personnel to continue to work pending
culture results, but stress proper handwashing and aseptic techniques. There are no
data that indicate one option is superior. Certainly, the first option would be the conservative approach. Once culture results are available and the numbers of persons possibly implicated are reduced, then an additional option becomes available: treat all
culture positive persons. The risk of treatment vs. the option of removal from work
pending antibiogram/phage typing results again must be addressed. Once all epidemiologic and clinical data are available, the following should be considered for each
implicated individual: a. therapy aimed at eradication of the organism, if possible and
b. long-term follow-up to determine if the carrier state has been eradicated. If the
carrier state cannot be eradicated, the person should be studied to determine if he or
she is a disperser. If the patient is not a disperser, then education designed to reduce
the risk of transmission may be tried. If the person is found to be a disperser that is
resistant to therapy, a job change may be necessary. Probably as important as what
options and courses of action are taken is the working together of the employee health
team and the infection control team and the formulating of reasonable options prior
to the time when their use is required.

Streptococcus pyogenes Carriers

The term "carrier", as applied to the individual from whom *Streptococcus pyogenes* is cultured, has varied widely in its usuage in the medical literature. Some have used the term broadly to apply to any person from whom this organism has been recovered. Hamburger et al. used the term in this manner in describing the epidemiology of streptococcal disease in the military during World War II.[38] Others more recently have reserved the usage of the term for those individuals from whom the organism can be recovered, but in whom there is no evidence of active symptomatic infection. This confusion of terms may be partially due to the uncertainty in clinically differentiating streptococcal pharyngitis from pharyngitis due to other causes (e.g., a pharyngitis due to a viral agent in a patient who chronically harbors S. pyogenes in his pharynx.).[39] In the hospital setting, the broader definition of carriage may be the more useful since nosocomial outbreaks of disease due to S. pyogenes have been traced to both symptomatic, as well as asymptomatic carriers of this organism.

S. pyogenes has been recovered from nearly every external body surface and orifice. The pharynx, skin, vagina, and anus are epidemiologically the most important body sites from which this organism can be recovered in terms of transmission of this organism in the hospital setting.

Pharyngeal Carriage

The prevalence of pharyngeal carriage of *S. pyogenes* may vary according to degree of crowding, age, and season of the year. Crowding, as is often seen in institutional settings and in the military, is associated with high prevalence of carriage as well as explosive outbreaks. Streptococcal pharyngitis is usually seen in the winter and early spring and is associated with more northern regions of the U.S. School-age children more frequently carry the organism than infants. During the winter as many as 30% of children will harbor this organism, while carrier rates among adults are thought to be generally quite low. Streptococcal pharyngitis, usually manifested by fever, sore throat, cervical adenitis, and pharyngeal exudate, is clinically difficult to differentiate from other causes of the same symptom complex, such as pharyngitis due to the Epstein-Barr virus, diphtheria, various respiratory viruses, *Mycoplasma pneumoniae*, and in some cases, unknown agents. Nearly one third of patients with documented streptococcal pharyngeal infections may have no symptoms, and an equal number will have such mild symptoms that they do not seek medical advice. The diagnosis of streptococcal pharyngitis usually rests with the recovery of the organism from the throat. One must remember, however, that if only one pharyngeal culture is performed, approximately 10% of positive cases will be missed compared to results if two cultures had been taken.[40] Many experts feel that a diagnostic antibody titer rise to the Streptolysin O antigen (or DNAse B antigen) are necessary for diagnosis of infection as opposed to carriage.

Skin Carriage

The frequency with which *S. pyogenes* can be recovered from the normal skin is probably low. Streptococcal skin infections may be classified as superficial or deep. The former include impetigo, pyoderma, and secondary infections of traumatic skin lesions, such as abrasions and eczema or other chronic skin disorders. Deeper skin infections are usually associated with cellulitis, wounds, and burns. Staphylococci are frequent secondary invaders in many superficial infections and occasionally can produce confusion in diagnosis. Additionally, staphylococci may inhibit the growth of streptococci on a sheep blood agar plate, but the addition of one part per million crystal violet to the agar will alleviate this problem. The diagnosis is facilitated by culturing the lesions in their early stages when the streptococci are more abundant. Superficial skin infections with *S. pyogenes* are more common in the summer and fall and are associated with more southern regions in contrast to pharyngeal infections. In common with pharyngeal infections, however, superficial skin infections are more commonly found in crowded conditions, and among young children. Many streptococcal skin infections, both superficial and deep, are related to specific predisposing factors such as trauma or chronic skin disorders.

Vaginal Carriage

Vaginal carriage of *S. pyogenes* in adult women seems to be of low incidence. On the other hand, Hedlund[42] reorted that 10 to 15% of his patients with streptococcal sore throats had vaginal infections with the same strain, and Boisvert[43] found that one half of his patients with vaginitis due to this organism also had *S. pyogenes* in a nasopharyngeal cultures.[44] Vulvovaginitis due to this organism usually produces local irritation and a moderate amount of yellow discharge. The discharge is frequently described as blood tinged and may be quite thick. The diagnosis usually rests with the recovery of the organism, and serological tests are apparently of no value. An asymptomatic vaginal carrier of *S. pyogenes* was implicated in an outbreak of hospital acquired infection. She worked in an operating room and on testing was found to be a good disperser of organisms.

Anal Carriage

S. pyogenes can be recovered from the stool, particularly of individuals suffering from scarlet fever. Anal carriage of this organism may be symptomatic, mildly symptomatic, or asymptomatic. Symptomatic infection often involves a cellulitis of the anal and perinanal areas. Children with this disease often complain of painful defecation and may have secondary constipation. Adults on the other hand may only complain of severe pruritus. Symptomatic infections are seen at the same time of year that respiratory streptococcal infections are prevalent. Frequently other members of the families of these patients will be harboring *S. pyogenes*. The diagnoses can be made usually with a culture of the erythematous skin in the perinanal region. Mildly symptomatic cases usally are seen in adults, and these patients usually complain of mild pruritus. Asymptomatic individuals, on careful examination, may have an anatomical abnormality noted. This abnormality may be a small fissure, a slightly erythematous tag, or excoriations indicating chronic pruritus. There have been several reports of nosocomial *S. pyogenes* infections that have been traced to anal carriers.[45-47] Operating room personnel were implicated in each case and on testing were found to be good dispersers of the organisms. In several cases the organisms could not be recovered from other body sites. Anal carriage should be considered whenever hospital outbreaks of *S. pyogenes* infections are occurring.

Transmission

Transmission of *S. pyogenes* is usually human to human and only in rare instances are animals involved in the spread of this organism. The possible modes of transmission of this organism include the following: aerosols (airborne droplet nuclei), droplets, direct contact, and vectors. Airborne droplet nuclei is not thought to be a major mechanism for the transmission of these organisms. Droplets appear to be one of the more common mechanisms of transmission. Crowding is a significant epidemiologic factor in disease caused by this organism, suggesting the airborne route as a major means of transmission. Direct contact certainly plays a significant role in the transmission of skin infections due to *S. pyogenes*. In various parts of the world, it has been

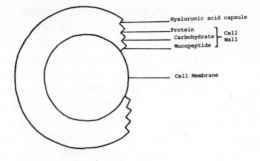

FIGURE 8. Schematic diagram of the *Strepto-coccus pyogenes.* The protein layer contains the M, T, and R antigens, and the carbohydrate layer contains the group-specific antigens.

thought that vectors, such as flies and mosquitoes, may play a role in transmitting streptococcal skin infections.

Epidemiologic Markers of Streptococcus pyogenes

Structural and immunological characteristics of this organism play an important role in studying the disease in a hospital setting. *S. pyogenes* is the taxonomic designation for the Lancefield group A streptococcus. Figure 8 is a schematic diagram of the capsule, cell wall, and cell membrane. Not all group A streptococci have a capsule that appears to have some antiphagocytic properties. From a clinical and epidemiological point of view, the cell wall is probably the most important structal component of the organism. The carbohydrate layer contains the group-specific substance, on which the grouping of streptococci are based. This polysaccharide reacts in a precipitin reaction with group specific antisera to differentiate group A from other groups, such as B, C, D, etc. Epidemiologically it is important to group streptococci because the usual presumptive tests for classification used clinically (presence of beta-hemolysis, sensitivity to a 0.02 unit bacitracin disk, and identify with fluorescence-tagged antibody) are too inaccurate for epidemiologic purposes. Other beta-hemolytic streptococci belonging to groups B, C, G, etc. also may be found in various body sites. One should also be aware that not all group A streptococci are beta-hemolytic. James and McFarland[48] reported an outbreak of pharyngitis, involving several cases of subsequent rheumatic fever, due to a group A streptococcus that was not beta-hemolytic.

The protein layer contains several different protein antigens. The M protein antigens, of which there are over 50, appear to be virulence factors and antibody to these proteins confer type-specific, long-lasting immunity. The T and R protein antigens (although they apparently do not have a significant biolgical role for the organism) and the M antigen serve as epidemiologic markers. The M and T antigens are epidemiologically the more important of the protein antigens and in addition to the group-specific carbohydrate, should be determined in any epidemiologic work-up involving group A streptococci. As with any typing system, it is useful to remember that even though the same type of group A streptococci are recovered from two or more persons, this does not "prove" one actually acquired this organism from the other person. Typing information must be used in conjunction with all other clinical and epidemiological information.

Management of Carriers

It is epidemiologically useful to think of *S. pyogenes* as "a people pathogen". Group

A streptococcal infections usually are acquired from people, not from the environment. Although pharyngeal and skin infections are the most common group A streptococcal infections and these are the most common sites cultured when investigating an outbreak of strepcoccal disease in a hospital, other body sites, such as the vagina and anus, should not be overlooked as possible sources for the outbreak.

In a hospital setting, the treatment of individuals who are found to be harboring *S. pyogenes* is reasonably straight forward. Once an individual or group of individuals have been implicated epidemiologically as being possibly important in an outbreak, they should be cultured from multiple sites, including all obvious lesions, pharynx, rectum, and vagina. Two swabs from each site would enhance the possibility of recovering the organism. Those individuals from whom the organism is recovered should be treated appropriately. Patients who harbor group A streptococci in their pharynx should be treated with 1.2 millon units of benzathine penicillin. Smaller doses should be used for children, and in the penicillin-allergic individual, erythromycin is an appropriate second drug of choice. Similar drugs may be used for streptococcal skin infections, even if staphylococci are present in the lesions. Experience with treating pyoderma in children has indicated that the presence of staphylococci does not interfere with the response to penicillin preparations.[49] Although there are no controlled studies indicating the best drugs for treating anal and vaginal carriage, penicillin has been used in both situations, with reasonably good results. Vancomycin given orally was used in treating some of the anal carriers.[47,48] The vancomycin was given in anticipation of penicillin inactivation by the penicillinase producing bowel flora.

Although the incidence of infections due to *S. pyogenes* seems to have decreased somewhat in recent years and cheap, relatively nontoxic drugs are available to treat these infections, those persons concerned with hospital acquired infections in both patients and employees will occasionally encounter problems caused by this organism. Such persons should be aware of the usual and unusual sources of this organism, its mode of transmission, and the various clinical syndromes associated with infection, otherwise important facts relative to an epidemic may be overlooked and the problem unnecessarily prolonged.

FOOD HANDLERS

Nearly all state and local governments have laws regarding food establishments. The laws usually include specifications for storage, preparations, and serving of food and for sanitation of utensils involved in the preparation and serving of foods. The laws focus on minimizing intrinsic contamination (microorganisms already present in food) and extrinsic contamination (microorganisms innoculated into food during the preparation and serving process). In addition, statutes are included concerning the health of those persons engaged in the preparation and serving of food. An example of such statues can be found in Title 10, Section 4, of the Department of Health and Mental Hygiene, Environmental Health Administration, State of Maryland.

> While affected with a disease in a communicable form, or while a carrier of a disease, or while afflicted with boils, infected wounds, or an acute respiratory infection, a person may not work in a food service facility in an area and capacity in which there is a likelihood of transmission of disease to patrons or to fellow employees, either through direct contact or through contamination of food or food contact surfaces with pathogenic organisms. The manager or person in charge of the establishment shall notify the approving authority when any employee of a food service facility is known to have or is suspected of having a disease in a communicable form.

Employee health personnel should familarize themselves with state and local laws, the mechanisms of inspection and enforcement of these laws, and work with the hos-

Table 10
FACTORS CONTRIBUTING TO 493
FOODBORNE OUTBREAKS

Factor	Outbreaks (%)
Inadequate refrigeration	68
Food preparation far in advance of serving	32
Infected persons and poor personal hygiene	31
Inadequate cooking or heating	28
Food kept warm at wrong temperature	23
Contaminated raw materials in uncooked foods	17
Inadequate reheating	13
Cross-contamination	12
Inadequate cleaning of equipment	11
Other conditions	32

Adapted from Bryan, F. L., *Food Technol.*, 28, 52, 1974.

pital administration to formulate hospital policies and procedures compatible with these local and state codes.

Many microorganisms and chemical agents have caused contamination of food that has lead to foodborne outbreaks.[50] In addition, a variety of factors have contributed to the contamination of foods by microorganisms as shown in Table 10. Although many of these factors are important, the following discussion will be limited to the management of food handlers with salmonellosis, shigellosis, hepatitis, and certain parasitic diseases.

Salmonellosis

Salmonellae are aerobic, Gram-negative nonincapsulated, nonspore-forming, motile, rod-shaped bacteria. Three species are included in the genus *salmonella*: a. *typhi*, b. *choleraesuis*, and c. *enteritidis*. Some 1400 different serotypes are included in the last species. Except for *Salmonella typhi*, salmonellae are found in a wide variety of animals. *S. typhi* is almost exclusively found in humans, either carriers or those with active disease.

Epidemiology

Contaminated food or water is the primary mode of transmission of salmonellosis, although direct person-to-person spread has been reported, and the airborne and vector routes are at least potential mechanisms of transmission. Since 1900 there has been a decreasing incidence of disese because of *S. typhi*. Approximately 85% of chronic carriers of *S. typhi* are over 50 years of age, and carriers are the major source of infection. Carriers may excrete more than 10^6 organisms per gram of feces, and urinary carriage may also occur. Females are more than three times as likely to be carriers as males.

The major source of infection with salmonellae other than *S. typhi* is animals. Meat, particularly beef and fowl, eggs and egg products, pharmaceutical products, and water are common sources of salmonellae. Asymptomatic carriers have been less commonly implicated as sources of disease. Food handlers, probably by virtue of their constant exposure to contaminated food stuffs, seem to have a somewhat higher carrier rate than the general population. Carriers, in addition to contaminating food, have been a source of person-to-person spread, particularly in institutions.[51]

Pathogenesis

The primary portal of entry of salmonellae is the oral route. Most people probably ingest salmonellae daily, but in quantities insufficient to produce infections. Natural host defenses, such as gastric acidity, intestinal motility, and gut flora, prevent infection (see chapter entitled "Gastrointestinal Infections"). Depending on the infecting organism, the pathogenesis can vary. Those organisms producing a typhoidal syndrome reenter the bloodstream from their intracellular sites in the reticuloendothelial system, produce a sustained bacteremia which infects the biliary tract, and then repopulate the GI tract. This bacteremia in and of itself may cause a wide variety of clinical signs and symptoms. Those species of salmonella that produce a gastroenteritis syndrome cause a local inflammatory response in the GI tract approximately 6 to 48 hr following ingestion, and bacteremia is an uncommon event.

Isolation of the organism from stool, blood, urine, or other clinically involved sites is the only definitive diagnostic maneuver. A fourfold rise in agglutinins against somatic and flagellar antigens is presumptive evidence of infection, as long as there is no history of recent immunization. A single high titer is of no value in diagnosis. *S. typhi* can be isolated from the blood in nearly all cases during the first week of illness, in about one half of cases by the third week, and rarely after the fourth week of illness. Isolation of *S. typhi* from the stool can best be achieved during the fourth week of illness. After 6 weeks, GI shedding of the organism decreases, and by 1 year, 3% of cases are still culture positive. Patients still positive 1 year after illness are termed chronic carriers. Chronic carriers shed large numbers of organisms and most have chronic biliary tract infections. Patients with gastroenteritis syndromes rarely have *Salmonella* organisms cultured from the blood, but nearly all will be shedding organisms in the stool. In 2 weeks following onset of illness, approximately one half of cases will no longer have positive stool cultures, and by 4 weeks, only about 10% are still culture positive. Rarely will fecal carriage last 6 months or more.

Chloramphenicol is the drug of choice for treating salmonellosis due to *S. typhi*. Antimicrobial susceptibility testing should be performed to determine if a chloramphenicol-resistant strain is involved, in which case ampicillin or trimethoprim sulfamethoxazole should be used. Regardless of in vitro susceptibility to other agents (e.g. cephalosporins), agents other than chloramphenicol, trimethoprim sulfamethoxazole, or ampicillin have been of no clinical value.

Management of Food Handlers

The management of the food handler with salmonellosis must be guided by the clinical situation, local and state laws, and hospital policy. The following guidelines may be helpful in the management of food handlers.

1. Symptomatic or asymptomatic infected individuals should be removed immediately from food handling responsibilities.
2. Antimicrobial therapy will be determined by clinical findings.
3. Hospital policy should not financially penalize the employee. Such policies will encourage employees to refrain from reporting possible serious illnesses.
4. When clinically indicated the employee may return to work in a nonfood-handling capacity; personal hygiene and handwashing practices should be stressed.
5. Frequency of culturing and follow-up examinations are usually determined by

law, but, if not, it seems reasonable that the employee may handle food after three negative cultures, performed on different days, are obtained.

Shigellosis

Shigellae are aerobic, Gram-negative, nonmotile, rod-shaped bacteria. They are divided into four major groups, A to D, that encompass nearly 50 serotypes. Group A consists of *Shigella dysenteriae* and is uncommon in this country, as is group C which includes *Shigella boydii*. *Shigella flexneri*, a member of group B, is less commonly found at present in the U.S. compared to the early 1960s. Group D consists of *Shigella sonnei*, the most common cause of shigellosis in the U.S. today. *Shigella* is rarely found outside of the human, and there is no important animal or inanimate reservoir. Acids destroy the organism, but under ideal conditions, the organism can persist in foods or water.

Epidemiology

Human-to-human transmission by the fecal-oral route is the major mode of spread, but foodborne and waterborne outbreaks of disease have been reported.[52] Vectors such as flies have been suspected of having a role in transmission, but there is no evidence that they are an important mechanism in the U.S. In contrast to salmonellosis, general sanitation improvement has not resulted in a dramatic decrease in shigellosis. In fact, shigellosis has been reported in increasing numbers in the U.S. in the past decade. Three fourths of all cases are in children, and children are epidemiologically the most important age group in maintaining a human reservoir. Institutional settings account for many cases.

Pathogenesis

In contrast to salmonellosis, relatively few organisms need be ingested to produce infection. Two hundred organisms will cause illness in approximately one fourth of volunteers, and three fourths will become ill following ingestion of 10^5 organisms: organisms that reach the small bowel and colon, penetrate the epithelial cells, and replicate in the lamina propria or submucosa without further dissemination in the body. Bloodstream invasion is extremely rare. Microabscesses form in the submucosa, and the colonic mucosa becomes friable, with small ulcers that bleed easily. Antacids seem to increase the risk of infection, but unlike salmonellosis, there are few systemic illnesses that predispose patients to shigellosis. The role of exotoxins and endotoxins in the pathogenesis is unclear.

The diagnosis rests with isolation of the organism from the stool. Culture techniques are key in maximizing the recovery of shigellae from the stool. Rectal swabs are not as satisfactory as stool specimens. Delay in innoculating specimens reduce the efficiency of recovery of the organism. Flecks of blood or mucous in stool specimens have high concentrations of organisms and are ideal material for culture. Serological testing is usually of little value in establishing diagnosis.

Very mild or asymptomatic infections of persons who can maintain good personal hygiene and who are at low risk of transmission to others need not be treated.[53] Those with moderate or severe symptoms should be treated, as should those who are at particular risk of transmitting the disease to others. These persons include young children, food handlers (including those who prepare food in the home), institutionalized persons, or those in whom personal hygiene is in question. Widespread resistance, particularly to ampicillin and tetracycline, demand that antimicrobial susceptibility testing guide therapy. Trimethoprim sulfamethoxazole has been shown to be as effective as ampicillin in treating shigellosis in an ambulatory setting.

Management of Food Handlers

The management of the food handler with shigellosis should be approached in a fashion similar to that as described earlier for salmonellosis. The following guidelines may be helpful in the management of such food handlers.

1. Symptomatic or asymptomatic persons should be removed from food handling responsibilities.
2. Food handlers should be treated.
3. Hospital policy should not financially penalize the employee. Such policies will encourage employees to avoid reporting serious illnesses.
4. Return to work should be allowed when clinically feasible and when allowed by law. In the absence of such laws, three negative cultures (adequately performed — see above) on different days is probably reasonable.
5. Individuals in close contact, such as family members of the food handler, should be cultured so as to identify human reservoirs that may reintroduce infection in the food handler.

Foodborne outbreaks of hepatitis A traced to food handlers are not uncommon. To date, there is no evidence that food handlers with hepatitis B constitute a significant risk to consumers of the food they have prepared, and transmission of hepatitis B by food has not been documented.[55] There are insufficient data regarding non-A, non-B hepatitis to determine whether such an illness in a food handler can be transmitted by food to other persons. It is important therefore when a food handler develops signs and symptoms compatible with viral hepatitis, that the particular type of hepatitis be determined.

Since the HBsAg is present in infected patient's serum for several weeks before onset of clinical illness, testing of the serum of a food handler in whom clinical hepatitis is present for HB,Ag, using radioimmunoassay or reversed passive hemagglutination, should be performed as soon as the diagnosis is suspected. If HbsAg is present in the serum, it can mean either that the patient is acutely ill with hepatitis B or that the patient is a chronic carrier (persistently antigenemic) of HBsAg in whom a superimposed hepatitis of another etiology is present. To resolve this dilemma, Anti-HBs can be determined using passive hemagglutination or radioimmunoassay. This antibody does not appear in the serum until several weeks (occasionally months) after clinical illness has resolved and the antibody persists for years. Therefore, if a patient is serotested early in his/her clinical illness and found to be HbsAg "positive" and HBs "negative", one can be reasonably certain that the patient is acutely ill with hepatitis B.

If, on the other hand, serological tests indicate that HbsAg is not present in the food handler's serum, then hepatitis A or hepatitis non-A, non-B must be considered. The diagnosis of hepatitis non-A, non-B is made on the basis of history and by excluding other diseases that can present as clinical hepatitis. Historically, many individuals with hepatitis non-A, non-B report a recent exposure to blood transfusion (or blood products) or to other types of parenteral exposure (e.g., parenteral drug abuse). However, in others no such history is elicited. Infections with CMV and Epstein-Barr virus must be excluded before a diagnosis of hepatitis non-A, non-B can be entertained.

Techniques for confirming a diagnosis of hepatitis A are just becoming available at the present time. The virus can be detected in stool specimens using immune electron microscopy, and serum antibody to the virus can be detected using the modified hepatitis A virus antibody test (differential radioimmunoassay). Hepatitis A virus has been demonstrated in the stool of infected persons several weeks prior to the onset of clinical illness. By the time the patient develops clinical illness, virus excretion in the stool diminishes, and by the time the patient's liver enzymes peak, virus can no longer be detected in stool. Antibody to hepatitis A usually appears early in clinical illness and reaches a peak several months later.

The three types of hepatitis usually cannot be distinguished one from another on clinical grounds alone. History and the epidemiological factors surrounding any particular case (other ill family members; or preference for seafood, such as clams, mussels, etc.) can be helpful, but can only suggest a presumptive diagnosis. Definitive diagnosis rests on laboratory studies, many of which are not widely available, and all of which take from several days to several weeks to perform. Therefore, each hospital's employee health program must modify its approach to a food handler who develops clinical hepatitis depending on its available resources. The following is an "idealized" set of suggested guidelines:

1. Remove the individual from food handling responsibilities.
2. Notify appropriate public health authorities and apprise them of the facts involved in the case.
3. Obtain stool specimen for immune electron microscopy (hepatitis A virus).*
4. Obtain serum specimens for radioimmunoassay or reversed passive hemagglutination (HbsAg), differential radioimmunoassay (anti-hepatitis A).*
5. Obtain appropriate specimens to rule out CMV and Epstein-Barr virus infections.*
6. The food handler can return to work when clinically feasible and when allowed by law. In the absence of such laws, when the patient feels clinically well enough to work and liver enzymes are returning toward baseline, it is probably safe to return to work. If 2 weeks have elapsed since onset of clinical illness, the chances of the patient being infectious (hepatitis A) are almost nil.
7. Personal hygiene must be stressed upon returning to work.

Parasites

To date, there have been no reports in the U.S. of foodborne outbreaks due to parasitic disease among food handlers.[57] There are, however, several parasites found in the U.S. that potentially could be transmitted by foods: *Enterobius vermicularis*, *Entameba histolytica*, and *Gardia lamblia*. The magnitude of the risk of transmission by food handlers of these organisms is unknown.

Conclusions

It is obvious from examing these four diseases that prevention of transmission is important because in all cases, by the time clinical illness occurs, transmission has probably already occurred. Personal hygiene, particularly handwashing, will minimize the risk of transmission. Routine microbiological surveillance, unless required by local or state law, is probably not cost beneficial. Preemployment screening is probably also not cost beneficial, except possibly in the case of *S. typhi* carriers. Management of food handlers with infectious disease requires a team approach: someone to care for the food handler's clinical problem; somebody to perform surveillance for secondary cases among patrons at the food establishment, as well as fellow employees and other contacts; and someone to make the administrative decisions necessary to protect the public. The employee health team is the focal point for coordinating these activities in the hospital setting.

---

* These steps may be deleted if such tests are not available. In that case, a conservative approach would be to remove the patient from food handling responsibilities for 2 weeks.

REFERENCES

1. Atuk, N. O. and Hunt, E. H., Serial tuberculin testing and isoniazid therapy in general hospital employees, *JAMA,* 218, 1795, 1971.
2. Craven, R. B., Wenzel, R., and Atuk, N. O., Minimizing tuberculosis risk to hospital personnel and students exposed to unsuspected disease, *Ann. Intern. Med.,* 82, 628, 1975.
3. Atuk, N. O., Hart, A. D., and Hunt, E. H., Close monitoring is essential during isoniazid prophylaxis, *South. Med. J.,* 70, 156, 1977.
3a. Thompson, J. J., Glassroth, J. L., Snider, D. E., and Farer, L. S., The booster phenomenon in serial tuberculin testing, *Am. Rev. Respr. Dis.,* 119, 587, 11979.
3b. Center for Disease Control, Guidelines for prevention of TB transmission in hospitals, DHEW Publ. CDC 79-8371, 1979.
3c. McGowan, J. E., Jr., The booster effect — a problem for surveillance of turberculosis in hospital employees, *Infect. Control,* 1, 147, 1980.
4. Seeff, L. B., Wright, E. C., Zimmerman, H. J., et al., Type B hepatitis after needlestick exposure: prevention with hepatitis B immune globulin. Final report of the Veterans Administration cooperative study, *Ann. Intern. Med.,* 88, 285, 1978.
5. Alter, H. J., Seeff, L. B., Kaplan, P. M., McAuliffe, J., Wright, E. C., Gerin, J. L., Purcell, R. H., Holland, P. V., and Zimmerman, H. J., Type B hepatitis: the infectivity of blood positive for e antigen and DNA polymerase after accidental needlestick exposure, *N. Engl. J. Med.,* 295, 909, 1977.
6. Melnick, J. L., Dreesman, G. R., and Hollinger, F. B., Approaching the control of viral hepatitis type B, *J. Infect. Dis.,* 133, 210, 1976.
7. Center for Dieease Control, Morbidity and Mortality Weekly Report, Supplement: Perspectives on the Control of Viral Hepatitis, 25: (17), May 7, 1976.
8. Center for Disease Control, Morbidity and Mortality Weekly Report, Immune Globulin for Protection Against Viral Hepatitis, 26: (52) Dec. 30, 1977.
9. Feldman, H. A., Some recollections of the meningococcal diseases. The first Harry F. Dowling lecture, *JAMA,* 220, 1107, 1972.
10. Center for Disease Control, Morbidity and Mortality Weekly Report. 27: (38), 358, 1978.
11. Center for Disease Control, Morbidity and Mortality Weekly Report. 17: (18), 147, 1978.
12. McCormick, J. B. and Bennett, J. V., Public health considerations in the management of meningococcal disease, *Ann. Intern. Med.,* 83, 883, 1975.
13. Munford, R. S., Taunay, A. E., DeMorais, J. S., Fraser, D. W., and Feldman, R. A., Spread of meningococcal infection within households, *Lancet,* 1, 1275, 1974.
14. Beam, W. E., Newberg, N. R., Devine, L. F., Pierce, W. E., and Davies, J. A., The effect of rifampin on the nosopharyngeal carriage of *Neisseria meningitidis* in a military population, *J. Infect. Dis.,* 124, 34, 1971.
15. Center for Disease Control, Meningococcal meningitis — United Kingdom, Morbidity and Mortality Weekly Report, 1, Jan. 3, 1976.
16. Center for Disease Control, Analysis of endemic meningococcal disease by serogroup and evaluators of chemoprophylaxis. The meningococcal disease surveillance group, *J. Infect. Dis.,* 134, 201, 1976.
17. Center for Disease Control, Vestibular reactions to minocycline after meningococcal prophylaxis. Morbidity and Mortality Weekly Report, 24: (2), Jan. 11, 1975, 9.
18. Jacobson, J. A., Prohylaxis of meningococcal infections, (correspondence) *N. Engl. J. Med.,* 294, 843, 1976.
19. Assri, M. and Raisanen, S., Transmission of acute toxoplasma infection, the survival of trophozoites in human tears, saliva, and urine and in cow's milk, *Acta Opthalmol.,* 52, 847, 1974.
20. Schiff, G. M. and Dine, M. S., Transmission of rubella from newborns, *Am. J. Dis. Child.,* 110, 447, 1965.
21. Harty, J., Monif, G., Medearis, D., and Sever, J., Postnatal transmission of rubella virus to nurses, *JAMA,* 191, 1034, 1965.
22. Schiff, G. M., Smith, H. D., Dignan, P. S. J., and Sever, J., Rubella: studies on the natural disease, *Am. J. Dis. Child.,* 110, 366, 1965.
23. Yeager, A. S., Longitudinal, serological study of cytomegalovirus infections in nurses and in personnel without patient contact, *J. Clin. Microbiol.,* 2, 448, 1975.
24. Cox, F. and Hughes, W. T., The value of isolation procedures for cytomegalovirus infections in children with leukemia, *Cancer,* 36, 1158, 1975.
25. Hamory, B.H., Osterman, C. A., and Wenzel, R. P., Herpetic whitlow, *N. Engl. J. Med.,* 292, 268, 1975.
26. Francis, D. R., Henman, K. L., MacMahon, J. R., Chavigny, H., and Santerlin, K. C., Nosocomial and maternally acquired herpesvirus hominis infections, *Am. J. Dis. Child.,* 129, 889, 1975.

27. Linneman, C. C., Light, I. J., Buchman, T. G., Ballard, J. L., and Roizman, B., Transmission of herpes-simplex virus Type 1 in a nursery for the newborn: identification of viral isolates by D.N.A. "fingerprinting", *Lancet,* 1, 964, 1978.

28. Nahmias, A. J. and Rickhoff, T. C., Staphylococcal infections in hospitals: recent developments in epidemiologic and laboratory investigations, *N. Engl. J. Med.,* 265, 74, 120, 177, 1961.

29. Williams, R. E. O., Healthy carriage of *Staphylococcus aureus*: its prevalence and importance, *Bacteriol. Rev.,* 27, 56, 1963.

30. Shinefield, H. R., Ribble, J. C., and Boris, M., Bacterial interference between strains of *Staphylococcus aureus, Contrib. Microbiol. Immunol.,* 1, 541, 1973.

31. Noble, N. C., The cutaneous distribution of the Micrococcaceae, *Contrib. Microbiol. Immunol.,* 1, 537, 1973.

32. Hill, J., Howell, A., and Blowers, R., Effect of clothing on dispersal of *Staphylococcus aureus* by males and females, *Lancet,* 2, 1131, 1974.

33. Mitchell, N. J. and Gamble, D. R., Clothing design for operating room personnel, *Lancet,* 2, 1133, 1974.

34. Heczko, P. B., Pryjma, J., Kasprowicz, A., and Krawiec, H., Influence of host and parasite factors on the nasal carriage of staphylococci, *Contrib. Microbiol. Immunol.,* 1, 581, 1973.

35. Nahmias, A. J. and Eickhoff, T. C., Epidemiologic aspects and control methods, in *The Staphylococci,* Cohen, J. O., Ed., John Wiley & Sons, New York, 1972, 494.

36. Wenzel, R. P., unpublished data, 1979.

37. Wilson, S. Z., Martin, R R., and Putman, M., In vivo effects of josamycin, erythromycin, and placebo therapy on nasal carriage of *Staphylococcus aureus, Antimicrob. Agents Chemother.,* 11, 407, 1977.

37a. Bryan, C. S., Wilson, R. S., Meade, P., and Sill, L. G., Topical antibiotic ointments for staphylococcal nasal carriers: survey of current practices and comparison of bacitracin and vancomycin ointments, *Infect. Control,* 1, 153, 1980.

38. Hamburger, M., Green, M. J., and Hamburger, V. G., The problem of the dangerous carrier of hemolytic streptococci, *J. Infect. Dis.,* 77, 68, 1945.

39. Wannamaker, L. W., Perplexity and precision in the diagnosis of streptococcal pharyngitis, *Am. J. Dis. Child.,* 124, 352, 1972.

40. Kaplan, E. L., Unresolved problems in diagnosis and epidemiology of streptococcal infections, in *Streptococci and Streptococcal Diseases,* Wannamaker, L. W. and Matsen, J. M., Eds., Academic Press, New York, 1972, 557.

41. Dillon, H. C., Impetigo Contagiosa: suppurative and nonsuppurative complications, *Am. J. Dis. Child.* 115, 530, 1968.

42. Hedlund, P., Acute vulvovaginitis in streptococcal infections, *Acta Pediatr.,* 42, 388, 1953.

43. Boisvert, P. L. and Walcher, D. N., Hemolytic streptococcal vaginitis in children, *Pediatric,* 2, 24, 1948.

44. Stamm, W. E., Postoperative Streptococcal Wound Infections Traced to a Vaginal Carrier, paper presented at the 25th Ann. Epidemic Intelligence Service Conf., Center for Disease Control, Atlanta, April 5, 1976.

45. Richman, D. D., Breton, S. J., and Goldman, D. A., Scarlet fever and Group A streptococcal surgical wound infection traced to an anal carrier, *J. Pediatr.,* 90, 387, 1977.

46. Schaffner, W., Lefkowitz, L. B., Goodman, J. S., and Koenig, M. G., Hospital outbreak of infections with Group A streptococci traced to an asymptomatic anal carrier, *N. Engl. J. Med.,* 280, 1224, 1969.

47. McKee, W. M., DiCaprio, J. M., and Sherris, J. C., Anal carriage as the probable source of a streptococcal epidemic, *Lancet,* 2, 1007, 1966.

48. James, L. and McFarland, R. B., An epidemic of pharyngitis due to a non-hemolytic Group A streptococcus at Lowry Air Force Base, *N. Engl. J. Med.,* 284, 750, 1971.

49. Dillon, H. C., The treatment of streptococcal skin infections, *J. Pediatr.,* 76, 676, 1970.

50. Black, R. E., Cox, R. C., AND Horwitz, M. A., Outbreaks of food-borne disease in the United States, 1975, *J. Infect. Dis.,* 137, 213, 1978.

51. Steer, A. C., Hall, W. J., Wells, J. G., Craven, P. J., Leotsakis, N., Farmer, J. J., and Gangerosa, E. J., Person-to-person spread of *Salmonella typhimurium* after a hospital common-source outbreak, *Lancet,* 1, 319, 1975.

52. Rosenberg, M. L., Wiessman, J. B., Gangerosa, E. J., Reller, L. B., and Beasley, R. P., Shigellosis in the United States: ten year review of nationwide surveillance, 1964-1973, *Am. J. Epidemiol.,* 104, 543, 1976.

53. Weissman, J. B., Gangerosa, E. J., Dupont, H. L., Nelson, J. D., and Haltalin, K. C., Shigellosis: to treat or not to treat, *JAMA,* 229, 1215, 1974.

54. **Nelson, J. D., Kusmiesz, H., and Jackosn, L. H.,** Comparison of trimethoprim-sulfamethoxazole and ampicillin therapy for shigellosis in ambulatory patients, *J. Pediatr.,* 89, 491, 1976.
55. Center for Disease Control, Mortality and Morbidity Weekly Report, Vol. 25, No. 17, Suppl., May 7, 1976.
56. **Bradley, D. W. and Maynard, J. E.,** Serodiagnosis of viral hepatitis A by radioimmunoassay, *Lab. Manage.,* 16, 29, 1978.
57. **Juranek, D.,** personal communication.
58. *Isolation Techniques for Use in Hospitals,* 2nd ed., U.S. Departmnt of Health, Education and Welfare, U.S. Public Health Service, Center for Disease Control, Atlanta, Ga.

INFECTION CONTROL IN SMALL HOSPITALS

Michael R. Britt

INTRODUCTION

There are a number of unique circumstances in the small hospital which require modification of the traditional approaches to nosocomial infection control. I will attempt to outline the nature of these unique circumstances and their impact on infection control programs applicable to small hospitals.

In 1977, 50% of 6447 hospitals in the U.S. contained fewer than 100 beds. These hospitals have 16% of 1,062,416 hospital beds and admitted 15% of the 36,097,109 total acute care hospital patients.[1]

Small hospitals have the dilemma of needing to provide a full range and a similar quality of hospital services as large hospitals, but the actual demand for these services is only occasionally required. Small hospitals must be prepared to handle many illnesses that only rarely actually occur. Public expectation of quality health care is rising and is not limited to those populous areas where larger hospitals are possible. One proposed solution to the above dilemma is to merge small hospitals into larger ones which is applicable for urban and suburban areas, but not practical or possible for rural areas. Many of these rural hospitals are located in remote, sparsely populated regions and serve as the only hospital available for a considerable distance and simply cannot be eliminated. Thus, we must meet this demand for high-quality and available hospital services within the fiscal and personnel limitations of the small rural hospital, and this includes nosocomial infection control.

In the remainder of this chapter, I will review the philosophical perceptions on infection control activities which serve as a foundation for the proposed program, then the available information on infections in small hospitals, and finally some approaches on how to order priorities in an infection control program for the limited resources of a small hospital to maximize the potential benefits to the patient.

NOSOCOMIAL INFECTIONS — BACKGROUND AND COMMON MISCONCEPTIONS

Nosocomial infections are not a new or recent entity. They have existed as long as hospitals have existed. Florence Nightingale's nursing reforms were largely aimed at proper management and prevention of nosocomial infection. Semmelweis introduced the use of antiseptic handwashing techniques and reduced nosocomial puerperal fever deaths of his hospital from over 9 to 3.6% of maternity patients.[2] The current emphasis on hospital acquired infection dates from the mid-1950s and the emergence of the epidemics of the penicillin-resistant *Staphylococcus aureus*. Multidisciplinary committees were organized to assist in the control of these antibiotic resistant endemic and epidemic nosocomial pathogens. During the 1960s and early 1970s, two early-warning or monitoring systems for nosocomial infections were developed: (1) routine bacteriologic monitoring of the hospital environment and (2) surveillance of patient infections. With each approach, the idea was to use the information gathered to identify potential remedial problems which could be corrected. In the surveillance approach, the counting is usually done by a medically trained (usually a nurse or microbiologist) nonphysician surveillance officer supervised by a physician (chairman of the infection committee or hospital epidemiologist). The surveillance team then reports to multidisciplinary infection committees that establish infection control policy. Studies reveal that there is a persistant background of endemic occurrence of nosocomial infections.[3-6] The most common sites of these endemic nosocomial infections are the urinary tract; especially those associated with indwelling bladder catheters, lower respiratory tract, and incisional surgical wound infections. These endemic infections are the majority of nosocomial infections found in most institutions.[7]

On occasion, there are clear-cut outbreaks of epidemics within the hospital. These epidemics can be a cluster of single-site infections or multiple sites of infection secondary to a single epidemic strain of bacteria. The epidemic may be due to a common source, breakdowns in routine techniques, emergence of an especially virulent or antibiotic-resistant organism, clustering of very susceptible hosts, or to a combination of these factors. Many epidemics or clusters of nosocomial infections spontaneously stop, with no apparent reason for first occurring of the cluster or for its disappearance.

There is a common misconception that all nosocomial infections are preventable. It is clear that all hospital acquired infections are not preventable. Modern medical care has inherent risks of infection which can be minimized, but not eliminated. The only absolute way to prevent surgical wound infection is not to do surgery. The risk of wound infection can be minimized by the use of proper surgical techniques, sterile instruments, clean operating room environment, prophylactic antibiotics, etc., but all of these do not ever reduce the risk of nosocomial infection to zero.

This misconception that all nosocomial infections are preventable is only a problem when it interferes with the surveillance and recognition of nosocomial infections that are occurring. If the expectation within the hospital is that there will be no nosocomial infections, then those that occur are often explained away rather than studied. This denial may interfere with the development of practical approaches that minimize the occurrence of nosocomial infection. The proper perception is that some occurrence of nosocomial infection is inevitable when modern medical care is given, but the rate of such infections can and should be minimized.

Another common misconception is that the risk of nosocomial infection for patients is relatively uniform. Since the incidence of nosocomial infection is between 3 and 5%, therefore the risk of nosocomial infection for each patient is commonly perceived as about 3 to 5%. This is not true. Figure 1 presents a graphic representation of how the risk of nosocomial infection varies among hospitalized patients. Most patients are at no risk for many types of nosocomial infection, i.e., patients who are not operated on have no risk of surgical wound infection, patients without indwelling bladder catheters are not at risk of catheter associated urinary tract infection, patients without an I.V. do not get I.V.-associated infections, etc.

The smaller second and third levels of the pyramid in the figure represent the fact that among patients exposed to given risk factors, only some are colonized with potential pathogenic bacteria. It should be noted that many of our effective infection control activities (use of sterile supplies, use of good handwashing techniques, etc.) are aimed at the prevention of colonization. The next level of the pyramid reveals that only some of the patients colonized will become clinically ill. The development of clinical illness depends upon the host's immunological status, the basic virulence of colonizing organisms, and the size of inoculum. Infection control practices may influence only the latter two aspects. In fact many medical care practices as well as the number of underlying diseases adversely affect the host's immune status.

The severity of the patient's underlying conditions has a marked influence on the risk of hospital acquired infectons. In a recent study,[8] physicians rated the severity of patients' underlying condition at time of admission. This study showed that patients considered to be at risk of dying during the current admission ("fatal") have a tenfold

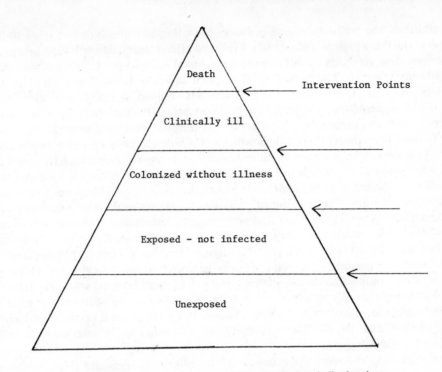

FIGURE 1. Pattern of nosocomial infections in hospitalized patients.

higher rate of nosocomial infection than patients with "nonfatal" illnesses. Patients with "ultimately fatal" illnesses (life expectancy 3 to 5 years) had a four- to fivefold higher rate of nosocomial infection that "nonfatal" patients. This study suggests that simple clinical assessments can be used to identify the subgroup of patients at high risk of being clinically ill when colonized in the hospital.

The final two layers of the pyramid reveal that traditional curative medicine's intervention is designed to prevent death from occurring among clinically ill patients. Thus, the rate of nosocomial infection within an institution is influenced by the degree of illness of the patient population, their therapies, and the environmental reservoir of potential flora, as well as the routine practices of the individual caring for the patient.

Surveillance systems which measure clinical illness do provide a systematic method for quantifying some aspects of the magnitude and nature of the nosocomial infections within an institution. However, they do not measure directly the quality of the routine preventive practices of the staff of the hospital.

BACKGROUND ON CONTROL OF NOSOCOMIAL INFECTION

Control of nosocomial infection is a very complex issue. Nosocomial infections are not a single entity or disease. Current surveillance systems do not identify only preventable infections. There is the need for all members of the hospital care team to use good techniques concurrently in the care of individual patients. However, good techniques by some individuals will not offset the bad techniques of others. Also, bad techniques by personnel do not lead to immediate problems for the patient, and for most patients, some may never result in infection. Even when infection results from bad techniques, it is difficult for the individuals with the bad techniques to relate their bad techniques to the infection because of the incubation period. Thus, the hospital staff person receives little reinforcement of either the benefit of good infection control techniques or harm to the patient from poor techniques. Finally, there are not available effective established methods of prevention for all types of nosocomial infections.

In addition, the well-established practices are often not distinguished from those practices which are logical, but not of established effectiveness. Many logical practices are proposed as methods of controlling nosocomial infections which have not been critically investigated. The failure to distinguish carefully between proven effective practices and logical, but unproven practices has resulted in many institutions' attempting or implementing the unproven practices before the established effective procedures. This is an especially critical error in a hospital with only limited resources. Priority must be in doing those things which are clearly effective first and then implementing the logical but unproven practices later if there are any resources left.

Another problem in the control of nosocomial infection has been a focus on the recognition and control of hospital epidemics as the major activity of a hospital infection control program. The training of surveillance officers in the past had often emphasized this activity. The number and percentage of nosocomial infections which are part of definable epidemics is very small. One study estimates that there is only one epidemic for every 10,000 discharges.[9] To become effective in solving epidemics, most new surveillance persons must acquire many new skills through additional training. These skills are only valuable if epidemics occur. In a small hospital with only 1000 to 2000 discharges annually, it will be years between epidemics. In addition, our experience in training infection control persons suggests that the interval between epidemics is often longer than the likelihood of many small hospital infection control persons remaining on the job.

The relationship between the existence of surveillance systems and effective control programs is often a point of confusion. The existence of a surveillance program which is very effective at identifying and cataloging nosocomial infections does not mean the institution has an effective control program. The availability of a surveillance system does allow the institution to establish and document its unique infection problems, to monitor for outbreaks, and to evaluate the success or failure of proposed control measures. The proposed control measures and their implementation are not the same activity as the surveillance system. There are many hospitals that have catalogued their nosocomial infections for years without ever instituting a control program.

There are a number of debates about how much surveillance is necessary for an effective control program. The answer is different for each hospital and depends upon unique circumstances of the institution. One needs enough surveillance to decide what is happening and to evaluate whether the control measures that have been implemented are doing what is expected. This evaluation is necessary, so that ineffective measures can be stopped and replaced. Surveillance systems have a number of intrinsic limitations which should be understood. Routine environmental monitoring has been largely dropped because the environment is not sterile and therefore cultures are usually positive. The significance of most positive environmental cultures was usually impossible to interpret and did not lead to meaningful control programs in most institutions.

The systematic measurement of the incidence of clinically apparent nosocomial infections by surveillance individuals is dependent to a great extent on the quality and quantity of the available bacteriology within the institution. To illustrate, the recognition within the institution of an epidemic of antibiotic-resistant *Staphylococcus aureus* infection in a newborn nursery can only occur if cultures are obtained on sick newborns and if the laboratory can identify *S. aureus* consistently and perform reproducible antibiotic susceptibility tests. The usefulness of surveillance systems counting the incidence of clinical nosocomial infections in a hospital is dependent on the majority of clinically apparent infections being cultured and the laboratory's successfully providing reproducible reliable results. Both are potential problem areas in small hospitals. While many small hospitals attempt to adapt large hospital infection control systems

Table 1

COMPARISONS OF PREVALENCE SURVEY DATA FROM 18
SMALL HOSITALS,[10] 1972—73, AND THE LDS HOSPITAL
(LDSH), 1971[11]

	18 small hospitals		LDS hospital	
	Number	Percent	Number	Percent
Total patients	525	100	566	100
Medical	268	51	179	31
Surgical	257	49	387	68
Patients with infections	140	27	107	19
Community acquired	107	20	60	11
Medical	85	32	34	19
Surgical	22	9	26	7
Hospital acquired	38	7	48	9
Medical	15	6	10	6
Surgical	23	9	38	10
Hospital acquired infections — sites				
Lower respiratory tract	13	3	6	1
Urinary tract	13	3	21	4
Skin and s.c. tissue	4	1	2	0
Wounds	5	1	12	2
Others	4	1	11	2
Community acquired infections — sites				
Lower respiratory tract	55	11	18	3
Urinary tract	15	3	13	2
Skin and s.c. tissue	13	3	9	2
Wounds	0	0	0	0
Others	24	5	22	4
Patients receiving antimicrobials	153	29	130	23

to their institution, including the use of formal surveillance programs, most have not dealt with the question of how their microbiology laboratory performance and/or physician culture practices will limit the usefulness of their data.

There are a number of problems that are common to all infection control programs, regardless of institution size, that can be especially critical to programs in small hospitals. The approach to the solution of these same problems will need to be different in the small hospital from the approach in large hospitals.

NOSOCOMIAL INFECTION IN SMALL HOSPITALS

A major question for this paper, however, is whether the size of the institution has any unique influence on the incidence of nosocomial infection. It is clear that most physicians practicing in small hospitals recognize the potential hazard of nosocomial infections, but most do not believe there is any serious problem in their institution. There is only a limited amount of information on the rate of occurrence of nosocomial infection in small hospitals.

In 1972 we conducted a 1-day prevalence survey in 18 small hospitals[10] in 5 Mountain States using a protocol similar to a 1971 study of the largest hospital in our region.[11] The results (see Table 1) revealed that the prevalence of infection was remarkably similar for similar types of patients (the risk of being a surgical patient was much higher in the larger hospital). This study suggests that the endemic risk of nosocomial infection for similar patients is not likely to be different in various sized hospitals. However, it also shows that there are clearly differences in the likelihood of certain patient types being found in different sized hospitals.

A survey of five small hospitals conducting their own surveillance in 1977 revealed a combined incidence rate of 2.1%.[12] The individual hospital rates ranged from 4.3 to 0.7%. The distribution of infection sites was similar to the findings in the prevalence survey.

Antibiotic usage was also studied during the 1972 prevalence study. This study revealed that 29.3% of the patients were receiving systemic antibiotics, but only 68% had evidence that bacterial infection was being treated. The finding that 13% of all noninfected patients were receiving antibiotics for prophylactic purposes was similar to the rate found in several other prevalence surveys.[5,13]

ADEQUACY OF BACTERIOLOGY IN SMALL HOSPITALS

We also conducted a third study in the majority (16) of the same 18 hospitals.[12] Using a specially developed survey form, we measured the steps in performing routine cultures in an attempt to determine whether the microbiology services of small hospitals were likely to provide clinically useful information. The results of this survey (see Table 2) reveal that the routine approach used in many of the laboratories would not allow in many specimens for the isolation and/or proper identification of genus or species of many potential pathogens.

Pathogenic organisms whose growth or identification required special media or incubation conditions were those most likely not to be considered. In addition, most laboratories did not comply with the five major process steps in performing antibiotic disc diffusion studies as recommended by Bauer and Kirby[14] and the National Committee for Laboratory Standards.[15]

These data and information gathered in a similar survey in 1978 suggest that the probable quality and reproducibility of bacterial culture results reported in many small hospitals may be open to question. This question must be answered before any useful formal surveillance system can be established. If it is not, the data gathered by the surveillance system may only be measuring variability in the laboratory rather than what is occurring among the patients in the hospital.

PHYSICIAN CULTURING PRACTICES IN SMALL HOSPITALS

One additional observation made during our small hospital survey[12] which has potential bearing on small hospital infection control programs was the pattern of physician culturing practices. In the small hospitals, a culture was ordered in only 53% of the community-acquired infections judged likely to be bacterial in etiology. For infections nosocomial in origin, only 41% were cultured. This pattern of only occasionally using cultures in the management of bacterial infections had two potential adverse effects. These practices led to the very low volume of cultures performed in the microbiology labs of these hospitals. The low volume leads technologists to modify standard approaches which result in errors of both commission and omission which then result in findings like what our survey of the laboratories revealed. In addition, this low frequency of culturing potential bacterial infections will limit the usefulness of any formal surveillance system to identify clusters or epidemics of nosocomial pathogens.

These studies suggest the following general conclusions about nosocomial infection and its control in small hospitals:

Table 2

ADEQUACY OF ROUTINE BACTERIOLOGICAL
PROCEDURES IN 16 SMALL HOSPITAL
LABORATORIES

	Number of laboratories adequate
By specimen	
Throat	7
Sputum	10
Urine	6
Wounds	8
Cerebrospinal fluid	8
Stool	6
Vagina	7
By organism[a]	
Haemophilus influenzae[a]	
Cerebrospinal fluid	10
Sputum	6
Pathogenic *Neisseria*	
Cerebrospinal fluid	8
Vagina	10
Streptococcus pyogenes	
Group A	9
Enterococcus	9
Pneumococcus	10
Enterobacteriaceae	12
Staphylococcus aureus	14
Antibiotic snesitivity tests	
Inoculum	
Inoculum properly standardized	5
Inoculum direct from clinic specimen	3
Inoculum direct from original isolation plate	8
Using Mueller Hinton agar	4
Zone diameters measured	12
Antibiotic disks properly stored	14
All four above procedures acceptable	6

[a]   Species identification not required.

From Britt, M. R., *Ann. Intern. Med.*, 89, 757, 1978. With permission.

1. The risk of nosocomial infection for similar patients is approximately the same as the risk in larger hospitals.
2. The types of patients likely to be found in small hospitals are different from those found in large hospitals (fewer complex surgical patients, fewer medical immuno-compromised patients, and more acute short-term illnesses).
3. Antibiotic usage by small hospital physicians tends to be similar, but not identical to their large hospital colleagues.
4. The quantity and quality of available microbiological laboratory services are less in small hospitals. This potentially limits the usefulness of formal surveillance systems. Formal surveillance systems should only begin after review of physician culturing practices and procedures in the microbiology laboratory to assure the usefulness of surveillance data.

ADDITIONAL DIFFERENCE BETWEEN LARGE AND SMALL HOSPITALS WITH IMPLICATIONS FOR INFECTION CONTROL PROGRAMS

There are just fewer patients in small hospitals. So while the rate of infection is similar, there will still be fewer infections, and those infections which occur will be spread over time. This means that monthly tabulation of nosocomial infection will be characterized primarily by their absence. Tabulation at longer intervals will more likely describe the actual situation.

It is our experience and the experience of others that successful infection control programs are more the result of the personal efforts of an interested, concerned surveillance person working with an interested, committed, and supportive physician and hospital administration than with the detailed adherence to a performance of preselected proper components of an infection control program. The dilemma for the small hospital is that there are fewer individuals available in the small hospital, and therefore there is much greater risk that the person with the necessary interest may not exist within the hospital employee pool or community. In addition, the same individual characteristics that make a good infection control person also define the characteristics needed in many other leadership positions within the hospital. Finally, even if the proper individual exists, and there is the necessary interest and support for infection control activities among the hospital administration and medical staff; the job still will require only a part time effort.

The surveillance person working part time creates additional potential problems for developing an effective infection control program in a hospital. The other duties assigned to the infection control person may consume all of that person's available time. This is especially true if, as is often the case, the infection control activities are assigned to an existing leader in nursing services whose day is already full. Even when limited to individuals assigned only to patient care activities, the day-to-day mini-crises which are the staple of caring for hospitalized patients tend to consume all the available time. The remote long-term benefits of infection control are more difficult to appreciate than benefits of solving the day-to-day immediate patient crises of bedside nursing. Infection control is an unfamiliar activity, while the other duties are often well-understood, familiar activities. It is not surprising that the familiar is done, and the infection control activities may remain perpetually on tomorrow's list of things to do.

There is another very real constraint on the small hospital administrator who wishes to implement an effective infection control program. Since few individuals exist who already possess the body of information necessary to perform infection control activities, it has been efficient to have the individual assuming infection control responsibilities receive some specialized training in a formal workshop, usually a training course and/or brief 1- to 2-week apprenticeship with a functioning infection control person. This expenditure is easier to justify for full-time infection control persons that are expected to influence the care of 5,000 to 15,000 patients each year (200 hospital beds, with an average patient length of stay of 7 days is equivalent to approximately 10,000 discharges per year). It is difficult to justify 1 to 2 weeks of training for the part-time surveillance persons who may influence the care of only 750 to 2000 patients per year.

The total cost for this formal training for the small hospital is also higher because the part-time individual who is away from the hospital at a workshop is not only not performing the infection control functions, but also is not performing the other part time noninfection control functions. In general, one can understand that long, formal infection control training programs may be marginally cost efficient or beneficial for small hospitals.

PREREQUISITES TO EFFECTIVE INFECTION CONTROL PROGRAM

Personnel

The necessary components for effective infection control in any institution, large or small, is the existence of three interested individuals:

1. A physician member of the hospital staff
2. A surveillance person with a clearly defined responsibility for infection control and regular amount of time concommitant to this activity
3. An administrator willing to commit some of the institution's fiscal resources

Without all three of these individuals, there is little likelihood of the infection control programs having any impact on the quality of the care provided.

Institutional Receptiveness to Change

Institution of infection control programs imply change. No matter how good an institution already is, some improvement can be made. Commitment by the rest of the institution personnel, but especially its medical and nursing staff, to improve the institution is needed. If the only commitment is to preserve and justify the existing order, then the infection control program will not significantly improve existing patient care practices. Resistence to change is very common because all need to change, even to make something good into something better, carries with it implicit criticism. One could always ask, "If this change is so good, how come we didn't do it yesterday?" In general, professionals in hospitals view their previous routine activities as effective, efficient, and motivated by their desire to do the best job possible. The suggestion to change may be consciously or unconsciously interpreted as suggesting their previous activities were ineffective, inefficient, or harmful. Rather than admit this, there is an undercurrent of opposition to any proposed changes to "improve patient care". An effective infection control program will require many institution personnel to change. This should be understood and accepted in advance by at least the powerful and influential leaders of the institution.

INFECTION CONTROL PROGRAM FOR SMALL HOSPITALS

Once it is determined that the necessary prerequisites for a successful program are present, the following graded program may be instituted:

1. Basic level — establish control of common endemic nosocomial infections and establish an "informal" surveillance network
2. Intermediate level — add a formal surveillance system
3. Advanced level — add an in-hospital epidemic investigation and control capability

Basic Level

This plan makes the assumption that the nosocomial infection patterns in most small hospitals will be similar to those described above. The plan acknowledges that it is the control of nosocomial infections that is the ultimate goal. Thus, the hospital should concentrate first on assuring that the routine day-to-day patient care includes those practices which have been shown to control nosocomial infections effectively. Institution of formal surveillance systems is delayed because of the potential limitations of physician culturing practices and available microbiology services on achieving the formal surveillance's goal of determining the unique infection control problems of the hospital.

Control of Endemic Nosocomial Infections

The following is a list and discussion of infection control practices that are of established effectiveness and deal with infections commonly seen. These should be routine hospital procedures in all hospitals.

1. Closed sterile drainage for indwelling bladder catheters should be used and strictly maintained. Comment — It is possible to reduce the daily rate of acquisition of bacteriuria from the 25% seen with open systems (i.e., all infected by the fourth day), to rates in the order of 2 to 4%/day using closed sterile drainage. Since in acute care hospitals 50% of indwelling bladder catheters are removed each day of catheterization (i.e., most catheters are in only a few days), the impact of delayed acquisition of bacteriuria on the absolute number of catheter-associated infections can be enormous.

2. Use indwelling bladder catheters only when necessary. Comment — There are no catheter-associated infections if there are no catheters used. While total elimination is not possible, one should remember to remove them as soon as possible and avoid using them for solely nursing convenience. In males, external condom drainage should be used whenever possible.

3. Change peripheral I.V. sites every 48 to 72 hr: a. use scalp vein needles rather than plastic catheters whenever possible; and b. Heparin locks need to be changed only every 4 days. Comment — Data on this subject suggest that the risk of problems at the I.V. site increases geometrically with time. For peripheral I.V. sites, regular site changes eliminate the majority of problems. There is conflicting information available on effectiveness of regular I.V. site care with topical antibacterial agents. Site care is expensive and probably only of marginal benefit if sites are changed regularly. In-line filters are also expensive and of marginal benefit. Site care and filters are probably justified for central lines which often cannot be changed at short intervals and/or when hyperalimentation fluids are used.

4. Change large volume I.V. solutions at least every 24 hr. Comment — While it is uncommon to contaminate I.V. solutions during use, it is still reasonable that the bottle not hang more than 24 hr. When contamination occurs, maximum bacterial growth occurs in 12 to 18 hr. This policy of changing sterile solutions after being open 24 hr should be carried out for all sterile solutions used directly on patients (i.e., fluid used for wound irrigations).

5. Be sure that the solutions used in nebulizers of venilators, IPPB machines, etc. do not contain bacteria. Comment — Blowing organisms into patients' lungs certainly increases the patients' risk of pneumonia.

6. Nursing techniques to prevent aspiration episodes should be routinely employed.

7. Prevent atelectasis in postsurgical and comatose individuals. Comment — The relative value of IPPB treatment vs. blow bottle vs. cough and deep-breathing exercises remains the subject of some debate. Simple and inexpensive approaches should routinely be employed.

8. Tracheal suction of nasotracheal tubes or tracheostomy sites should be done using sterile techniques and sterile catheters and solutions.

9. Use effective sterilization techniques for instruments, etc. Comment — Cold sterilization should be absolutely minimized. Heat or gas sterilization should be carried out whenever possible. When cold sterilization is used, the most effective agents and proper contact time should be used. This usually means use of glutaraldehyde agents. Quaternary ammonium products should be avoided.[16]

10. Wash hands when approaching patients with decreased resistance to infection. Comment — The most common way that patients are colonized by nosocomial bacteria is from transient bacterial contamination carried by the hands of the hospital personnel. On clinical grounds alone, there are easily identifiable patients who are likely to be more susceptible to infection then others. Hands should be washed when approaching the following types of patients: those who have underlying illnesses which compromise the immune system (such as many types of cancer), those who are receiving medication which compromise the immune system (such as radiation therapy, steroids, and cancer chemotherapy), and those who are on high-dose, broad-spectrum antibiotics. Hands should be washed after handling material likely to be contaminated with bacteria (such as wound dressings, bed pans, etc.).

11. Use therapeutic antibiotics properly. Comment — When antibiotics are used therapeutically, the most specific (narrowest spectrum), effective antibiotic should be selected — and the lowest effective dose utilized. This reduces the risk of superinfections.

12. Use antibiotics in prophylaxis of surgical wounds properly. Comment — Antibiotics used in surgical prophylaxis (antibiotics designed to prevent infection — not antibiotics used to treat existing or inevitable clinical infections) should be begun before the operations (no more than 1 to 2 hr) and may be discontinued after the wound has sealed (usually within 6 to 12 hr after the operation). Prophylactic antibiotics are generally indicated in contaminated surgery. (In dirty surgery, the use is therapeutic.) Prophylactic antibiotics are generally not indicated in clean surgery unless plastic or steel prostheses are inserted.

13. Use proper techniques in the well-baby nursery.

14. Use proper techniques in operating and delivery suites and while doing invasive procedures, such as inserting I.V. and indwelling bladder catheters.

15. Use pragmatic and limited isolation techniques and facilities. Comment — Isolation techniques should be aimed directly at interrupting the transmission of the pathogen causing clinical disease in one patient in order to prevent illness in other patients. In many hospitals, isolation is commonly either under- or overdone. It is necessary that hospital policy and practice should reflect the need to protect the patients, i.e., an attending physician should not be able to prevent a patient needing isolation from getting it; nor, on the other hand, should all patients with even the remotest potential need for isolation be isolated. Common sense and good judgment must be employed. Graded isolation as recommended by the Public Health Service may avoid a lot of unnecessary, expensive isolation procedures.

This list focuses on activities that are generally already established policy in most large and small hospitals. What is usually needed is only a method of assuring that day to day patient care activity actually reflects the established policy.

Thus, for the small hospital, infection control activities should first focus on assuring that routine hospital care is provided in such a way that the patients have a chance to benefit from these effective methods of infection control.

2. Informal Surveillance

The second activity of the basic level is the establishment of an informal surveillance system. Surveillance systems allow the hospital to determine if there are unique infection control problems in that institution. This is how suspected epidemics or poor compliance with established policy are identified. In small hospitals, informal systems can be very effective because communication between all members of the hospital community are better and simpler than in large institutions. The infection control person should easily know essentially all that is occurring throughout a small hospital on a routine (almost daily) basis — a task that is much more difficult in a large hospital. While this informal system may be effective, it is often difficult to document its existence for outside accreditation and licensing agents. Development of methods of documenting of the number and nature of problems identified and remedial action taken will usually satisfy these agencies. The more important modification of the usual informal surveillance system (hospital grapevine) is the institution of a problem solving capacity in response to what is learned. The problems are often identified by the informal hospital system, but rarely does the information lead to action attempting to solve the problems. Establishment of an effective informal surveillance system will give the infection control program needed flexibility to solve the unique problems of the hospital. One other way of stating this would be to say that the second component of the basic program should be fo find effective ways to solve the problems that everyone already knows about.

Intermediate Level: Establishment of a Formal Surveillance System

Formal surveillance systems provide sensitive measurements of the unique status of nosocomial infections within an institution. Formal surveillance systems are useful, especially for changing influential members of the hospital community perception of nosocomial infections within an institution. Other nosocomial infections are not perceived as a problem, and this prevents any remedial action from being undertaken. Formal surveillance will document the existence of problems in a way that makes denying its existence much more difficult. This formal surveillance system requires the use of standard definitions of infections [suggestions of the Center for Disease Control (CDC) are reasonable], systematic review of patient records, periodic analysis, and formal presentation of findings to the medical, nursing and administrative staff. As mentioned earlier, in small hospitals because of the small number of infections, the data should be tabulated only quarterly, otherwise it is difficult to interpret (i.e., the epidemiologic and biologic significance of one infection in a category does not create much excitement or action).

Before instituting a formal surveillance system in a small hospital, one should obtain a concensus among the medical staff that at least the majority of nosocomial infections should be cultured. If some physicians do not think that cultures are needed for clinical management, they might be done as part of the infection control program at the hospitals expense.

The second prerequisite before setting up a formal surveillance system is a complex problem, i.e., assuring reproducible microbiology. A complete discussion of how to do this is beyond the scope of this article. However, it is our impression that many of the technical problems encountered by the technologists doing bacteriology in small hospitals are exaggerated by the low volume of clinical cultures performed. Very low volume, i.e., one culture per day or less, creates problems in having available the necessary media and in performing the needed quality control procedures. In smaller institutions, clinicians must be more aware of the need for the bacteriology lab to process a certain minimum number of cultures (probably at least one culture daily) in order to assure the results are likely to be accurate. The concomitant improvement in clinical microbiology services may be the major patient care benefit of instituting a formal surveillance system in small hospitals.

Advanced Level: Epidemic Investigation and Control Capability

The ability to investigate and control nosocomial infection epidemics properly within an institution requires special information and skills beyond the usual background of individuals assigned to become the infection control person. This additional knowledge includes the bacteriology and epidemiology of various nosocomial infections and epidemiologic methodology used to solve epidemics. As discussed earlier, although the risk of epidemics is approximately the same in both large and small hospitals, the risk is small.

Therefore epidemic investigation skills are probably a luxury for small hospital infection control persons. All that is needed is the ability to recognize that an epidemic might be occurring. At that point, consultants from either nearby large hospitals with an infection control program, the state medical school hospital, state health department, or CDC. (See chapters entitled "The State Health Department", "The Center for Disease Control", and "Association for Practitioners in Infection Control".) could be contacted to assist in solving the epidemic. In this manner, learning epidemic investigation skills could be delayed until needed. Omitting this training from the formal workshops in infection control for small hospitals would greatly shorten the existing training programs.

WHICH HOSPITALS SHOULD USE WHICH PROGRAM LEVEL

I believe standards of good patient care dictate that basic level activities be carried out in every hospital. Intermediate-level activities should be added in those institutions desiring to obtain Joint Commission Accreditation. It might be possible to obtain their certification with a well-documented, basic-level program, but it would be easier with a more formal surveillance system. The institution of intermediate level activity when done as outlined should have many direct implications for improved care of all infected patients beyond its obvious implications for nosocomial infection control. Small hospitals will only develop advanced level programs on rare occasions.

REFERENCES

1. *Hospital Statistics,* American Hospital Association, Chicago, 1977.
2. Lilienfeld, A. M. and Lilienfeld, D. E., What else is new?, *Am. J. Epidemiol.,* 105, 169, 1977.
3. Eickhoff, T. C., Hospital infections, Disease-a-Month, Year Book Medical Publishers, 1972.
4. Scheckler, W. E., Garner, J. S., Kaiser, A. B., and Bennett, J. V., Prevalence of infections and antibiotic usage in eight community hospitals, in *Proc. Int. Conf. Nosocomial Infection,* C.D.C., Brachman, P. S. and Eickhoff, T. C., Eds., American Hospital Association, Chicago, 1972, 299.
5. McGowan, J. E., Jr. and Finland, M., Infection and antibiotic usage at Boston City Hospital: changes in prevalence during the decade 1964—1973, *J. Infect. Dis.,* 129, 421, 1974.
6. Eickhoff, T. C., Brachman, P. S., Bennett, J. V., and Brown, J. F., Surveillance of nosocomial infections in community hospitals, I. Surveillance methods, effectiveness, and initial results, *J. Infect. Dis.,* 120, 305, 1969.
7. Scheckler, W. E., Nosocomial infections in a community hospital, 1972 through 1976, *Arch. Intern. Med.,* 138, 1792, 1978.
8. Britt, M. R., Schleupner, C. J., and Matsumiya, S., Severity of underlying disease as a predictor of nosocomial infection, *JAMA,* 239, 1047, 1978.
9. Tenney, J. H., Outbreak of Nosocomial Infection with Report of Study in 5 Community Hospitals, Abstract, Epidemic Intelligence Services Conference, Center for Disease Control, Atlanta, Ga., 1974.
10. Britt, M. R., Burke, J. P., Nordquist, A. G., Wilfert, J. N., and Smith, C. B., Infection control in small hospital, prevalence surveys in 18 institutions, *JAMA,* 236, 1700, 1976.

11. **Moody, M. L. and Burke, J. P.,** Infections and antibiotic use in a large private hospital, January 1971, *Arch. Intern. Med.,* 130, 261, 1972.
12. **Britt, M. R.,** Infectious diseases in small hospitals, prevalence of infections and adequacy of microbiology services, *Ann. Intern. Med.,* 89, 757, 1978.
13. **Adler, J. L. and Shulman, J. A.,** Nosocomial infection and actibiotic usage at Grady Memorial Hospital, *South. Med. J.,* 63, 102, 1970.
14. **Bauer, A. W., Kirby, W. M. M., Sherris, J. C., and Turck, M.,** Antibiotic susceptibility testing by a standardized single disc method, *Am. J. Clin. Pathol.,* 45, 493, 1966.
15. Performance standards for antimicrobial disc susceptibility tests, National Committee for Clinical Laboratory Standards, 1975.
16. **Sanford, J. P.,** Disinfectants that don't, *Ann. Intern. Med.,* 72, 282, 1970.

Medical-Legal Policies

MANAGEMENT OF MEDICAL-LEGAL PROBLEMS

Harry C. Nottebart, Jr.*

INTRODUCTION

When one thinks about being admitted to a hospital, it is one's first thought that it is a place to go to get well: to have an operation, to restore function and health, to convalesce there, and to return home whole and well. One does not think of a hospital as a place to go to be exposed to some infectious disease: to come home with more problems, with perhaps a disease that one did not have when one initially entered the hospital, or to possibly die of some infection acquired while in the hospital. It is important to note that lawsuits are often predicated on the failure of someone or something to meet one's expectations. Since most people associate going to a hospital with eventual improvement of health, any infection acquired there is a failure in their expectations which may then become the nidus (or the background) for a future lawsuit against a hospital and possibly against one or more physicians.

INFECTION CONTROL PRACTITIONERS

In an effort by the hospital to prevent hospital acquired infections and to monitor those that are present, modern hospitals employ one or more infection control practitioners (ICP). These people may come from diverse backgrounds. They may be clinical microbiologists or nurse-epidemiologists, and in a very few hospitals, there may even be a physician who is the hospital epidemiologist. In many hospitals, unfortunately, these people (or person) may be assigned infection control duties as a part-time or ancillary function. For the rest of the time, they may report to another department rather than to the hospital administration. It is my opinion that in order for ICPs to function in the best possible way for the benefit of the patients and to protect the hospital's interests in controlling infections, they should be independent of the various clinical departments and should report directly to the hospital administration. Additionally, ICPs should be full time and paid directly by the hospital rather than through one or more of the hospital's departments. In this manner, a hospital can protect the independence of the ICPs and insure that they are not subject to any conflicting loyalties. For example, if an ICP is a nurse-epidemiologist and still reports to and is paid by the department of nursing, it may be very difficult for him to point out errors in procedures within the department of nursing. In general, it would be particularly difficult to identify specific nursing areas or nurses who customarily did not adhere to infection control practices. Likewise, if there is a hospital epidemiologist and if he depended upon consultations for his support, it might be very difficult to identify departments, services, or individual physicians who may not adhere to infection control practices, isolation procedures, or antibiotic usage if there was any likelihood, either implicitly or explicitly, that such identification might result in fewer or no consultations. Thus, the ICP should be a full-time employee reporting directly to the hospital administration in order to protect him from undue pressures which might work to oppose the hospital's own interest in monitoring hospital acquired infections. Such

---

* Prior to his present position as Director, Bureau of Communicable Diseases, Virginia State Department of Health, Dr. Nottebart was Assistant Professor of Medicine at the Medical College of Virginia; Chief of Infectious Diseases, McGuire V. A. Hospital; and Chairman of the Infection Control Committee at the McGuire V. A. Hospital, Richmond, Virginia.

independence may help avoid bias in identifying possible sources of breaks in technique or in identifying other problem areas of which the hospital may be held later to have had knowledge. With respect to the latter point, such charges may be made even though that knowledge was not communicated; alternatively, information may have been suppressed because of possible intradepartmental problems that such information would have caused the ICP.

HOSPITAL INFECTION COMMITTEE

The hospital infection committee has representatives from most of the departments within the hospital. It is by means of the hospital infection committee that the hospital monitors hospital acquired infections, analyzing information as to various situations throughout the hospital that may be associated with increased risk of infections. It is not only the monitor, the receiver, and accumulator of all the information acquired within the hospital by the ICP, with respect to various patients who are found to have hospital acquired infections, but also the committee prepares various reports and analyses dealing with hospital acquired infections and possible risk factors. The hospital infection committee is also the source of information disseminated throughout the hospital to establish policy for isolation, to improve common hospital procedures, and to disseminate any other information which may decrease the risk of acquiring nosocomial infections by the patients. Some states have exempted by statute those committees and their reports involved in peer review. Of course, infection committees are not involved in peer review in the sense that professional performance is reviewed, but if there is an attempt to improve patient care by means of self-analysis, criticism, and the institution of reforms and changes in policy, these things all might bring the infection control committee within the statutes; however, in one state, even though the minutes and reports of committees were not subject to disclosure by statute, still the information considered by those committees could be subpoenaed as in the *Tucson Medical Center, Inc. vs. Misevch*, 545 P.2d 958 (1976).

There are two cases in which the courts allowed access to hospital infection committee reports. In *Spears vs. Mason*, 303 S.2d, 260 (1974), a plaintiff was allowed access to the hospital infection committee reports as they related to the plaintiff's case and to the period he was hospitalized. The other case, *Young vs. King*, 344 A.2d 792 (1976), the plaintiff was allowed access to the records from the hospital infection committee that related to the patient and his death. Clearly this is not any significant problem to date, but one might consider this when one is preparing a report for the hospital infection committee or when the minutes for the committee are being written.

LEGAL BACKGROUND

In trying to understand the legal process and how it applies to hospital acquired infections, it may be helpful to have a brief, superficial view of the legal process. First, in a litigious society such as ours, it is obvious that there are a great many claims made of possible injury. The party who is alleging injury may present this claim either himself or by way of letter or other communication to the party that he is alleging to have done the injury. A claim may be equally as well presented by an attorney for the party. Many of these claims are settled very quickly at this stage.

If no settlement is reached and if the injured party feels strongly enough about his injury and the need for compensation, he will obtain the services of an attorney-at-law, who will formalize the complaint and initiate a lawsuit against the party. At this point, the injured party becomes a plaintiff, and the party who is alleged to have done the injuring is the defendant. There then may follow a period of varying length during which time the defendant may by way of pleadings answer the plaintiff's allegations. Various processes of what are called discovery may take place. These may include affidavits, depositions, and interrogatories, all of which are ways of eliciting the facts of the circumstances surrounding the alleged injury and of narrowing the scope of the issues in contention. If the case gets to trial, neither of the parties will have to prove that which is not in controversy. The facts as acknowledged by both sides will be taken as admitted, and only those issues on which there is conflict will have evidence presented for proof.

At this stage, it is possible that the lawsuit may be settled between the plaintiff and defendant, usually by some sort of settlement payment being given by the defendant to the plaintiff in exchange for discontinuing the lawsuit at this point. The lawsuit may also be terminated during this period by a court decree. For example, the defendant may file a demurrer to the plaintiff's allegations. This motion essentially says that even if one assumes that all the facts that the plaintiff alleges are true, that he (plaintiff) still has not stated a basis for recovery from the defendant and the defendant has not violated any law or any duty owed to the plaintiff. The legal phrase used to describe this is that the plaintiff does not have a cause of action against the defendant. Even if the defendant's motion on demurrer is overruled, he can then produce various affidavits and might move for a summary judgment. This would be a final judgment in the case and would only be granted if there was no substantial disagreement in the facts or the details of evidence, and the court could then say as a matter of law that the plaintiff could not recover. If none of these pretrial motions end the case at that point, there will then be time for pretrial discovery in which more details would be elicited and the issues narrowed and a trial date will be set. Of course a settlement might be effected between the two parties at any point in time, and the case would be ended immediately. Because all of this is time consuming and expensive, a great many of the cases are settled before trial. Obviously then, those cases that even get to trial are a very small percentage of the number of original claims and a small percentage of those in which a suit was filed. Even during the course of a trial, the two parties may get together on a settlement and end the case right there, without going through the long process of trial and jury verdict.

After the presentation of the evidence by both the plaintiff and the defendant, the defendant (it does not have to be the defendant, but he is the usual party) may move for a directed verdict. This motion, if granted, would take the case out of the hands of the jury, and the judge would say as a matter of law that there was not sufficient evidence to support the allegations of the plaintiff. If granted, it would mean a verdict entered for the defendant.

After all the evidence has been presented by the plaintiff and the defendant and after the judge has instructed the jury as to the law, then it is the jury's province to determine the facts of the case, if there is any conflict, and to render a decision. It should be emphasized that a decision is a verdict on the basis of facts found by the jury in the framework of the law as given to the jury by the judge. After the jury has returned and rendered their verdict, the losing party can request a new trial or can ask for a judgment notwithstanding the verdict. In either case, the basis would be that the losing party would ask the judge to say that as a matter of law, the jury's verdict was not substantiated by the evidence presented. Whether the judge grants either of those motions or enters judgment based on the jury's verdict, the judgment or motions can then be appealed to a higher appellate court. The appeal is made at the time when an appellate court can review the lower court's decisions. In general, something is appealable when it essentially terminates the proceedings. Those motions made during the course of a trial on whether evidence is to be admitted or not are not appealable in the following sense: the party who is ruled against cannot stop the trial and go through the lengthy process of appeal just to review a specific motion. However, after the case is terminated some other way and if it is appealed to a higher court, then those motions ruling on the admission of evidence can be reviewed by the higher court.

After a judgment is rendered by a jury, many cases end there. Cases may go further, but even if the case is appealed, it is still possible for the two parties to reach a settlement while waiting for the appellate court to hear the case. Thus, still fewer cases get to the appellate courts. Therefore, by the time a case gets to an appellate court level, there are very, very few of those complaints that were initially voiced or even those cases which were originally filed.

The general rule is that the appellate court will review only issues of law. The fact questions decided by the jury or the trier of fact — the judge if not tried before a jury — will not be reviewed unless there are obvious or gross errors in fact determinations. The appellate court will then consider reviewing the motions on which the trial judge ruled to determine whether they were correct as a matter of law. However, when the case below has been terminated by summary judgment, directed verdict, judgment notwithstanding the verdict or the granting of a new trial, which are all made by the trial judge by determining as a matter of law that there was not sufficient evidence to support the allegations of the other party, the appellate court on review then may get into the question of whether the trial court was right in ruling as a matter of law on the sufficiency of the evidence. In such cases, the appellate courts will consider the legal sufficiency of the evidence.

It is also important to understand that because of the volume of litigation and because the appellate courts deal with questions of law which have general applicability rather than dealing with only the specific facts in a particular case, only the appellate decisions are published so that there is general access to them. Therefore, the law reports that are readily and publicly accessible contain only a very small percentage of original claims or cases filed, and these reports are more concerned with the principles of law than with specific factual situations, except as they may impinge upon the principles of law. Therefore, it is obvious that if one goes to law reports looking for cases involving hospital acquired infections, there will be very few cases to begin with that reach the appellate level and are reported. Most of the cases that have reached the appellate level and are reported involve some general principle of law rather than specific questions of hospital infection control.

One will also note that there is often a distinction made in the law between procedure and substance. Procedure deals with the mechanics of bringing a complaint from filing to pretrial motions, discovery, trial, judgment, and appeal. Substantive aspects are essentially all those other aspects which deal with causes of action, kinds of proof, how much is needed to prove the allegations brought by the plaintiff, what sort of defenses are available to the defendant, and what kind and how much evidence is needed to be presented by the defendant to prove those.

The substantive area that we are most concerned about with respect to hospital acquired infections is that area referred to as the law of torts. This covers wrongs committed by one person against another person. This is as opposed to those wrongs which are violations of the state's laws which are all lumped together under the heading of criminal law. Under the larger heading of torts, there are the two main areas of intentional torts and unintentional torts. Examples of intentional torts are assault, battery, and false imprisonment. Under the unintentional torts, perhaps the largest category is that of negligence. Under the tort law of negligence, there have to be four elements present for there to have been legally compensable negligence. These are all well known, but for sake of completeness, they will be mentioned briefly. The four elements necessary for negligence are

1. There has to be a standard of care (duty).
2. There has to be a failure to meet the standard of care or perform the duty.
3. The injury complained of must be the direct result of the failure to meet the standard of care or to perform the duty (this failure to meet the standard of care or to perform the duty is the proximal cause of the injury).
4. There must be actual damages which can be assessed in terms of monetary loss.

These actual damages include such things as medical expenses, e.g., physicians' bills, hospital bills, and pharmacy bills for medications. There are such ancillary expenses as expenses for housekeepers, maids, and babysitters. These are all relatively easy to quantitate. Other actual damages include loss of income, both current and future. As long as there are actual damages, there can be an award for pain and suffering. This of course is the hardest of the elements to quantitate.

There were times and situations in which a plaintiff could not prove each of these specific elements of negligence in order to gain a recovery for an injury. There were certain situations in which it seemed obvious that the injured party ought to recover because he had nothing to do with the injury, and the event that occurred was so far beyond the ordinary course of events that it seemed that it could not have happened unless there had been negligence on someone's part, yet the injured party could not show specific negligence on the part of any particular person. In these situations, the courts have announced certain criteria which enable the plaintiff to still go forward against the defendant in these cases in which specific negligence cannot be proved. The courts will still allow the jury to consider the possible negligence of the defendant on this basis. This has been given the name of *res ipsa loquitur* which means "the thing speaks for itself". The elements that must be present are the following:

1. Whatever occurred causing injury to the plaintiff must be something that ordinarily does not happen unless there is negligence.
2. The agents or instrumentalities that caused the incident to take place were under the complete control of the defendant.
3. The plaintiff did nothing in any way to contribute to the injury.

There has been a reluctance on the part of the courts to apply this to medical situations. Perhaps the area in which this doctrine is most widely applied in the medical field is that situation in which some injury occurred to a plaintiff during the time of an operation. During that period, the plaintiff may well have been under anesthesia and could not tell who was there or what happened to him. So as long as he shows that whatever occurred was something that ordinarily does not occur without negligence and that he was unconscious at the time and that all the instrumentalities and agencies involved were those of the defendant and that he did nothing to contribute to his injury, then this will be enough of a presentation to allow the judge to let the jury decide in that situation whether the plaintiff's injury was due to the defendant or not and whether the plaintiff could recover. In a way, this may be looked at as a special exception to the ordinary elements of negligence enabling the plaintiff to get to the jury without having to bring forth quite so much in the way of evidence.

THE EXPERT WITNESS

There is one area of the presentation of evidence in a case involving negligence that should be emphasized, and that is the role of the expert witness. In cases not involving medical negligence, the duty owed one person to another person is often described in terms of what a reasonable man would have done under the same or similar circumstances. The jury having been instructed by the judge on this point as a matter of law is then free to decide in the particular fact situation whether the defendant behaved in accordance with the standard of care toward the plaintiff. The jury can bring to this decision their own knowledge of circumstances in everyday life. However, when the case involves questions of medical negligence, then the courts are almost universal in their statements to the effect that the jury is not free to speculate as to what the standards of care are, what the duties are, and whether the injury complained of could be causally linked to the duty that the plantiff is alleging that the defendant failed to perform and which was owed to the plaintiff by the defendant. There are, of course, some situations in which the court will say that it is obvious to ordinary men whether the injury which occurred, and the alleged behavior of the defendant was such that no expert testimony was needed. As an example, it would not take an expert witness to testify to the fact that if a plaintiff went to an operating room to have a tonsillectomy performed, the occurrence of a burn on the foot was something that would ordinarily not occur and should not be considered a routine risk of the procedure. Such an event is something that even nonmedical laymen would understand was not part of the contemplated procedure. The role of the expert can be crucial in that if the plaintiff cannot find experts to testify as to the standard of care, then his case may fail. If the plaintiff cannot find experts to testify that the defendant's actions failed to meet the standard of care owed to the plaintiff, then the plaintiff's case will fail. If the plaintiff cannot find experts who will testify that the defendant's failure to meet the standard of care directly resulted in the injury that the plaintiff incurred, then again the plaintiff's case will fail. It is apparent that it is very important to the plaintiff's case to be able to find experts who will testify to these various elements in order to establish negligence. On the other hand, it is just as important for the defendant to find experts willing to testify on the opposite side of those issues. In fact, in reading through some of the cases, if one only superficially considers the fact situations, one will note that there will be cases in which the fact situations seem to be identical, but the results are diametrically opposed. In many of these cases, the difference can be traced back to the fact that in one case, one might have expert testimony saying that a particular defendant's behavior violated the standard of care and that this failure to meet the standard of care was the direct cause of the plaintiff's injury, while in the other cases, the testimony of the experts may be all on the other side. This is particularly apparent in those cases involving *res ipsa loquitur* and the question of whether the occurrence of a certain event necessarily means negligence. There are some cases with virtually the same fact situation in which the plaintiff has found an expert witness who testifies that such an event cannot happen without negligence being present. If the opposing side does not present any evidence to the contrary, then this is what the court has to accept in that case (medical facts or objective reality notwithstanding). In other cases with the same fact situation, the testimony may be that the event that occurred can occur quite naturally without the presence of any negligence. If this is not opposed by some contrary evidence, then this is what the court has to accept. Of course, there is an exception when the facts in question are so obvious or well known, and the court can take judicial notice of those facts, but in situations involving medical judgment, the courts have to rely strictly and solely on the medical experts' testimony. One can imagine the possible bizarre results which may occur, depending on the accuracy of the medical expert testimony involved. Therefore, it is extremely important for those with expertise in the fields of infectious disease, infection control, and hospital epidemiology to be willing to testify as experts in cases involving such questions. Such involvement will prevent medically inaccurate testimony to be thrust upon the courts by those who do not have the same knowledge or expertise in these areas.

HOSPITAL ACQUIRED INFECTIONS

It is interesting and helpful to look at the phrase "hospital acquired", both from a medical viewpoint and a legal viewpoint. One definition which is equivalent to the phrase "nosocomial infection" appears in *Control of Communicable Diseases in man*:[5] "An infection originating in a medical facility; e.g., occurring in a hospitalized patient in whom it was not present, or incubating at the time of admission, or is the residual of an infection acquired during a previous admission. Includes infections acquired in the hospital but appearing after discharge; it also includes infections among staff."

Obviously then, there are several different kinds of hospital acquired infections. There can be those acquired by a patient from another patient because of something the hospital either did or did not do. It may be an infection acquired by a patient from an employee, particularly a nurse, or it may be an infection acquired by the patient from a visitor. It may be an infection acquired by an employee. It may be an infection acquired by a visitor to the hospital, presumably either from a patient or an employee. One should note that this does not include patients who are seen as outpatients or patients who were seen only in the emergency room, nor does it include the possibility of someone acquiring an infection through some action or inaction on the part of the hospital, even though the person so infected had no contact with the hospital (as far-fetched as this sounds, see the Derrick case *infra*).

From this, one might say that hospital acquired infections are viewed in one of three possible ways: temporally, geographically, or causally. Obviously the definition of the hospital acquired infection is not based on the temporal aspects in the sense that one is only looking at infections which appear during the time of hospitalization, since a hospital acquired infection is not any infection that appears during the time of the hospitalization; specifically excluded from hospital acquired infections are those infections that occur during the time of hospitalization, but which were incubating at the time of admission. On the other hand, included in hospital acquired infections are those that began while still in the hospital and yet were not manifest until after discharge; those are to be counted as hospital acquired infections. If the basis for a hospital acquired infection is not based on the time in which it is acquired, then most people would probably assume that it related to causation, i.e., a hospital acquired infection was one caused by the hospital. As attractive as this idea may be some people, particularly attorneys and plaintiffs, it is not my views of what is meant by a hospital acquired infection. The true etiology of some infections is very difficult, if not impossible, to pinpoint. I do not believe that the definition looks specifically to causation. One will note from the definition that it is possible to have an infection that may have been caused, in an absolute sense, by a hospital to a patient in the emergency room, by an outpatient, or perhaps to someone not even associated with the hospital, and yet that would not be considered as hospital acquired. On the other hand, it is quite possible for a visitor to a patient to bring some infection in with him and thus infect the patient. That would not necessarily be caused by the hospital, but yet it would be considered a hospital acquired infection. Therefore, I believe that the definition of hospital acquired infections pertains to the geographic aspects of whether an infection is hospital acquired or not. This is reasonable, since hospitals are concerned about those infections that occur in patients while they are hospitalized which may prolong their hospitalization and which may be due to some environmental factors which the hospital may be able to identify and to eliminate. One looks at hospital acquired infections not to determine liability or blame, nor for the etiology of every single infection (unless a very unusual or rare one). Hospital acquired infections are viewed for epidemiologic purposes. If one were concerned specifically with causation, then every single hospital acquired infection would have to be traced back to its etiology, if possible. However, a study of hospital acquired infections looks at the overall picture of infections acquired within a hospital and observes trends for several months to get a standard or baseline. Such a standard yields an understanding of those infections that are commonly and ordinarily found in a particular hospital. It is then, and only then, with that baseline data on which to base one's perspectives that one can appreciate any increase in infections in one area of the hospital or in patients who undergo one type of procedure or patients who have any particular factors in common. When the hospital surveillance done by the ICP identifies an increase in infections above the baseline, there is an attempt made to find the factor or factors in common, and when these are identified, to then try to find a remedy and effect that remedy. This must be done individually for each specific hospital, and the results at one hospital often cannot be compared with the results at another hospital. If there are any factors found in common, these often can be traced to changes in handwashing, isolation, disinfection, or sterilization techniques. Since we exist in a sea of organisms, it is highly unlikely that there will ever be a time or place when there will be a zero incidence of infection following any procedure. Whether it be an operation, a catheterization, drawing bloods, giving injections, or whatever, there will be a certain percent who will develop some infection no matter how careful one is. Also, since human bodies will continue to have infections even outside of hospitals, it is reasonable to assume that a certain percentage of human beings will develop similar infections while they are in a hospital, so that for epidemiological purposes, we may consider these as nosocomial or hospital acquired. There should be no fault merely because such infections occur.

Of course, hospitals may be liable for hospital acquired infections if reasonable procedures and standards have not been met in sterilizing equipment, maintaining proper isolation techniques, and maintaining other standards that deal with patients and infections. Most hospital acquired infections will probably not result in litigation unless there has been some breakdown in isolation or sterilization techniques and unless such failure is the direct cause of the hospital acquired infection. The definition of standards of care can be as important as following established policies and procedures.

CASES INVOLVING HOSPITAL ACQUIRED INFECTIONS

In considering all of the summaries in the section entitled Table of Cases, one can see that approximately half are cases involving postoperative or postprocedure infections. One can note the extremely important place of expert testimony in almost all of these cases. In some of the cases involving similar events, the results seem to be very closely tied to whether there was expert testimony establishing a standard of care, establishing whether there had been a violation of that standard of care and whether that violation was the proximal cause of the injury. For example, refer to the Casey case in which gangrene developed in an arm after open reduction. There was indication that defendant's neglect to inspect the wound for 4 days despite indications of possible infection and embarassment to the circulation violated the standard of care to the plaintiff and that this was the proximal cause of her injury. Yet in the Smith case, there was staphylococcal osteomyelitis following open reduction of a fractured left femur. No medical expert testimony was produced by the plaintiff, and therefore the defendant received a directed verdict in his favor, since the mere presence of an infection was not evidence of negligence per se. In the case of Perrin after a slot graft fusion on plaintiff's leg, an infection developed. In this case, the defendant produced a medical expert, who testified to the fact that the care given to the plaintiff was reasonable, even though the bandage and cast had not been inspected for 14 days. This just emphasizes the fact that appropriate medical expert testimony which is sufficient to create a fact issue will then become a jury question, but that if no such medical expert testimony is forthcoming, then plaintiff may very well lose before even getting to the jury.

Perhaps it is even clearer to see what happens in the postinjection cases in which the plaintiff is complaining of some infection which appeared after receiving an injection. There are the cases like Kalmus, where the expert testimony was that the infection that occurred after the injection could have been due only to severe bruising or to an infected needle. Since there was no evidence of bruising, therefore there must have been an unsterile needle, and everyone had agreed that the use of an unsterile needle violated the standard of care to the plaintiff. There is also the Southern Florida Sanitarium and Hospital case, where the medical expert testimony was that infectious thrombophlebitis would have occurred if there were no departure from the medical standard of sterility, but that this condition could occur from a failure to maintain sterility. In these cases, of course, the plaintiff won. However, in the Kaster case, there was no expert testimony that plaintiff's infection after the injection was caused by anything done by the defendant or its emloyees, and there was no evidence of any causal connection between the injection and the subsequent infection. Without the necessary expert testimony, the plaintiff lost. In the Sommers case, the evidence was that the needles involved were sterile and disposable. There was no evidence that the needle was contaminated prior to the injection, and there was undisputed medical expert testimony that bacteria were not only on the surface of the skin, but under the surface where they might not always be killed by antiseptics and that it was impossible to inject without carrying some bacteria along with the injection. In these cases, it is easy to see the effect that the difference in the medical expert testimony had on the various outcomes. It is not too difficult then to conclude that the medical expert testimony is one of the very most important parts of a case involving any medical malpractice, but particularly when it comes to hospital acquired infections. If the plaintiff's medical experts testify to something and it is undisputed by the defendant's experts, then that is accepted as a fact. The same thing of course, can occur with defendant's medical experts' testimony. With respect to the cases involving newborn infants, it is interesting to note how many of them seem to involve skin infections of one sort or another. (There seem to be fads in lawsuits as well as in many other areas.)

In those cases involving the transmission of an infection to a patient from either another patient or from a staff member, the two most widely cited cases are those of Helman and Kapuschinsky in which both of the infections were staphylococcal, and in both cases there was a question of whether the strain of staphylococci found in the plaintiff was identical to the same strain found in the plaintiff's roommate in the Helman case and in one of the nursing aides in Kapuschinsky. This again involved matters of medical expert testimony. In neither of these two cases was Phage typing available, and the evidence dealt with a comparison of the antibiotic sensitivities of the different staphylococci. In the Helman case, the court noted that since there was evidence on both sides of the question as to whether the staphylococcus that infected Helman was the same as the staphylococcus that his roommate had, it was a jury question to decide. In spite of the fact that there were different antibiotic sensitivities, the jury apparently decided that these two staphylococci were the same. In the Kapuschinsky case, the staphylococci grown from the nose culture of the nursing assistant showed a different pattern of antibiotic sensitivities as compared to those from the plaintiff's left hip. Again the jury said that the two organisms were the same, and the hospital was found liable for the transfer of the staphylococcal infection from the nursing assistant to the newborn plaintiff.

In the Thigpen case, it was established that a nurse's aide did have a cause of action against the hospital for the acquisition of a staphylococcal infection. In part, the hospital's negligence was alleged because the hospital had knowledge of the presence of the staphylococcal infections which had been documented by the infectious disease committee some months before the plaintiff became ill.

Finally, there are the cases in which the plaintiffs were indirectly related to the defendant. In the Gill case, the plaintiff was said to have a valid cause of action against his roommate's physician because the roommate's physician did not warn either his patient or the plaintiff or the hospital that the physician's patient had a contagious disease. Such failure to communicate was said to subject the plaintiff to an unreasonable risk of catching that disease. One would think that such a precedent would encourage many physicians to put patients on isolation now, since their failure to do so might occasion a lawsuit from another patient in the same room who might be unreasonably exposed to whatever disease had not been isolated. In the Derrick case, the plaintiff was neither a patient in the hospital nor a patient of the doctor and had no connection with the hospital, yet the court held that the plaintiff had a cause of action against the defendant hospital, since it did not notify the local health officer that one of the patients in the hospital had a contagious disease and that the plaintiff subsequently contracted the contagious disease. One wonders about the possible broad applicability of such a precedent, particularly in the field of venereal diseases. If the doctors and hospitals who do not report gonorrhea and syphilis to the health department as required by law and if their infected patients or perhaps their contacts continue to spread the disease, then would one who contracted the disease subsequently have a valid cause of action against the doctor or hospital who failed to report, thus setting up a chain of failing to identify all the contacts and failing to have them treated and cleared of their infections? Following the Derrick case, such a chain of causation might well establish a valid cause of action. In this way, it is somewhat similar to the Missouri, Kansas, and Texas Railway case in which a nonhospitalized member of the community was exposed to small pox because of the defendant hospital's action or inaction.

MANAGEMENT OF MEDICAL-LEGAL PROBLEMS

It is obvious that as with many infectious diseases, the best treatment is prevention. One must continually review the obligation of the hospital to its patients which comes under the broad heading of "duty". Of course, the duty of reasonable care and behavior is something that will always be present. One would want that maintained on the basis of appropriateness and reasonableness, if for no other reason. With respect to the duties which may be imposed by policies and procedures, then perhaps one should be realistic. Some seem to like to write policies and procedures that may be theoretically ideal, but which are not practically attainable because of either the time, personnel, or costs involved. However, to put a policy or procedure like this in one's manuals just because it is thought that it might look good to any inspecting group that might later inspect, can be detrimental if such policy or procedure is not followed and if it is possible that expert testimony might link a patient's injury to the failure of the hospital to follow such a policy or procedure. Also, one's policies and procedures ought to be workable and enforceable. If adherence to the policy cannot be monitored, then one should think very seriously about whether such a policy or procedure should appear in one's official policy and procedure manuals. A hospital may find to its regret that such a procedure was not being followed, and yet because it did not monitor the adherence to that policy, it may be found negligent in its care of its patients. In this respect, there should be frequent monitoring of the policies and procedures to make sure that they are being followed. In particular, those involving infection control probably should be surveyed or monitored at some regular interval by the ICP.

One could detect any failure to follow such a policy or procedure and to correct it, but also prove, even if retrospectively, that the hospital was interested and concerned in that area, that it was actively monitoring infection control procedures, that nonadherence was being corrected, and that the hospital was pursuing a reasonable course in protecting its patients from infection.

In doing this, it is my opinion that one should not try to hide problems. If a hospital infection committee's minutes reflect that problems within the hospital are recognized and that active attempts are made in trying to correct those situations, such evidence would not be harmful to a hospital. If, however, none of that information appears in the hospital infection committee's minutes, then some people might try to draw the conclusion that the hospital either tried to hide problems or was not concerned enough to even attempt to identify problems or deal with them.

Although in most of the cases there has been no duty imposed on the hospital to warn patients coming into it that there were various infections present within the hospital, one might attempt to inform entering patients of the possibility of a hospital acquired infection by means of one of the hospital informational booklets that some hospitals give to all entering patients. Or perhaps the hospital's attorney might consider putting such warning or notice in the informed consent form which most hospitals get entering patients to sign acknowledging consent to hospitalization.

If litigation does arise, then the best procedure would be to thoroughly brief the attorney representing the hospital as to the medical aspects, particularly the infectious disease and microbiological aspects of the particular case. As noted above, the medical expert testimony may be the key to the hospital's presentation of its side of the case. With good medical expert testimony, good documentation of an active, conscientious infection control committee that is actively seeking out problem areas and dealing with those problems consistently and in an appropriate manner, and with a competent attorney who is thoroughly grounded in the medical aspects of the case and the implications, then the hospital will be able to present the best possible case for its side. Failure to do so may be not only disasterous for the hospital, but may allow medically inaccurate statements, opinions, and information to be perpetuated and to influence future litigation.

TABLE OF CASES

Adams vs. Eye, Ear, Nose, and Throat Hospital, 346 So.2d 327 (1977). Plaintiff was scheduled for the removal of a cataract from his left eye on September 11, 1972. Preoperatively, his ophthalmologist cultured his eye and gave prophylactic antibiotics. Antibiotics were also used postoperatively. On September 14, an eye infection was noted. The antibiotics were increased, and new ones were added. The infection progressed and the left eye had to be removed on September 20. The plaintiff was subsequently discharged from the hospital on September 24, 1972, after an uneventful recovery. The infecting organism was *Citrobacter diversus.* The expert testimony indicated that there were no reported cases of eye infection due to that organism, that the defendant, hospital, and doctor had met or exceeded the standard of care, and that infection could occur, no matter how meticulous or cautious the surgeon had been. The hospital pathologist said, "There was no evidence of the organism found in the hospital, and there were no reports of any of the other patients developing a similar infection." In addition, there was no expert testimony indicating how the organism might have gotten into the plaintiff's eye. The plaintiff's suit was dismissed, and that was affirmed on appeal. It is interesting that the court thought that the organism might have come from the patient himself.

Adams vs. Poudre Valley Hospital District, 173 Colo. 98, 476 P.2d 565 (1970). Plaintiff was operated on December 17, 1963, and he alleged that he contracted a staphylococcal infection about the time of the operation. The court held that the claims based on negligence and *res ipsa loquitur* were barred by a 2-year statute of limitations, but that a third claim based on a breach of contract would not be barred because there was a longer statute of limitations for contracts. Since there was no evidence as to whether there was an express contract or not, the case was remanded for retrial. At the retrial, 31 Colo. App. 252, 502 P.2d 1127 (1972), it was determined by the trial court that there was no express contract, and a summary judgment was granted. That was affirmed by the appellate court.

Aetna Casualty and Surety Company vs. Pilcher, 244 Ark. 11, 424 S.W.2d 181 (1968). Plaintiff had his leg operated upon on September 21, 1962. He was discharged from the hospital 8 days later. Two months later, he was admitted to another hospital with a fever and reddened throat and was diagnosed as having a streptococcal respiratory infection and was subsequently discharged on December 10, 1962. Four days later, he was seen by his surgeon who saw no sign of leg infection. On January 25, 1963, he was re-examined and found to have a bone infection. The infection was said to be due to a *Staphylococcus epidermidis.* Plaintiff first alleged that the hospital failed to warn the plaintiff of the presence of organisms within the hospital. The court held that the hospital's failure to warn the plaintiff was not the proximal cause of his injury. There was no testimony that the paintiff would have refused the operation if he had been so apprised or that he would have done anything about it if he had the knowledge. Also, plaintiff's physician knew of the presence of the organism, and if the physician did not use reasonable care to guard against infection from those organisms, then the physician was negligent and not the hospital. Plaintiff also alleged negligence in that the hospital failed to discover the presence of the organisms in the hospital. The court held that the hospital did discover them and had made efforts to guard against them. Plaintiff also alleged that the hospital had failed to discover that the plaintiff had developed an infection with those organisms. The court said that this was the duty of his physician and not of the hospital, but in addition, since the infection apparently developed 4 months later and he had not been in the hospital since 8 days after his operation, the hospital could not discover the subsequent infection. Finally, the plaintiff claimed that the hospital had been negligent in failing to keep the operating room and the surgical instruments free from infecting organisms and that this was the proximate cause of his infection. The court held that since there was undisputed testimony that the organism could have entered the plaintiff in so many different ways and from so many different sources and in view of the difficulty in controlling it, the court held that the jury's verdict for the plaintiff was based on mere speculation and not on substantial evidence. The court also noted that there was no expert testimony that the hospital was negligent; therefore, the judgment for the plaintiff was reversed.

Anderson vs. Lutheran Deaconess Hospital, 257 N.W.2d 561 (1977). In this case, plaintiff alleged negligence of the hospital in failing to diagnose and treat *Hemophilus parainfluenza* endocarditis. The court held that the action was barred by the statute of limitations.

Aurelio vs. Laird, 352 Mass. 1, 223 N.E.2d 531 (1967). Plaintiff was born October 6, 1960 and discharged with his mother October 10, 1960, at which time at least one of the nurses had noted a small red area on the right hip. For the next few days, the mother described pus and blood draining from this area and attempted to see their family doctor. Finally on October 18, plaintiff was seen by a pediatrician, who immediately referred him for hospitalization for a cellulitus due to *Staphylococcus aureus.* Defendant doctor's liability was based on how he responded to treatment of the plaintiff when he was informed of the pus draining from the area 2 to 3 days after he was discharged from the hospital. The court apparently felt that good and prudent care would have required culturing the red area that had pus on October 10 and then either start antibiotics at that time or await the culture report.

Bartlett vs. Argonaut Insurance Companies, 258 Ark. 221, 523 S.W.2d 385 (1975). Following back surgery, the plaintiff developed infection with *S. aureus.* A summary judgment in favor of the hospital was affirmed on appeal. The court noted that *res ipsa loquitur* did not apply, since the hospital was not in complete control of the staphylococcal organisms which might be brought into the hospital by the patient himself. Also the plaintiff presented no expert testimony showing that the hospital used substandard housekeeping procedures. There were depositions from the plaintiff to the effect that the hospital floors were not swept every day and some of the nurses wore their hospital uniforms from home, but there was no proof as to how these events were the proximal cause of the plaintiff's injuries.

Beeck vs. Tucson General Hospital, 18 Ariz. App. 165, 500 P.2d 1153 (1972). During a myelogram the X-ray screen struck the needle in the plaintiff's back causing an injury to the plaintiff and subsequent pneumonia (the court said, " . . . she had contracted pneumonia from the extravasation of the dye from the myelographic procedure."). It was assumed that the radiologist was negligent. Thus, the question was really whether the hospital was liable on the principle of respondeat superior or whether the radiologist was an independent contractor, thus exonerating the hospital. It was decided that the hospital was liable for the assumed negligence of the radiologist.

Brown vs. Shannon West Texas Memorial Hospital, 222 S.W.2d 248 (1949). Plaintiff gave a blood donation at defendant hospital and within a day developed an infection in the arm from which the blood was drawn. The expert testimony indicated that there was no way of telling the source of the infection and there was no expert testimony that the needle in blood-drawing was infected. Judgment for the defendant hospital was affirmed.

Burchfield vs. Geitz, 516 S.W.2d 299 (1974). Plaintiff was operated on for a herniated disk August 11, 1969. Subsequently he developed drainage from the incision and was treated off and on for this for several months. Finally in March 1970, he went to another city to another physician at which time he had another operation, and the infection was found centered around two sutures deep in his incision. Subsequently his incision healed without complications. The medical expert who testified for the plaintiff indicated that the defendant had not failed in his standard of care. The plaintiff also alleged that the use of a Hubbard tank after her incision began to drain was negligent. The court noted that the plaintiff already had her infection before she had been put into the Hubbard tank. There was no proof of any causal connection between the defendant's actions and the plaintiff's injury. The defendant obtained a directed verdict at the trial and this was affirmed on appeal.

Bush vs. Board of Managers of Binghamton City Hospital, 251 App. Div. 601, 297 N.Y.S. 991 (1937). Plaintiff's wife and child were admitted to the defendant hospital on June 19, 1926, for the treatment of measles. Plaintiff's wife died July 6, 1926. Plaintiff sued the defendant hospital for the death of his wife, and the court held that there was too little evidence to support finding that plaintiff's wife contracted diphtheria and died from it. The judgment for the plaintiff was reversed and the case was remanded for a new trial. Plaintiff's only expert based his opinion that plaintiff's wife had diphtheria on a smear from the nose, throat culture being negative.

Capelouto vs. Kaiser Foundation Hospitals, 7 Cal. 3d 889, 103 Cal. Rptr. 856, 500 P.2d 880 (1972). Plaintiff was born on July 30, 1964. Plaintiff and her mother were both discharged on August 2. Subsequently plaintiff developed projectile vomiting, severe diarrhea, dehydration, and she was hospitalized six times during her first year of life. Stool culture grew *Salmonella newport*; it was treated and she ultimately recovered with no permanent disability. In the lower court, there was evidence presented that the defendant hospital did not meet its duty with respect to newborn infants and that its standard of care fell below the standards of care for hospitals in the area; furthermore, there was evidence that *Salmonella* infections did not spread if the standards of care were met. There was evidence that the plaintiff contracted the *Salmonella* infection shortly after birth from another newborn infant, who apparently contracted the disease at birth from his mother who was an asymptomatic carrier. On appeal, the question was not whether the hospital was liable for the *Salmonella* infection transmitted to the plaintiff, but whether the plaintiff as a newborn infant could collect for pain and suffering as well as medical expenses, and the appellate court held that the plaintiff could so collect.

Casey vs. Penn, 45 Ill. App.3d 573, 360 N.E.2d 93 (1977). Plaintiff, a 15-year-old girl, fell from a pony and broke her left wrist. On June 5, 1967, an open reduction of that fracture was performed by the defendant. For the next 5 days her arm was swollen, there was seepage and foul odor because of the infection that developed. On June 30, she had to have her left arm amputated below the elbow. At the trial, there was a jury judgment for the defendant which was reversed by the appellate court which held that defendant was negligent in that he failed to inspect the wound for 4 days postoperatively despite indications of possible infection or embarassment to the circulation. Also, it was negligent not to follow up on the Gram stain and culture performed June 8. The defendant also contributed to her problem by the use of a compressive bandage on her left arm postoperatively.

City of Shawnee vs. Jeter, 96 Okla. 272, 221 P. 758 (1923). Plaintiff's wife entered defendant's hospital in January 1922 and died on January 22. Plaintiff alleged that his wife contracted smallpox in the hospital and that that disease was the cause of her death. Judgment for the plaintiff at the trial court was reversed and remanded for a new trial. The only evidence showed that the plaintiff's wife was in a section entirely separate from where there was a patient with smallpox, and there was no evidence that either of the two nurses who worked in the isolation section with the smallpox patient ever left that section of the hospital or visited any of the other wards. Also, because of the incubation period of smallpox, it was believed that the plaintiff's wife already had been exposed to smallpox at the time of her admission, and thus, even if the hospital had been negligent in isolating the patient with smallpox, that was not the proximate cause of the plaintiff's wife contracting smallpox and dying.

Contreras vs. St. Luke's Hospital, 78 Cal. App.3d 919, 144 Cal. Rptr. 647 (1978). In 1970, plaintiff developed a knee injury while water skiing. It was diagnosed as a torn medial collateral ligament of the right knee. After consultation with several orthopedic surgeons who advised operation, plaintiff decided to have the operation. He was apprised by the surgeon of possible complications of the operation, including infection; postoperatively the patient developed an enterococcal infection of the knee and was hospitalized for 40 days and a second operation was required. At the trial, plaintiff presented evidence only by himself, his wife, and an intern. At the trial, a nonsuit was granted in favor of the defendants, the court holding that the plaintiff had not presented any substantial evidence as to the negligence of the defendant hospital or surgeon.

Criss vs. Angelus Hospital Association of Los Angeles, 13 Cal App.2d 412, 56 P.2d 1274 (1936). Plaintiff sued for the death of his 12-day-old child, alleging that the hospital negligently permitted the newborn infant to become infected with impetigo, negligently treated the infant after the infection developed, and negligently discharged the mother and the infant at the time when the infant was suffering from impetigo. No facts were related with respect to either the diagnosis or the treatment. Plaintiff won.

DeFalco vs. Long Island College Hospital, 393 N.Y.S.2d 859 (1977). Plaintiff had a cataract removed from an eye on May 14, 1970, and on May 26 or 27, it was noted that he had developed an eye infection with *Enterobacter* and *Staphylococcus albus.* Plaintiff alleged that this resulted in his losing his eye on January 21, 1976. There was a jury verdict for the plaintiff, but on appeal, the defendant's motion to set the verdict aside was granted, the court holding that the presence of the infection in late May 1970 did not give rise to an inference of negligence per se, that there was no medical expert testimony that the plaintiff's infection was the result of negligence, or that there was any negligence on the part of the defendant which resulted in the plaintiff's losing his eye some 6 years later.

Denneny vs. Siegel, 276 F. Supp. 281 (1967), 407 F.2d 433 (1969). Plaintiff had had past medical history that revealed multiple abdominal operations and was admitted for a vaginal hysterectomy and anterior and posterior repair. This was performed on June 6, 1961. Consequently the right uterine artery tore loose from the surgical clamp and a laparotomy was necessary. There was an infection in the surgical wound postoperatively that was said to have been expected. On June 17, the abdominal incision opened and part of the intestinal tract protruded. Again, another infection was found in the incisional site, and her physicians attributed it to the same etiology as her previous infection. On July 2, she began to hemorrhage from the vagina and was rushed to the operating room to find the bleeding site. At that time, it was alleged by the plaintiff that a person in street clothes assisted in taking her to the operating room, went into the operating room, and that it was the negligence of the hospital in allowing this person in street clothes into the operating room which caused a postoperative incisional wound infection a week after this operation. There was a considerable dispute as to whether anyone in street clothes had ever entered the operating room. The trial court held that even if this occurred, there needed to be some expert medical testimony establishing a relationship between this act and the subsequent wound infection. Since there was no such expert testimony, a jury's verdict could only be based on speculation and conjecture; the courts will not permit this, and the trial court directed a verdict in favor of the defendant.

Derrick vs. Ontario Community Hospital, 47 Cal.App.3d 145, 120 Cal.Rptr. 566 (1975). This case does not specifically involve a hospital acquired infection, but it has many implications in the area of hospital infection control. The plaintiff, who was never a patient in the defendant hospital sued the hospital, a hospital patient (a minor girl), the patient's mother, the patient's attending physician, and some fictitious doctors. The defendants demurred, and the trial court sustained the demurrer. The Court of Appeals reversed, saying that although there was no breach of a common law duty, there was a breach of the statutory duty to report to the local health officer any infectious or communicable disease. The defendant patient was admitted to the hospital on May 28, 1971, following an automobile accident. She was hospitalized from May 28, 1971 to June 16, 1971. While she was a patient in the hospital, she apparently developed what was said to be an infectious, highly contagious, communicable disease (which is never named). The patient apparently was discharged from defendant hospital. This is the "poisonous, infectious, contagious communicable disease" the plaintiff alleged that he had contracted from the defendant patient and that he suffered extensive surgery to his face and great mental and physical pain and permanent damages to the extent of $1 million. The statute said that the defendant hospital had a duty to report to the local health officer any infectious or communicable disease. This the hospital did not do. The court held that " . . . a presumption of negligence arises from the violation of a statute which was enacted to protect a class of persons of which the plaintiff is a member against the type of harm which the plaintiff suffered as a result of the violation of the statute." Since the statute was enacted to protect the public against the spread of communicable diseases, the hospital had a duty to inform the local health officer, and the hospital violated that duty in failing to report the case to the local health officer. The court noted in passing that there would be a real problem in proving proximate causation, i.e., it was the hospital's failure to inform the local public health officer of the defendant patient's contagious disease that was the direct cause of the plaintiff's injury. That was said to be a problem of proof and not that there was no cause of action. The case was remanded for trial. The plaintiff had stated a cause of action, whether he could prove his case or not was a different question to be resolved at trial.

Esposito vs. New York State Willowbrook State School, 38 App.Div.2d 985, 329 N.Y.S.2d 355 (1972), 46 App.Div.2d 969, 362 N.Y.S.2d 54 (1974). The first action was a workman's compensation claim for hepatitis developed by plaintiff as a food service worker at a state school where he was employed for 1½ days July 3 and 4, 1969, with the development of infectious hepatitis on August 25, 1969. In the first case, there was no evidence that he had come in contact with any particular patient or patients who had infectious hepatitis, and the only evidence presented was from the hospital director, who said that infectious hepatitis was endemic at the school. On this basis, the award to the plaintiff was reversed. In the second case, there was said to be substantial evidence to support the workman's compensation board's determination that plaintiff had contracted infectious hepatitis as a result of his exposure to the disease while employed at the state school. Although there was conflicting medical opinion, there was substantial medical evidence of a causal relationship and therefore the determination of the board was upheld.

Foley vs. Bishop Clarkson Memorial Hospital, 185 Neb. 89, 173 N.W.2d 881 (1970). Plaintiff was administrator of the estate of the deceased patient, who died 31 hr after delivering a child at the defendant hospital. The patient died of a beta hemolytic streptococcal infection. At the end of plaintiff's evidence, defendant requested a directed verdict. It was granted, but was reversed on appeal, the appellate court relying on the standard of care as shown by the rules of the defendant hospital. The court held that a hospital must guard against not only known physical and mental conditions of its patients, but also against such conditions as it should have discovered with the exercise of reasonable care. The court relied on the fact that before the deceased was admitted into the hospital, she had a sore throat. Plaintiff's medical expert attributed her death to failure to obtain a history of a cold prior to admission, failure to give more than aspirin at 14 hr postpartum when she had an increased temperature, pulse, and respiration, failure to notify the attending physician of this change in vital signs, and the administration of codeine and ice on her lower abdomen. It was also noted that several days after she died, one of her surviving children was treated in the hospital for a strep throat.

Folk vs. Kilk, 53 Cal.App.3d 176, 126 Cal.Rpt. 172 (1975). Plaintiff developed a brain abscess 5 days after a tonsillectomy. At the trial, there was a jury verdict in favor of the physicians and a nonsuit for the hospital. These verdicts were affirmed. The experts who testified had never heard of a brain abscess occurring immediately after a tonsillectomy, and it was the unanimous medical opinion that throat cultures were not standard preoperative before tonsillectomies. Since the etiology of brain abscess and the standard of care with respect to tonsillectomies were not a matter of common knowledge, medical expert testimony was necessary. If that was true, the court was correct in refusing to give a *res ipsa loquitur* instruction to the jury, the court saying, " . . . it is not even common knowledge that the abscess was probably caused by the tonsillectomy, let alone that the abscess was probably caused by a negligently performed tonsillectomy."

Gadsden General Hospital vs. Bishop, 209 Ala. 272, 96 So. 145 (1923). Plaintiff was administratrix for the deceased patient, her husband. Patient was hospitalized in defendant hospital March 1, 1920 to March 6, 1920. He developed a high fever on March 14 or 15. Four days later, he had a rash which was diagnosed as smallpox, and on April 1, he died. Plaintiff alleged that the death of the deceased was due to negligence of the defendant hospial in exposing him to smallpox. The court held that for the plaintiff to recover, five things had to be established: (1) plaintiff's intestate died of smallpox; (2) he contracted the disease while a patient in defendant hospital; (3) this resulted from an infection communicated to the deceased from another patient, who was in the hospital during the deceased's presence; (4) the defendant hospital's nurses, agents, or servants, who controlled or managed the hospital, knew that such other patient was afflicted with smallpox; and (5) they so negligently handled the patient with smallpox that they negligently exposed the deceased to the infection. The court noted that there was no evidence that there was a patient at the time that the deceased was in the hospital who had smallpox, nor could any of the hospital employees be held to have knowledge of the existence of any case of smallpox in the hospital. The plaintiff not having met her burden of proof, the trial court judgment for the plaintiff was reversed.

Garafola vs. Maimonides Hospital of Brooklyn, 22 App.Div.2d 85, 253 N.Y.S.2d 856 (1964). The patient, who was deceased, had a Caesarean section performed on June 7, 1954. On June 10, she developed a fever. On June 13, she developed a pain in her jaw and neck. On June 14, it was noted that she had difficulty opening her mouth, there was rigidity of neck and spasm of the jaws, and a tentative diagnosis of possible tetanus was made. On June 15, she died. The defendant hospital was held liable because it knew through its agents (a nurse and house officer) on June 13 of the deceased's complaints that she could not open her jaw and that not only was the diagnosis not made, but the attending physician was not informed of this. In an interesting dissent, it was noted that there was no medical expert testimony showing that the defendants, either doctors or hospital, were negligent in the performance of her Caesarean section, there was no suggestion made that there was any deviation from proper medical practice, and there was no evidence that the steps to insure adequate asepsis at the time of surgery were not done. The dissenters also noted that there was no expert testimony showing that if the attending physician had been notified on June 13 of the deceased's symptoms that anything different would have been done or that it would have made any difference in the outcome. (In other words, there was no showing that the hospital's failure to notify the attending physician was the proximate cause of her death.)

Garrison vs. Hotel Dieu, 319 So.2d 557 (1975). Plaintiff was operated on December 18, 1969 for a herniated disk which was removed. On December 19, plaintiff got up and showered. On December 24, plaintiff left the hospital. In mid-July 1970, plaintiff collapsed at home, and X-rays revealed an infection in the lumbar area in the space where the disk was removed. Plaintiff alleged that the infection in his back was due to bacteria forming on the surgical dressing which was dampened by the shower that he took on December 19. Plaintiff alleged that the defendant hospital's personnel negligently harassed him into taking a shower on the day after his surgery and that this resulted in his staphylococcal back infection. At the trial, plaintiff won; it was reversed on appeal. The court held that the evidence failed to establish a standard of care by the hospital, that the evidence failed to establish that the hospital personnel harassed the plaintiff into taking a shower, and that the evidence failed to establish that his back infection was caused by or even related to the shower incident. It was further noted that the skin incision was well healed and never showed any evidence of infection or drainage. The court also held that *res ipsa loquitur* did not apply.

Gill vs. Hartford Accident Indemnity Company, 337 So.2d 420 (1976). Plaintiff sued the defendant surgeon who was not the plaintiff's doctor, but the doctor of the patient in the same room as the plaintiff. Plaintiff alleged that the defendant knew or should have known that defendant's patient had a highly contagious infection, but that the defendant failed to take any steps to prevent its spread to the plaintiff, failed to warn the plaintiff of such infection, and failed to warn the plaintiff's physician or the hospital of these things, causing an unreasonable increase in the risk of injury to the plaintiff. The trial court granted a motion to dismiss for failure to state a cause of action. On appeal, the court said that this did state a cause of action, since it alleged a duty and a breach of that duty. The trial court's action was thus reversed and remanded for trial.

Gino vs. Syracuse Memorial Hospital, Inc., 38 App.Div.2d 887, 329 N.Y.S.2d 272 (1972). Plaintiff was born July 22, 1956. Four days later, it was noted that plaintiff had some weight loss and some jaundice, so blood was drawn from his femoral vein. Four days after that, plaintiff went home, and at home it was noted that he would scream when touched on the left leg. An appointment was made to see his physician on the following day. The parents of plaintiff went to the hospital and were told to return on the following day. They returned and were again told that plaintiff could not be seen. They returned 2 days later with the plaintiff, and he was treated with penicillin with no effect. The plaintiff was brought in the following day and was left in the hospital, and it was not until the following morning that a doctor examined the plaintiff and removed purulent material from his hip which grew *S. aureus*. At the time the operation was performed, the infection had damaged the head of the femur, and the left leg was said to be 2¼ in. shorter than the right. The defendant hospital was sued for not having timely and properly treated the plaintiff for his infection. Judgment for the plaintiff in the trial court was affirmed on the appellate level, the hospital being found negligent in its delay in examination.

Greenstein vs. Meister, 368 A.2d 451 (1977). Plaintiff sued for the death of her husband, who died on March 12, 1969, 2 days after his fourth spinal fusion. At the time that he died, it was apparently thought that it was secondary to a transfusion reaction. Subsequently it was decided that his death was due to a clostridial infection apparently developing at the site of the bone donation in the hip. There was medical expert testimony on behalf of the plaintiff which indicated that the defendant had not met the standard of care.

Griffin vs. Miles, 553 S.W.2d 933 (1977). Patient developed an infection postoperatively because of a sponge left within the abdomen. Plaintiff entered a voluntary nonsuit against his physician and recovered in judgment against the hospital. Later, plaintiff wanted to reinstate the claim against the physician which was not allowed. The plaintiff had already taken a voluntary nonsuit.

Hall vs. City of Huntsville, 278 So.2d 708 (1973). Plaintiff was admitted to defendant hospital June 7, 1964 for a GI ailment and required injections in her left hip for pain. On June 16, 1964, plaintiff had an operation for GI problems. Subsequently the left hip became hard, swollen, and painful, with red streaks down the leg, and the diagnosis was made of staph infection. The plaintiff was then not discharged from the hospital until August 1. The plaintiff's theory of the negligence of the hospital was that there was an implied contract to keep the plaintiff safe from infection, and that since an infection occurred, there was a breach of contract. The trial court directed a verdict for the defendant which was affirmed by the appellate court. The court on appeal said that if the plaintiff's theory was adopted, this would make the hospital an insurer against infection. Plaintiff also testified that the defendant hospital used non-disposable syringes and asked the court to submit the case to the jury on the basis of a *res ipsa loquitur* instruction that such use was negligence per se. The court on appeal held that even if the defendant hospital did use nondisposable syringes (and there was a dispute about this fact), even so this was not negligence per se.

Hanna vs. U.S. Veterans Administration Hospital, 514 F.2d 1092 (1975). Plaintiff had a spinal fusion in defendant's hospital on August 26, 1969. There was a postoperative infection which lasted for 3 months. Subsequently on June 10, 1971, there was a recurrence of the infection and the action was filed on February 25, 1974. The trial court dismissed the action as being barred by the statute of limitations. This was reversed on appeal because there was a fact issue as to when the statute of limitations started running since there was at least some medical testimony that the osteomyelitis was not diagnosed until June 1972. Since there was a fact issue, it would not be said as a matter of law that the statute of limitations had run on this cause of action, so it was remanded to the trial court for further proceedings.

Hanrahan vs. St. Vincent Hospital, 516 F.2d 300 (1975). Plaintiff had a cholecystectomy in defendant hospital, and while recuperating plaintiff developed a perianal abscess. Plaintiff alleged that it was caused by the negligence of the hospital by the improper administration of an enema. Plaintiff wanted the *res ipsa loquitur* instruction to be given to the jury. The trial court refused and on appeal the appellate court agreed. The question of whether a perianal abscess would occur in the ordinary course of events, even if reasonable care was used, was not within the common experience of the jury, so there must be medical expert testimony. There was medical expert testimony that such perianal abscessees were highly unusual, but the court held that the mere rarity of the occurrence was not sufficient in and of itself to apply *res ipsa loquitur.*

Harmon vs. Rust, 420 S.W.2d 563 (1967). Plaintiff had burns to his right leg and some skin was transplanted from his left leg to his right leg. Subsequently both legs became infected. At the trial, the plaintiff presented no expert witness that testified that the defendant failed to meet the standard of care in caring for the plaintiff, so the trial court directed a verdict in favor of the defendant. This was affirmed on appeal, the court saying that there was no inference of negligence from the presence of an infection following an operation or in an area under treatment.

Hart vs. Fielden, 295 S.W.2d 911 (1956). Plaintiff injured her left index finger on February 11, 1954. On February 19, she went to see the defendant, whose exam revealed a fracture, and this fracture was set. In June, she noted a drooping of the distal phalanx of her finger, and an X-ray revealed a bone spur. On September 15, 1954, she had surgery done to remove the spur. After the surgery an infection developed in the finger. This became dry gangrene, and on October 12, her left index finger was amputated at the second joint by a different physician. At the trial court, the jury found the defendant negligent on several counts, but for most of these, the jury said that such negligence was not the proximal cause of the loss of the plaintiff's finger.

Nevertheless, the jury found for the plaintiff. On appeal, the court said that there was no evidence that showed any causal connection between the failure of the defendant to examine the plaintiff's finger and the gangrene which caused the loss of the finger. The jury's decision for the plaintiff was reversed and judgment was entered for the defendant.

Helman vs. Sacred Heart Hospital, 62 Wash.2d 136, 381 P.2d 605 (1963). This is one of the most frequently cited cases with respect to a hospital's liability for a hospital acquired infection. Plaintiff was injured in an automobile accident on July 4, 1957 and sustained a crushed chest, a dislocated left hip, and multiple fractures in the area of the left pelvis. He spent nearly a month in the hospital in Idaho before being transferred to the hospital in Washington. Plaintiff was put in the same room with another patient, who had been admitted July 9, 1957 with a fractured back and was paralyzed from the waist down. On August 1, surgery was performed on plaintiff's hip. On August 2, plaintiff developed spiking septic fever. On August 9, the other patient in the room complained of a boil under his right arm, and hot compresses were applied. On August 10, purulent drainage was noted coming from the other patient's boil, and this was cultured. On August 13, the other patient's culture grew *S. aureus,* and he was transferred to another room. On that same day, plaintiff's surgical wound erupted yielding a large amount of purulent drainage which also grew *S. aureus.* This was an infection from his hip, and subsequently plaintiff had a hip operation on October 28 with a hip fusion and was ultimately discharged from the hospital on March 14, 1958. There was evidence on both sides of the question on whether the *Staphylococcus* from the other patient was the same as the *Staphylococcus* that had infected the plaintiff. Since there was evidence on both sides of this issue, it therefore became a jury question of fact, and the jury decided in favor of the plaintiff who was awarded $67,839.97. This was affirmed on appeal.

Howell vs. Industrial Commission, 13 Ariz.App. 68, 474 P.2d 75 (1970). Plaintiff worked as a janitor for a hospital, and he alleged that his coccidioidomycosis was aggravated by his work. The industrial commission found that this was noncompensable. The Court of Appeals of Arizona said that the evidence supported the Industrial Commission's finding, so it was affirmed.

Hurley vs. Nashua Hospital Association, 88 N.H. 469, 191 A. 649 (1937). Plaintiff sued defendant hospital, alleging that a nurse who had a severe cold attended the plaintiff and plaintiff caught this cold which developed into pneumonia and subsequently empyema. At the trial, there was a jury verdict in favor of the plaintiff, but the court on appeal directed the verdict in favor of the defendant, saying that there was no causal connection between the harm complained of and any negligence of the defendant, if any. The court mentioned in passing that the only evidence as to the presence of the sick nurse was the plaintiff's testimony. The nurse could not be named or described. Circumstantial statements by the plaintiff indicated that the plaintiff's symptoms began December 26, 1928. Treatment began on December 27, but the sick nurse apparently attended the plaintiff on December 27 or 28. Since at that point the condition had already begun, there could be no causal connection between a nurse's illness and the condition of the plaintiff whose symptoms had begun at least a day earlier. Therefore, judgment was entered for the defendant.

Inderbitzen vs. Lane Hospital, 124 Cal.App. 462, 12 P.2d 744 (1932). It was alleged that a doctor of the defendant hospital performed a rectal and vaginal exam without washing or sterilizing his hands. It was also alleged that a younger man (a medical student?) examined the plaintiff in the same way, and he did not sterilize his hands either before examining her. It was also said by the plaintiff that she was examined in the delivery room by 10 to 12 young men. The physician who examined the plaintiff some 2 months after her delivery said that she had a tear in her uterus, that it was infected, and that it was discharging profusely. The trial court granted a nonsuit at the end of the plaintiff's evidence. This was reversed on appeal, the appellate court noting that usually one needed expert testimony, but where it was a matter of general knowledge, expert testimony was not necessary, and the court could take judicial knowledge of the danger of infection to a pregnant woman from a vaginal exam performed with unsterilized hands. (Subsequently, because plaintiff did not pursue this lawsuit, a judgment was entered dismissing the suit against the defendant, and this was affirmed on appeal for failure to prosecute, 61 P.2d 514 (1936).)

Johnson vs. Myers, 118 Ga.App. 773, 165 S.E.2d 739 (1968). (Previous opinions in the same case were 113 Ga.App. 648, 149 S.E.2d 378 (1966), 116 Ga.App. 232, 156 S.E.2d 663 (1967).) Plaintiff's left knee was operated on by the defendant on August 29 or 30, 1958. Beginning September 2 and for about 4 weeks, plaintiff's knee was infected with *S. aureus.* Plaintiff alleged that defendant was negligent in discovering and treating the postoperative infection. The question was whether the defendant should have cultured the knee in exercising a reasonable degree of skill and care in the management of the plaintiff's infection. Eventually there was a jury decision in favor of the defendant, and this was affirmed on appeal.

Jones vs. Sisters of Charity of the Incarnate Word, 173 S.W. 639 (1914). Plaintiff's wife was hospitalized in defendant hospital on January 14, 1913, and she died February 6, 1913 of smallpox. Evidence presented showed that when the plaintiff's wife was in the hospital, there was another patient in the hospital at the same time with smallpox, but this other patient with smallpox was in another wing and on a different floor. Neither the plaintiff nor his wife knew of the other case of smallpox in the hospital, but apparently the physician did. After plaintiff's wife entered the hospital, three more cases of smallpox developed, but on the same floor as the original case and in the same wing. Plaintiff's wife had an operation, and 14 days postoperatively, while convalescing from her operation, she developed smallpox and died shortly thereafter. Evidence was presented that no patient that ever previously occupied that room had had smallpox, nor had anyone had smallpox in that wing of the building. Evidence was also presented that only the nurse and the doctor were allowed into the room to see the smallpox patient, and this nurse was not allowed to see other patients in the hospital and did not even go into the wing of the building in which the plaintiff's wife was. At the trial, there was a directed verdict in favor of the defendant hospital. On appeal, the court affirmed this decision saying, "Plaintiff's wife in some unaccountable way may have contracted the disease from cases which occurred in the hospital, but the hospital authorities could not, in the circumstances, have reasonably anticipated that she would contract the disease, and cannot therefore be held to have been guilty of negligence in failing to inform her when she applied for admission that there was a case of smallpox in the hospital."

Joplin vs. U.S., 441 F.Supp. 1142 (1977). Plaintiff had an exploratory hernia operation at a Veterans Administration (VA) hospital, and plaintiff alleged the VA physician was negligent and severed his sperm cords and the muscle on the right side of his penis, resulting in impotency and tuberculosis. A government physician examined the plaintiff and his records and testified that there was no negligence by the Veterans Administration physician, the sperm cords and penis muscle were not severed and that there was no evidence of tuberculosis. The plaintiff did not present any medical evidence whatsoever. The trial court held that the plaintiff had completely failed to prove his claim and dismissed suit.

Kalmus vs. Cedars of Lebanon Hospital, 132 Cal.App.2d 243, 281 P.2d 872 (1955). Plaintiff alleged that one of the nurses of defendant hospital used an unsterile needle and syringe in giving an injection. This was manifest by redness around the injection area and pain the morning after the injection was given. Two days later when the plaintiff went home, there was an abscess formation at the location of the injection. The plaintiff's temperature reached 101°. A culture was taken which grew *S. aureus*. The defendant's expert witness testified that two things might have caused the abscess: severe bruising or an infected needle and nothing else. Since there was no evidence of bruising in this case, therefore an unsterile needle must have been involved. Many witnesses had testified to the fact that the use of an infected needle violated the standard of care, therefore there was a reasonable medical certainty that the infection had been caused by the injection. Judgment for the plaintiff was affirmed on appeal.

Kapuschinsky vs. U.S., 248 F. Supp. 732 (1966); 259 F.Supp. 1 (1966) (on question of damages only). This is one of those classic cases that is always mentioned when the question of a hospital's liability for infection control is mentioned. Plaintiff was a premature infant born in a U.S. Naval Hospital. Plaintiff was born November 14, 1961, and at birth her weight was 2 lb, 15 oz. She was kept in an isolette in the premature nursery which was separate from the newborn nursery. Plaintiff became jaundiced after birth. By November 18, her condition was such that she was put on the critical list. Because of the jaundice, it was necessary to perform several femoral taps for blood on November 17, 18, and 21. On November 22, this was discontinued, since she seemed to be improving. On November 21, it was noted that the umbilical cord was falling off and there was some redness around the cord, and a culture of this grew *Proteus vulgaris*. On November 23, it was noted that plaintiff cried when she was disturbed, her lower extremities seemed rigid, and she kept her legs and hips wide apart. On November 25, she was removed from the critical list and the abnormality of her hips was again noted. On November 26, she was put back on the critical list, some swelling was noted in both hip areas, and her temperature was 101°F. Subsequently she was seen in consultation by an orthopedic surgeon, who found bulging in the area of both hip joints. He incised both the hip joints and drained them, sterilely, obtaining 1 to 2 oz of grossly purulent material from the hips. Subsequently she began to recover, to progress and to gain weight. The X-rays showed osteomyelitis involving both right and left femurs, pelvic girdle, and some involvement of the right humerus. Culture of the material from the left hip grew *S. aureus*; pus from the right hip grew *Pseudomonas*. The court noted that it had been suspected that the *Pseudomonas* was an overgrowth and that this pus probably also contained the *S. aureus*. Subsequently nose and throat cultures were taken from all the personnel in the nursery. One nursing assistant was found to have a nose culture positive for *S. aureus* sensitive to Aureomycin®, Terramycin®, tetracycline, Chloromycetin®, and Furadantin®. (The plaintiff's *S. aureus* was sensitive only to Chloromycetin® and Furadantin®.) Subsequently the plaintiff remained in the hospital some 4 to 5 months before discharge. She improved and her infection was controlled, but she had developed permanent damages as a result of that infection. An orthopedic surgeon who examined her on December 31, 1963 said that she had limitation of motion in the elbow, her right hip was permanently dislocated, and that there was a destructive process in the left hip joint which would probably cause her pain later in life. There was damage to the left femur, so that it would be approximately 2 in. shorter than the right when she was fully grown. Plaintiff at the time of trial walked with a sway and a limp and had to wear a special orthopedic brace. The court held that a higher standard of care was required of the hospital in caring for a child than an adult and that a premature infant was entitled to the highest possible degree of care consistent with good medical practice because of its precarious toehold on life and its helplessness. The court held that the Naval Hospital violated its duty to the plaintiff in two respects; the court said either one of which would have been sufficient to sustain its cause of action. First, it permitted an inexperienced nursing assistant to come into critical contact with a plaintiff whose susceptibility to infection was well-known, in violation of proper medical standards, and second, that it permitted this critical contact without a complete physical examination of the nursing assistant, including appropriate laboratory tests before she began to work in the premature nursery. The court held that each of those failures resulted in the communication of the pathogenic organism to the plaintiff. The Naval Hospital and subsequently the U.S. government was held to be liable for injuries to the plaintiff. In the later separate trial on damages, plaintiff was awarded $175,000.

Kaster vs. Woodson, 123 S.W.2d 981 (1938). Plaintiff sued defendant doctors on the basis that they failed to properly sterilize the needle used for an injection, they failed to properly sterilize the skin where the needle entered, and that they failed to use a solution for injection that was properly sterilized. Verdict was directed for the defendants. It was affirmed on appeal, the court saying that there was no expert testimony that the infection in the plaintiff's arm was caused by anything done by the defendants; there was no expert testimony showing a causal connection between what the plaintiff complained that the defendants did and the injury that plaintiff had sustained. The court said, "What is an infection and from whence did it come are matters determinable only by medical experts."

Kirchoff vs. St. Joseph's Hospital, 194 Minn. 436, 260 N.W.509 (1935). On March 13, 1933, plaintiff's wife entered the defendant hospital, and on March 14, she delivered a male infant. Several days later, during feeding time, a nurse brought a baby to feed, but in a few minutes the nurse returned saying that the baby was not hers. Plaintiff claimed that the baby had impetigo and that subsequently plaintiff's son developed impetigo due to the mother's temporarily nursing the wrong child. There was evidence that while in the defendant hospital, plaintiff's son did develop impetigo on his ear. Plaintiff won at the trial court. This was affirmed, the court saying that the plaintiff presented sufficient evidence to find that the wrong child was brought to the mother, the wrong child did have skin disease, and that plaintiff's son contracted impetigo from coming into contact with his mother shortly after the infected baby had been taken away. The court also noted that the defendant hospital was negligent in taking the wrong baby to the mother.

Lane vs. Calvert, 215 Md. 457, 138 A.2d 902 (1958). Plaintiff's wife had cancer of the descending colon, and she was first operated upon on May 5, 1953. Subsequently she had fever for 6 weeks postoperatively, and she had several subsequent draining procedures on May 25, when an abscess was drained, and on June 11, when no pus was found, although a fistula later developed. Subsequently a third procedure was done in which a loculated pocket of pus was found and drained. At that time, drains were left in place which drained the pus, and eventually the fistula closed. Plaintiff claimed negligence in that the defendant did not use dye studies in the fistula early enough and thus the plaintiff's wife's hospitalization was prolonged. This prolonged the pain and suffering as well. The court held that there was no evidence to support such a finding, there was no common knowledge by which the jury could make such a finding, and that the expert testimony presented did not require that conclusion. Judgment was in favor of the defendant doctor and hospital.

Lang vs. Abbott Laboratories, 398 N.Y.S.2d 577 (1977). Plaintiff had already obtained the hospital records on septicemias which occurred during the plaintiff's hospitalization. Then the plaintiff asked for the hospital records on septicemias in general and Gram-negative sepsis for the 2 years prior to hospitalization. The hospital refused to release those records, and the trial court sustained the hospital in this. On appeal, this protection of the hospital records was denied, the court saying that these records were not exempted under the law protecting the performance of the medical review function.

Lee vs. Andrews, 545 S.W.2d 238 (1976). Plaintiff's husband had a hemorrhoidectomy performed on June 4, 1975. On June 5 at 6 pm, it was noted that the patient was retaining urine, and he was catheterized, At 10:45 pm, it was noted that his scrotum was swollen to three or four times normal. On June 6 and June 7, no treatment was given for any infection. On June 8, a scrotal infection was diagnosed, and on June 9, the patient died of Gram-negative sepsis and shock. Judgment for the plaintiff was affirmed, the court saying that there was sufficient evidence to support the jury finding that the defendant had not met the standard of care owed to the patient. There was medical expert testimony that he would have survived if there had been a consultation earlier or if there had been appropriate therapy earlier.

LeFort vs. Massachusetts Bonding and Insurance Company, 358 F.2d 741 (1966). Plaintiff developed a *S. aureus* infection in the incision of his hernia operation 3 to 4 days postoperatively. The plaintiff did not establish any causal connection between the claimed deviations from accepted professional standards and his infection; therefore the trial court directed a verdict for the defendant and the Court of Appeals affirmed.

McCall vs. St. Joseph's Hospital, 184 Neb. 1, 165 N.W.2d 85 (1969). On January 28, 1963, plaintiff was operated on for a herniated disk. Postoperatively he developed a staphylococcal infection at the site of surgery. Plaintiff alleged no specific acts of negligence and based his claim on *res ipsa loquitur.* A summary judgment was granted to the defendant. This was affirmed, the court saying that infection at the site of a surgical incision is not negligence, nor could one reasonably infer negligence merely from the presence of infection. The court further noted that there was no expert testimony or any offer of proof to the effect that the mere presence of a staphylococcal infection would automatically lead to an inference of negligence by the people in control of the operation or in the treatment of the patient.

Miller vs. U.S., 431 F.Supp. 988 (1976). Plaintiff told defendant hospital that he was allergic to antihistamines, yet on discharge he was treated with Vistaril®; it was admitted that Vistaril® had some antihistaminic properties. Subsequently he developed infection in his prostate, epididymides, and right testicle. Judgment was rendered on behalf of plaintiff.

Missouri, Kansas, and Texas Railway Company of Texas vs. Wood, 95 Tex. 223, 66 S.W.449 (1902). The evidence was that the defendant railway ran a hospital for its employees. At the end of July 1899, a patient was injured and sent to one of defendant's hospitals. The patient was placed on a ward where there were some other patients who were said to have chicken pox (actually it was smallpox). This patient was then discharged on August 2, 1899, and he left to go back home. Subsequently, when it was found that the patients in the hospital had smallpox, the hospital was quarantined. Subsequently on August 19, the patient broke out in a rash and was diagnosed as having smallpox. On August 20 this patient was put into a tent and quarantined, and an attendant was hired to watch over him. On August 22, this patient escaped, wandered onto the property of the plaintiff, and communicated to plaintiff husband, wife, and child the disease smallpox. The plaintiff won, the court holding " . . . when the duty to prevent the spread of a contagious disease rests upon a private corporation or person, an obligation arises in favor of each member of the community, and a right of action exists in favor of him who suffers from its breach."

Montana Deaconess Hospital vs. Gratton, 169 Mont. 185, 545 P.2d 670 (1976). In this case, the hospital was the plaintiff, suing to collect its bill and the defendant patient counterclaimed alleging malpractice due to his suffering a staphylococcal infection. The patient fractured his right shoulder June 14, 1970 and was hospitalized at the hospital from June 14 to June 30, and he was subsequently discharged with his surgical wound which was healed. Subsequently on September 10, he was rehospitalized for a boil in the area of the surgical incision, and cultures grew *Staphylococcus* and subsequently a *Pseudomonas*, and he was eventually discharged October 16, 1970. He was rehospitalized November 18 to November 24, 1970 and eventually treated at the Mayo Clinic. He claimed that his right arm was still disabled. The patient's counterclaim was dismissed, since he did not present any evidence of any standard of care against which the acts or admission of the hospital or doctors could be measured in order to establish negligence. There was no evidence that the instrumentality causing his infection was within the exclusive control of the hospital or the doctors.

Mosley vs. U.S., 405 F.Supp. 357 (1974), 499 F.2d 1361 (1974), 538 F.2d 555 (1976). Plaintiff was the estate of a patient, who had rheumatic heart disease with mitral stenosis and who died of pneumonia, while awaiting open heart surgery at a Veterans Administration hospital. The court seemed to say that the hospital's negligence was based on failure to provide intensive care and treatment and not the acquisition of the pneumonia. Judgment on behalf of the plaintiff was affirmed on appeal.

Mullins vs. Bexar County Hospital District, 535 S.W.2d 44 (1976). Plaintiff was bleeding from his GI tract, secondary to an ulcer, and required a blood transfusion. An I.V. needle in his left arm became inflamed, and he developed what was diagnosed as infectious thrombophlebitis caused by a *Staphylococcus*. The expert testimony did not relate his infection to the blood being used, and there was no testimony pointing toward unsterile I.V. catheters. However, there was testimony that the probable source of his infection was either the blood or the I.V. equipment; therefore the jury could speculate as to the cause of infection, and there was no evidence to support the jury finding that the defendant hospital failed to provide uncontaminated I.V. instruments. The jury gave a verdict in favor of the plaintiff, but this was not allowed to stand. A judgment was entered for the defendant hospital notwithstanding the verdict. On appeal this was affirmed.

Mutschman vs. Petry, 46 Ohio App. 525, 189 N.E. 658 (1933). On January 18, 1929, plaintiff's husband became ill. He had a duodenal ulcer. On January 22, he had a blood transfusion, and a tooth was removed. That night he showed twitching and a hypersensitivity to noise. On January 23, he had an operation performed for his ulcer. On January 25, he died of tetanus. The source of the tetanus was thought to be the tooth socket. It is interesting that the court found the two general surgeons liable, but not the dental surgeon, who removed the tooth. The judgment for the plaintiff at the trial was affirmed on appeal, the court saying that the operation destroyed the patient's resistance, it hastened and directly contributed to his death, and therefore was a proximate cause of his injury.

O'Connor vs. Boulder Colorado Sanitarium Association, 107 Colo. 290, 111 P.2d 633 (1941). Plaintiff had a common cold, and she entered the defendant sanitarium on January 2, 1937 about 9 p.m. After her condition was diagnosed, she was started on hydrotherapy. She was treated that night with hot baths and hot water treatments. She alleged that she was not thoroughly dried before being put into an extremely cold hospital room. She further alleged that the cold progressed to pneumonia which progressed to tuberculosis. At the trial, there was a jury verdict for the defendant sanitarium, and this was upheld on appeal. The question was, even if the treatment on the night of admission were negligence, was this a proximal cause of the pneumonia and tuberculosis? The court said that there was no evidence on which the jury could have made a determination that the treatment on the night of admission was the proximate causation of her subsequent pneumonia and tuberculosis. Plaintiff's expert only testified that the treatment on the night of admission might possibly have been the cause of her pneumonia and tuberculosis. The court held that possibilities were not probabilities and that for a basis for legal remedy, there must be a reasonable certainty which would not leave the question open to conjecture or speculation. The court further indicated that defendant should have been granted a directed verdict as a matter of law.

Peck vs. Charles B. Towns Hospital, 275 App.Div. 302, 89 N.Y.S.2d 190 (1949). Plaintiff alleged that he had contracted an infection secondary to a nonsterilized hypodermic needle. At the trial, a directed verdict was rendered for the defendant. On appeal this was reversed, and a new trial was awarded, the court saying that there was medical expert testimony showing that the defendant hospital failed to provide the usual and customary facilities for the sterilization of hypodermic needles in that it did not provide a closed appliance using steam under pressure for sterilization. Furthermore, there was expert testimony that the boiling of hypodermic needles in the open air was an inadequate means of sterilization.

Perrin vs. St. Paul Fire and Marine Insurance Company, 340 So.2d 421 (1976). Plaintiff shot himself with a 12-gauge shotgun on March 5, 1972. The pellets entered his leg, and in the emergency room, most of these were removed. Subsequently he developed problems, and an operation was performed on October 9, 1972. Subsequently on June 20, 1973, another operation was performed. The leg was bandaged and put into a cast. These were not removed until July 3, 1973, at which time an infection was noted. The plaintiff chose to have his leg amputated rather than have further surgery. Plaintiff sued based on this last infection that he developed. He alleged that the doctors failed to note his rising temperature after the operation, they failed to perform a white blood cell count, and they failed to check his lymph glands. Plaintiff also alleged that the nurses failed to note the odor from the wound which would have indicated an infection. Plaintiff's expert had not treated a patient with this sort of problem, and he did not know the body's responses to a bone graft. The defendant's experts indicated that the treatment and care were reasonable and that it was common practice to leave a bandage and cast in place for 14 days. The jury judgment in favor of the defendant was affirmed on appeal.

Pollard vs. Goldsmith, 117 Ariz. 363, 572 P.2d 1201 (1977). Plaintiff was the estate of a woman, who sustained a compound comminuted fracture of the ankle in an automobile accident. She was treated in an emergency room and transferred to another hospital; 10 days later she developed tetanus and died. The trial court granted a summary judgment in favor of the physician defendant. The appellate court reversed, saying that the affidavit from plaintiff's expert raised questions which could not be disposed of by a summary judgment.

Posthuma vs. Northwestern Hospital, 197 Minn. 304, 267 N.W. 221 (1936). Plaintiff was admitted to defendant hospital for 1 day, May 30, 1932. On the morning of admission, she was treated with an injection of morphine, and subsequently she developed an infection in the arm in which she had received the injection. Plaintiff alleged that the nurse who gave the injection sterilized the area of her arm, but then negligently inserted the needle outside of the area that had been prepared, and that this caused the infection in the arm. The trial court directed a verdict in favor of the defendant, and this was affirmed on appeal. The court noted that the plaintiff's husband did not know which area had been sterilized and that he did not testify that the needle was inserted outside the area sterilized. Since the only claim of negligence was on the basis that the needle was inserted outside of the area sterilized and since there was no evidence to that specific point, then there was no evidence to justify a jury finding of negligence, and a directed verdict was proper.

Prewett vs. Philpot, 142 Miss. 704, 107 So. 880 (1926). Plaintiff was operated upon for appendicitis on a hot night in June, and during the operation one or more windows were left open. Although the windows were screened, a large number of bugs came through and were in the operating room while the operation was being performed. Ten days later, plaintiff was discharged from the hospital, and a few days after that, his wound became inflamed, and pus formed. He was rehospitalized, and the wound was reopened and drained. Plaintiff's mother testified that two of the kinds of bugs that were in the operating room were gotten out of his wound. The trial court verdict directed in favor of the defendant. This was reversed by the appellate court which said that a jury could have believed that the bugs got into the wound during the operation.

Rimmele vs. Northridge Hospital Foundation, 46 Cal.App.3d 123, 120 Cal. Rptr. 39 (1975). On August 24, 1969, plaintiff was in defendant hospital for delivery of a child. On August 27, patient was discharged from the hospital. On August 30, patient experienced pain in her right hip, with fever and chills, and was hospitalized again. Diagnosis made was acute peripheral neuritis secondary to previous injections. Subsequently she was diagnosed as having spinal osteomyelitis and probable involvement of the sciatic nerve due to an infection originating in the right buttocks and spreading to the bone. All the plaintiff's medical experts agreed that the probable cause of her infection was the injections she received during her hospitalization; furthermore, there was medical expert testimony indicating that an injection in the buttocks would not without negligence result in the conditions from which she suffered. The appellate court affirmed the directed verdict for the doctors, but reversed the jury verdict for the hospital. The court said that it was prejudicial to the plaintiff to let the jury consider whether the hospital had exclusive control over the injections and whether the plaintiff could have been contributorily negligent. An interesting dissent in favor of affirming the judgment for the hospital referred to an infectious disease expert's testimony with respect to the origination of the plaintiff's spinal osteomyelitis.

Roberts vs. Young, 369 Mich. 133, 119 N.W.2d 627 (1963). Plaintiff had a Caesarean section and subsequently developed a postoperative pneumonia. Plaintiff did not present any expert testimony that the defendants did not follow the proper standards. The trial court directed a verdict in favor of the defendants and the appellate court affirmed. The court noted that after any major surgical procedure, there was a risk of infection, and the development of such infection is not actionable unless it was caused by the failure of the plaintiff's doctors to observe proper care in the care and treatment of the patient. The court also noted that there was no duty to warn of possible postoperative infections.

Robey vs. Jewish Hospital of Brooklyn, 280 N.Y. 533, 20 N.E.2d 6 (1939). Plaintiffs alleged that the defendant hospital was negligent in admitting to the hospital the mothers of the plaintiffs prior to their birth while there was in the hospital a malady infecting infants without giving notice of said malady to the plaintiffs' mothers. The trial court rendered judgment for the defendant, indicating that there was no actionable negligence on the part of the defendant. The intermediate appellate court reversed this judgment and ordered a new trial. On further appeal to the higher appellate court, the intermediate court's order was reversed and the trial court was affirmed.

Rhody vs. James Decker Munson Hospital, 17 Mich.App. 561, 170 N.W.2d 67 (1969). Plaintiff alleged that defendant hospital negligently administered an injection in May 1961. The injection reacted differently than other injections in that the next day, plaintiff's arm swelled up, and this was the area in which the subsequent infection first occurred. It was noted that after June 19, 1961, a staphylococcal infection erupted on her arm, but that she had been in and out of the hospital almost the entire month of June for treatment of eczema and the birth of a child without any complaint concerning her arm. At the trial, there was a jury verdict in favor of the plaintiff, but the trial court granted the defendant's motion for judgment notwithstanding the verdict. The Michigan Court of Appeals affirmed. The court noted that the plaintiff had failed to satisfy the conditions for the application of *res ipsa loquitur* because the infection occurred a month after the injection and the plaintiff had been in the hospital for other reasons in the meantime. The court noted that the mere occurrence of an infection is not enough to imply negligence. One could only speculate or conjecture that an infection occurred as the result of negligence. There was no expert testimony linking the staphylococcal infection to the injection.

Russell vs. Camden Community Hospital, 359 A.2d 607 (1976). This case involved a workman's compensation claim by a nurse's aide who developed tuberculosis, allegedly from applying an ointment to a caseating tuberculous ulcer. The plaintiff had applied the ointment to the patient's tuberculous ulcer on several occasion during the 20 days that the patient was in the hospital from March 24, 1972 to April 12, 1972. On August 1, 1973, plaintiff coughed up some blood, chest X-ray revealed a lung infiltrate, culture revealed no tuberculosis, and skin test was positive. Her physician thought that she had tuberculosis and treated her for it. The court affirmed the award to the plaintiff, saying that it was more probable than not that her infection with tuberculosis was a result of her care of the patient with the tuberculous ulcer.

Sebree vs. U.S., 567 F.2d 292 (1978). Plaintiff had a laceration near his left eye, and he had general surgery under anesthesia in order to suture the wound. While under the anesthesia, he vomited and subsequently developed fever; he was diagnosed as having aspiration pneumonia and was treated with ampicillin and acetaminophen. He was discharged from the hospital 5 days later afebrile. The following day he returned lethargic, irritable, and unresponsive. Subsequently, he was transferred to another hospital and diagnosed as pneumococcal meningitis. Subsequently he had muscle atrophy and partial permanent paralysis of both legs and left arm as a residual from this infection. At the trial, the court noted that the physician's diagnosis of aspiration pneumonia conformed to the accepted standards of care in the locality and therefore there was no showing that an earlier diagnosis and therapy would have resulted in any lessening of his injuries. Judgment was in favor of the defendant. On appeal, the appellate court affirmed noting that evidence supported the decision and that the trial court was not clearly erroneous (the trial court believed that the plaintiff developed the meningitis while he was at home).

Shields vs. King, 40 Ohio App.2d 77, 317 N.E.2d 922 (1973). Plaintiff was estate of deceased, who had chronic glomerulonephritis and who was undergoing chronic hemodialysis at the defendant hospital. On July 5, 1966, dialysis began. Thirty minutes after his own blood was administered, he went into shock; he died July 8. The cause of death was listed as *Escherichia coli* septicemia. At the trial, a verdict was directed for the defendant, but on appeal this was reversed. The court on appeal noted that *res ipsa loquitur* could be applied where there were two or more defendants who were in collective and concurrent control of the only instrumentalities which the evidence established caused the injury. In this case, the court noted that the plaintiff's deceased had been dialyzed before without any problems. The court said that the septicemia that developed was due to some problem and that the defendant doctor and defendant hospital had the control over the dialysis equipment and the blood, and the plaintiff's expert testified that the septicemia was due to contaminated blood.

Shurpit vs. Brah, 30 Wis.2d 388, 141 N.W.2d 266 (1966). Plaintiff injured his right hand on November 14, 1958, and several fingers had to be amputated. Because his hand was useless, plaintiff and defendant doctor agreed that an amputation would benefit the plaintiff. On May 12, 1959, defendant amputated the right hand above the wrist. On May 13, plaintiff's temperature went up to 104°F, the wound was red and swollen, and there was bloody drainage with blebs at the suture line. On May 15, his temperature was 99°F, there was an area of necrosis at the suture line, and the laboratory report was gas-forming organisms. Defendant doctor called in another doctor, and massive doses of gas gangrene antitoxin and penicillin were given. After consultation with several other doctors, defendant amputated plaintiff's arm just below the shoulder to save his life. Plaintiff recovered. A jury verdict for the defendant was affirmed on appeal. The medical expert witnesses noted that gas gangrene spores could come from anywhere, a variety of sources. The medical experts also testified that defendant's preoperative and postoperative care met the standard of care. They also testified that there was no delay in the diagnosis of plaintiff's gas gangrene. The court noted that one could not infer negligence merely from the fact that the plaintiff contracted gas gangrene and that rarity was not a basis for allowing a jury to infer negligence.

Smith vs. Curran, 28 Colo.App. 358, 472 P.2d 769 (1970). Plaintiff developed a staphylococcal osteomyelitis after an open reduction of a fractured left femur. Plaintiff produced no medical expert testimony and *res ipsa loquitur* was held not to apply. The court noted that the mere presence of an infection following an operation was not prima facie evidence of negligence. The court also noted that the cause of an infection or its source were matters in the field of medical experts. Directed verdict in favor of the defendant was affirmed.

Sneath vs. Physicians and Surgeons Hospital, 247 Or. 593, 431 P.2d 835 (1967). Plaintiff had a cranial operation, and postoperatively a wound infection involving *Staphylococcus* developed. At the trial, there was a judgment for the defendant hospital which on appeal was affirmed. The appellate court noted that the clinical microbiologist, who ran the microbiology lab, who had worked for 11 years as a clinical microbiologist, and who helped the infection control committee "trace the source of infections", was competent to give testimony. Her testimony had been excluded at the trial, but the court held that that was not prejudicial error, since two expert witnesses, physicians, gave substantially the same testimony as that which was excluded.

Sommers vs. Sisters of Charity of Providence in Oregon, 277 Or. 549, 561 P.2d 603 (1977). Plaintiff was injured in an automobile accident and was treated in the emergency room in April 1973. An indwelling I.V. catheter was placed in the right lower arm, and 3 days later plaintiff developed a fever. A culture of the site of infection revealed staphylococci. The infection continued for 8 days. Two medical experts testified that plaintiff's infection was caused by the entry of the needle into the bloodstream, but there was no testimony that the needle itself was the source of infection. The evidence presented was that the needles were sterile disposable needles. There was no evidence that the needle was contaminated prior to insertion into the plaintiff's arm, but this was plaintiff's theory of defendant's negligence. There was undisputed testimony that staphylococcal bacteria were not only on the surface of the skin, but under the surface in the pores, where they could not always be killed by antiseptics. It was also held that *res ipsa loquitur* was inapplicable, since the medical testimony was that it was impossible in all cases to prevent the bacteria which were under the skin or in the pores from being introduced into the bloodstream through the insertion of an I.V. needle. The trial court directed a verdict in favor of the defendant, and this was affirmed on appeal.

Southern Florida Sanitarium and Hospital vs. Hodge, 215 So.2d 753 (1968). Plaintiff developed thrombophlebitis after an I.V. injection, and plaintiff alleged infection as the result of the injection. At the trial, there was a judgment for the plaintiff which was affirmed on appeal. The medical expert testimony at the trial was that infectious thrombophlebitis would not occur if the medical standard of sterility was not departed from, but that infectious thrombophlebitis could occur from a failure to maintain sterility; therefore, the *res ipsa loquitur* instruction was applicable. The court also noted that there was some proof that specific negligence was also involved, since the chief of staff of the defendant hospital did not know whether it was hospital practice to have people giving these I.V. injection clean their hands prior to the procedure, that the injection site was not covered by a bandaid, and that the infection was introduced in injecting or withdrawal of the needle.

Stone vs. Lutheran Deaconess Home and Hospital, 203 Minn. 124, 280 N.W. 178 (1938). On June 18, 1935, plaintiff was born at the defendant hospital. About 5 days after birth, plaintiff developed a rash which was treated with silver nitrate. By June 27, the rash had improved, and plaintiff and mother were discharged from the hospital. At home, plaintiff's rash spread; he was treated by one doctor for 4 to 5 days and then switched to another doctor. On July 6, 1935, plaintiff was said to have pemphigoid impetigo over the body and that erysipelas subsequently developed. There was then a secondary infection in his hip joint, and osteomyelitis destroyed the hip joint; the leg on that side would be about 4 in. shorter than the other. Plaintiff alleged that a nurse attending the children in the nursery broke hospital routine and handled another baby that had impetigo and then the plaintiff without changing her apron or sterilizing her hands. The evidence for this was based on the fact that there were visitors who said they did not see the nurses change aprons or sterilize their hands. The court noted that there was no competent evidence that the other baby had the same disease which affected the plaintiff. In fact, there was medical expert testimony that the other baby did not have the disease which the plaintiff complained that he did. The court held that the plaintiffs had failed to meet their burden of proof because they had not shown competently that the other baby had the disease which subsequently afflicted the plaintiff. Also, they did not competently show negligence on the part of the defendant in the handling of the two babies. The jury gave a verdict for the plaintiff, but the trial court entered a judgment for the defendant notwithstanding the verdict. The verdict was affirmed on appeal.

Suburban Hospital Association Incorporated vs. Hadary, 22 Md.App.186, 322 A.2d 258 (1974). Plaintiff had psoriasis beginning in 1964 or 1966. In November 1967, methotrexate was begun. Because of the possibility of liver damage, a liver biopsy was performed on June 5, 1970. On June 6, plaintiff was discharged to go home, but that afternoon the defendant doctor who had done the biopsy called, saying that the needle used at the time of the biopsy might not have been sterile. Subsequently gamma globulin injections were begun which lasted from June 1970 to November 1970. Unfortunately the methotrexate treatment had to be suspended until December 1970, when it was finally resumed. The court said that no medical expert testimony was needed where a hospital's negligence was of such to be within the comprehension of laymen and required only common knowledge and experience to understand and judge it. There was a Maryland statute in the Department of Health regulations stating that sterile supplies and equipment should be stored in a suitable enclosed space providing separation from unsterile supplies. The court held that a jury could determine whether a hospital had provided suitable separation of sterile supplies from the nonsterile ones and no medical expert testimony was needed. The plaintiff won at the trial level, and this was affirmed on appeal, even though there was no proof that the plaintiff ever had any infection.

Taaje vs. St. Olaf Hospital, 199 Minn. 113, 271 N.W. 109 (1937). This is another case which is frequently cited with respect to hospital liability for hospital acquired infections. Plaintiff was the administrator for the estate of his deceased son, who died at the age of 2 months. Deceased was born June 19, 1935, 1 month premature. He was hospitalized on the maternity ward of defendant hospital which was staffed by three regular nurses and two substitute nurses. The particular nurse in question was one of the two regular day nurses. On June 25, this nurse saw her physician because she had had a severe cold and cough for over 6 weeks. Chest X-ray at that time was negative, and a sputum test was said to be positive for tubercle bacillus (test not said to be either a smear of the sputum or a culture of the sputum). It was said that this nurse was immediately sent to a sanitorium where she was still confined at the time of the trial. On June 30, the plaintiff's wife and son left the hospital, but within 2 weeks the child became ill. He returned to the hospital on August 10 and died August 22. The cause of death was acute miliary tuberculosis. At the trial, there was expert medical testimony to the effect that during the 6 days that the nurse helped to take care of the premature infant, she was infective. There was also testimony that the other nurses were free of tuberculosis. There was also medical testimony to the effect that the child was infected with tuberculosis shortly after birth. At the trial, there was a jury verdict for plaintiff. On appeal this was affirmed, the court noting that besides the medical expert testimony, there was evidence of negligence on the part of defendant hospital, since the hospital superintendent visited the maternity ward at least once each day and should have known about the nurse's chronic cough and should have removed her from duty, even if she only had a common cold. The other nurses and some of the patients even knew of the nurse's chronic cough, so this knowledge was widespread. It was also noted that there was a hospital policy requiring nurses who were ill to report that fact and to be taken off duty; therefore, there were two bases of the hospital's negligence: (1) that it knew or should have known that the nurse had a chronic cough, yet nothing was done about it, and (2) since nurses who were ill were required to report the fact, this was a violation of the hospital policy; since the violation of this policy was the direct cause of the injury to the deceased child, this in itself would be negligence on the part of the hospital. With respect to the verdict for the plaintiff of $1,500, the court said, "The child was but 2 months old. The verdict is substantial but, we think, not excessive."

Thigpen vs. Executive Committee of Baptist Convention of State of Georgia, 114 Ga.App. 839, 152 S.E.2d 920 (1966). Plaintiff was a nurse's aide employed by defendant's hospital in June 1956. Plaintiff alleged that she contracted staphylococcal disease in the hospital's nursery for premature infants in December 1958. She alleged that she had no knowledge, notice, or warning of the danger of the staphylococcal disease in the hospital or in the nursery in which she worked. She alleged that the hospital did have such knowledge, alleging that the knowledge of the danger of the staphylococcal infection had been brought to the attention of the Infectious Disease Committee in June 1958 after outbreaks of the staphylococcal disease in other hospitals throughout the U.S. which the defendant hospital knew about. There had been an outbreak of the staphylococcal disease in the nursery in November and December 1958, of which the plaintiff was not aware and that the defendant hospital failed to take the precautionary measures which it knew were necessary to prevent the entry of the staphylococcal disease into the nursery. The defendant hospital knew that hospitals generally and in that community were taking such precautionary measures. She further alleged that because of the alleged negligence of the hospital, she contracted the staphylococcal disease while carrying out her duties and that she was incapacitated for about 5 months. The hospital demurred, and the trial court sustained the demurrer. On appeal, the Court of Appeals of Georgia reversed, saying that the plaintiff had stated a cause of action and the issues of negligence — diligence, assumption of the risk, and proximate cause — would have to be tried before a jury. The trial court's judgment was reversed and the case was remanded for trial.

Thompson vs. Methodist Hospital, 211 Tenn. 650, 367 S.W.2d 134 (1962). Plaintiffs were father, mother, and child. On February 28, 1958, plaintiff child was born in defendant hospital. On March 3, the child and his mother went home, and that day a rash and pimples were noted on the baby by the father. Subsequently the mother, who nursed the child, also developed this, and subsequently the father developed the same problem. At the trial, all the plaintiffs obtained a judgment against the defendant hospital. The intermediate Court of Appeals reversed this decision and the Supreme Court of Tennessee affirmed the Court of Appeals, reversing the trial court decision. It was admitted that there was substantial evidence that the baby acquired his staphylococcal infection while in the hospital and that subsequently the mother and father acquired the infection from the child; however, there was undisputed medical expert testimony that staphylococcal infections occurred both inside and outside of hospitals and could occur without negligence on the part of anyone, since the organism was carried by countless numbers of people without their knowledge. It was further noted that one of the people in the defendant hospital who was found to be a staphylococcal carrier was an intern and that this intern examined the mother on admission to the hospital, but there was no evidence that he ever came into contact with the baby. There was also evidence that a practical nurse from time to time had a boil, but she was sent home. It was noted that she had been in the newborn nursery for a total of 3 days throughout her employment of more than 1 year in the hospital. There was no evidence that she was ever in the nursery during the time that the plaintiff baby was there or that the baby was ever exposed to her. A nurse testified to the fact that there were infractions of the hospital rules in keeping with aseptic techniques. There was testimony that these were occasional violations of the rules rather than the hospital practice, and there was no evidence that these rule infractions occurred while the baby was in the hospital. Therefore, the court held that there was no evidence of negligence on the part of the defendant hospital at the time that the baby was there, and if there were any such negligence, it was not the cause of the baby's infection. Since there was no proof that the baby's infection was the direct result of anything the hospital did and since the infection could have come from one of many different sources for which the hospital was not responsible, liability of the hospital would be purely conjecture. This was not sufficient to allow the jury's verdict.

Tulsa Hospital Association vs. Juby, 73 Okla. 243, 175 P. 519 (1918). On February 15, 1915, plaintiff entered defendant hospital for an appendectomy. At the operation, there was a finding of an infected gall bladder, as well as an infected appendix. On February 20, there was a heavy rain, the roof leaked, the patient's bed and blankets got wet, and part of the bed was changed, but the patient stayed wet from 5:30 to 8:30 or 9:00 am. Plaintiff got chilled, and 5 days later she developed pneumonia from which she suffered a long time. Plaintiff alleged that the leaky roof was the direct and proximate cause of her subsequent pneumonia. There was medical expert testimony that pneumonia might be superinduced by exposure; therefore this presented a question of fact for the jury, and thus the judgment for the plaintiff (which was not against the evidence) was affirmed. The appellate court also felt the hospital was negligent in leaving the plaintiff in a wet bed for 2 hr and by putting the plaintiff in the charge of a student nurse.

Uter vs. Bone and Joint Clinic, 184 So.2d 304 (1966). Plaintiff fractured her leg in 1955. On June 14, 1961, she entered defendant hospital for correction of her right knee problem. On June 15, an operation was performed. She developed an infection in the operative area, but was discharged on July 1. Subsequently she was admitted on several occasions in July and August for more therapy and skin grafts. Judgment for the defendant hospital was affirmed. The evidence was that the sterilization procedures used at the time of the operation were those of the community standards, and there was no expert medical testimony linking her subsequent staphylococcal infection with any negligence by the hospital. There was no medical expert testimony indicating that the defendant doctors did not meet the standard of care.

Utter vs. United Hospital Center, Inc., 236 S.E.2d 213 (1977). On August 25, 1973, plaintiff injured his right wrist, elbow, and back, suffering a comminuted compound fracture of the right wrist, posterior dislocation of the right elbow, and a compression fracture of L2. A cast was applied to the right arm. On August 28, he was transferred to a medical center, but was subsequently transferred to another medical center in another state for hyperbaric oxygen, and his right arm was subsequently amputated. Apparently there were changes in his right arm under the cast on August 27 and early August 28. There was medial expert testimony that time was of the essence in treating plaintiff's wound. There was some testimony that plaintiff's physician was not aware of or ignored changes reported to him by the nurses. At the trial, plaintiff gained a judgment against both the doctor and hospital. The hospital's motion to set aside the verdict was granted, but on appeal, this was reversed, reinstating the jury verdict against the hospital. The appellate court noted that there was a hospital policy in the department of nursing manual requiring the nurses to follow up the failure of a doctor to act by calling the departmental chairman which was not done in this case. Since time was so important in the care of plaintiff's injury, this failure on the part of the nurses to take timely action was a proximal cause of the plaintiff's injury.

Valentin vs. La Societe Francaise de Bienfaisance Mutuelle de Los Angeles, 76 Cal.App.2d 1, 172 P.2d 359 (1946). Plaintiff's son was admitted to defendant hospital for an operation on August 19, 1940. Subsequently on August 27, he had a temperature of 101°, with right pleuritic pain. On August 28 and 29, his temperature was 102.6°. On August 30, he was less talkative. On August 31, he had an inability to chew and pain on attempting to open his mouth. He died on September 1, 1940. Death was attributed to tetanus. The trial court rendered judgment in favor of the plaintiff. The court entered judgment notwithstanding the verdict in favor of the defendant. On appeal the court reversed and entered judgment for the plaintiff. The court noted that there was medical expert testimony to the effect that tetanus was curable and that the delay in instituting therapy was the proximal cause of the death of the patient.

Valentine vs. Kaiser Foundation Hospitals, 194 Cal.App.2d 282, 15 Cal. Rptr. 26 (1961). Plaintiff was circumcised at the age of 2 days; subsequently he lost the glans penis from what was thought to be gangrene. There was some evidence that there was thought to be a black spot on his penis before he left the hospital. There was some evidence that plaintiff's loss was due to an infection which occurred after he left the hospital and that had progressed so far as to be uncurable by the time he returned to the hospital. Judgment was for the plaintiff.

Woodlawn Infirmary vs. Byers, 216 Ala. 210, 112 So. 831 (1927). On March 5, 1926, plaintiff's daughter entered the defendant hospital with appendicitis. She had an appendectomy. On March 16, she died with tetanus. Judgment for the plaintiff at the trial court was reversed and remanded for a new trial because the appellate court held that it was prejudicial to the defendant to admit in evidence the fact that in the year in which plaintiff's daughter died, of three deaths from tetanus, two were in the defendant hospital. This was prejudicial to the defendant (it did not go to the issue of whether defendant was negligent with respect to this specific patient). The plaintiff's evidence against the hospital included such things as the cleanliness of the floor, the method of sweeping, proper sterilization of instruments, insufficient heating of the rooms, and improper postoperative wound care.

ACKNOWLEDGMENTS

Mrs. Marjorie D. Kirtley and Mrs. Cecile C. Taylor of the Virginia State Law Library of the Supreme Court of Virginia were invaluable in helping me obtain various legal references. The T. C. Williams School of Law Library was also gracious in allowing me to use its facilities.

REFERENCES

1. Dornette, W. H. L., Legal aspects of hospital-acquired infections, *J. Leg. Med.,* 1(2), 37, 1973.
2. Hayt, E., Legal Considerations in control of hospital infections, *J.A.H.A.,* 40, 75, October 16, 1966.
3. Nottebart, H. C., Legal aspects of infection control, in *Infection Control in Health Care Facilities: Microbiological Surveillance,* Cundy, K. R. and Ball, W., Eds., University Park Press, Baltimore, 1977, 189.
4. Rivkind, R. J., Legal responsibilities in infection control, *APIC J.,* 6, 23, March 1978.
5. Benenson, A., Ed., *Control of Communicable Diseases in Man,* 12th ed., American Public Health Association, Washington, D.C., 1975.
6. Morris, R. C., Legal aspects of nosocomial infections, in *Hospital Infections,* Bennett, J. V., and Brachman, P. S., Eds., Little, Brown, Boston, 1979, 181.
7. Cram, S., The hospital's obligation to protect patients from carriers of infectious diseases, *Medico-legal News,* 7(3), 8, Fall 1979.
8. Morris, C., Nosocomial infections and the law, in *Proc. Int. Conf. on Nosocomial Infect.,* Brachman, P. S., and Eickhoff, T. C., Eds., American Hospital Association, Chicago, 1971, 322.

Investigating an Epidemic

POSTOPERATIVE WOUND INFECTIONS

Robert C. Aber and Julia S. Garner

BACKGROUND

Postoperative wound infections represent approximately 20% of all nosocomial infections and occur in approximately 1 of every 100 patients admitted to hospitals.[1,2] Approximately 5 to 7% of all surgical wounds become infected postoperatively.[3,4]

Estimated costs attributable to postoperative wound infections vary, depending on the techniques and assumptions of the investigators, but most agree that duration of hospitalization is prolonged by approximately 6 to 13 days, at a cost varying from $500 to $3000 per infection.[3,5,6] Hence, of approximately 40 million patients admitted to acute care hospitals in the U.S. annually, 400,000 will develop postoperative wound infection, at a total estimate cost ranging between $200 million and $1.2 billion. Although these estimates are crude, they provide some measure of the magnitude of the problem. At the present time, it is uncertain what proportion of these infections is preventable or associated with detectable outbreaks.

There is general agreement in the literature for the definitions of an infected wound, a possibly infected wound, and an uninfected wound (see Table 1).[4,6] Hence, the numerator comparability of published investigations is generally good. In contrast, the denominators (patients at risk for developing postoperative wound infection) vary considerably among reported investigations, ranging from all patients admitted to or discharged from hospital (or hospitals) to patients having specific operative procedures or risk factors associated with wound infections. Selected operative procedure-specific rates of postoperative wound infection have been reported by only a few investigators, but the data illustrate considerable differences in the rates, depending upon the operative procedure and the institution (see Table 2).[3,4,7]

Comparison of reported postoperative wound infection rates requires careful consideration of the factors demonstrated to influence the risk of infection (see Table 3). Of these factors, the degree of microbial contamination of the wound during the operative procedure is perhaps one of the most widely reported. The Ad Hoc Committee of the Committee on Trauma, National Academy of Sciences — National Research Council, devised a classification (see Table 4) based upon degree of microbial contamination at the time of surgery and used it extensively in conducting its study on postoperative wound infections (see Table 5).[4] Subsequent experience, however, suggests that the precision and accuracy of such classification depends upon direct observation of the operative procedure. *Post facto* classification is less precise, and resulting data are less accurate. It should be noted that risk factor comparability is especially important when the case-control method of analytic epidemiology is used for hypothesis testing.

RECOGNIZING AND INVESTIGATING AN OUTBREAK

Recognizing an Outbreak

The foundation for detecting an outbreak or epidemic is routine surveillance of acceptable sensitivity and specificity (see chapter entitled "Surveillance and Reporting of Hospital Acquired Infections"). A special feature of surveillance for postoperative wound infections is provision for adequate follow-up after the procedure. Such follow-up is increasingly important as 1-day admissions for surgery and outpatient surgery are becoming more prevalent. A number of methods have been described to achieve

Table 1
EVALUATION OF POSTOPERATIVE WOUND INFECTION

Definitely infected — postoperative wound which drains purulent material, whether or not microorganisms are recovered by culture

Possibly infected — postoperative wound which is inflamed or which drains serous fluid from which microorganisms are recovered

Uninfected — postoperative wound which heals per primum without discharge

Note: Stitch abscesses are generally excluded from definitely or possibly infected categories if localized and if healing occurs within 72 hr after stitches are removed.

Table 2
PROCEDURE-SPECIFIC POSTOPERATIVE WOUND INFECTION RATES

	Infection rates (%)		
Procedure	University of Virginia[7]	National Research Council[4]	Foothills Hospital[3]
Appendectomy	6.0	11.4	6.4
Cholecystectomy	5.8	6.9	2.0
Herniorrhaphy	2.7	2.0	0.5
Colon resection	10.0	10.0	17.6
Transabdominal hysterectomy	3.0	6.1	4.2
Caesarean section	4.8	—	7.8
Laminectomy	2.4	1.4	2.0
Menisectomy	0.6	—	0.5
Coronary artery bypass graft	6.0	—	—
Femoral-popliteal bypass graft	8.7	—	7.9
Nephrectomy	7.0	17.3	6.1
Thyroidectomy	—	2.2	1.2
Breast biopsy (excisional)	—	2.2	0.3

Table 3
FACTORS WHICH INFLUENCE THE RISK OF POSTOPERATIVE WOUND INFECTION[4,6]

Degree of bacterial contamination of the wound
Duration of the operative procedure
Prophylaxis with antimicrobial agents
Length of preoperative hospitalization
Age of patient
Obesity
Nutritional state
Presence of infection at a remote site
Drains
UV light in the operating room (clean-refined procedures only)
Skill/experience of the surgical team
Timing of the preoperative shave
Preoperative shower
Corticosteroid therapy (possibly)

Table 4
CLASSIFICATION OF OPERATIVE WOUNDS BY DEGREE OF MICROBIAL CONTAMINATION[4,6]

Clean wounds — nontraumatic, uninfected operative wounds in which neither the respiratory, alimentary or genitourinary tracts, nor the oropharyngeal cavity are entered. Clean wounds are elective, primarily closed, and undrained. No breaks in aseptic surgical technique occur.

Clean-contaminated wounds — operative wounds in which the respiratory, alimentary, or genitourinary tract is entered without unusual contamination or wounds that are mechanically drained. Minor break in aseptic surgical technique.

Contaminated wounds — include open, fresh traumatic wounds, operations with a major break in aseptic surgical technique, and incisions encountering acute, nonpurulent inflammation.

Dirty wounds — include old traumatic wounds and those involving clinical infection or perforated viscera.

Table 5
POSTOPERATIVE WOUND INFECTION RATES ACCORDING TO DEGREE OF MICROBIAL CONTAMINATION OF THE WOUND

Category	Infection rate (%)	
	National Research Council[4]	Foothills Hospital[3]
Clean	5.1	1.7
Clean-contaminated	10.8	8.8
Contaminated		17.5
	21.9	
Dirty		41.6
Overall	7.4	5.0

follow-up, including postcards which are completed by patient or physician, and postoperative follow-up clinics. Each epidemiologist must develop the system of optimal efficiency and utility to his institution and patients.

The epidemiologist's index of suspicion for an outbreak is perhaps greatest when he identifies one or more wound infections caused by organisms previously associated with outbreaks. Organisms such as Group A streptococcus (*Streptococcus pyogenes*) and *Staphylococcus aureus* elicit such suspicion. A single case of Group A streptococcal postoperative wound infection warrants intensified surveillance and suspicion of an outbreak.

When microorganisms which are more ubiquitous or more commonly associated with patient infections are isolated from infected wounds, one relys upon more specialized analyses, such as temporal or spatial clustering or typing (fingerprinting) of the microorganism, to help determine whether an outbreak exists. Clustering of microorganisms possessing "markers", such as an unusual antimicrobial susceptibility pattern or biochemical reaction, may be easily recognized and may facilitate detection of an outbreak. When the organisms do not possess "markers" which are readily recognized, clustering may be detected by more sophisticated statistical analyses. In general, such analyses use surveillance data to establish a "baseline" or usual rate of occurrence of a particular antimicrobial susceptibility pattern (antibiogram) or biochemical reaction pattern (biotype), and then compare the recent (usually monthly) rate of occur-

Table 6
MICROORGANISMS THAT CAUSE NOSOCOMIAL INFECTION AND FOR WHICH SELECTED EPIDEMIOLOGIC TYPING SYSTEMS ARE MOST USEFUL AND APPLICABLE

Typing system	Microorganisms
Biotype	*Salmonella, Shigella*, other Enterobacteriaceae, *Pseudomonas*, fungi
Antibiogram	Enterobacteriaceae, *Pseudomonas*, and other nonfermentative bacteria, *Staphylococcus*
Serotype	Viruses, Enterobacteriaceae, *Pseudomonas*, streptococci, *Legionella, Chlamydia*
Bacteriocin type	*Shigella, Pseudomonas, Serratia*
Bacteriophage type	*Staphylococcus, Pseudomonas, Salmonella*, mycobacteria
Restriction enzyme analysis	Herpes simplex virus, adenovirus, plasmids

rence of the pattern to the established baseline. A significant increase in the recent rate of occurrence may warrant investigation to determine whether an outbreak exists. This type of analysis may be applied to postoperative wound infection rates in general, regardless of the microorganisms isolated from the wounds. It is claimed, for instance, that monitoring the clean wound infection rate reflects surgical technique in an institution.[3] Significant increases in this rate may indicate a need for review of aseptic technique being used by the operating team, operating room personnel, and others.

Laboratory typing or fingerprinting of microorganisms of the same genus and species (e.g., *S. aureus*) may be used to define the genetic relatedness or identity of these organisms; the epidemiologic implication being that organisms which are genetically related or identical by these techniques are more likely to have arisen from a common source in the hospital environment and that control measures which remove the source or interrupt transmission of the organism are likely to reduce the rate of infection.[49,50] A variety of such typing systems are available (see Table 6), but in general they are performed only in special laboratories.

The ability to detect outbreaks of postoperative wound infections may be quite variable, depending upon the types of analyses which are performed in a given institution. Few institutions currently employ the most sophisticated statistical methods for detecting clusters or significant increases above baseline of infection rates (i.e., threshold analysis) but the efficiency and cost-effectiveness of these techniques have not been fully explored.

Investigating an Outbreak
General Measures

Epidemiologic investigation of an outbreak or suspected outbreak of disease entails a logical sequence of steps or procedures and should proceed in an orderly fashion. Approaches to such investigations, irrespective of the particular site or microbiologic cause of infection, have been published and are briefly outlined in Table 7.[8-10]

It is usually relatively easy to verify the diagnosis of postoperative wound infection by adhering to the definitions in Table 1. If specific microorganisms appear to be causing the outbreak, it is important to begin saving all such isolates at the outset, anticipating that special typing of the organisms may be helpful (see Table 6).

Case definition in this setting is usually not difficult. Case finding, however, may be limited by inefficient surveillance, incomplete or inaccessible laboratory records, inadequate culturing of infected wounds, or inaccessibility to a portion of the population at risk because of early discharge from hospital or outpatient surgery.

The initial line-listing of cases should include enough information to enable the in-

Table 7
OUTLINE OF AN OUTBREAK INVESTIGATION

1. Verify the diagnosis and laboratory identification of the etiologic agent (if applicable).
2. Define what is meant by a case (may be appropriate to group into definite, probably, possible, etc.).
3. Implement case finding and initiate a line listing (or equivalent) of cases.
4. Make preliminary determination as to whether an outbreak or epidemic exists, i.e., compare to baseline or previous rate of occurrence.
5. Review descriptive characteristics of the cases, i.e., orient as to time, person, place, morbidity, etc. and develop appropriate rates of disease.
6. Perform "quick and dirty" analyses of cases employing available rates of disease to develop impressions as to the nature of the outbreak, desirability for further investigation and desired speed of investigation.
7. Formulate tentative hypotheses which include source or reservoir of etiologic agent, mode of transmission, or other potentially remediable factors contributing to the outbreak.
8. Initiate appropriate control measures based upon likely hypotheses while preparing to test the hypotheses.
9. Initiate special investigations to test hypotheses, i.e., analytic epidemiologic techniques (cohort or case control studies), epidemiologic typing of microorganisms, culture surveys, intensified case finding, modification of denominators (persons at risk) to increase specificity.
10. Revise and refine control measures as hypotheses are either accepted or rejected and continue surveillance of the high-risk populations.

vestigator to orient the cases as to time, place, and person, as well as any special risk factors which seem appropriate, the site of infection, operative procedure, and results of the wound culture.

A preliminary determination as to whether an outbreak exists is facilitated by existing surveillance data. In developing rates of postoperative wound infection the numerator is the number of such infections (or the number of patients having such infections) for a given time period, and the denominator reflects, with as much accuracy as feasible, the number of patients or operative wounds at risk for developing postoperative wound infection during the same time period. Crude estimates of the population at risk (denominator) include the number of patients admitted to or discharged from hospital or the number of patients admitted to or discharged from the surgical services during the given time period. These estimates may be sufficient to establish the existence of an outbreak. More specific estimates of the population at risk for developing postoperative wound infection include the number of patients actually operated upon or the number of surgical wounds created during the time period. If review of the line-listing suggests that a particular operative procedure precedes the infections, then the denominator should reflect the number of patients having the particular procedure or the number of wounds created by the procedure. Other estimates of the population at risk may be appropriate and should be used at times as well, such as all patients operated on by a specific surgeon or attended by a specific member of the operating or postoperative team.

The "quick and dirty" analysis of cases and available rates of infection may suggest the source or reservoir of infection, the mode of transmission, or other potentially remedial factors contributing to the outbreak, especially when considered in the light of previous outbreaks of similar nature. For example, the reservoir of Group A streptococcus in recently reported outbreaks of postoperative wound infection is usually an infected or colonized member of hospital staff, and transmission of the organism usually occurs by direct contact of the wound with hands or objects recently in contact with the source.

Hypotheses represent "straw men" and serve mainly to determine the nature and direction of subsequent investigative activity and control measures. With respect to postoperative wound infections, such hypotheses might consider:

1.   Whether the infecting organism is endogenously (part of the infected patient's flora) or exogenously (from the animate or inanimate environment) acquired
2.   How and when the infecting organism entered the surgical wound site
3.   What specific factors (host, organism, or other) tipped the balance of the interaction between host and microorganism in favor of the microorganism

Endogenous microflora may include "hospital strains" acquired after hospitalization, but before the operative procedure. *S. aureus* colonization of the skin or anterior nares, for example, may be acquired in the hospital. Similarly, nosocomial aerobic Gram-negative rods may become part of the oropharyngeal, skin, or gastrointestinal (GI) microflora after admission to hospital, but prior to the creation of the surgical wound, and then subsequently infect the wound.

Initial control measures depend somewhat on the early impressions of the outbreak and should be directed at minimizing the risks of infection in the uninfected population at risk. Such measures as wound and skin precautions for infected patients, spatial segregation of infected patients from uninfected patients at risk, segregation of hospital personnel caring for such groups of patients, and appropriate therapeutic measures for the infected patients, may be initiated early while the investigation continues. More specific control measures may be indicated as more information becomes available.

Complete discussion of hypothesis testing is beyond the scope of this chapter, but several excellent discussions have been published.[11,12] Probably the most frequently used technique is the case control study. In essence, "control" patients are selected (preferably at random) from the uninfected population at risk for comparison with "cases" to determine which characteristics of cases are associated with infection or which characteristics of controls are associated with absence of infection. It is difficult (some say impossible) to establish causation of disease using case-control analysis, but some associations may be suggestive enough to warrant implementation of control measures aimed at altering the risk factors so identified.

A type of special investigation which is often inappropriately utilized is the culture survey. The less-experienced epidemiologist often has a compelling urge to culture everything when confronted with an outbreak. This is often inappropriate because simply finding the organism in the patient's environment (animate or inanimate) does not establish either the flow of the organism (patient to environment or vice versa) or causation (such surveys are usually *post facto*) and may lead to inappropriate actions, such as sending an employee home (with or without pay) or making expensive alterations in the physical plant. Culture surveys often make very valuable contributions, however, when conducted for specific purposes in well-designed investigations. Such surveys may improve case finding, define the extent of an animate or inanimate reservoir of the organism, and help to assess the effect of control measures.

In summary, investigation of an outbreak of postoperative wound infections should be conducted in an orderly fashion as outlined in Table 7. Each investigation, however, is unique, and the investigator must adapt these principles and techniques to the investigation.

Outbreaks Caused by Staphylococci

Staphylococci, particularly *S. aureus*, were the most frequent cause of infection in hospitalized patients in the 15-year period 1950 to 1965, and the postoperative surgical wound was among the most common sites of infection. This stimulated intensive investigation by the medical community to define the sources, reservoirs, modes of transmission, and effective methods of control of these infections. Much of the information in Table 8 about *S. aureus* postoperative wound infection outbreaks reflects these ear-

Table 8

EPIDEMIOLOGIC CHARACTERISTICS OF POSTOPERATIVE WOUND INFECTION OUTBREAKS CAUSED BY SELECTED MICROORGANISMS

Organism	Incidence[a] and relative frequency[b]	Source or reservoir	Transmission	Host factors	Special epidemiologic typing	Control measures	Ref.
Staphylococcus aureus	16.3,[a] approximately 15%[b]	Human: a. infected b. colonized: 1. respiratory shedders 2. dermatitis; Local environment often heavily contaminated, but role as reservoir appears limited	Primarily direct contact of wound by hands or objects recently in contact with source or reservoir: 1. endogenous and 2. exogenous; airborne also documented, but probably less important	Colonization with S. aureus prior to surgery	Bacteriophage susceptibility	1. Wound and skin precautions or strict isolation as appropriate 2. Search for persons with overt infection — remove from patient contact and treat 3. Spatial segregation of cases and uninfected patients at risk 4. Cohorting of cases and personnel may be necessary 5. Good hygienic practices 6. Appropriate treatment of infected and epidemiologically implicated reservoirs 7. Hexachlorophene bathing pre- and postoperatively may be helpful during the outbreak	1, 13—19, 29
Group A streptococcus	0.9[a] approximately 0.7%[b]	Human: a. infected b. colonized: 1. anal/rectal 2. nasal dispersers 3. vagina 4. pharynx	Direct contact or airborne	Colonization with group A streptococci prior to surgery	Serologic typing with M and T antisera	1, 20—29
Group C streptococcus	Rare	Human: a. colonized: 1. perianal 2. nasal	Uncertain — probably direct contact or airborne	None known	None	1. Identification and treatment of source 2. Treatment of cases	30
Clostridium perfringens (welchii)	Rare	Human, colonized, GI tract Inanimate environment Elastic bandages	Direct contact, usually endogenous, rarely exogenous Role of airborne route unclear	Devitalized tissue	None	1. Wound and skin precautions 2. Spatial segregation as above 3. Review aseptic and sterilization techniques 4. Appropriate treatment of cases 5. Sterilization of elastic bandages	31—33, 52

Table 8 (continued)
EPIDEMIOLOGIC CHARACTERISTICS OF POSTOPERATIVE WOUND INFECTION OUTBREAKS CAUSED BY SELECTED MICROORGANISMS

Organism	Incidence[a] and relative frequency[b]	Source or reservoir	Transmission	Host factors	Special epidemiologic typing	Control measures	Ref.
Pseudomonas multivorans	Rare	Disinfectant solution	Direct contact of vehicle with wound	None	Antibiogram, serotyping with *Pseudomonas aeruginosa* antisera	1. Removal of reservoir 2. Appropriate treatment of cases	37
Aeromonas hydrophilia	Rare	Infected patients	Direct contact with wound via hands during dressing change	None	Biotype	1. Improve wound dressing techniques 2. Handwashing between patient contacts	1
Aerobic Gram-negative bacilli (see text)	42.9[a] approximately 37%[b]	Human infected, colonized; inanimate vehicle	Usually direct contact, endogenous: hands, contiguous spread, exogenous: hands, common vehicle,	Degree of illness; antimicrobial agents colonization/infection at another site	See below	See text	1, 38—42
Escherichia coli	17.3[a] approximately 16%[b]	Especially GI tract	—	—	Biotype, antibiogram, serologic type, R-factors	—	1
Klebsiella spp.	6.2,[a] approximately 5%[b]	Especially GI tract, disinfectants, hand creams, and lotions	—	—	Biotype, antibiogram, capsular serotype, R-factors	—	1, 39, 41, 42, 53
Enterobacter spp.	4.0,[a] approximately 4%[b]	Hand creams	—	—	Biotype, antibiogram, R-factors	—	1, 39
Proteus, providencia	7.8,[a] approximately 7%[b]	—	—	—	Biotype, antibiogram, R-factors	—	1, 47

P. aeruginosa	5.2,[a] approximately 4%	Especially disinfectants and other liquid vehicles	—	—	Biotype, antibiogram, serologic type, pyocin production and susceptibility, bacteriophage susceptibility, R-factors	—	1, 35, 36, 39
Serratia spp.	1.1,[a] approximately 1.2%[b]	Especially infected or colonized patients, disinfectants	Direct contact with wound	None	Biotype, antibiogram, serologic type	—	1, 38, 39
Rhizopus rhizopodiformis (mucormycosis)	Rare	Elastic adhesive dressing	Direct contact with wound	None	Biotype	Removal of source	43, 44
Mycobacterium fortuitum complex	Rare	Uncertain	Probably direct contact	Open heart surgery via sternum	Biotype	1. Recognition of the organism 2. Appropriate treatment of cases 3. General review and "clean-up" of all or and postoperative care units 4. Temporary suspension of surgery	45, 46

[a] Incidence is number of isolates reported per 10,000 patients discharged from hospital.

[b] Relative frequency is expressed as percent of all isolates from infected surgical wounds.

lier experiences.[13-17] Since 1967, only three outbreaks of surgical wound infection caused by *S. aureus* have been intensively investigated by the Center for Disease Control (CDC), although additional outbreaks have been reported and less intensively investigated. *S. aureus* represents 15% of all pathogens isolated from wound infections reported to the National Nosocomial Infections Study (NNIS).[1] Several additional outbreaks have been reported in the literature.[18,19] Outbreaks are usually detected by temporal or spatial clustering of infections and confirmed by bacteriophage susceptibility typing of the organisms and by epidemiologic investigation. Recent outbreaks have invariably been traced to a human source, usually a member of the surgical team with anterior nasal colonization (presumably a heavy shedder) or one with active dermatitis. Transmission is presumed to occur primarily by direct contact with the wound by hands or objects recently in contact with the source, but the role of airborne spread is usually not convincingly excluded. Control measures outlined in Table 8 are usually successful when combined with careful epidemiologic investigation. Mass culture surveys are not recommended as the initial or exclusive approach to an outbreak. Selective culture surveys as indicated by epidemiologic investigation are usually necessary to confirm the source and to document eradication of the organism.

Although *Staphylococcus epidermidis* is considered a pathogen in 4.8% of surgical wound infections reported to the NNIS,[1] little is known about the epidemiology of such infections. No *S. epidermidis* wound infection outbreaks were investigated by the CDC during the period 1967 to 1977, and none have been located in the English literature since 1965.

Outbreaks Caused by Streptococci

Group A streptococci (*S. pyogenes*) are implicated as pathogens in only 0.7% of surgical wound infections reported to NNIS,[1] but such infections often occur in clusters or outbreaks. A single case warrants attention and careful surveillance, and two cases occurring in temporal or spatial relationship within an institution warrant investigation. The CDC epidemiologists investigated three such outbreaks during the period 1967 to 1977, and several more outbreaks have been reported in the literature since 1965.[20-27,51] Such outbreaks have been traced to an infected or colonized human source. Although pharyngeal colonization with *S. pyogenes* is relatively common, epidemiologically important disseminators of the organism are usually colonized in the nose,[28] peri-rectal area,[20-25,51] or vagina,[26] or have active infection. As with *S. aureus*, transmission is presumed to be primarily by direct contact, but airborne transmission may occur.[29] Suggested control measures are similar to those for *S. aureus* outbreaks.

Group C streptococci (*Streptococcus equisimilis*) have been reported to cause one outbreak (two cases) of postoperative wound infections.[30] The source proved to be a member of the surgical team colonized in the nose and rectal area. Eradication of the organism from this source was temporally associated with termination of the outbreak.

Group B streptococci are implicated as pathogens in 1.8% of surgical wound infections reported to the NNIS.[1] There are no reported outbreaks of postoperative wound infections caused by these organisms as yet. The organism occurs endogenously in the vagina, GI tract, and pharynx, and may be expected to produce wound infections in these areas.

Group D streptococci are commonly isolated from postoperative wound infections, accounting for 10% of pathogens from this site reported to the NNIS.[1] The organism is part of the normal GI and vaginal flora and frequently occurs in association with surgical procedures in these areas. Epidemiologic investigation of these organisms has been hindered by lack of special typing systems.[49]

Outbreaks Caused by Clostridia

Clostridial myonecrosis or gas gangrene originating in a postoperative wound is a rare, but dramatic, disease. Sporadic cases occur from time to time in surgical practice. The causative organism, *Clostridium perfringens (welchii)*, is a normal GI tract inhabitant which is commonly found in the environment.[31] Most isolated cases probably result from endogenous organisms which gain access to the wound.[32] At least one outbreak (three cases) of *Clostridium perfringens* surgical wound infections has been reported since 1962.[33] The source of the organism was presumed to be endogenous in the first patient, with transmission to two subsequent cases by direct contact. These reflections were retrospective, and therefore, may have been in error. Since the organism has been isolated from the air and the inanimate environment during investigation of isolated cases, airborne or indirect contact transmission may occasionally occur. Control measures have not been adequately tested. A primary consideration is to avoid the panic which sometimes occurs in response to this dramatic disease.

More recently, *C. perfringens* wound infections were associated with the use of nonsterile elastic bandages in five diabetic patients. The bandage material was found to contain *C. perfringens* and other clostridial species.[52]

Outbreaks Caused by Aerobic Gram-Negative Bacilli

As a group, aerobic Gram-negative bacilli are the most frequent bacteria isolated (approximately 37%) from surgical wound infections reported to the NNIS.[1] Indeed, 68% of surgical wound infections reported to the Comprehensive Hospital Infections Project, 1971 to 1973, were caused by aerobic Gram-negative bacilli, either alone or in combination with other pathogens.[34] Discrete outbreaks of postoperative wound infections caused by these organisms have been reported only rarely. During the period 1967 — 1977, CDC epidemiologists investigated eight outbreaks of infections due to aerobic Gram-negative bacilli among surgical patients; however, only one of the eight involved predominantly or exclusively wound infections (see Table 8, *Aeromonas hydrophilia*). The majority of outbreaks involved bacteremias, usually without associated infection of the surgical wound. Review of literature since 1965 yielded few such outbreaks as well.[35-37]

The surgical wound may be one of several sites infected during more general outbreaks of infections caused by aerobic Gram-negative bacilli. Hence, an outbreak of surgical wound infections caused by these organisms must be suspected, at least initially, of being part of a more generalized outbreak. Case finding efforts should be broadened to define the magnitude of problem and general control measures may be appropriate early in the investigation.

A detailed discussion of the epidemiology of aerobic Gram-negative bacilli in the hospital is beyond the scope of this chapter; however, several general principles are pertinent. Sources or reservoirs of these organisms include colonized or infected persons (almost always patients, seldom personnel),[38,48] or a portion of the inanimate environment favoring persistence, and usually, multiplication of the organism.[39,48] Some common inapparent sites of colonization or infection of patients serving as reservoirs include the urinary tract (especially with an indwelling urinary catheter),[38] the oropharynx,[40] and the GI tract.[41,53] Asymptomatic GI colonization with epidemic strains of aerobic Gram-negative bacilli has been discovered in several outbreaks investigated by CDC epidemiologists or reported in the literature.[41,42,53] Such colonization may occur preoperatively even though infection develops postoperatively, and the importance of this reservoir in perpetuating such outbreaks has not been fully explored. The inanimate reservoirs are usually moist or liquid in nature and often superficially deceptive, such as antiseptic or disinfectant solutions, ice machines, skin creams or lotions, "bacteriostatic" irrigating solutions, medications, or "sterile" fluid for parenteral use.[39] Transmission of these organisms usually occurs by direct contact on the hands of personnel, contiguous spread, or by common vehicle.[48] The organisms may be endogenous or exogenous in origin. Factors which appear to predispose the host to colonization or infection with aerobic Gram-negative bacilli include severity of illness (especially intensive care), administration of antimicrobial agents (usually broad spectrum), and procedures which violate normal host defense mechanisms (surgery, urinary catheter, I.V. catheter, and tracheal intubation).[48]

Control measures which may be applicable to an outbreak of infections (including wound infections) caused by aerobic Gram-negative bacilli include the following:[38,39,42,53]

1.   Spatial segregation of infected (colonized) patients and uninfected (noncolonized) patients at risk, ranging from isolation of individual patients to cohorting of patients and personnel as appropriate
2.   Intensified surveillance and case finding to define the human reservoir(s)
3.   Emphasis and implementation of good personal hygiene, especially handwashing, among patient and personnel
4.   Review of appropriate patient care practices with personnel, e.g., care of the urinary and I.V. catheters, sterile dressing technique, etc., as determined by the nature of the outbreak and sites of infection
5.   Removal or modification of the selective pressure of antimicrobial agents if applicable (i.e., organism is multiply resistant)
6.   Identification and removal of the inanimate source or reservoir (lessons from previous outbreaks, directed environmental culture surveys, etc.)

It may also be appropriate to review plans for disposition of all colonized or infected patients to prevent transferring the epidemic organism to another facility. It appears that the risk of colonization or infection with the organism among healthy family members in the home environment is minimal, although few such followup investigations have been reported.

In outbreaks involving only surgical wound sites of infection by aerobic Gram-negative bacilli, an inanimate reservoir and transmission via common vehicle which is directly applied to the wound should be suspected early,[35,37] since transmission by hands usually results in inoculation of other sites as well.

Outbreaks Caused by Other Microorganisms

Outbreaks of surgical wound infections caused by *Rhizopus rhizopodiformis*[43,44] (mucormycosis, 23 cases) and organisms of the *Mycobacterium fortuitum* complex[45,46] have been reported recently and are in Table 8.

REFERENCES

1. Center for Disease Control, National Nosocomial Infections Study Report, Annual Summary 1977 (issued November 1979), Atlanta.
2. **Wenzel, R. P., Osterman, C. A., and Hunting, K. J.,** Hospital-acquired infections. II. Infection rates by site, service and common procedures in a university hospital, *Am. J. Epidemiol.,* 104, 645, 1976.
3. **Cruse, P. J. E.,** Incidence of wound infection on the surgical services, *Surg. Clin. North Am.,* 55, 1269, 1975.
4. National Academy of Sciences — National Research Council, Division of Medical Sciences, Ad Hoc Committee of the Committee on Trauma, Postoperative Wound Infections, The influence of ultraviolet irradiation of the operating room and of various other factors, *Ann. Surg.,* 160 (Suppl. 2), 1, 1964.
5. **Green, J. W. and Wenzel, R. P.,** Postoperative wound infection: a controlled study of the increased duration of hospital stay and direct cost of hospitalization, *Ann. Surg.,* 185, 264, 1977.
6. Committee on Control of Surgical Infections, American College of Surgeons, Incidence and cost of infections, in *Manual on Control of Infection in Surgical Patients,* J. B. Lippincott, Philadelphia, 1976, chap. 2.
7. **Wenzel, R. P., Hunting, K. I., and Osterman, C. A.,** Postoperative wound infection rates, *Surg. Gynecol. Obstet.,* 144, 749, 1977.
8. **Dixon, R. E.,** Investigation of endemic and epidemic investigations, in *Hospital Infections,* Bennett, J. V. and Brachman, P. S., Eds., Little, Brown, Boston, 1979, chap. 5.
9. **Castle, M. and Mallison, G. F.,** Effective investigations of nosocomial outbreaks, *Association for Practitioners in Infection Control Newsletter,* 5, 13, 1977.
10. **Agate, G. H.,** The epidemiological investigation of institutionally-acquired infections, in *Control of Infections in Hospitals,* Berlin, B. S. and Hilbert, M., Eds., The University of Michigan, Ann Arbor, 1966, 183.
11. **MacMahon, B. and Pugh, T. F.,** *Epidemiology: Principles and Methods,* Little, Brown, Boston, 1970.
12. **Armitage, P.,** *Statistical Methods in Medical Research,* John Wiley & Sons, New York, 1973, chap. 16.
13. **Williams R. E. O.,** Healthy carriage of *Staphylococcus aureus:* its prevalence and importance, *Bacteriol. Rev.,* 27, 56, 1963.
14. **Nahmias A. J. and Eickhoff, T. C.,** Staphylococcal infections in hospitals: recent developments in epidemiologic and laboratory investigation, *N. Engl. J. Med.,* 265, 74, 120, 177, 1964.
15. **Fekety, R., Jr.,** The epidemiology and prevention of staphylococcal infection, *Medicine,* 43, 593, 1964.
16. U.S. Department of Health, Education, and Welfare, Communicable Disease Center, Proceedings of the National Conference on Hospital-Acquired Staphylococcal Disease, U.S. Government Printing Office, Washington, D.C., 1958.
17. **Calia, F. M., Wolinsky E., Mortimer, E. A., Jr., Abrams, J. S., and Rommelkamp, C. H., Jr.,** Importance of the carrier state as a source of *Staphylococcus aureus* in wound sepsis, *J. Hyg. Camb.,* 67, 49, 1969.
18. **Ayliffe, G. A. and Collins, B. J.,** Wound infections acquired from a disperser of an unusual strain of *Staphylococcus aureus, J. Clin. Pathol.,* 20, 195, 1967.
19. **Payne, R. W.,** Severe outbreak of surgical sepsis due to *Staphyloccus aureus* of unusual type and origin, *Br. Med. J.,* 2, 17, 1967.
20. **McKee, W. M., DiCaprio, J. M., Roberts, J. E., Jr., and Sherris, J. C.,** Anal carriage as the probable source of a streptococcal epidemic, *Lancet,* 2, 1007, 1966.
21. **McIntyre, D. M.,** An epidemic of *Streptococcus pyogenes* puerperal and postoperative sepsis with an unusual carrier site — the anus, *Am. J. Obstet. Gynecol.,* 101, 308, 1968.
22. **Schaffner, W., Lefkowitz, L. B., Jr., Goodman, J. S., and Koenig, M. G.,** Hospital outbreak of infections with group A streptococci traced to an asymptomatic anal carrier, *N. Engl. J. Med.,* 280, 1224, 1969.
23. **Gryska, P. F. and O'Dea, A. E.,** Postoperative streptococcal wound infection — the anatomy of an epidemic, *JAMA,* 213, 1189, 1970.
24. Center for Disease Control, Hospital outbreak of streptococcal wound infection — Utah, Morbidity and Mortality Weekly Report 25 (No. 18), 141, 1976.
25. **Richman, D. D., Breton, S. J., and Goldmann, D. A.,** Scarlet fever and group A streptococcal surgical wound infection traced to an anal carrier, *J. Pediatr.,* 90, 387, 1977.
26. **Stamm, W. E., Feeley, J. C., and Facklam, R. R.,** Wound infections due to group A streptococcus traced to a vaginal carrier, *J. Infect. Dis.,* 138, 287, 1978.

27. **Quinn, R. W. and Hillman, J. W.,** An epidemic of streptococcal wound infections, *Arch. Environ. Health,* 11, 28, 1965.

28. **Hamburger, M., Jr., Green, M. J., and Hamburger, V. G.,** The problem of the "dangerous carrier" of hemolytic streptococci. II. Spread of infection by individuals with positive nose cultures who expelled large numbers of hemolytic streptococci, *J. Infect. Dis.,* 77, 96, 1945.

29. **Rammelkamp, C., Jr., Mortimer, E. A., Jr., and Wolinsky, E.,** Transmission of streptococcal and staphylococcal infections, *Ann. Intern. Med.,* 60, 753, 1964.

30. **Goldmann D. A. and Breton, S. J.,** Group C streptococcal surgical wound infections transmitted by an anorectal and nasal carrier, *Pediatrics,* 61, 235, 1978.

31. **Lowbury, E. J. L. and Lilly, H. A.,** The sources of hospital infection of wounds with *Clostridium welchii, J. Hyg. Camb.,* 56, 169, 1958.

32. **Pyrtek, L. J. and Bartus, S. H.,** *Clostridium welchii* complicating biliary-tract surgery, *N. Engl. J. Med.,* 266, 689, 1962.

33. **Eickhoff, T. C.,** An outbreak of surgical wound infections due to *Clostridium perfringens, Surg. Gynecol. Obstet.,* 114, 102, 1962.

34. **Stamm, W. E., Martin, S. M., and Bennett, J. V.,** Epidemiology of nosocomial infections due to gram-negative bacilli: aspects relevant to development and use of vaccines, *J. Infect. Dis.,* 136 (Suppl.), S151, 1977.

35. **Ayliffe, G. A. J., Lowbury, E. J. L., Hamilton, J. G., Small, J. M., Asheshov, E. A., and Parker, M. T.,** Hospital infection with *Pseudomonas aeruginosa* in neurosurgery, *Lancet,* 2, 365, 1975.

36. **Moore, B. and Forman, A.,** An outbreak of urinary *Pseudomonas aeruginosa* infection acquired during urological operations, *Lancet,* 2, 929, 1966.

37. **Bassett, D. C. J., Stokes, K. J., and Thomas, W. R. G.,** Wound infection with *Pseudomonas multivorans, Lancet,* 1, 1188, 1970.

38. **Schaberg, D. R., Weinstein, R. A., and Stamm, W. E.,** Epidemics of nosocomial urinary tract infection caused by multiply-resistant negative bacilli: epidemiology and control, *J. Infect. Dis.,* 133, 363, 1976.

39. **Bassett, D. C. J.,** Common source outbreaks, *Proc. R. Soc. Med.,* 64, 980 1971.

40. **Johanson, W. G., Pierce, A. K., and Sanford, J. P.,** Changing pharyngeal bacterial flora of hospitalized patients *N. Engl. J. Med.,* 281, 1137, 1969.

41. **Selden, R., Lee, S., Wang, W. L. L., Bennett, J. V., and Eickhoff, T. C.,** Nosocomial *Klebsiella* infections: intestinal colonization as a reservoir, *Ann. Intern. Med.,* 74, 657, 1971.

42. **Curie, K., Speller, D. C. E., Simpson, R. A., Stephens, M., and Cooke, D. I.,** A hospital epidemic caused by a gentamicin-resistant *Klebsiella aerogenes, J. Hyg. Camb.,* 80, 115, 1978.

43. **Gartenberg, G., Bottone, E. J., Keusch, G. T., and Weitzman, I.,** Hospital-acquired mucormycosis (*Rhizopus rhizopodiformis*) of skin and subcutaneous tissue: epidemiology, mycology and treatment, *N. Engl. J. Med.,* 299, 1115, 1978.

44. **Center for Disease Control,** Nosocomial outbreak of *Rhizopus* infections associated with Elastoplast wound dressings — Minnesota, Morbidity and Mortality Weekly Report, 27, 33, 243, 1978.

45. **Robicsek, F., Daugherty, H. K., Cook, J. W., Selle, J. G., Masters, T. N., O'Bar, P. R. Fernandez, C. R., Mauney, C. U., and Calhoun, D. M.,** *Mycobacterium fortuitum* epidemics after open-heart surgery, *J. Thorac. Cardiovasc. Surg.,* 75, 91, 1978.

46. **Center for Disease Control,** Atypical mycobacteria wound infections — North Carolina, Colorado, in National Nosocomial Infections Study Report, Annual Summary 1974 , U.S. Public Health Service, U.S. Department of Health, Education and Welfare, Atlanta, Ga. (issued March 1977, 12.

47. **Iannini, P. B., Eickhoff, T. C., and LaForce, F. M.,** Multidrug-resistant *Proteus rettgeri:* an emergent problem, *Ann. Intern. Med.,* 85, 161, 1976.

48. **Maki, D. G.,** Control of colonization and transmission of pathogenic bacteria in the hospital, *Ann. Intern. Med.,* 89 (Part 2), 777, 1978.

49. **Aber, R. C., Mackel, D.,** Epidemiologic Typing of Nosocomial Microorganisms, 2nd Int. Symp. on Nosocomial Infect., Atlanta, August 5-8, 1980.

50. **Goldman, D. A. and Macone, A. B.,** A microbiological approach to the investigation of bacterial nosocomial infection outbreaks, *Infec. Control,* 1, 391, 1980.

51. **Schrack, W. D., Jr., Miller, G. B., Parkin, W. E., Fontana, D. B.,** Four streptococcal infections traced to an anal carrier, *P. Med.,* 82, 35, 1979.

52. **Pearson, R. D., Valenti, W. M., Steigbigel, R. T.,** *Clostridium perfringens* wound infection associated with elastic bandages, *JAMA,* 244, 1128, 1980.

53. **Aber, R. C.,** Nosocomial Infection with Gentamicin-resistant Tribe Klebsielleae Organisms, Epidemic Intelligence Serv. Conf., Atlanta, April 15-19, 1974.

INFECTIONS IN BURN PATIENTS

C. Glen Mayhall

INTRODUCTION

Patients hospitalized with serious burns frequently have a prolonged course and may die from one or a combination of complications. Of the 42,755 burn cases submitted to the National Burn Information Exchange (NBIE),[1] 5,730 (or 13.4%) ended fatally. Death was due to organ system failure in 45.9% and to infection in 40.1%; death occurred as a direct result of accident (primary pulmonary injury, burn over 90%, or concurrent injuries) in 13.9% of cases and was iatrogenic in 0.1%. Thus, infection is one of the most important causes of death in burn patients.

The NBIE has reliable data on complications for only 15,531 cases, unfortunately. Therefore, absolute incidence rates for the vaious complications (based on 42,755 cases) cannot be computed. However, "relative rates" (those based on the 15,531) can be determined, and they indicate the relative importance of the different types of complications. Thus, the relative rates for infection at different sites are 11.4% for septicemia, 7.6% for pneumonia, 3.7% for wound sepsis, 1.3% for urinary tract infection, and 0.4% for septic phlebitis. Thus, there are 1.5 times as many nosocomial bloodstream infections as nosocomial pneumonias and almost 6 times as many nosocomial pneumonias as nosocomial urinary tract infections in burn patients. The rates given above based on a subset of cases submitted underestimate the absolute rate of infectious complications. When the latter consideration is combined with the facts that about 40% of deaths in burn patients are due to infection and that most infections in burn patients are hospital acquired, the importance of infection control in burn care facilities can be placed in perspective.

INFECTIONS IN BURN PATIENTS

Although the burn wound may be contaminated at the time of thermal injury, the overwhelming majority of infections in burn patients occur several days after admission and are therefore hospital acquired by definition. Patients who have sustained thermal injury are particularly susceptible to nosocomial infection. In addition to the instrumentation required by most critically ill and injured patients, the burn patient also has a burn wound with all its attendant risks. The burn eschar is always colonized by bacteria and provides an excellent culture medium of necrotic tissue and serum.

The burn wound may be colonized by *Staphylococcus aureus*, *Pseudomonas aeruginosa*, or members of the family Enterobacteriaceae, such as *Enterobacter* and *Klebsiella*. The wound surface may also be colonized by fungi, such as *Candida* and *Aspergillus*. Although organisms growing on the burn wound surface may not cause serious infection, they provide a large reservoir for contamination and infection of other body sites or other patients. In some patients, the microorganisms on the wound surface may invade the burn wound, multiplying to large numbers and involving subjacent viable tissue.

The most reliable method for diagnosis of burn wound infection is wound biopsy. Although not all investigators agree,[2] a generally accepted criterion for burn wound infection is the presence of $\geqslant 10^5$ organisms per gram of tissue.[3] In addition to bacteria, *Candida* sp., *Aspergillus* sp., members of the family Zygomycetes (formerly Phyco-

Table 1
BACTERIA AND FUNGI THAT
COMPRISED ≥1.0% OF 1894 ISOLATES
FROM 1267 BURN WOUND INFECTIONS:
NATIONAL NOSOCOMIAL INFECTIONS
STUDY (NNIS) OF THE CENTER FOR
DISEASE CONTROL (CDC) — JULY 1974 to
JULY 1978

Species	Percent of total isolates
Staphylococcus aureus	22.9
Pseudomonas aeruginosa	20.9
Pseudomonas sp.	7.2
Escherichia coli	6.7
Streptococci, group D	5.0
Streptococcus faecalis	4.2
Klebsiella pneumoniae	3.7
Serratia marcescens	3.1
Enterobacter cloacae	3.0
Proteus mirabilis	2.8
Enterobacter sp.	2.5
Klebsiella sp.	2.2
Staphylococcus epidermidis	1.4
Streptococci, Group A	1.1
E. aerogenes	1.0
Candida albicans	1.3

mycetes), and *Herpes simplex* virus may also cause invasive burn wound infection. Table 1 shows data from the National Nosocomial Infection Study (NNIS)[4] of the Center for Disease Control (CDC) on microorganisms isolated from over 1200 burn wound infections for the period July 1974 to July 1978. Note that bacteria, particularly *S. aureus* and *P. aeruginosa*, were, by far, the most important causes of burn wound infection. Fungi accounted for 2.4% of the isolates.

Another serious infection in burn patients is that of bacteremia. Bacteremia, particularly when due to Gram-negative bacilli, is difficult to treat and carries a high mortality. The burn wound[5,6] is the most important source for organisms that cause bacteremia. Urinary tract infections and septic thrombophlebitis[7] may also give rise to bloodstream invasion. I.V. catheters may easily become contaminated and infected by the large reservoir of microorganisms growing on the surface of the adjacent burn wound. I.V. catheters may be a source of bacteremia, even when signs of local inflammation or purulence are absent. Invasion of all the venous wall with evidence of intraluminal pus[7] may develop, resulting in continuous seeding of the bloodstream with microorganisms. Septic thrombophlebitis and bacteremia may also lead to infection of heart valves or endocarditis. Bacterial endocarditis in burn patients is difficult to diagnose and, in one series, had a mortality of 96%.[8]

Urinary tract infections in burn patients[5,8] are related to frequent use of indwelling urinary catheters and to the large reservoir of microorganisms on the patients' burn wounds. Pneumonia also occurs frequently in burn patients, and predisposing factors include endotracheal intubation, frequent suctioning of the tracheobronchial tree, and, in many patients, the presence of inhalation injury. Pneumonia may develop through bacteremic seeding of the lungs or by the airborne route.[10] In either case, the microorganism(s) recovered from sputum is frequently identical to the one colonizing the burn wound surface.

EPIDEMIOLOGY OF INFECTIONS IN BURN PATIENTS

Information on the epidemiology of infections in burn patients is derived from descriptions of outbreaks as well as from studies of endemic infections in burn care facilities. Although most of the information presented in this section is from reports of outbreaks, data from publications on endemic infections do not appear to conflict with published accounts of epidemics in burn care facilities. Most of the literature on the epidemiology of infections in burn patients relates to infections caused by *P. aeruginosa*. However, there are reports of outbreaks due to other microorganisms including *S. aureus*,[11,12] *Enterobacter cloacae*,[6] *Providencia stuartii*,[9] and *Salmonella typhimurium*;[13] and differences in the epidemiology of infections caused by the various organisms will be noted where appropriate.

Colonization of the Burn Wound by Microorganisms from Feces

Although there is evidence that the burn wound may be colonized by organisms from the patients' stools, the frequency of colonization by this route is uncertain. It is also difficult to determine whether microorganisms that colonize the burn wound by way of stool are part of the patients' normal fecal flora or are acquired from a hospital source after admission. Most of the data implicating the GI tract as a reservoir for bacteria that cause hospital acquired infections has been derived from studies of *P. aeruginosa* isolated from human bowel contents or feces. On the basis of available data, it is unlikely that patients' burn wounds are colonized frequently by *P. aeruginosa* from the normal bowel flora prior to admission. Lowbury and Fox[14] found *P. aeruginosa* in the stools of only 3% of students, and Stoodley and Thom[15] recovered *P. aeruginosa* from only 4% of normal people who applied for jobs in their hospital Catering Department.

P. aeruginosa is isolated much more frequently, however, from stools of patients in the hospital. Shooter et al.[15] found that 24% of all patients on a surgical ward cultured within 2 days of admission had *P. aeruginosa* in their stools, and 26% of patients cultured after 3 days in the hospital had stools positive for *P. aeruginosa*. Thirty-eight percent of their patients had *P. aeruginosa* isolated from stool at some time during their hospitalization. In a later study, Shooter et al.[17] reported that 26% of a group of patients from a surgical and a medical ward had *P. aeruginosa* in their stools at some time while in the hospital. Stoodley and Thom[15] isolated *P. aeruginosa* from stools of 18.3% of patients who had specimens submitted to their hospital microbiology laboratory for investigation of diarrheal diseases.

Several factors which may predispose hospital patients to a higher stool carriage rate of *P. aeruginosa* have been identified. Shooter et al.[16] found higher rates of fecal carriage in patients who had been hospitalized in the 6 months prior to culture, in patients who had been treated with antibiotics, and in those with colostomies, ileostomies, or cecostomies. Stoodley and Thom[15] confirmed the high stool *P. aeruginosa* carriage rate in patients with ileostomies and also noted higher isolation rates from stools of patients with symptoms of GI disease.

The source of *P. aeruginosa* in stools of hospitalized patients has not been conclusively identified. However, it is clear that patients may develop bowel colonization with *P. aeruginosa* after admission to the hospital, and there is evidence highly suggestive of food being a major source. First, Buck and Cooke[18] demonstrated that *P. aeruginosa* fed to normal volunteers could be recovered in stool within 12 hr of ingestion. Recovery in stool required a dose of at least 10^4 organisms, and isolation from stool occurred regularly after doses of 10^6 organisms. *P. aeruginosa* persisted in stools for up to 6 days after ingestion. In one volunteer, who also took ampicillin, *P. aeruginosa* could be recovered from stool for 14 days after ingestion.

Second, *P. aeruginosa* has been recovered from hospital food and kitchens, hospital water, and medications. Shooter et al. isolated *P. aeruginosa*[17] and *Escherichia coli*, *P. aeruginosa*, and *Klebsiella* sp.[19] from hospital food and from the environment of hospital kitchens. Kominos et al. recovered *P. aeruginosa* from raw vegetables in a hospital kitchen, the hands of dietary personnel, knives, and cutting boards,[20] from vegetable salads, milkshakes, feeding formulas, and a Waring® blender.[21] Shooter et al.[17] also cultured *P. aeruginosa* from kitchen water taps and peppermint water.

Third, *Pseudomonas* ingested in hospital food has been recovered from the stools of patients. Shooter et al.[17] recovered strains of *P. aeruginosa* from the feces of five patients that were indistinguishable from strains isolated from food eaten by the patients. Fourth, Kominos et al.[20] found that the four most common pyocine types isolated from vegetables in their hospital were identical to four of the six most common pyocine types of clinical isolates. Fifth, Kominos et al.[21] were able to reduce the rate of *P. aeruginosa* infections in their burn patients from 32 to 6.25% after institution of a diet that eliminated *P. aeruginosa* from the food.

Evidence that *P. aeruginosa* in stool may colonize the burn wound in close proximity is provided by Barclay and Dexter.[22] Citing a personal communication with Sachs (1966), they applied his concept to a study of fecal contamination of burn wounds as a source of *P. aeruginosa* colonization. According to Sachs, burns of the buttocks, perineum, lower abdomen, and upper thighs are prone to *Pseudomonas* infection ("pyocyaneus-prone burns"), and burns of other areas are less likely to be colonized ("non-pyocyaneus-prone" burns). In a 12-month period, Barclay and Dexter found that 27 of 36 patients with "pyocyaneus-prone" burn wounds in their unit developed *P. aeruginosa* colonization of their wounds, whereas *P. aeruginosa* was found on none of 30 patients with "nonpyocyaneus-prone" wounds.

In addition to hospital food, water, medications, and environment, patients colonized with *P. aeruginosa* may themselves also be a source of the organism for bowel colonization of nearby patients. Shooter et al.[16] observed on 18 occasions in a surgical ward that a strain in the stool of one patient would later appear in the feces of one or more other patients on the ward. Lowbury et al.[23] showed that burn patients acquired *P. aeruginosa* on their wounds in the hospital by cross-infection, but that the organism sometimes appeared in feces first, from whence it spread to the burn wound. Thus, although *P. aeruginosa* may be spread directly from the wound of one patient to that of another *(vide infra)*, it would appear that spread may occur from the bowel or wound of one patient to the GI tract of another, with subsequent colonization of the second patient's wound from feces.

In two studies,[14,24] it was suggested that cross-infection with *P. aeruginosa* in burn units occurred by direct transfer between wounds and that contamination of wounds by stool was unimportant. However, neither of these studies was designed in such a manner that would allow cross-infection by way of the GI tract to be ruled out. On the other hand, in two reports,[25,26] there was evidence that cross-infection by *P. aeruginosa* among burn patients occurred rarely, if at all, by way of the GI tract.

Whether or not the GI tract plays a role in transmission of other microorganisms to the burn wound is largely unknown. Lowbury et al.[23] studied cross-infection in a burn unit with patients treated in plastic isolators and air curtains and observed that coliform bacilli were transmitted to burns from the fecal flora and that many of these Gram-negative bacteria were acquired from the hospital environment on food and fomites. In an outbreak of *Enterobacter cloacae* infections in the burn center at the author's hospital,[27] the epidemic strain was recovered from 9 of 16 rectal swabs and from salads collected from the hospital kitchen in concentrations of 2×10^4 to $2.9 \times$

10^7 bacteria per gram of salad. However, in the absence of an epidemiologic marker for *E. cloacae*, it could not be proven that salads from the hospital kitchen were the source of the outbreak. Also, it was not possible to determine whether *E. cloacae* appeared in the feces first and then on the burn wound or vice versa because burn wound and stool cultures were not taken daily from the time of admission of each patient. In a small outbreak of *S. typhimurium* infections in a burn unit, McHugh et al.[13] isolated the epidemic strain from the stools of two patients and suggested that the burn wound of the index case was infected from contaminated feces. This observation is consistent with the fact that the portal of entry for almost all *Salmonella* infections is the GI tract. Thus, although it may be difficult to determine exactly what role fecal contamination of burn wounds plays in a given outbreak, it is clear that the GI tract as a possible route for infection of burn wounds cannot be ignored.

Reservoirs of Infection

The reservoirs or sources of microorganisms in a burn care facility may be numerous and include inanimate surfaces and objects (particularly when moist), health care personnel, the patients themselves, and food, water, and medications.

One of the most important environmental sources of bacteria is the hydrotherapy equipment used in burn units. In three outbreaks due to *P. aeruginosa*, hydrotherapy equipment was found to be at least one of the environmental reservoirs.[28-30] In two outbreaks,[28,29] it was noted that cultures from cleaned tanks were positive for *P. aeruginosa*, and in one report,[28] the water aerators and agitators were culture positive and very difficult to clean. A water hose used to fill a hydrotherapy tank was implicated in an outbreak due to *E. cloacae*.[6]

Although it would appear unlikely, sink drains and traps may be an environmental reservoir for *P. aeruginosa*. Kohn[26] cultured *P. aeruginosa* from sinks and traps in a burn unit, even when there was no other demonstrable clinical or environmental reservoir. Without giving details, he stated that the hands of nursing and medical staff could be infected under experimental conditions from wash basins, sinks, and brushes. MacMillan et al.[30] isolated *P. aeruginosa* from sinks and drains and implemented measures designed to prevent spread of organisms from this source, but they did not prove that the sinks and drains were a source for the *P. aeruginosa* that infected their patients. Holder[31] observed that two serotypes commonly isolated from burn wounds were also frequently recovered from sink basins and drains and that *P. aeruginosa* could be disseminated as far as 48 in. from sinks by splashing water. However, he did not demonstrate that splashing water from sinks was the source of *P. aeruginosa* that infected patients. Wormald[32] and Kominos et al.[33] concluded from their studies that sinks and drains were not reservoirs for *P. aeruginosa* that colonized the wounds of burn patients. Likewise, workers searching for the source of *P. aeruginosa* that caused infections in a premature nursery[34] and in an injuries unit[35] were unable to implicate sinks as an environmental reservoir of organisms that colonized patients. Thus, the bulk of evidence suggests that sinks and drains are not common reservoirs for *P. aeruginosa* that infect burn patients. The importance of sinks and drains as reservoirs for other microorganisms in burn care facilities is unknown.

Other areas in the environment of burn patients from which epidemic strains have been isolated include faucets,[29,30] faucet handles, towel racks, bars of soap,[29] bed rails,[30,36] and a chair[6] used by ambulatory patients waiting for hydrotherapy. Although not implicated as a reservoir during an epidemic, "blanketrol" units for warming and cooling patients may be a reservoir for *Pseudomonas* in burn care facilities.[36] Microorganisms may be isolated from the water circulated through the units.

Personnel who work in burn care facilities may also act as reservoirs for microorganisms that infect burn patients. Since Gram-negative bacilli are easily removed from hands by soap and water,[37] hands are usually considered as vectors for transmission and not reservoirs. However, it has been demonstrated in a clinical setting other than that of the burn unit,[38] that *Klebsiella* may colonize the hands of personnel for long periods. Thus, although uncommon, the hands may be a reservoir. Other body sites in medical personnel that are potential reservoirs for microorganisms that colonize and infect patients include the nasopharynx, hair, and rectum. In the one report of an outbreak in a burn unit in which rectal cultures were taken from personnel,[29] none were positive for the epidemic organism. Hair may have been a reservoir in one outbreak,[32] but was ruled out as a source of the epidemic strain in two other epidemics.[31,39] Although several investigations have shown that the nasopharynx of burn unit personnel is not an important source of Gram-negative bacilli,[14,28,29,31,39] Gram-positive cocci have been recovered from nasopharyngeal cultures of burn unit personnel. Group A streptococci may colonize the throats of personnel and may even spread between members of the burn unit staff.[32] *S. aureus* have also been isolated from the nares of health care personnel during outbreaks of infection in burn units.[11,40]

Another important reservoir for microorganisms that infect burn patients are the patients themselves. Patients may carry epidemic strains on their wounds, in the nares in the case of *S. aureus*, or perhaps in their stools. Several studies indicated that patients were the likely reservoirs for epidemic microorganisms because other reservoirs could not be identified. In most reports,[6,11,12,14,26] the burn wound appeared to be the reservoir. Shooter et al.[16] implicated the bowel as a possible reservoir of *Pseudomonas* in burn patients.

Food, water, and medications may also be sources of microorganisms that infect burn patients. These microorganisms could reach the burn wound by way of the GI tract; as noted above, this appears to be a plausible route for colonization of the burn wound. *P. aeruginosa* has been isolated from raw vegetables, particularly salads,[17,20,21] from milkshakes and feeding formulas,[21] from cold foods other than salads, hospital water, and medications.[17] *E. cloacae*[27] has been isolated from salads, and other coliform bacilli have been isolated from unspecified types of food.[23] *S. aureus* has rarely been isolated from food.[23]

Modes of Transmission

Several vectors for transmission of microorganisms in burn units have been identified. These include hands of personnel, fomites, hydrotherapy treatments, food, and possibly, airborne transfer. Transmission may occur directly from patient to patient or to patients from reservoirs in the environment.

The most important mode of spread would appear to be by contaminated hands of health care personnel. Most of the studies that have examined hands as a vector have been carried out during outbreaks of *P. aeruginosa* infection. Although a few studies[30,39] have been unable to implicate hands as a means of transmission, most studies[14,20,21,28,29,31] have found hand contamination by the epidemic organism in from a few to 38% of personnel sampled. In an outbreak due to *P. stuartii*,[9] the epidemic strain was recovered from 8% of hospital personnel hands, and 50% of the personnel had positive hand cultures in an outbreak due to *E. cloacae*.[6]

Several additional factors involving hand transmission should be noted. First, Holder[31] observed that *P. aeruginosa* that contaminate hands may not be recoverable after the hands have become completely dry. Therefore, identifying hands as a vector for transmission may depend on timing of the cultures. Second, spread by hands of personnel may be direct or indirect; in some studies,[14,29,31] hands could have been contaminated from environmental reservoirs, and in others[6,20] spread appeared to be direct from patient to hands of personnel to patient. Third, transmission may take place via hands, even when gloves are worn.[27,28,30] This may occur from contaminated surfaces of gloves[11] or may be due to water entering the tops of short gloves while personnel are working with patients in hydrotherapy tanks.[27]

In addition to acting as reservoirs for hand contamination, fomites may also transmit microorganisms by direct contact with patients. Fomites that have been implicated in the possible spread of bacteria to patients include beds, blankets, bedjackets, bedpans,[14] urine bottles, clean pillows,[23] toys,[14,23,32,39] bedrails,[30,36] a chair,[6] papers and books,[14,23] and crockery and glassware.[23]

Although hydrotherapy equipment could be classified as a fomite, it will be discussed separately because this mode of transmission is more complex than simple contact of a contaminated surface with the patient's wound. It is obvious that patients with burn wounds colonized with large numbers of bacteria may contaminate hydrotherapy water, surfaces of equipment, and hands of hydrotherapy personnel. Transmission to patients treated subsequently could then occur via water, surfaces of equipment, and hands of personnel. In an outbreak described by Stone and Kolb,[28] hydrotherapy water was contaminated with *P. aeruginosa* after 83% of patient treatments. They also observed that hydrotherapy water was contaminated prior to patient treatments, probably due to difficulty in disinfecting the equipment after use, particularly the aerators and agitators. Transmission by hands of personnel also appeared to play a role, as 26.7% of hand cultures were positive for *P. aeruginosa* prior to patient contact. Stone and Kolb found that more than one half of patients whose burn wounds were free of *P. aeruginosa* prior to hydrotherapy became colonized during the treatments. Mayhall et al.[6] demonstrated transmission of *E. cloacae* in a burn center by way of hydrotherapy water and personnel. Even though plastic liners were used in the tubs and all surfaces of the equipment were culture negative for *E. cloacae*, 50% of samples of hydrotherapy water taken prior to patient contact with the water were positive for *E. cloacae*. Cross-contamination of consecutive tanks of water appeared to take place by way of contaminated hands of personnel and a contaminated filling hose. This study demonstrates that, even when reservoirs of contamination are removed from hydrotherapy equipment, contamination of hydrotherapy water may still occur. Maley[41] also found contamination of hoses used to fill hydrotherapy tanks and demonstrated that fissures in the luminal surface of rubber hoses harbor bacteria that are impossible to remove by soaking in a disinfectant solution. In another study,[11] it appeared that surfaces of hydrotherapy equipment contaminated with *S. aureus* served as a source of contamination for the gloved hands of personnel, with subsequent transfer of organisms to patients' burn wounds.

Another possible mode for dissemination of microorganisms in burn care facilities is that of airborne spread. There is little evidence that Gram-negative bacilli are transmitted between burn patients through the air. One investigation of a *P. aeruginosa* outbreak failed to find the organism in the air of the burn unit.[30] In other reports, *P. aeruginosa* was recovered from the air rarely,[26] was found in large numbers in the air during dressing changes,[14] and was recovered from the air of the rooms of all patients who developed *Pseudomonas* wound colonization, even up to a height of 9 ft.[22] However, none of the latter studies proved that *P. aeruginosa* was transmitted between patients through the air. In a report of an outbreak due to *P. stuartii*,[9] there appeared to be a relationship between positive air samples for *P. stuartii* and the number of patients from which the organism could be recovered within 7 days of sampling. Even though air samples were positive only during periods of patient colonization, the data were not convincing for airborne spread. Mayhall et al.[6] were unable to isolate *E. cloacae* from air of a burn unit during an outbreak due to that organism. In a study of cross-infection conducted with patients in plastic isolators and air curtains, Lowbury et al.[23] concluded that Gram-negative bacilli are not transmitted between burn patients by the airborne route.

Although airborne transmission of *S. aureus* has been demonstrated in other settings,[42] there is little evidence that this is an important mode of spread in treatment facilities for burn patients. Cason et al.[43] noted higher *S. aureus* counts in rooms ventilated by windows than in those ventilated by air conditioners, but there was no difference in infection rates due to *S. aureus* in these two types of rooms. Hambraeus and Laurell[40] were able to demonstrate dispersal of *S. aureus* in the air of a burn unit, but were unable to prove airborne transmission from patient to patient. Hambraeus[44] also isolated *S. aureus* from air of a burn unit and correlated dispersal with burn wound size, but could not establish an airborne pathway from patient to patient. In an outbreak of *S. aureus* infections in a university-affiliated hospital burn unit,[11] no evidence for airborne spread could be found. Lowbury et al.[23] concluded from their study that *S. aureus* was likely spread between burn patients by both direct contact and the airborne route. When all the evidence is considered, it would appear that airborne spread is not an important mode of transmission of infection between burn patients or from personnel or the environment to burn patients.

As noted above, food may be a reservoir for microorganisms that infect burn patients. Because the food is ingested, it is also a vector for transmission. However, food may be a vector without being a reservoir; when food enters the hospital free of microorganisms and is contaminated in the course of handling and preparation, it becomes purely a vector. Such an occurrence was documented by Kominos et al.[21] in which a Waring® blender contaminated with *P. aeruginosa* appeared to play a role in contamination of hospital prepared milkshakes and feeding formulas.

It is clear that contact with contaminated hands of personnel and fomites are the most important modes of spread of microorganisms in burn treatment facilities. Although the role of hydrotherapy equipment and water in the transmission of microorganisms among patients in burn care facilities has not been studied extensively, hydrotherapy would appear to be a potentially important vector in this setting. Contaminated food and the GI tract appear to be important vectors, but more data are needed on their role in transmission. Airborne dissemination plays a minor, if any, part in spread of microorganisms among patients in burn treatment facilities. Two other important considerations must be kept in mind. First, after microorganisms have been deposited on a particular body site, infection may spread to other sites. This has been observed to take place from wound to urinary tract and respiratory tract,[9] nose to wound,[12] or alimentary tract to wound.[16] Second, microorganisms are more likely to be transmitted when aseptic technique deteriorates during periods of absolute staff shortage[6] or when there is a relative shortage of personnel[11] during times of a very high patient census.

Factors that Affect Colonization of the Burn Wound by Microorganisms

After microorganisms have been transported directly or indirectly to the burn wound surface, several local factors may, singly or in combination, determine whether microorganisms are able to colonize the wound. The virulence characteristics of the microorganisms may play a role, but are beyond the scope of this chapter. Discussion will be limited to burn wound size, whether wounds are dressed or exposed, and to the influence of topical and systemic antimicrobial agents.

Several investigators have demonstrated a relationship between burn wound size and colonization rate by microorganisms. Lowbury and Fox[14] and Kohn[26] showed that a majority of patients with burns of greater than 10% body surface area became colonized by *P. aureginosa*, and Wormald[32] found that the colonization rate of his patients by *P. aeruginosa* was much greater for those with burns larger than 30% than for those with burns of less than 30% body surface area. Of the patients reported by Kohn, all of them with a burn of ≥40% became colonized by *P. aeruginosa*. Studies of two *S. aureus* outbreaks in burn units have also shown a relationship between percent surface burned and colonization rate.[11] In one of the studies, patients with colonization or infection had mean burn wound sizes about two to four times greater than that of noncolonized patients. In the other study, there was a progressive increase in the colonization rate with increasing burn wound size; patients with burn wounds <20% had a 21% colonization rate, and those with burn wounds of 60 to 70% had a 100% colonization rate.

Another variable that could, conceivably influence burn wound colonization is the method of treatment with respect to whether the wound is covered with a dressing or left exposed. Wallace[45] suggested that burn wounds be treated with the exposed method because bacteria grow poorly on the dry surface of the uncovered wound. Lowbury and Fox[14] noted growth of *P. aeruginosa* on 38% of exposed facial wounds, but usually in scanty amounts. Alexander and Moncrief[46] point out that, while bacteria grow less well on a dry eschar, the exposed surface lends ready access to bacteria. On the other hand, while covered wounds decrease access to microorganisms from outside, bacteria multiply more rapidly in the warm moist environment beneath the dressings in wounds treated by the closed method. Thus, it is not clear what role, if any, the method of local treatment of the burn wound plays in the epidemiology of burn wound infections.

The third local factor affecting burn wound colonization is the use of systemic and topical antimicrobial agents. In many burn care facilities, newly admitted patients are given antimicrobial prophylaxis with parenterally administered semisynthetic penicillins or cephalosporins for prevention of wound infections due to staphylococci and streptococci. Although this appears to have prevented burn wound infections due to these organisms, outbreaks of infection due to methicillin-resistant *S. aureus* have been reported from three centers.[11,12,47] Even in those units where methicillin-resistant *S. aureus* has not appeared, prevention of Gram-positive wound infections with antibiotics has occurred at the expense of selecting out Gram-negative bacilli which commonly colonize the burn wounds of most patients currently admitted to burn units in this country. Therefore, when outbreaks in burn treatment facilities are investigated, the antimicrobial agent(s) used for prophylaxis and the susceptibility of the epidemic strain to the agent(s) must be taken into consideration.

In addition to systemic antimicrobials, topical agents are also used for prophylaxis against burn wound colonization and infection. The introduction of agents, such as silver nitrate, mafenide acetate, and silver sulfadiazine, brought about a significant decrease in mortality due to burn wound sepsis.[73] Topical antimicrobial preparations suppress the growth of microorganisms on the burn eschar and lessen the chance for wound invasion.

Since microorganisms may become resistant to topical preparations, the susceptibility of an epidemic strain to the topical agent in use at the time of an outbreak must be determined. If the epidemic organism is resistant to the topical antimicrobial, it may be selected out by continued application of the agent to the patients' burn wounds. Cason et al.[43] and Lowbury[48] noted that several coliform bacteria including *Klebsiella* and *Enterobacter* sp. were resistant to silver nitrate. Cason also found that silver nitrate had only moderate activity against *S. aureus*. McHugh et al.[13] observed that *S. typhimurium* that caused an outbreak in their unit was resistant to 0.5% silver nitrate solution. There are three reports of organisms resistant to silver sulfadiazine. Rosenkranz et al.[49] reported the results of in vitro studies on two silver sulfadiazine resistant isolates of *E. cloacae* from burn patients. Gayle et al.[50] found that isolates of *E. cloacae* recovered from patients during an outbreak were resistant to silver sulfadiazine, while isolates of *E. cloacae* from patients on other services in the same hospital were susceptible to silver sulfadiazine. Wenzel et al.[9] described an outbreak due to *Providencia stuartii* in which the epidemic strain was resistant to silver sulfadiazine.

Infections Caused by Nonbacterial Microorganisms

Several species of fungi and viruses may cause burn wound infections. Burn wounds may be colonized by *Candida* sp.,[51-54] Phycomycetes and *Aspergillus*,[53] *Cladosporium*,[52] *Cephalosporium*,[52,53] *Penicillium*,[52,53] *Trichophyton*,[52,53] *Rhodotorula, Trichosporum, Fusarium,* and *Fonsacea*.[53] However, the overwhelming majority of nonbacterial burn wound infections are caused by Phycomycetes,[51,52,55-57] *Aspergillus*,[51,52] and *Candida*[54,58] sp.

In a prospective study of burn wound colonization, Bruck et al.[53] found that wound colonization was unusual before the seventh day postburn, but after that time, colonization increased with a peak incidence in the third and fourth week. Fungal colonization was detected in 58.8% of patients with third-degree burns, but in only 16.7% of those with second-degree burns. They found that *Candida* species were the fungi that most commonly colonized burn wounds. In another study by Bruck et al.,[52] it was noted that invasion of the burn wound by Phycomycetes or *Aspergillus* occurred most frequently between the 9th and 15th postburn days, with a range of 5 to 64 days. The average area of burn injury in patients with fungal burn wound infection was 53%. Infections occurred in areas of second- and third-degree burns with equal frequency. After burn wound invasion, fungi may invade blood vessels and cause disseminated disease.[52,54] The most important factor influencing burn wound colonization by fungi that has been identified to date is the use of topical antimicrobial agents. In a study at the U.S. Army Institute of Surgical Research in San Antonio, Nash et al.[51] found that fungal burn wound infections increased tenfold after mafenide acetate topical therapy was introduced in 1964. Environmental reservoirs for fungi, modes of transmission, and other factors that affect colonization and invasion of the burn wound are unknown. *Candida albicans* is found in the normal flora; this is probably the source for infection in many patients. However, there is no information about possible cross-contamination between patients or from environment to patients.

Foley et al.[59] reported six cases of burn wound infection due to *Herpesvirus hominis*. Two patients developed disseminated infection. The most notable involvement occurred in areas of healing second-degree burns and in donor sites. All patients had burns involving the face, the most common area of the body for latent and recurrent infections. It was not possible to determine whether infections were primary or represented reactivation of latent infection. The investigators noted that herpetic burn wound infection was often complicated by secondary bacterial invasion resulting in conversion of partial-thickness to full-thickness skin loss. There is no information on reservoirs, modes of transmission, or facilitating factors for viral burn wound infections or whether all or some infections are due to reactivation of latent infection.

IDENTIFYING AN OUTBREAK

Recognition of an outbreak depends on recognition of an increased incidence of infection. The increase in incidence of infection may be identified by personnel working in the burn care facility and this information passed on to hospital infection control personnel. A more reliable method of detection is a good surveillance program which may be part of hospital-wide surveillance activity. Another approach to surveillance is to monitor all culture reports including in vitro susceptibility tests from patients in the burn unit. Most burn care facilities perform frequent routine cultures of the burn wound surface, and these data combined with all other culture results, provide a sizable body of information that may constitute an early warning system. In the burn center at the author's hospital, all culture reports from patients are entered daily in a log book kept in the center. There are sections for burn wound cultures, blood cultures, urine cultures, and sputum cultures. Each culture report is accompanied by results of susceptibility tests. The data are reviewed daily and allow hospital infection control personnel to identify an increased prevalence of a given species of microorganism with a characteristic susceptibility pattern from one or more body sites. Also entered in the log book are the results of cultures of burn wound surface taken on admission prior to debridement. This makes it possible to monitor the flora being introduced into the unit by new patients.

INVESTIGATION OF THE OUTBREAK

The approach to work up of an outbreak should be carefully thought out and well organized. Lines of communication must be established with the burn unit staff, the hospital microbiology laboratory, medical record personnel, the chairperson, and members of the hospital infection control committee, and the hospital administration.[60] Effective communication with the latter groups is key to conducting a successful outbreak investigation.

The objectives of an investigation should be to determine the cause of the outbreak and to institute control measures as soon as possible. Figure 1 outlines the sequential steps in an extensive epidemiologic investigation. Not every investigation need be that extensive nor follow the sequence presented in the figure. In many instances, the source(s) and mode(s) of spread of the epidemic organism may be discovered early in the investigation, and control measures may be derived and applied after a very limited investigative effort. Even when an investigation is more prolonged, it may become obvious early on that certain preliminary control measures should be applied immediately. Thus, control measures should be instituted as the investigation progresses when they appear appropriate. In Figure 1, control measures have been included only at the end of the diagram because it is difficult to determine for every outbreak when they may be indicated.

The first step in an investigation is to derive case definitions. These definitions will be used when documentation of infection is sought from the medical charts of patients who have cultures positive for what would appear to be the epidemic organism. Thus, a case of burn wound infection could be defined as a patient with clinical signs of sepsis (hyper- or hypothermia, altered mentation, adynamic ileus) and a burn wound biopsy that contained $\geqslant 10^5$ microorganisms of the epidemic species per gram of burn eschar. Although burn wound infection can be definitely diagnosed only when biopsy indicates that there are $\geqslant 10^5$ microorganisms per gram of burn eschar, biopsy data may not always be available. In the absence of biopsy data, a case of burn wound infection might be defined as a patient with clinical signs of sepsis, evidence of purulence beneath the eschar, and a burn surface culture positive for the epidemic organism. The definitions for infections at other sites can be found elsewhere[61,62] (see chapter entitled "Surveillance and Reporting of Hospital Aquired Infections").

The general approach to investigation has been stated in the chapter entitled "Postoperative Wound Infections", but it is important to document that patients are infected and not just colonized with the epidemic strain. Nevertheless, it should be stated that an increase in the incidence of infection, whether caused by one or many strains,

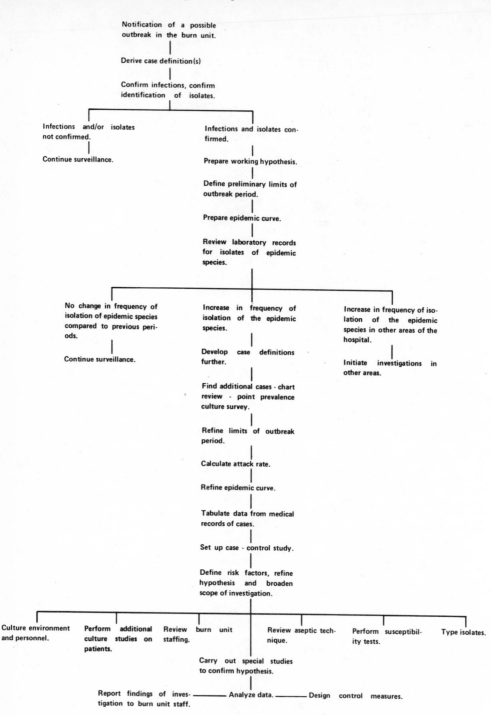

FIGURE 1.   Outline for an extensive epidemiologic investigation of an outbreak in a burn care facility.

requires an investigation. The next step is to confirm the identity of isolates of the epidemic species. Pseudoepidemics have occurred in hospitals because of incorrect identification of microorganisms by the hospital laboratory.[63] If infections with an epidemic strain are confirmed, the next step is to prepare a working hypothesis and to define the preliminary limits of the outbreak period. It may be possible to develop a working hypothesis at this point using early clues as to source and mode of spread of the epidemic species. The outbreak period is defined as the time between the first isolation of the epidemic strain and the most recent isolation. The epidemic curve should be prepared for the outbreak period. It must be established that the apparent increase in frequency of isolation of the epidemic species (isolates per month) is real. If laboratory record review indicates that there is not an increased number of isolates of the epidemic species during the outbreak period compared to a similar period just prior to the outbreak or to a similar period in the previous year, surveillance of burn patients should be intensified to insure early detection of an impending outbreak or to confirm a high rate of endemic infections.

If it is established that an outbreak is in progress, further case finding should be carried out among the patients currently hospitalized in the burn unit. This can be accomplished by review of each patient's medical record and by a point prevalence culture survey. Cultures should be taken from the burn wound, other body sites, such as the urinary or respiratory tract, and from areas that are frequently important sites of colonization in burn patients, such as the nose (*S. aureus*) or feces (Gram-negative bacilli). Although cultures of burn wound surfaces, nose and feces do not identify new infections, they provide important information on the sites and numbers of patients colonized by the epidemic strain. When case definitions are applied to patients with isolates of the epidemic species identified by chart review and culture survey, most if not all, of the cases of infection will have been discovered by this point in the investigation.

With all the cases known, the limits of the outbreak period can be refined and the attack rate of infection by the epidemic strain can be determined. Attack rate (AR) is determined by the following formula.

$$AR = \frac{total\ cases}{number\ of\ patients\ at\ risk} \qquad \text{Un. eq. A}$$

If more than one type of case occurred, the attack rate can be refined by determining site specific attack rates for infections at specific sites such as burn wound or urinary tract. Thus, the attack rate for burn wound infections can be determined as follows:

$$AR\ (burn\ wound) = \frac{total\ burn\ wound\ infections}{number\ of\ patients\ at\ risk} \qquad \text{Un. eq. B}$$

At this point, with all cases known and the limits of the outbreak period firmly established, the epidemic curve can be refined.

The medical records of all cases should be reviewed and appropriate data tabulated. Data recorded should include name, hospital number, age, sex, date of admission, area of burn unit to which the patient was admitted, all areas in the unit where the patient has received care, date of discharge or death, area of total and third-degree burns, associated injuries (including inhalation injury), underlying diseases, types of instrumentation, all treatments (including corticosteroids, systemic, and topical antimicrobial agents), hydrotherapy, other types of physical therapy, surgical procedures (including skin grafting), and all culture results. After tabulation, the data should be analyzed for common associations between the various epidemiologic parameters and occurrence of infection. Such an analysis may suggest risk factors for infection that will be helpful in guiding further investigative efforts.

At this point, using clues as to risk factors and source and mode of spread of infection derived from data tabulated from medical records, the investigation could be broadened as shown in Figure 1. However, more definitive conclusions may be drawn from the patient data if a case-control study is carried out. In the case-control study, data for cases and controls are compared to determine if there are significant differences between the two groups with respect to the various epidemiologic characteristics tabulated from medical charts. Control patients are selected from among patients admitted to the burn unit during the outbreak period who have no evidence of infection with the outbreak organism. An attempt is made to match cases and controls with respect to age, sex, and time of admission. Except for culture results, the data listed above for cases are also recorded for controls, and cases and controls are compared using statistical tests to identify significant differenes between the groups with respect to the various epidemiologic parameters. With risk factors identified by the case-control study, the hypothesis may be refined and the scope of the investigation can be broadened.

Using the data generated up to this point in the investigation, a protocol for culturing environment and personnel can be derived. In addition to cultures indicated by the case-control study, other areas that may be cultured are shown in Tables 2, 3, and 4. Although these tables are not meant to be all inclusive, they list areas commonly sampled in investigations. The method of culture and the selection of culture media depend on the source of the culture and the growth requirements of the epidemic organism. Dry surfaces may be cultured by sterile swabs moistened in sterile saline or broth and planted on culture media as soon as possible. Dry swabs may be used for moist surfaces. Liquid can be cultured by filtration and culture of the filter on agar or by adding a liquid sample to an equal volume of double-strength broth. Solid foods and medications can be cultured by grinding weighed portions of sample with a sterile mortar and pestle, diluting with sterile saline, and culturing of aliquots of the dilutions on agar plates for colony counts. Air samples may be taken with settling plates or any one of several commercially available air samplers. Selective media may be used by incorporating antibiotics or other substances in the media to inhibit the growth of contaminating microorganisms and allow isolation of the epidemic strain. When samples cultured in broth may contain residual disinfectant, neutralizers, such as 0.07% lecithin and 0.5% polysorbate-80, should be incorporated into the media.[64] When the protocol for culture of environment and hospital staff is being devised, personnel in the hospital microbiology laboratory should be consulted for assistance in selecting media and application of appropriate culture techniques.

Besides cultures of environment and burn unit personnel, additional cultures of patients may be desirable. Studying the kinetics of colonization may provide helpful clues to the mode of transmission. This type of study is carried out by culturing a group of patients daily from the time of admission. Multiple sites, such as nose, pharynx, burn wound, and rectum, are cultured. Such a study may help determine how rapidly new patients acquire the epidemic organism, which body site becomes culture positive first, whether colonization spreads from one site to another in a given sequence, or the epidemic strain colonizes all sites simultaneously. Data from a kinetics of colonization study may then be correlated with such epidemiological factors as burn wound size and instrumentation.

Another important facet of the investigation is review of burn unit staffing characteristics. Many hospitals have established standards for the number of personnel needed in each area for good patient care. Personnel time records should be reviewed for several months before and during the outbreak to determine whether or not staffing levels were adequate during these periods. In addition to total numbers, the relative numbers of registered nurses, licensed practical nurses, nurses' aides, attendants, and

Table 2
SUGGESTED SITES FOR ENVIRONMENTAL CULTURES IN PATIENT CARE AREAS OF THE BURN UNIT

Sites	Methods	Comments
Surfaces	Sterile swabs	Moisten with saline or broth
Bedside tables		
Bedrails		
Bed cradles		
Cubicle curtains		
Sphygmomanometers		
Dopplers		
EKG electrodes		
Stethoscopes		
I.V. poles		
Toys		
Door handles		
Bed scales		
Wheelchairs		
Stretchers		
Hydraulic lift		
Lift seats		
Faucet handles		
Counter tops		
Equipment		
Faucet aerators	Drop disks in broth	Remove disks from aerator with sterile forceps
Respiratory therapy equipment	Culture respirator output on agar plates	Ryan and Mihaly[72] have described a simple technique
	Culture water from nebulizers and humidifiers in broth or by filtration	Add water to equal volume of double strength broth or filter water and culture filters on agar or in broth
Cooling-warming blanket		
Surfaces	Sterile swabs	
Liquid	Broth or filtration	
Liquids		
Saline for irrigation	Broth or filtration	
Soap from dispensers	Inoculate sample into Letheen broth (normal strength)	Mix well with broth
Hand lotion	Inoculate sample into Letheen broth (normal strength)	Mix well with broth; for quantitative cultures, an aliquot of broth may be added to pour plates prior to incubation

Table 3
SUGGESTED SITES FOR ENVIRONMENTAL CULTURES IN HYDROTHERAPY TREATMENT AREA

Sites	Method	Comments
Equipment	Sterile swabs	Moisten swabs if surface is dry
Inside walls and floors of tanks		
Outside walls of tanks		
Tank drains		
Headrests		

Table 3 (continued)
SUGGESTED SITES FOR ENVIRONMENTAL CULTURES IN HYDROTHERAPY TREATMENT AREA

Sites	Method	Comments
Agitators		
Sling above tank		
Plastic liners		Culture new liners prior to use
Filling hoses	Flush with broth	May also flush with sterile water into equal volume of double strength broth
Stools and counters	Sterile swabs	
Liquids		
Tap water	Broth or filtration	Add water to equal volume of double strength broth or filter water and culture filters on agar or in broth
Tank water after patients' treatments	Broth or filtration	Use neutralizers if water contains antiseptic agents
Tank water just prior to patients' entry	Broth or filtration	
Liquid soap	Inoculate sample into Letheen broth (normal strength)	Mix well with broth

Table 4
SUGGESTED SITES FOR CULTURES FROM PERSONNEL

Sites	Method	Comments
Nares	Sterile swabs	Swab anterior ⅓ of both nares
Pharynx	Sterile swabs	
Hair	Rodac plates	
Vagina	Sterile swabs	
Stool	Standard procedure for collection of stool specimens	Rectum may also be cultured by sterile swab, personnel may obtain their own cultures
Hands	Sterile swabs	Use moistened swabs, swab palmar surfaces of both hands
	Large (150 × 15 mm) agar plates	Press palmar surface of each hand lightly to the surface of the agar
	Broth rinse	Rub hands together in broth contained in sterile plastic bag or pan

burn technicians should be tabulated. Such a survey can help determine the overall quality of patient care in the unit. The number and location of nursing personnel pulled to and from the burn unit with respect to other areas of the hospital should be determined. This could provide a clue to the source of the epidemic strain. Turnover in nursing personnel should be examined. Such data may indicate the overall level of experience among personnel and may be an index to personnel morale. Personnel should be interviewed and employee health records reviewed to identify burn unit personnel who may have had recent skin eruptions or infections of the hands or other areas.

Patient care practices should be reviewed. Both written protocols and actual technique used by personnel should be reviewed to detect deficiencies that could account for cross-infection between patients or for infection of patients from environmental reservoirs. Examination of written policies may identify errors in technique incorporated into the policies at the time they were written. Even when written protocols are correct, personnel may not adhere to proper technique due to lack of training and proper supervision or for lack of time when staffing levels are inadequate. Thus, it is necessary for investigators to do an onsite review of aseptic technique to identify improper practices that may account for transmission of infection.

Important information may be derived from susceptibility tests of isolates of the epidemic species with antibiotics and topical antimicrobial agents. As mentioned above, a common antibiogram can be used as an epidemiologic marker to help trace the source and mode of spread of the epidemic strain. Therefore, susceptibility tests should be performed with all epidemic isolates not tested earlier in the investigation. It is also important that antimicrobial susceptibility patterns be examined with respect to antibiotic prophylaxis and therapy administered to burn patients before and during the outbreak. Such data may indicate that use of one or more antibiotics provided a selective advantage for the epidemic species. Laboratory tests to determine the susceptibility of the epidemic strain to the topical antimicrobial agent in use at the time of the outbreak may indicate that the epidemic organism is resistant to the agent in use. Thus, resistance to the topical antimicrobial may also have provided a selective advantage for the epidemic strain, and such knowledge may be important in designing control measures for the epidemic.

Other laboratory tests of importance include various procedures for typing the epidemic species. Such tests include phage typing, serologic typing, and bacteriocin typing. These techniques provide a better epidemiologic marker for the epidemic species than do susceptibility tests. Since these tests are not readily available in most hospital laboratories, it will ordinarily be necessary to send isolates of the epidemic species to local or state health department laboratories.

Special studies to confirm a suspected source and mode of spread may be carried out. For example, if information generated earlier in the investigation indicated that spread of the epidemic organism probably occurred by way of hydrotherapy, a special study could be designed to further substantiate this mechanism of transmission. All patients would be cultured before and after hydrotherapy. Cultures would be taken from hydrotherapy water and equipment after each patient, from the equipment after cleaning, from the hydrotherapy water prepared for the next patient, and from the hands and forearms of hydrotherapy personnel before and after each patient. Technique used during hydrotherapy would be carefully observed and errors in technique recorded. Such a study may indicate that patients who were culture positive for the epidemic species contaminated the water and equipment and that cross-contamination of the hydrotherapy water for the next patient occurred due to inadequate cleaning of equipment. Alternatively, it may be determined that personnel were responsible for cross-contamination of hydrotherapy water or that cross-contamination of patients did not occur by way of hydrotherapy water, but that personnel transmitted the organism directly by hand contact.

When all the data have been collected, they should be carefully analyzed, and appropriate statistical tests should be applied to demonstrate significant relationships. Based on the analysis, conclusions should be drawn with respect to the source and mode of spread of the epidemic organism and other factors that may have influenced the course of the outbreak or that were important in perpetuating the epidemic. Accurate analysis of data and appropriate conclusions based on data analysis are critically important for the formulation of effective control measures.

As noted above, not every investigation will need to be as extensive as the one outlined in Figure 1. All steps may not be included or the exact sequence may not be followed. It is intended that the investigative protocol presented here be a suitable framework for design of protocols for limited or extensive investigations that may be tailored to provide effective plans for the conduct of investigations in units of varying size and in varying epidemiologic settings. In any case, even the limited investigation should include preparation of case definitions, confirmation of infections and the epidemic species, tabulation of data from medical records of cases, an initial working hypothesis, definition of the outbreak period, review of laboratory records, preparation of an epidemic curve, calculation of the attack rate, review of aseptic technique, appropriate cultures of patients, personnel and environment, analysis of data, appropriate conclusions, feedback of results of the investigation to burn unit personnel, and design of control measures.

CONTROL OF THE OUTBREAK

After data have been tabulated, analyzed, and conclusions drawn as to the source(s) of the epidemic microorganism, its mode(s) of transmission, and other factors that influenced the onset and course of the epidemic, it is important that this information be conveyed in detail to the burn unit medical and paramedical staff. Control measures should be formulated in cooperation with the burn unit staff. Approaches to control may take one or more of several forms. A control program may require that new protocols for aseptic technique be devised. It may be necessary to modify guidelines for usage of topical and systemically administered antimicrobial agents. New equipment may be needed or existing equipment may need modification. The staffing level may need to be raised. Whatever the approach to control, it will almost invariably be necessary to reeducate personnel who work in the burn unit. In some instances, inservice education of the staff may be the only control measure needed. In addition to helping design control measures the infection control team should help the burn unit staff procure the needed resources. This may be done through communication of information derived from the investigation to the hospital administration or through the hospital infections committee.

At the time control measures are initiated, the infection control team should be available for consultation and should provide the inservice program for burn unit staff. The infection control team will also need to monitor the effect of control measures. This may be done by intensive surveillance of the patients in the unit for infections and by appropriate cultures. Repeat cultures may be taken from environmental reservoirs uncovered by the investigation (including personnel), and point prevalence cultures surveys may be taken from patients to determine whether or not control measures are preventing colonization of patients by the epidemic organism. After corrective measures have been instituted and the epidemic controlled, follow up activities should include ongoing surveillance, periodic observation of aseptic technique, in-service programs, and perhaps culture of the environmental site, if any, that harbored the reservoir for the previous outbreak.

Although it is not possible to provide information on how all outbreaks can be controlled, control measures for the most commonly encountered reservoirs, modes of transmission, and facilitating factors for outbreaks in burn care facilities will be discussed.

If the investigation indicates that the burn wound was colonized by way of feces, control measures should be aimed at preventing colonization of the GI tract by the epidemic species. If the source of GI colonization is food, water, or medications, these items must be removed from the patients' diets or treatment regimens. Further corrective measures may be needed in the hospital kitchen or pharmacy if these areas have been implicated in contamination of food or medications.

If cross-contamination appears to have taken place between patients by transfer of the epidemic organism from one patients' wound or stool to the GI tract of another, good barrier technique will be needed to prevent this type of transmission. Each patient should be provided with his own environment separate from that of all other patients.[65] Handwashing between patients must be emphasized, and gloves must be worn by personnel when direct patient contact is necessary. Gloves should be changed between certain procedures in the same patient, such as urine testing and mouth care. A logical sequence should be followed in the care of each patient, so that the cleanest areas, such as I.V. catheters, are manipulated first and the dirtiest, such as collecting urine, last. When gloves have become contaminated by contact with a patient, items which will later be touched by ungloved hands should not be handled. All inanimate objects that are placed at one patient's bedside or that have come into contact with that patient are considered to be contaminated for other patients. All patients must have certain items, such as stethoscopes and blood pressure cuffs, assigned to them and not used on other patients. For those items that must be used on more than one patient, adequate decontamination between patients is extremely important. Medical personnel working with a patient are also considered contaminated by that patient and must decontaminate themselves prior to the next patient contact. In addition to handwashing, soiled or wet clothing must be changed or soilage must be prevented by wearing a gown or disposable plastic apron while carrying out patient care. Other important environmental control measures include prompt disposal of soiled dressings, gloves, and other disposable items in plastic bags, prompt bagging of soiled linen, and disposal of partially used solutions. Cubicle curtains should not be touched with gloved or contaminated hands. Curtains should be changed when soiled and when patients are discharged or transferred. Furniture at the patient's bedside should be cleaned frequently with a disinfectant solution. These barrier techniques may also be used with other control measures including those described below.

If contaminated hands of personnel are vectors for transmission, control measures may depend on several other variables. Prevention of dissemination of microorganisms by hands hinges on the effective decontamination of hands between patient contacts. Effective removal of microorganisms from hands depends on awareness by staff of the need and proper technique for handwashing, availability of properly functioning handwashing devices, and adequate staffing levels to provide time needed for handwashing. Therefore, corrective measures may be aimed at education of personnel in proper handwashing technique, increasing the number of handwashing devices, or increasing the number of burn unit staff. In addition, supervisory personnel must assume the responsibility for reminding other members of the staff of the need for frequent handwashing. Sterile gloves must be worn when burn wound treatments are being carried out or when endotracheal tubes or tracheostomies are suctioned.

Health care personnel may be implicated in the spread of microorganisms by means other than contaminated hands. They may be nasal carriers of *S. aureus* or pharyngeal, rectal, or vaginal carriers of beta hemolytic Group A streptococci. Personnel may also disseminate *S. aureus* and Group A streptococci from lesions on their hands and arms. If personnel are found to be the source as well as the vector for spread, control measures will involve removal of the implicated personnel from duty and treatment with topical and systemic antimicrobial agents to eliminate the carrier state or infective lesions.

When fomites have been implicated in transmission of the outbreak organism, control measures may provide for removal of the implicated device from patient contact, for replacing it with a disposable device or for effective decontamination. For instance, toys implicated in transmission of microorganisms can be eliminated from the unit, particularly if they cannot be effectively decontaminated. Disposal EKG electrodes can be used to avoid dissemination of bacteria by these implements which are difficult to disinfect under ordinary working conditions. Objects made of metal, such as faucets and bedrails, can easily be disinfected. When faucet aerators have been identified as a source of the epidemic species, they should be removed. Maley[36] eliminated bacterial contamination of the fluid in warming-cooling blankets by replacing the water with 40% propylene glycol. Morris[66] demonstrated that the decontamination program recommended by the American Thoracic Society[67] was effective for nebulizers used for respiratory therapy in a burn unit.

When hydrotherapy equipment has been identified as a reservoir or vector of transmission, it may be due to absence of an effective cleaning and disinfection protocol. Effective disinfection requires that residual material be cleaned from all surfaces, an effective disinfectant be applied to all surfaces, and that disinfectant be circulated through the agitators. However, in some instances, it is difficult, if not impossible, to decontaminate agitators. Therefore, it may be necessary to remove these devices and change to a system in which the tub is lined with a new disposable plastic liner for each patient. Agitation of the water is provided by compressed air forced through channels in the bottom of the liner. However, as noted above,[6] cross-contamination may still occur by way of filling hoses or inadequate technique of personnel. We have solved these problems by requiring that hydrotherapy attendants wear disposable shoulder-length gloves and aprons which are changed between each patient. Our filling hoses have been replaced by new fixtures which prevent contact of the plumbing with hydrotherapy water and equipment and patients. Water is delivered to each tank by a long filling spout, and a separate metal hose which cannot reach the tank is used for rinsing patients and washing equipment. The hose is hung up on the wall when not in use. It is soaked in a phenolic disinfectant and rinsed with tap water once a week. In some burn care facilities, sodium or calcium hypochlorite or iodophor solutions are added to hydrotherapy water to prevent contamination of patients from this source.[28,36,68,69] Although it may be possible to eliminate hydrotherapy as a reservoir and vector for transmission by adequate cleaning and disinfection of equipment and good aseptic technique during patient treatments, the question still remains whether or not antiseptics added to the water prevent spread of infection from one area of the burn wound to another or from rectum to burn wound. If a decision is made to add antimicrobial agents to hydrotherapy water, these agents should not be used as a substitute for good technique. Iodophors do not invariably prevent contamination of equipment,[28] and when calcium hypochlorite is used, the pH of the water must be maintained between 7.2 and 7.6.[69] Below pH 7.0, hypochlorite may cause irritation, and above pH 7.6, it loses much of its antimicrobial activity.

If the epidemic species has been found resistant to the topical antimicrobial agent in use at the time the outbreak began, it may be necessary to change to an alternate agent. Although Lindberg et al.[70] demonstrated that mafenide acetate penetrates burn eschar very effectively, there is no evidence that any topical agent can effectively treat established burn wound sepsis. One hundred percent of animals experimentally burned and infected are protected only when mafenide acetate is applied within 48 hr of burning.[71] Gayle et al.[50] found in a small number of patients involved in an *E. cloacae* outbreak that switching from silver sulfadiazine to mafenide acetate after infection was established was ineffective in controlling infection. Therefore, when designing control measures, if the epidemic species was found to be resistant to the topical antimicrobial agent in use at the time of onset of the outbreak, it would appear that a new topical antimicrobial should be selected for application to patients from the time of admission. Selection of a new agent should be guided by in vitro susceptibility tests.

FUTURE

Much remains to be learned about the epidemiology of nosocomial infections in burn patients. Most of the published data are on the epidemiology of *P. aeruginosa* infections. Relatively much less is known about the epidemiology of infections due to other species of bacteria. More information is needed on environmental reservoirs and the exact route of transmission of these other species, so that optimal barrier techniques may be designed to protect patients from all microorganisms. A particularly intriguing area for future research is that of the role of food as a reservoir and vector for transmission of microorganisms to the burn wound by way of the GI tract. New topical antimicrobial agents are needed because there are few suitable agents at present. If resistance to these preparations continues to develop, it may be difficult in the future to provide adequate topical prophylaxis. One of the most serious deficiencies in our knowledge at present is about the epidemiology of fungal and viral burn wound infections, particularly if the incidence of these infections continues to rise.

REFERENCES

1. Feller, I., The National Burn Information Exchange, University of Michigan, Ann Arbor, 1978.
2. Loebl, E. C., Marvin, J. A., Heck, E. L., Curreri, P. W., and Baxter, C. R., The method of quantitative burn-wound biopsy cultures and its routine use in the care of the burned patient, *Am. J. Clin. Pathol.*, 61, 21, 1974.
3. Pruitt, B. A., Jr. and Foley, F. D., The use of biopsies in burn patient care, *Surgery*, 73, 887, 1973.
4. Allen, J. R., personal communication, 1978.
5. Rabin, E. R., Graber, C. D., Vogel, E. H., Finkelstein, R. A., and Tumbusch, W. A., Fatal pseudomonas infection in burned patients. A clinical, bacteriologic and anatomic study, *N. Engl. J. Med.*, 265, 1225, 1961.
6. Mayhall, C. G., Lamb, V. A., Gayle, W. E., Jr., and Haynes, B. W., Jr., *Enterobacter cloacae* septicemia in a burn center: epidemiology and control of an outbreak, *J. Infect. Dis.*, 139, 166, 1979.
7. O'Neill, J. A., Jr., Pruitt, B. A., Jr., Foley, F. D., and Moncrief, J. A., Suppurative thrombophlebitis — a lethal complication of intravenous therapy, *J. Trauma*, 8, 256, 1968.
8. Baskin, T. W., Rosenthal, A., and Pruitt, B. A., Jr., Acute bacterial endocarditis: a silent source of sepsis in the burn patient, *Ann. Surg.*, 184, 618, 1976.
9. Wenzel, R. P., Hunting, K. J., Osterman, C. A., and Sande, M. A., *Providencia stuartii*, a hospital pathogen: potential factors for its emergence and transmission, *Am. J. Epidemiol.*, 104, 170, 1976.
10. Pruitt, B. A., Jr., DiVincenti, F. C., Mason, A. D., Jr., Foley, F. D., and Flemma, R. J., The occurrence and significance of pneumonia and other pulmonary complications in burned patients: comparison of conventional and topical treatments, *J. Trauma*, 10, 519, 1970.
11. Dixon, R. E., personal communication, 1978.
12. Everett, E. D., Rahm, A. E., Jr., McNitt, T. R., Stevens, D. L., and Petersen, H. E., Epidemiologic investigation of methicillin resistant *Staphylococcus aureus* in a burn unit, *Mil. Med.*, 143, 165, 1978.
13. McHugh, G. L., Hopkins, C. C., Moellering, R. C., and Swartz, M. N., *Salmonella typhimurium* resistant to silver nitrate, chloramphenicol, and ampicillin, A new threat in burn units?, *Lancet*, 1, 235, 1975.
14. Lowbury, E. J. L. and Fox, J., The epidemiology of infection with *Pseudomonas pyocyanea* in a burns unit, *J. Hyg.*, 52, 403, 1954.
15. Stoodley, B. J. and Thom, B. T., Observations on the intestinal carriage of *Pseudomonas aeruginosa*, *J. Med. Microbiol.*, 3, 367, 1970.

16. Shooter, R. A., Walker, K. A., Williams, V. R., Horgan, G. M., Parker, M. T., Asheshov, E. H., and Bullimore, J. R., Faecal carriage of *Pseudomonas aeruginosa* in hospital patients. Possible spread from patient to patient, *Lancet*, 2, 1331, 1966.

17. Shooter, R. A., Cooke, E. M., Gaya, H., Kumar, P., Patel, N., Parker, M. T., Thom, B. T., and France, D. R., Food and medicaments as possible sources of hospital strains of *Pseudomonas aeruginosa*, *Lancet*, 1, 1227, 1969.

18. Buck, A. C. and Cooke, E. M., The fate of ingested *Pseudomonas aeruginosa* in normal persons, *J. Med. Microbiol.*, 2, 621, 1969.

19. Shooter, R. A., Faiers, M. C., Cooke, E. M., Breaden, A. L., and O'Farrell, S. M., Isolation of *Escherichia coli*, *Pseudomonas aeruginosa* and *Klebsiella* from food in hospitals, canteens and schools, *Lancet*, 2, 390, 1971.

20. Kominos, S. D., Copeland, C. E., Growiak, B., and Postic, B., Introduction of *Pseudomonas aeruginosa* into a hospital via vegetables, *Appl. Microbiol.*, 24, 567, 1972.

21. Kominos, S. D., Copeland, C. E., and Delenko, C. A., *Psuedomonas aeruginosa* from vegetables, salads, and other foods served to patients with burns, in *Pseudomonas aeruginosa: Ecological Aspects and Patient Colonization*, Young, V. M., Ed., Raven Press, New York, 1977, 59.

22. Barclay, T. L. and Dexter, F., Infection and cross-infection in a new burns centre, *Br. J. Surg.*, 55, 197, 1968.

23. Lowbury, E. J. L., Babb, J. R., and Ford, P. M., Protective isolation in a burns unit: The use of plastic isolators and air curtains, *J. Hyg. Camb.*, 69, 529, 1971.

24. Davis, B., Lilly, H. A., and Lowbury, E. J. L., Gram-negative bacilli in burns, *J. Clin. Pathol.*, 22, 634, 1969.

25. Sutter, V. L. and Hurst, V., Sources of *Pseudomonas aeruginosa* infection in burns: study of wound and rectal cultures with phage typing, *Ann. Surg.*, 163, 597, 1966.

26. Kohn, J., A study of *Ps. pyocyanea* cross infection in a burns unit. Preliminary report, in *Research in Burns*, Wallace, A. B. and Wilkinson, A. W., Eds., E. and S. Livingstone, Edinburgh, 1966, 486.

27. Mayhall, C. G., Lamb, V. A., Gayle, W. E., Jr. and Haynes, B. W., Jr., unpublished data, 1976.

28. Stone, H. H. and Kolb, L. D., The evolution and spread of gentamicin-resistant pseudomonads, *J. Trauma*, 11, 586, 1971.

29. Shulman, J. A., Terry, P. M. and Hough, C. E., Colonization with gentamicin-resistant *Pseudomonas aeruginosa*, pyocine type 5, in a burn unit, *J. Infect. Dis.*, 124 (Suppl.), S18, 1971.

30. MacMillan, B. G., Edmonds, P., Hummel, R. P., and Maley, M. P., Epidemiology of *Pseudomonas* in a burn intensive care unit, *J. Trauma*, 13, 627, 1973.

31. Holder, I. A., Epidemiology of *Pseudomonas aeruginosa* in a burns hospital, in *Pseudomonas aeruginosa: Ecological Aspects and Patient Colonization*, Young, V. M., Ed., Raven Press, New York, 1977, 77.

32. Wormald, P. J., The effect of a changed environment on bacterial colonization rates in an established burn centre, *J. Hyg. Camb.*, 68, 633, 1970.

33. Kominos, S. D., Copeland, C. E., and Grosiak, B., Mode of transmission of *Pseudomonas aeruginosa* in a burn unit and an intensive care unit in a general hospital, *Appl. Microbiol.*, 23, 309, 1972.

34. Jellard, C. H. and Churcher, G. M., An outbreak of *Pseudomonas aeruginosa* (pyocyanea) infection in a Premature Baby Unit, with observations on the intestinal carriage of *Pseudomonas aeruginosa* in the newborn, *J. Hyg. Camb.*, 65, 219, 1967.

35. Lowbury, E. J. L., Thom, B. T., Lilly, H. A., Babb, J. R., and Whittall, K., Sources of infection with *Pseudomonas aeruginosa* in patients with tracheostomy, *J. Med. Microbiol.*, 3, 39, 1970.

36. Maley, M. P., Comprehensive strategy reduces burn unit infection risks, *Hosp. Infect. Cont.*, 5, 139, 1978.

37. Steere, A. C. and Mallison, G. F., Handwashing practices for the prevention of nosocomial infections, *Ann. Intern. Med.*, 83, 683, 1975.

38. Knittle, M. A., Eitzman, D. V., and Baer, H., Role of hand contamination of personnel in the epidemiology of gram-negative nosocomial infections, *J. Pediatr.*, 86, 433, 1975.

39. Edmonds, P., Suskind, R. R., MacMillan, B. G., and Holder, I. A., Epidemiology of *Pseudomonas aeruginos* in a burns hospital: surveillance by a combined typing system, *Appl. Microbiol.*, 24, 219, 1972.

40. Hambraeus, A. and Laurell, G., Infections in a burns unit. An attempt to study the airborne transfer of bacteria, in *Staphylococci and Staphylococcal Infections*, Polish Medical Publishers, Warsaw, 1973, 464.

41. Maley, M. P., personal communication, 1978.

42. Williams, R. E. O., Epidemiology of airborne staphylococcal infections, *Bacteriol. Rev.*, 30, 660, 1966.

43. Cason, J. S., Jackson, D. M., Lowbury, E. J. L., and Ricketts, C. R., Antiseptic and aseptic prophylaxis for burns: use of silver nitrate and of isolators, *Br. Med. J.*, 2, 1288, 1966.

44. Hambraeus, A., Dispersal and transfer of *Staphylococcus aureus* in an isolation ward for burned patients, *J. Hyg. Camb.*, 71, 787, 1973.

45. Wallace, A. B., Treatment of burns, *Br. J. Plast. Surg.*, 1, 232, 1949.

46. Alexander, J. W. and Moncrief, J. A., The control of infection in severely burned patients, *Surg. Clin. North Am.*, 47, 1039, 1967.

47. Taplin, G., Allyn, P., Nolan, M., Garland, J., Bartlett, R., and Thrupp, L., Contrasting Epidemiologic Virulence of Methicillin-Resistant *Staph. aureus* (MRSA) in Hospital and Community: Persistence in a Burn Unit but Lack of Spread to Family Contacts of Discharged Patient Carriers, presented at 17th Interscience Conf. Antimicrobial Agents and Chemotherapy, New York, October 12 to 14, 1977, 424.

48. Lowbury, E. J. L., Advances in the control of infections in burns, *Br. J. Plast. Surg.*, 20, 211, 1967.

49. Rosenkranz, H. S., Coward, J. E., Wlodkowski, T. J., and Carr, H. S., Properties of silver sulfadizine-resistant *Enterobacter cloacae*, *Antimicrob. Agents Chemother.*, 5, 199, 1974.

50. Gayle, W. E., Jr., Mayhall, C. G., Lamb, V. A., Apollo, E., and Haynes, B. W., Jr., Resistant *Enterobacter cloacae* in a burn center: the ineffectiveness of silver sulfadiazine, *J. Trauma*, 18, 317, 1978.

51. Nash, G., Foley, F. D., Goodwin, M. N., Jr., Bruck, H. M., Greenwald, K. A., and Pruitt, B. A., Jr., Fungal burn wound infection, *JAMA*, 215, 1664, 1971.

52. Bruck, H. M., Nash, G., Foley, F. D., and Pruitt, B. A., Jr., Opportunistic fungal infection of the burn wound with Phycomycetes and *Aspergillus*. A clinical-pathologic review, *Arch. Surg. (Chicago)*, 102, 476, 1971.

53. Bruck, H. M., Nash, G., Stein, J. M., and Lindberg, R. B., Studies on the occurrence and significance of yeasts and fungi in the burn wound, *Ann. Surg.*, 176, 108, 1971.

54. MacMillan, B. G., Low, E. J., and Holder, I. A., Experience with *Candida* infections in the burn patient, *Arch. Surg. (Chicago)*, 104, 509, 1972.

55. Rabin, E. R., Lundberg, G. D., and Mitchell, E. T., Mucormycosis in severely burned patients. Report of two cases with extensive destruction of the face and nasal cavity, *N. Engl. J. Med.*, 264, 1286, 1961.

56. Foley, F. D. and Shuck, J. M., Burn-wound infection with Phycomycetes requiring amputation of hand, *JAMA*, 203, 596, 1968.

57. Majeski, J. A. and MacMillan, B. G., Fatal systemic mycotic infections in the burned child, *J. Trauma*, 17, 320, 1977.

58. Nash, G., Foley, F. D., and Pruitt, B. A., Jr., *Candida* burn-wound invasion. A cause of systemic candidiasis, *Arch. Pathol.*, 90, 75, 1970.

59. Foley, F. D., Greenwald, K. A., Nash, G., and Pruitt, B. A., Jr., Herpes-virus infection in burned patients, *N. Engl. J. Med.*, 282, 652, 1970.

60. Castle, M. and Mallison, G. F., Effective investigations of nosocomial outbreaks, *Assoc. Pract. Infect. Control J.*, 5, 13, 1977.

61. Maki, D. G., Weise, C. E., and Sarafin, H. W., A semiquantitative culture method for identifying intravenous-catheter-related infection, *N. Engl. J. Med.*, 296, 1305, 1977.

62. Maki, D. G., Jarrett, F., and Sarafin, H. W., A semi-quantitative culture method for identification of catheter-related infection in the burn patient, *J. Surg. Res.*, 22, 513, 1977.

63. Weinstein, R. A. and Stamm, W. E., Pseudoepidemics in hospitals, *Lancet*, 2, 862, 1977.

64. Weinstein, R. A. and Mallison, G. F., The role of the microbiology laboratory in surveillance and control of nosocomial infections, *Am. J. Clin. Pathol.*, 69, 130, 1978.

65. Pruitt, B. A., Jr., Procedures used by U.S. Army Institute of Surgical Research, Brooke Army Medical Center, Fort Sam Houston, San Antonio, 1978.

66. Morris, A. H., Nebulizer contamination in a burn unit, *Am. Rev. Respir. Dis.*, 107, 802, 1973.

67. American Thoracic Society, Cleaning and sterilization of inhalation equipment: a statement by the Committee on Therapy, *Am. Rev. Respir. Dis.*, 98, 521, 1968.

68. Smith, R. F., Blasi, D., Dayton, S. L., and Chipps, D. D., Effects of sodium hypochlorite on the microbial flora of burns and normal skin, *J. Trauma*, 14, 938, 1974.

69. Center for Disease Control, Disinfection of Hydrotherapy Pools and Tanks, Atlanta, 1974.

70. Lindberg, R. B., Moncrief, J. A., Switzer, W. E., Order, S. E., and Mills, W., Jr., The successful control of burn wound sepsis, *J. Trauma*, 5, 601, 1965.

71. Moncrief, J. A., Lindberg, R. B., Switzer, W. E., and Pruitt, B. A., Jr., The use of a topical sulfonamide in the control of burn wound sepsis, *J. Trauma*, 6, 407, 1966.

72. Ryan, K. J. and Mihalyi, S. F., Evaluation of a simple device for bacteriological sampling of respirator-generated aerosols, *J. Clin. Microbiol.*, 5, 178, 1977.

73. Moncrief, J. A., Lindberg, R. B., Switzer, W. E., and Pruitt, B. A., Use of topical antibacterial therapy in the treatment of the burn wound, *Arch. Surg. (Chicago)*, 92, 558, 1966.

HOSPITAL ACQUIRED PNEUMONIA

James M. Veazey, Jr.

INTRODUCTION — INCIDENCE, MORBIDITY, AND MORTALITY OF HOSPITAL ACQUIRED PNEUMONIA

Incidence

The incidence of hospital acquired pneumonias will vary from institution to institution, but data obtained from the National Nosocomial Infections Study (NNIS) Report of 1976[1] suggest that nosocomial pneumonias occur in 0.56% of all patients discharged from U.S. hospitals. This makes hospital acquired pneumonia overall the third most common nosocomial infection, accounting for 15.7% of the total. Certain hospital areas appear to experience an increased incidence of hospital acquired pneumonia: over 7% in a newborn intensive care unit,[2] over 10% in a general medical intensive care unit,[3] and more than 20% in a respiratory intensive care unit.[4]

Morbidity

Morbidity related to hospital acquired pneumonia is somewhat difficult to estimate since no matched case-control studies have been performed. A nosocomial pneumonia due to a more easily treatable pathogen such as *Streptococcus pneumoniae* would likely cause less of a prolongation of hospitalization with its increased costs than one due to a more serious pathogen such as *Pseudomonas aeruginosa*. Some rough estimates of increased morbidity due to hospital acquired pneumonia have appeared in the literature: Hemming et al.[2] reported an increased duration of hospitalization of more than 5 weeks in infants in a newborn intensive care unit who developed a nosocomial infection at any site. Although pneumonia accounted for more than 29% of these infections, the presence of other risk factors such as lower birth weight and more severe underlying disease in infants with long hospital stays made it impossible to elucidate the exact role of pneumonia or any other nosocomial infection in prolonging the hospitalization.

A somewhat better estimate of excess hospitalization due to nosocomial respiratory syncytial virus (RSV) infections has been provided by Hall et al.[5] In two groups of hospitalized children with generally comparable underlying conditions, the group acquiring RSV had an estimated prolongation of hospital stay of an average of 11 days per patient. However, only about 30% of these children had pneumonia; the rest had upper respiratory infections, and the excess morbidity due to RSV pneumonia alone was not reported. In compromised hosts who developed nosocomial aerobic Gram-negative bacillary pneumonia, the median duration of therapy from onset to cure reported by Valdivieso et al.[6] was 10 days. This provides a crude estimate of increased duration of hospitalization from a single episode of hospital acquired pneumonia, although other factors also doubtlessly contributed to the longer hospitalization in this patient population.

Mortality

Mortality data are more readily available. Data from the Comprehensive Hospital Infections Project (CHIP)[7] show that hospital acquired pneumonia has a case-fatality ratio of 56% for bacteremic patients, 19% for nonbacteremic patients, and 20% for all patients. Bacteremia has the highest case-fatality ratio of all nosocomial infections at 39%. However, since hospital acquired pneumonia occurs more than three times as frequently as bacteremia, pneumonia is the leading cause of death among nosocomial infections.

Mortality may vary in different patient populations and with different etiologic organisms. In a university hospital, 50% of the patients who acquired pneumonia due to aerobic Gram-negative bacilli died.[8] In a cancer center, with use of the newest antibiotics and white cell transfusions, mortality from hospital acquired pneumonia due to these same organisms was held to 39%.[6] In a respiratory intensive care unit, mortality in patients with nosocomial pneumonia due to Gram-positive cocci was 5%.[4] In contrast, patients who acquired pneumonia due to aerobic Gram-negative bacilli other than *P. aeruginosa* experienced a mortality of 33%; this rose to 70% in nosocomial *P. aeruginosa* pneumonia.[4] In a newborn intensive care unit, there was a 26% mortality among infants who acquired pneumonia as compared to a 14% mortality among infants who did not become infected at any site.[2] In a group of patients at one hospital who were admitted with community acquired pneumonia and treated with antimicrobial agents for it, all of the patients who developed a secondary nosocomial pneumonia died either from the first or second episode of this illness.[105] However, this excessive mortality rate may reflect in part the generally aged and debilitated patient population admitted to the hospital.

Outbreaks of nosocomial viral illness involve varying proportions of upper respiratory illness and viral pneumonia, depending upon the report. Nevertheless, mortality data are readily available. There were no deaths in an outbreak of nosocomial RSV infections[5] or in an outbreak of nosocomial influenza infections (predominantly influenza A).[9] Viral illnesses acquired during the winter and spring months on a pediatric ward included RSV, rhinovirus, influenza A, influenza B, and parainfluenza type 3; and, in this report also, no deaths occurred.[10] In a study of hospital-acquired viral illnesses due to RSV, influenza A, and parainfluenza types 1, 3, and 4, apparently no deaths occurred in the hospital.[11] However, one child who died unexpectedly at home shortly after hospitalization for gastroenteritis and who was exposed to parainfluenza type 3 while in the hospital, had parainfluenza type 3 isolated at autopsy from his lungs, which showed histological changes of early bronchiolitis. The virus may therefore have played a role in his death. Thus, although hospital acquired viral pneumonias have been studied to a lesser extent than bacterial pneumonias, they probably do cause occasional deaths.

Pneumonias due to fungi or to parasites such as *Pneumocystis carinii* which first manifest themselves in the hospital may or may not be hospital acquired. In addition, reports on outbreaks due to such etiologic agents are sparse enough so as to make it difficult to render an accurate estimate of the mortality associated with them.

ETIOLOGY OF HOSPITAL ACQUIRED PNEUMONIA

The diagnosis of the etiologic agent of pneumonia is usually made through culture of coughed-up sputum or of secretions suctioned from nasotracheal, endotracheal, or tracheostomy tubes. All of these are contaminated by oropharyngeal flora which may potentially overgrow and obscure the identity of the true pathogen. Occasionally no effort is made to culture the etiologic organism. Cultures of transtracheal aspiration of sputum, percutaneous aspiration of empyemas or consolidated areas of lung, or blood in the absence of other sites of infection which could seed the bloodstream, are the best ways of determining the etiologic agent of pneumonia and are the only ways of proving an anaerobic etiology. No long-term studies of the etiologic agents of hospital acquired pneumonia using the latter techniques have been performed, so the potential inaccuracies of the former methods inevitably distort any listing of the presumed causes of nosocomial pneumonia. Nevertheless, these are generally the only data available.

The relative frequency of the pathogens causing hospital acquired pneumonia is shown in the chapter entitled "Surveillance and Reporting of Hospital Acquired Infections," Table 7C. Gram-positive cocci as a group caused less than 20% of the pneumonias, and aerobic Gram-negative bacilli, including *Pseudomonas aeruginosa,* caused over 40%. *Candida* species and other fungi comprised slightly more than 4% of reported pathogens. Anaerobes are probably underestimated in frequency as etiologic agents and may actually be involved in more than one third of hospital acquired pneumonias and may be the sole agent in 7 to 9%.[12,13] The lack of attention paid to viruses has likely led to an underestimation of their importance as etiologic agents of nosocomial pneumonia. Clearly, RSV, influenza A and B, rhinovirus, and various types of parainfluenza play a causative role in hospital acquired pneumonia.[5,9-11] More recently, it has become apparent that the recently-discovered etiologic agent of Legionnaires' disease,[90,91] *Legionella pneumophila,* is an increasingly important cause of nosocomial pneumonia.[92-98] The even more recent isolation of the related organism, the "Pittsburgh Pneumonia Agent" (*L. micdadei*), has led to the recognition of its role as an opportunistic pathogen in the cause of nosocomial pneumonia in immunocompromised patients.[99-101]

Certain circumstances may alter the frequency of occurrence of the etiologic agents of hospital acquired pneumonia. In a newborn intensive care unit, *S. aureus* alone caused almost 45% of the nosocomial pneumonias and was the leading etiologic agent in this setting.[2] In a cancer hospital, aerobic Gram-negative bacilli caused 90% of all episodes of hospital acquired bacterial pneumonia.[6] In compromised hosts, discussed below, unusual pathogens, including various fungi, parasites, viruses, and bacteria, assume a more prominent role in the etiology of hospital acquired pneumonia.[14,15] The exact incidence of these infections is not well defined, however, and it is often not clear if the infection is acquired from an exogenous source in the hospital or is an activation of a latent infection due to compromise of host defenses.

EPIDEMIOLOGY OF HOSPITAL ACQUIRED PNEUMONIA

The discussion of the epidemiology of any outbreak of infection invariably includes an examination of the reservoirs of infection, the vectors or modes of transmission of infection, and any risk factors or predisposing factors which increase the likelihood of acquisition of infection. Often there is an overlap of these areas, and hospital acquired pneumonia is no exception. Nevertheless, the epidemiology of nosocomial pneumonia will be discussed along these lines with an effort to minimize redundancy as much as possible. Reservoirs and modes of transmission will be discussed in terms of patients, hospital personnel, the inanimate environment, and air. Predisposing factors include admission to intensive care units, being in the immediate postoperative period, aspiration of gastric contents, reduction of host defense mechanisms, bronchoscopy, and the vast array of equipment used in anesthesia and respiratory therapy. The information in this section is derived from multiple sources: descriptions of large outbreaks, descriptions of small outbreaks, examination of indigenous infection rates in high-risk areas or high-risk patients, and evaluation of high-risk or potentially high-risk procedures and equipment in use on patients.

Reservoirs and Modes of Transmission of Infection

Pathogens may reach the lung and cause pneumonia by the hematogenous route or via the upper airways. Although pneumonia due to bacteremia from distant foci of infection such as *Escherichia coli* pyelonephritis[16] or *P. aeruginosa* burn wound infections[17] have been reported, acquisition of infection via the upper airways is far more likely. Pathogens may reach the alveoli through the upper airways by inhalation of spores of fungi such as *Aspergillus,* by inhalation of contaminated aerosols, or by aspiration of pharyngeal flora. A number of potential reservoirs for nosocomial pathogens exist. Some have been demonstrated to be of primary importance in hospital acquired pneumonias but not in other nosocomial infections. For other reservoirs, the converse is true, and these reservoirs may be of only theoretical importance in hospital acquired pneumonia. In addition, different reservoirs may be of varying import for different pathogens, as noted below.

Patients

Overall, the most common reservoir of the etiologic agents of hospital acquired pneumonia is probably the oropharynx of the patient, with aspiration as the mode of acquisition of pneumonia. Because of their predominant role as the etiologic agents in hospital acquired pneumonia, the best studied pathogens are the aerobic Gram-negative bacilli. Johanson et al.,[18] using an area sampling device for oropharyngeal culturing and performing repeated cultures on the subjects studied, found that about 6% of healthy individuals were colonized with aerobic Gram-negative bacilli and that colonization was transient. In contrast, Rosenthal and Tager,[19] using broth enrichment of swabs rubbed over the posterior pharynx, found that 18% of normal persons were colonized with Enterobacteriaceae or *P. aeruginosa* in a single culture survey. Likewise, Mackowiak et al.,[20] using saline gargles, found that 18% of normal persons were colonized with aerobic Gram-negative bacilli in a single culture survey.

Johanson et al.[18] also found that colonization rates with these organisms, when examined by repeat culturing, rose to 35% in moderately ill hospitalized patients and to 73% in moribund hospitalized patients. Mackowiak et al.[20] demonstrated that alcoholics and diabetics had significantly higher colonization rates with aerobic Gram-negative bacilli (35 and 36%, respectively) when compared to epileptics (17%), narcotic addicts (20%), and normal controls (18%). The predilection for episodes of unconsciousness among all of the groups except controls could therefore not be the explanation for the differences in colonization rates. Valenti et al.,[21] using broth enrichment of throat swabs, examined patients over age 65 and found increasing colonization rates with aerobic Gram-negative bacilli, ranging from 6 to 60% as the incidence of functional limitations due to respiratory disease or bed-to-chair or bedridden existence rose. In all of the above studies, the apparent reason for increased rates of colonization were decreased pharyngeal clearance mechanisms, possibly by decreased production of immunoglobulin A (IgA) which blocked bacterial attachment or by changes in buccal mucosa cell membranes allowing increased adherence of these pathogens.[20] More recent studies have demonstrated quantitatively the increased binding of certain aerobic Gram-negative bacilli to the buccal mucosal cells from the oropharynx of seriously ill patients[102] or patients who had recently undergone elective surgery.[103] Increased adherence in vitro correlated with increased oropharyngeal colonization with these organisms in vivo, but the exact mechanism remains unknown, nor does it occur in all of these patients. In any case, the significance of such an increased colonization rate is evident in a report from a medical intensive care unit, where 23% of colonized patients developed nosocomial pneumonia as compared to 3.3% of noncolonized patients.[3]

Although some evidence of patient-to-patient transmission of these organisms exists in the occurrence of clusters of patients colonized with the same species of Gram-negative bacilli, other clusters of patients in the same environment colonized with different species suggests acquisition of indigenous flora from the gastrointestinal tract.[22] Selden et al.[23] studied a hospital where there was endemic nosocomial infection due to multi-ply-resistant *Klebsiella pneumoniae* of eight different serotypes. There was a significantly increased risk of acquiring a nosocomial infection from a particular serotype if intestinal colonization with that serotype occurred first, and antibiotic therapy was shown to predispose toward such intestinal colonization. Although less than 10% of the hospital acquired infections described were pneumonias, the potential importance of this reservoir for pneumonia is clear. Schwartz et al.[24] looked at the sources of aerobic Gram-negative bacilli colonizing the trachea of patients requiring orotracheal intubation. All colonizing Enterobacteriaceae were isolated from the hypopharynx or hypopharynx and rectum simultaneously before being isolated from the trachea. Although hypopharyngeal isolations alone were more frequent, it was not possible to determine if rectal colonization came first in simultaneous isolations. In sharp contrast, non-Enterobacteriaceae were usually isolated from the trachea first, a highly significant difference and one which suggested other patient or environmental sources for these organisms.

An interesting study by Atherton and White[25] of ten patients who had paralytic ileus, and who were ventilated by oral endotracheal tubes, found that six were colonized in the stomach by the same aerobic Gram-negative bacilli found in their tracheal aspirates. In four of these patients, the stomach isolates preceded or coincided with the tracheal isolates, suggesting a previously unreported potential source of pathogens for hospital acquired pneumonia.

Rosendorf et al.,[26] after noting an 8.4% nosocomial infection rate (29% pneumonias) following open-heart surgery, predominantly caused by aerobic Gram-negative bacilli, prospectively examined multiple patient sites as potential reservoirs for these organisms in 22 patients. Over 90% of the patients became colonized at one or more of the following sites: nose, throat, axilla, groin, and rectum. Although the authors claimed to observe both spread of indigenous rectal flora and acquisition of hospital strains, or occasionally both, they did not say how, or which site was most important.

All of the above observations apply to situations in which patients contract nosocomial pneumonia from their indigenous flora, primarily oropharyngeal. The nasopharynx likewise appears to be relatively unimportant as a patient reservoir for indigenously acquired nosocomial pneumonia. One possible exception is *S. aureus*. Since approximately 30% of the general population may harbor this organism in the anterior nasopharynx at any one time, this is a potential (albeit unproved) reservoir for pneumonias in the newborn intensive care unit where *S. aureus* plays such a predominant role in hospital acquired pneumonias.[2]

However, in epidemics of hospital acquired pneumonia, the situation changes. The nasopharynx is the reservoir of infection in viral nosocomial pneumonias,[5,9,11] although one study has suggested that cross-infection due to the common viruses is quite rare.[10] Epidemics of bacterial nosocomial pneumonias are similar. Lowbury et al.[27] described a series of eight outbreaks of respiratory tract infections due to *P. aeruginosa* in which the reservoir appeared to be the tracheostomy tubes of infected patients. Sanders et al.[28] described a massive outbreak of *Serratia marcescens* infections which began with pneumonias and subsequently spread to cause urinary tract infections, surgical wound infections, and bloodstream infections. Although contaminated respiratory therapy equipment was the ultimate source of the outbreak, sputum of patients infected or colonized with *S. marcescens* played an important role in its propagation. Buxton et al.[29] described an outbreak of nosocomial respiratory tract infections and colonizations due to *Acinetobacter calcoaceticus* in which the sputum of colonized or infected patients could have played a minor secondary role as a reservoir of the epidemic organism. In this outbreak also, contaminated respiratory therapy equipment was the primary mode of transmission of the epidemic strain to patients.

Thus, a multiplicity of patient sites may serve as reservoirs for endemic or epidemic hospital acquired pneumonia, although most are of minor importance. Patients themselves have usually not been implicated as modes of transmission of infection, although the possibility of direct transmission of RSV by nosocomially infected infants who were not yet noticeably symptomatic has been noted.[5] Interestingly enough, the hands of patients have not been sufficiently evaluated to allow an adequate assessment of their potential role as reservoirs or modes of transmission of infection.

Personnel

The importance of various personnel sites as reservoirs of the etiologic agent of hospital acquired pneumonia has varied somewhat from one report to another. Although scalp colonization with Group A beta hemolytic streptococci was found in a woman felt to be the source of an outbreak of postoperative wound infections due to this organism,[30] this site has not been reported as a reservoir in nosocomial pneumonia. In this outbreak, the actual reservoir was felt to be the woman's vagina with aerosolization as the mode of transmission. The vagina has rarely been cultured in reported outbreaks of hospital acquired pneumonia. In the outbeak due to *A. calcoaceticus*, only one female had a positive vaginal culture, and this isolate had a different antibiogram from the epidemic strain.[29] Thus, neither scalp nor vagina appear to play an important role as reservoirs in hospital acquired pneumonia.

The rectum and stool likewise appear not to be important reservoirs. There were no positive rectal cultures among nurses and respiratory therapists in the *Acinetobacter* outbreak,[29] and neither physicians nor nurses in a *P. aeruginosa* outbreak in a premature nursery had stool cultures positive for this organism.[31] Even in the study suggesting intestinal colonization of patients as a reservoir of multiply-resistant *Klebsiella*, only 1 of 54 physicians and nursing personnel had this organism isolated on rectal culture.[23]

The pharynx of personnel has played a variable role as a reservoir of etiologic organisms in hospital acquired pneumonia. Throat cultures of personnel have usually been negative for the etiologic organisms sought.[23,26,31,32] In the *Acinetobacter* outbreak, only two persons had pharyngeal colonization with the outbreak strain, and this was transient.[29] In an outbreak of *K. pneumoniae* pneumonias resulting from use of contaminated aerosol solutions, only 1 of 48 throat cultures was positive for the epidemic serotype.[33] However, this one culture was from a respiratory therapist who sometimes prepared the aerosol solutions and who therefore presumably caused the contamination and the outbreak. Thus, although usually unimportant as a reservoir, the throat may be the key to an outbreak.

The nares of personnel likewise play a variable role as reservoirs. When examined for bacterial etiologic agents, cultures of the nares are generally negative[31,32,34] or positive only at a relatively low frequency (20%) without a clear-cut relationship to acquisition of nosocomial infections.[26] An obvious exception to this trend would be *S. aureus*. Where viral agents are concerned, nasopharyngeal carriage by personnel as a reservoir and a mode of transmission of the virus has been reported as unlikely in an RSV outbreak,[5] quite possible in an influenza outbreak,[9] and probable in the case of parainfluenza in a multiple virus outbreak.[11] In another multiple virus study where cross-infection between patients was not found, nasopharyngeal carriage and dissemination by visitors and personnel was considered highly suspect but not demonstrated.[10]

The site most consistently implicated as a mode of transmission of nosocomial infections overall is the hands of personnel. In a general culture survey, over 20% of hospital personnel had antibiotic-resistant *E. coli* and *Klebsiella-Aerobacter* species on their hands.[35] In a surgical intensive care unit, 70% of nurses had aerobic Gram-negative bacilli cultured from their hands in varying concentrations after handwashing with hexachlorophene-containing soap.[26] In an intensive care nursery, over 80% of hand cultures were positive for aerobic Gram-negative bacilli after hexachlorophene hand-washing, and about 50% were positive after povidone-iodine handwashing.[36] Of more concern in this study was the demonstration of active multiplication of the organisms on the hands of some personnel and the existence of a temporary carrier state on the hands of a few, suggesting that hands of personnel could serve as a reservoir for these organisms. This was confirmed in the *Acinetobacter* outbreak, where a respiratory therapist with chronic dermatitis had persistant colonization of his hands with the ep-idemic strain.[29] He contaminated the respiratory therapy equipment he handled, which in turn led to colonization and infection of the respiratory tract in patients treated with this equipment. He thereby was both the primary reservoir and the mode of trans-mission of the epidemic strain to the equipment, which in turn was the primary mode of transmission of the pathogen to patients.

In reports of outbreaks of hospital acquired pneumonia, the frequency of positive hand cultures has varied from study to study. In a *Serratia marcescens* outbreak traced to heavily contaminated ultrasonic nebulizers, none of the ward or inhalation therapy personnel had positive finger touch plate hand cultures.[32] In the study of intestinal colonization as a reservoir for *Klebsiella,* only 2 of 26 nurses cultured (8%) had positive finger impression cultures for one of the eight serotypes isolated in this endemic situa-tion, although both were of the same serotype as that most commonly isolated from all sources.[23] In the study of Lowbury et al.[27] of eight sequential outbreaks due to *P. aeruginosa,* using hand wash culturing, the organism was always found on the hands of some member of the staff, and nurses usually carried one or more of the epidemic strains causing the infections in each outbreak. In the *Acinetobacter* outbreak, just over 30% of nurses and respiratory therapists had at least one positive hand wash culture for the organism.[29] However, except for the persistently colonized respiratory therapist with dermatitis of the hands who was the source of the outbreak, only rarely did these personnel have a positive repeat culture, and in every case the subsequent isolates had different antibiograms, demonstrating that none of them were persistent carriers of the same strain. Nevertheless, their hands were felt to be a potential second-ary mode of transmission between patients, with colonized or infected patients serving as secondary reservoirs of the epidemic organism.

In outbreaks of viral nosocomial pneumonia, hands of personnel may also play a role. There is evidence suggesting that rhinoviruses may be spread by the hand-borne route;[37] spread by this route from infected personnel and visitors was implied in one multiple virus outbreak study.[10] In another multiple virus outbreak study[11] and in an influenza outbreak study,[9] this route of transmission from infected personnel was not specifically considered but was clearly possible. In an RSV outbreak, the likely mode of spread of infection between patients was felt to be by personnel — via their hands, clothing, or other objects.[5] A more recent study has provided clear evidence that the hands of personnel are probably the primary means of transmission of RSV.[104] Thus, the hands of personnel have been strongly implicated as modes of transmission of viral and bacterial pathogens causing hospital acquired pneumonia, and in the case of bac-teria at least, hands may also serve as a reservoir, even in the absence of dermatitis.

The Inanimate Environment

The inanimate environment of the hospital has been widely examined by various investigators to determine its role as a reservoir of pathogens causing hospital acquired pneumonia. Two special classes of equipment — fiberoptic bronchoscopes and the wide variety of equipment used in respiratory therapy — will be considered separately below in the section entitled "Predisposing Factors in the Acquisition of Pneumonia in the Hospital". The rest of the environment will be considered here.

Different investigators have found substantially different levels of contamination of the environment by the pathogens they were seeking and have attached varying degrees of significance to this contamination as a potential reservoir in the outbreaks they were reporting. In the *S. marcescens* outbreak described by Sanders et al.,[28] only 3 of 49 randomly performed environmental cultures were positive for the organism. These three sites — a sink, a mop bucket, and a spirometer tubing — were felt to be insignificant in view of the heavy contamination found in the bottles of inhalation therapy medications in use on patients. Impression plates recovered moderate numbers of *P. aeruginosa* from floor dust near the beds of infected patients in the outbreak reported by Phillips and Spencer,[34] but the dust was not felt to be a reservoir of infection. Heavy contamination with aerobic Gram-negative bacilli was found in the sinks and sink drains in the surgical intensive care unit examined by Rosendorf et al.[26] Other sites cultured in the unit and in the cardiac surgery operating room yielded little or no growth of the organisms, and the environment, including the sinks, was felt not to be an important reservoir. Selden et al.[23] cultured floors, sink drains, sink handles, bathtubs, horizontal surfaces (e.g., table tops or shelves), mops, inhalation and anesthesia equipment, sterile instruments, germicide solutions, and opened bottles of irrigating solution for the multiply-resistant *Klebsiella* they were seeking. The only positive cultures were from sink drains, floors, horizontal surfaces, inhalation equipment, and a bathtub in patient areas only; none were felt to be epidemiologically important as reservoirs.

Lowbury et al.[27] cultured the environment extensively during their series of eight outbreaks of *P. aeruginosa* infections. Isolates of strains causing infection were found in floor samples, floor mops, a kitchen draining board, plastic washing bowls, a bar of soap, a sink mop, a saucepan cleaner, a dish cloth, a syringe used for feeding, food mixers, mixed food, patient toothbrushes, a mouth-water container, protective felt cuffs, a nurse's uniform, and a bed rail. Sinks and washbasins consistently yielded an endemic strain which rarely caused infection. Occasionally they showed the transient presence of a strain causing current infection which was felt to have come from patients rather than being a reservoir for infecting patients. Multiple other environmental sites either yielded strains not causing infection or else no *P. aeruginosa* at all. *P. aeruginosa* was cultured from urine bottles and bedpans on several occasions, but only in samples taken after the eight outbreak periods were past. Failure to find the organism earlier during an outbreak was quite possibly due to the very small number of such samples taken.

Usually the epidemic strains of *P. aeruginosa* were found in the tracheostomies of patients before being isolated from the environment. However, in five of the outbreaks, at least one of the possibly multiple infecting strains was found in at least one environmental site before or simultaneously with its isolation from a tracheostomy site. Because of this and because of the widespread contamination of the environment with infecting strains, the inanimate environment was felt to be a likely reservoir of infection. Only sinks were inferred rarely to be a source of infection.

Other investigators have also focused close attention on sinks. Rubbo et al.[38] examined washbasins while investigating an outbreak of *P. aeruginosa* pneumonia and eye infections in a premature infant nursery. They found that the strains isolated from washbasin drains were of a different phage type than those causing infection and concluded that washbasins were not a reservoir. Fierer et al.,[31] in their investigation of a *P. aeruginosa* outbreak in a premature nursery, found that nearly half the sink drains in the nursery contained that organism and that all of the drains were heavily contaminated with a variety of other aerobic Gram-negative bacilli. However, the correlation between the location of the *Pseudomonas*-contaminated sinks and the location of infected infants was poor, and the epidemic strain as determined by pyocin typing was recovered only once from a sink drain. The authors concluded that this sink was probably secondarily contaminated and that sinks were not a reservoir of the epidemic strain.

Teres et al.[39] reported a 19-month study which looked for sources of *P. aeruginosa* in a respiratory/surgical intensive-therapy unit. Two pyocin types, 1 and 10, which were nearly always present in sinks, accounted for 75% of the *P. aeruginosa* colonizing or infecting the respiratory tract in patients who acquired the organism while in the unit. In addition, pyocin type 33 was occasionally isolated from sinks during the study, and 4 months after it ended, this strain was isolated for the first time from a patient who acquired the organism in the unit. Since no other environmental sources ever yielded *P. aeruginosa*, the preceding circumstantial evidence led the authors to conclude tentatively that sinks were the reservoir for this pathogen in the unit. They therefore instituted a daily decontamination procedure for all sinks which consisted of pasteurizing a 5% phenol solution in the sink for 90 min at 70°C, using an immersion coil. This reduced all bacterial contamination in the sinks virtually to zero and the authors hoped that by eliminating this reservoir, they could reduce the incidence of *P. aeruginosa* pneumonia in their unit. Unfortunately, this premise was not borne out, since some 2½ years later this same group admitted in another paper that the procedure had not affected the rate of *P. aeruginosa* pneumonia in the unit at all.[40] Ayliffe et al.[41] also examined sinks in a general hospital and in a burn unit for the presence of *P. aeruginosa*. Not surprisingly, the organism was more prevalent in burn unit sinks than in the general hospital sinks. The number of positive samples, as well as the level of contamination with *Pseudomonas*, was much greater in drain pipes and waste traps of sinks than in their basins or outlets. Directing water from the tap directly into or near the drain pipe did not disseminate *Pseudomonas* from the pipe into the basin or surrounding areas. These results, plus epidemiologic data on *P. aeruginosa* infections in the hospital, led the authors to conclude that although transmission of this pathogen from sinks might be possible, it was probably an uncommon event. They further concluded that a device they tested which effectively disinfected sink waste traps by boiling water in them would have at best an uncertain role in hospitals, even in special units.

It should not, however, be concluded that no part of a sink ever plays a role as a reservoir in an outbreak of hospital acquired pneumonia. In the *P. aeruginosa* outbreak in the premature nursery of Fierer et al.,[31] the aerator on the sink faucet in the delivery room was the reservoir for the epidemic organism. Resuscitation bags washed in this sink and used in the delivery room were heavily contaminated with the epidemic strain and delivered contaminated aerosols to the infants on whom they were used. In the *Acinetobacter* outbreak,[29] cultures of tap water in the hospital and at the home of the respiratory therapist who was the primary reservoir for the epidemic strain all failed to grow the organism. However, sink faucet handles in the respiratory therapy supply room grew *K. pneumoniae*. Although this organism was not causing an outbreak at that time, the finding suggests a potential reservoir which could contaminate the hands of personnel who could then pass on the *K. pneumoniae* (or similar organisms) to patients.

Other parts of the inanimate environment have been clearly implicated as reservoirs of infection. Mayhall et al.[42] reported an outbreak of *Enterobacter cloacae* infections in a burn unit, primarily involving burn wound colonizations and infections, and bacteremias, but also including four pneumonias and several respiratory tract colonizations with the epidemic strain.[43] The burn wound was the primary portal of entry of infection, and a chair on which patients sat in the hydrotherapy tank room was strongly implicated as a reservoir which directly transmitted *E. cloacae* to patients. In the *Acinetobacter* outbreak,[29] a washcloth used each morning by the respiratory therapist who was the primary reservoir of the infection, when cultured, grew out the epidemic strain in pure culture and did so again after a full week of air drying. This washcloth may have been responsible for reinoculating the therapist's hands each morning, since serial quantitative hand cultures performed on three consecutive days showed declining bacterial counts from morning to afternoon.

Several environmental sites have been implicated as sources of *Legionella pneumophila*. Circumstancial evidence has implicated the soil around hospitals as a potential source of *L. pneumophila* in patients contracting pneumonia due to this organism,[92,95] and it has been isolated from the shower bath on a renal transplant unit where two patients acquired *L. pneumophila* pneumonia. A contaminated cooling tower may be the environmental source of *L. pneumophilia* in an ongoing outbreak in one hospital,[96] and an auxillary air-conditioning cooling tower which was put into temporary use was clearly the source of *L. pneumophila* pneumonia in an outbreak at another hospital.[97]

Fireproofing material in a new hospital facility was implicated as the reservoir for *Aspergillus* species causing seven cases of pulmonary infection and one case of maxillary sinus infection with hematogenous spread in eight patients with acute leukemia.[44] Dust in the air-handling system outlets and above and on false ceiling panels also yielded positive cultures for *Aspergillus*. Dust above false ceilings was found to be a source of *Aspergillus fumigatus* causing pneumonia in two immunosuppressed renal transplant patients and tracheal colonization in a third.[45] Thus, although in general the environment is probably only rarely a reservoir for pathogens in outbreaks of hospital acquired pneumonia, under certain circumstances or with certain pathogens, an environmental site may turn out to be a major or even the sole reservoir. Therefore, the environment cannot be neglected in any extensive workup of an outbreak of nosocomial pneumonia.

Air

Even in hospitals, the bacterial density in air is very low and most of the bacteria suspended in air are not the Gram-negative bacilli which assume such a prominent role in hospital acquired pneumonia.[46] Under ordinary circumstances, therefore, air is not thought to be a reservoir of pathogens causing nosocomial pneumonia. Under outbreak situations, however, air has been examined by a number of methods as a possible mode of transmission of infection.

Using settle plates and a sieve air sampler, Mayhall et al.[42] were unable to detect *E. cloacae* in air in their burn unit outbreak. Using a slit air sampler, Buxton et al.[29] detected no *Acinetobacter calcoaceticus* in air in their outbreak. *P. aeruginosa* was not isolated from air by settle plates or a slit sampler in the outbreak of Phillips and Spencer,[34] and it was detected only rarely in air and only in extremely small numbers by a slit sampler in the series of eight outbreaks reported by Lowbury et al.[27] Rosendorf et al.[26] used settling plates to examine air for the presence of various aerobic Gram-negative bacilli in their surgical intensive care unit and cardiac surgery operating room. Air in the operating room was essentially free of these organisms, and in the unit in most places the settle plates either failed to grow any Gram-negative organisms or else grew only small numbers of them. Around sinks, however, the air was found to be heavily contaminated with aerobic Gram-negative bacilli. In contrast, Teres et al.[39] detected *P. aeruginosa* only in a settling plate placed on the rim of a sink; settling plates placed near the sink or elsewhere in their respiratory/surgical intensive-therapy unit did not grow the organisms. Ayliffe et al.[41] likewise noted that settle plates placed next to sinks only occasionally grew *P. aeruginosa*.

In a burn unit outbreak of multiple infections, including pneumonia, due to *Providencia stuartii*, the organism was detected significantly more often in air samples taken by a sieve air sampler than in individual hand washes obtained from personnel.[47] This finding, plus the direct temporal relationship that was detected between colonization of the air and colonization of nearby patients, led to the suggestion of airborne transmission of the organism. However, the number of air samples and hand washes obtained over the 6-month study period was too small, and the relationship between the times they were obtained was too unclear, to demonstrate convincingly the predominance of the airborne route of transmission. A subsequent study in the same burn unit of the reservoirs and modes of transmission of gentamicin-resistant *K. pneumoniae* and *Pseudomonas aeruginosa* reached the conclusion that patients were the reservoir, and the hands of personnel were the mode of transmission of these organisms.[48] The airborne route of transmission was felt to play little if any part.

Evidence of the importance of the airborne route of transmission of pathogens is not entirely lacking, however. It has been deomonstrated for *Staphylococcus aureus*,[49] although there is little evidence that this route is important in hospital acquired pneumonia caused by this organism. Grieble et al.[50] demonstrated that a chute-hydropulping system heavily contaminated hospital air with enteric bacilli and *P. aeruginosa* and circumstantially implicated this contamination as a cause of an outbreak of Gram-negative bloodstream infections due to these organisms. More importantly, they experimentally demonstrated widespread airborne dissemination of an *Escherichia coli* bacteriophage and, by implication, the potential airborne spread of other viruses.

In actual outbreaks due to viruses, the conclusions about the importance of the airborne route of spread have varied. In a study of nosocomial RSV infections, airborne transmission of small-particle aerosols from patient to patient was felt to be unlikely.[5] In one study of hospital acquired respiratory illness due to multiple viruses, it was concluded that aerosol spread from patient to patient was unlikely and that there was no need for isolation of patients with viral respiratory illness.[10] In another study involving multiple viruses, it was implied that airborne transmission was important and concluded that isolation of children with acute respiratory illnesses was necessary.[11] In a study of nosocomial influenza infections, no speculation regarding the mode of transmission was offered.[9] In all of these studies — regardless of the source of the virus acquired by the susceptible patient (ward personnel, visitor, or fellow patient) — airborne spread of large droplet aerosols over short distances from infected, shedding sources was conceivable.

In three reported outbreaks, one bacterial and two fungal, the airborne route was clearly the most likely mode of transmission. In the outbreak of Legionnaires' disease associated with a contaminated auxillary air-conditioning cooling tower, the airborne route was strongly suggested as the route of spread.[97] In one of the *Aspergillus* outbreaks, settling plates placed near outlets of the air-handling system and exposed to the air currents within the ductwork of the system grew *Aspergillus* species in the outbreak of pneumonia due to these organisms in patients with acute leukemia.[44] The contaminated fireproofing material was felt to be the ultimate source of the *Aspergillus* spores which invaded the respiratory tract of the patients via the airborne route. In the outbreak of *Aspergillus fumigatus* pneumonia and tracheal colonization in renal transplant patients, cultures failed to implicate the ventilation system, and there was no fireproofing material applied above the patients' ward.[45] *A. fumigatus* was found in high concentrations by an air sampler in air obtained at and below a hospital renovation site but not on two distant wards. The earlier renovation of the ward above the renal transplant ward presumably had contaminated the transplant ward air with *A. fumigatus* spores derived from the contaminated dust found above the transplant ward's false ceiling, and these spores then had invaded the patients' respiratory tracts via the airborne route. Accounts of this earlier renovation stated that visible quantities of dust had filtered down through pores in the false ceiling tiles and settled in the corridors and patient rooms of the transplant ward. Thus, although the air is usually not a prominent mode of transmission of infection in hospital acquired pneumonia, under certain circumstances it can be — and it should be — investigated in any extensive workup of an outbreak or when the situation in question clearly calls for such an investigation.

Predisposing Factors in the Acquisition of Pneumonia in the Hospital

The modern, complex hospital of today offers an array of potential risk factors for developing a hospital acquired pneumonia to patients entering it. These include admission to intensive care units, being in the critical period following general anesthesia for surgery, aspiration of gastric contents for a variety of reasons, compromise of host defense mechanisms from underlying illness or from treatment administered for an illness or condition, being bronchoscoped, or being exposed to the wide variety of equipment used in general anesthesia and respiratory therapy. Exposure to one or more of these risk factors significantly increases a patient's chances of contracting a hospital acquired pneumonia, as noted below. In addition, even entering the hospital with a community acquired pneumonia and being treated with antibiotics for it may increase a patient's risk of contracting a hospital acquired pneumonia. In a study in one hospital,[105] 59% of patients who were treated with antibiotics for community acquired pneumonia developed colonization of the respiratory tract with a new pathogen or pathogens. Seven percent of these colonized patients developed tracheobronchitis, and 18% developed one or more nosocomial pneumonias.

Intensive Care Units

Patients entering a medical intensive care unit were found to have a respiratory tract colonization rate by aerobic Gram-negative bacilli of 22% on the first hospital day.[3] This rate of colonization rose sharply over the first 4 days in the unit, then leveled off to a rate of about 45%. Colonization was shown to be significantly associated with the presence of coma, hypotension, expectoration of sputum, the use of endotracheal intubation, acidosis, azotemia, and either leukocytosis or leukopenia. The use of antimicrobial drugs was also significantly associated with colonization, but served primarily to increase the rate, since 70% of the patients who were colonized during or after antimicrobial therapy were already colonized before its institution. The incidence of hospital acquired pneumonia was much higher among colonized patients (23%) in comparison to noncolonized patients (3.3%).

In a newborn nursery, an additional risk factor was noted. Infants with low birth weight, defined as less than 1500 g, had a significantly higher rate of nosocomial infections overall, and 60% of the hospital acquired pneumonias were seen in this low-birth-weight group.[2] A number of host factors present in these smaller infants — including immature host-resistance mechanisms, the possible presence of such diseases as hyaline-membrane disease or congenital malformations, and the absence of a normal flora at birth to prevent or retard colonization with potential pathogens — may have contributed to their increased risk of acquiring nosocomial infections. As physical crowding of the nursery increased with less nursery space available per infant, the infection rate was noted to rise, perhaps related to clustering of high-risk infants or relative understaffing with resultant breaks in technique, increasing the risk of patient-to-patient spread of pathogens. When this increased infection rate was noted, the nursery was expanded with return of the space per infant to original levels; however, this did not lower the nosocomial infection rate.[2]

Postoperative Patients

Patients in the immediate postoperative period run an increased risk of hospital acquired pneumonia. Recent general anesthesia with its depressant effect on respiratory clearance mechanisms and the immobility, hypoventilation, sedation, and decreased cough and gag reflexes of postoperative patients all contribute to an increased likelihood of aspiration and development of pneumonia. Postoperative pneumonia is said to occur most frequently in patients with thoracic or high abdominal incisions, obesity, or chronic lung disease. Older patients and men are also at increased risk of developing postoperative pneumonia.[7] A more recent study suggests that only the extremes of very old age and massive obesity make these two risk factors important.[106] Additional risk factors delineated by this study were low preoperative serum albumin (less than 3.5 g/dℓ) and severity of other underlying diseases.

Aspiration of Gastric Contents

Patients who aspirate gastric contents with concomitant chemical insult to the tracheobronchial tree by stomach acid may subsequently develop pneumonia. The settings in which this event is most likely to occur are sedative drug overdose, obstetric or emergency general anesthesia, cerebrovascular accident, cardiopulmonary arrest, seizure disorder, alcohol intoxication, coma secondary to trauma, and metabolic cerebral dysfunction. When clear-cut aspiration of gastric contents occurs, signs of pulmonary derangement are virtually always present within 2 hr. If the chemical insult is sufficiently severe, death usually occurs within 24 hrs; those patients surviving the initial insult have clearing of pulmonary infiltrates in an average of 4 to 5 days. About 30% of these latter patients will go on to develop a superimposed bacterial pneumonia due to impaired pulmonary bacterial clearance from gastric acid damage to the tracheobronchial tree.[51]

The Compromised Host

A group of patients who are at special risk of contracting hospital acquired pneumonia due to unusual pathogens are those whose immune defenses are compromised. The immune defenses of these patients may be reduced due to their own underlying illnesses, such as leukemia, lymphoma, or diabetes mellitus, or may be iatrogenically reduced by administration of corticosteroids, cytotoxic drugs, or immunosuppressive agents used to treat various malignancies or to prevent rejection of organ transplants. Compromised hosts have been shown to be at increased risk of contracting pulmonary infections from herpes simplex virus, cytomegalovirus, and varicella-zoster virus; from fungi such as *Cryptococcus neoformans, Aspergillus, Phycomycetes, Candida albicans,* and *Coccidioides immitis;* from parasites such as *Pneumocytis carinii* and *Toxoplasma gondii;* and from higher bacteria such as Mycobacteria and Nocardia.[14,15] The exact incidences of these infections have not been defined nor has it been determined which are hospital acquired and which are community acquired but first manifest themselves in the hospital. In the case of *Legionella pneumophila,* it is clear that pneumonia due to this organism is solely hospital acquired in some cases, since the illness is contracted by both normal and compromised hosts.[93,95-98] To date, *L. micdadei* has been seen only in compromised hosts and its origin is still not clear.[99-101]

In some instances, the evidence for hospital acquisition has been relatively clear-cut. The *Aspergillus* outbreaks due to fireproofing material[44] and to hospital renovation[45] were clearly due to hospital acquisition of the organisms. Three cases of pulmonary Mucormycosis were seen in three patients, all of whom were receiving large doses of corticosteroids and were acidotic from acute renal failure and hyperglycemic from parenteral hyperalimentation.[52] Inhalation of airborne spores or aspiration of upper respiratory tract flora was thought probably to be the primary source of all three infections. Possible person-to-person spread of *P. carinii* infection was suggested in one cluster of 11 cases,[53] and the possibility of transmission of the organism within the hospital environment was cautiously proposed in another cluster of 10 cases.[54] Nevertheless, despite the propensity for compromised hosts to develop pulmonary infections due to unusual pathogens, it should not be forgotten that 90% of all episodes of hospital acquired pneumonia in these patients are caused by aerobic Gram-negative bacilli, virtually all of which are Enterobacteriaceae or *Pseudomonas* species.[6]

Bronchoscopy

A common hospital procedure which appears to carry with it some risk of hospital acquired pneumonia is fiberoptic bronchoscopy. Webb and Vall-Spinosa[55] reported three patients who developed pulmonary infections due to *Serratia marcescens* after multiple bronchoscopies with a flexible fiberoptic bronchoscope which had first been used on a patient with known *S. marcescens* pneumonia. All three patients infected by the bronchoscope had been receiving steroids and broad-spectrum antibiotics and had undergone tracheostomies for assisted ventilation prior to their bronchoscopies. The bronchoscope, which was routinely cleaned by suctioning of, first, sterile saline and then 70% alcohol through the aspiration channel, was clearly implicated as the cause of the outbreak. Switching to suctioning of an iodophor solution rendered the bronchoscope consistently culture negative. Pereira et al.[56] reported a series of 100 fiberoptic bronchoscopies performed in 95 patients and encountered a 16% risk of transient fever, a 6% risk of pulmonary infiltrates which may or may not have represented pneumonia, and one death due to a pneumonia distal to an obstructing carcinoma. Their cleaning method was similar to that of Webb and Vall-Spinosa, involving suctioning, first, of aqueous zephiran, then 70% alcohol.

On the other hand, Suratt et al.[57] reported no pneumonia in a retrospective examination of 103 patients bronchoscoped with an instrument presumably contaminated with *Pseudomonas aeruginosa,* as evidenced by an 80% culture positivity rate for the organism from the bronchial washings obtained from the patients. Their cleaning method consisted of an antibacterial soap-and-water-solution rinse, followed by a sterile water rinse. After a culture of the "disinfected" bronchoscope grew *P. aeruginosa,* they changed to an iodine-ethanol soak-cleaning method. After this change, the bronchoscope grew nothing, and 146 patients subsequently bronchoscoped and followed prospectively also developed no pneumonias.

Kellerhals[58] reported seven patients whose bronchoscopy cultures grew *S. marcescens* after the instrument was first used on a patient with an *S. marcescens* empyema; none of the seven developed pneumonia. The bronchoscope grew *S. marcescens* when tested after the eight patient cultures returned, suggesting that the iodophor cleaning method was ineffective and necessitating ethylene oxide gas sterilization of the instrument. However, it could not be determined if the iodophor cleaning method had been performed as recommended by the manufacturer. Thus, although trauma to the bronchial tree from the bronchoscope and impairment of host defenses by topical anesthetics and premedications would seem to increase the risk of hospital acquired pneumonia, the true rate is probably less than 1%.

Anesthesia and Respiratory Therapy Equipment

A great deal of attention has been focused on the equipment used in anesthesia and in respiratory therapy as risk factors in hospital acquired pneumonia. Wenzel et al.[59] have recently reviewed much of the literature on respiratory therapy equipment and outbreaks associated with it, with tables appended which analyze each article in detail.

The information in this section is derived in part from this source, which should be consulted if more detailed information on a particular topic is desired. Outbreaks of respiratory colonization, pneumonia, or infections at other sites, some of them fatal, have been associated with use of infant isolation incubators,[60] pulmonary resuscitation equipment,[31] oxygen analyzers,[61] respiratory tract suctioning equipment,[38,62] respirators,[34] various types of large-volume reservoir nebulizers,[32,63] and intermittent positive pressure breathing (IPPB) machines with medication nebulizers.[28,33] Close investigation of the outbreaks and examination of various types of equipment in clinical use have led to clarification of which practices and which pieces of equipment provide the greatest risks.

One outbreak associated with pulmonary resuscitation masks and Emerson bags resulted from failure to disinfect the equipment between patients.[31] The incidence of aerobic Gram-negative bacillary necrotizing pneumonia has been linked with the use of large-volume Venturi mainstream reservoir nebulizers, which inevitably and unavoidably become contaminated with these organisms and disseminate them to patients in the aerosols they deliver.[64,69] Spinning disk nebulizers[65] and ultrasonic nebulizers[32] have likewise been incriminated as delivering aerosols contaminated with these bacteria. Outbreaks associated with medication nebulizers on IPPB machines have resulted from introduction into the nebulizers of solutions from large-volume stock supply bottles which were contaminated with aerobic Gram-negative bacilli.[28,33] The IPPB machines then disseminated contaminated aerosols to patients.

Gases which enter respiratory therapy or anesthesia equipment do not influence the risk of hospital acquired pneumonia. When cultured, wall oxygen supplies, air from compressors, and oxygen and anesthesia gases from tanks are almost always sterile.[42,66-68] Hospital air contains small numbers of organisms,[46] but does not appear to contaminate ventilators sufficiently to cause them to disseminate significant numbers of bacteria to patients.[69] Gases exhausted from anesthesia machines do not appear to be significantly contaminated with bacteria.[68] Gases exhausted from ventilators in use on infected patients can spray out these organisms;[39] likewise, contaminated suction machines can emit heavy sprays of their contaminants,[38,62] and exhaust gases from IPPB machines can heavily contaminate the local environment with patient organisms.[70] This environmental contamination could theoretically lead to secondary transmission of infection via the hand-borne route, but it has never been conclusively demonstrated in a clinical situation.

The permanent internal parts of ventilators and anesthesia machines do not appear to become contaminated with pathogenic bacteria, probably because their dry surfaces do not promote bacterial growth.[68,71] The moisture which collects in the soda lime carbon dioxide absorbers of anesthesia machines does not appear to become contaminated, possibly because of the alkaline pH of the fluid.[68] The readily changeable parts of ventilators and anesthesia machines which connect to patients, such as flexible tubing, "Y" pieces, elbow unions, and face masks, do become contaminated with pathogenic bacteria,[72] and can transmit infection, including pneumonia, to patients if not sterilized — or at least disinfected — between patients.[71]

The greatest confusion about increased risk of hospital acquired pneumonia surrounds humidifiers and nebulizers simply because all too many workers in the field do not know the differences between the two. To avoid desiccating the tracheobronchial tree of patients receiving prolonged respiratory therapy, it is necessary to deliver moisture in the inspired gas. Humidifiers do this by producing moisture in vapor (i.e., molecular) form by passing gas over or bubbling it through liquid, which may or may not be heated. Nebulizers produce liquid in aerosol (i.e., droplet) form by use of the Venturi principle, by ultrasonic means using rapidly vibrating crystals, or by centrifugal force, using liquid dropped onto rapidly spinning disks. Nebulizers can therefore deliver more moisture than humidifiers. In addition, most humidifiers cannot be used in the very high flow rates achieved by IPPB machines.

Because pathogenic bacteria cannot be transported by molecules of water, humidifiers theoretically cannot carry pathogens to patients even if their reservoirs are heavily contaminated. In actual fact, some small amount of aerosol may be emitted by a humidifier, but actual measurements have demonstrated that the risk of a humidifier's emitting a contaminated effluent is extremely small.[67,73] Even the special Cascade humidifiers which can be used in the very high gas flow rates of IPPB machines emit effluents with a very low rate of contamination (comparable to ambient room air) unless their reservoirs are very heavily contaminated.[74] In contrast, the droplets of water in the aerosols generated by nebulizers in routine use tend to emit aerosols heavily contaminated with aerobic Gram-negative bacilli and would significantly increase the risk of hospital acquired pneumonia.[32,65,69] Whether or not a Venturi nebulizer emits a contaminated aerosol depends upon whether it is a large-volume mainstream reservoir nebulizer intended primarily for delivery of moisture to patients or whether it is a small-volume side-arm nebulizer intended only to deliver medications at intervals with IPPB therapy. The reservoirs of the large-volume mainstream Venturi nebulizers quickly become contaminated with aerobic Gram-negative bacilli and subsequently deliver heavily contaminated aerosols,[69] significantly increasing the risk of hospital acquired pneumonia in patients using them. The small-volume medication Venturi nebulizers do not pose any increased risk so long as the medications put into them are sterile.[75] Presumably they have time to dry out and thereby eliminate any acquired contamination between periods of use.

Patients receiving mechanical ventilatory assistance via nasotracheal, endotracheal, or tracheostomy tubes are not only devoid of upper airway defense mechanisms but also are predisposed to tracheal and bronchial injury from suctioning. The tubes may lead to inspissation and pooling of secretions, and to aspiration around the tubes of food, liquids, oral secretions, or gastric contents. Breaks in sterile technique during necessary suctioning also increase the risk of hospital acquired pneumonia. The overall risk of pneumonia for patients placed on respirators was 7% in one university hospital,[76] considerably higher than the 0.56% risk for all patients discharged from the NNIS hospitals.[1] By the nature of their combined risk factors, intubated patients on ventilatory assistance may prove to be the most fertile ground for an outbreak of hospital acquired pneumonia.

IDENTIFYING AND INVESTIGATING AN OUTBREAK OF HOSPITAL ACQUIRED PNEUMONIA

The recognition of the existence of an outbreak of hospital acquired pneumonia depends upon the recognition of an increased incidence of pulmonary infections in the hospital. This recognition may occur in several ways. Microbiology laboratory personnel may spot an increased incidence of pulmonary isolates of a particular pathogen. Alternatively, personnel in a given area of the hospital may note an increased incidence of pneumonia in patients in that area. However, both of these methods of recognition generally occur only with unusually alert personnel or in the face of grossly obvious situations. The best method of detecting an outbreak of hospital acquired pneumonia is to have an ongoing system of active surveillance for all hospital acquired infections in effect throughout the entire hospital (see chapter entitled "Surveillance and Reporting of Hospital Acquired Infections"). One or a number of methods[77,78] may be used.

Figure 1 shows an outline for an epidemiologic investigation of an outbreak of hos-

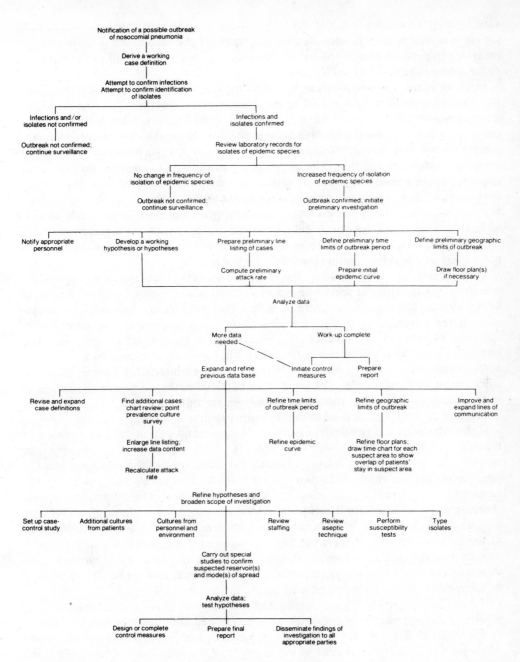

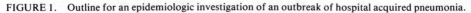

FIGURE 1.   Outline for an epidemiologic investigation of an outbreak of hospital acquired pneumonia.

pital acquired pneumonia. It is designed to describe the steps in the workup of an outbreak of bacterial nosocomial pneumonia, the usual situation which will be encountered. In the more unusual case of a viral, fungal, or parasitic nosocomial pneumonia, modifications may have to be made to fit the situation, based on reports in the literature of similar outbreaks or based on imagination and intuition if the situation is unique. The figure is divided roughly into two portions. The upper half outlines what is often informally referred to as a "quick and dirty" investigation, that is, one which is preliminary and not too detailed. This sort of investigation is often all that is necessary to bring an outbreak under control if the cause of the outbreak is a relatively simple one that is easy to identify and eliminate. If this is not the case, it may be necessary to perform most or all of the detailed steps in the lower half of the figure in order to bring the outbreak under control.

In either event, the investigation begins with the recognition or notification of the existence of a possible outbreak of hospital acquired pneumonia. The first step is to derive a working definition of a case of nosocomial pneumonia. Case definitions generally have both a clinical and a laboratory portion. Thus, the clinical portion might consist simply of a new pulmonary infiltrate on chest X-ray associated with new or increased sputum production. The laboratory portion might consist of an associated sputum culture growing a potential pathogen. Under certain conditions, the clinical portion may need to be more comprehensive. Recognition that up to 20% of severely neutropenic patients may not ever develop an infiltrate on chest X-ray during an episode of aerobic Gram-negative bacillary pneumonia[6] may lead to the inclusion of additional clinical criteria such as fever or the presence of rales and to the exclusion of production of a purulent sputum or of any sputum at all.

The next step is to confirm the existence of the outbreak. Pseudoepidemics do occur, primarily due to errors in specimen processing, but also due to clinical misdiagnoses or surveillance artifacts (e.g., failure to differentiate community acquired from hospital acquired infections or failure to review records carefully enough to show that an apparent increase in an infection rate is actually not an increase above endemic levels).[79] Using the working case definition, all apparent cases should be investigated by reviewing their charts to determine if they are indeed infected. Likewise, the identification of all known isolates of the suspect bacterial pathogen should be confirmed in the laboratory. If either infections or isolates are not confirmed, there is no outbreak, and no further steps need to be taken other than to continue surveillance.

If the infections and isolates are confirmed. the second step in the confirmation of the outbreak is to review the laboratory records for all recent isolates of the epidemic species. The definition of "recent" is somewhat arbitrary but should encompass the time period during which all known cases occurred. This review may reveal further cases and possibly enlarge the time span of the epidemic. The laboratory records should also be reviewed for a period of several months prior to the suspect epidemic period to determine if there has actually been an increase in the frequency of isolation of the epidemic species. If there has been no significant increase in frequency (and it may be necessary to do appropriate statistical tests to prove lack or presence of significance of change in frequency), then there is no outbreak, and no further steps need be taken other than to continue surveillance.

If there has been a significant increase in the frequency of isolation of the epidemic species, then the presence of the outbreak is confirmed and the preliminary investigation is initiated. Several steps must be taken virtually simultaneously. First, all appropriate personnel and groups must be made aware of the situation.[80] These include the microbiology laboratory staff and director, the hospital epidemiologist, the chairperson of the infection control committee, the Infectious Disease Service, the hospital administration, nursing personnel of the involved areas, and the infection control practitioners. Most — or even all — of these persons may already be involved to some extent, but all should be fully informed at this point and should be kept fully informed as the investigation progresses.

The microbiology laboratory should be asked to preserve all isolates of the epidemic species still in its possession and to preserve all future isolates collected. Records should be reviewed to detect all isolates of the epidemic species from all body sites, and the investigation may have to be broadened to include outbreaks in other body systems and in other areas of the hospital not previously known to be involved. The antibiotic susceptibility pattern, or antibiogram, should be recorded from all suspect epidemic species. An unusual or distinctive antibiogram may help differentiate the true epidemic species from other strains of the same bacterial species which have been isolated from patients during the same time period. Such a method of subtyping a bacterial species may help clarify the epidemiology of the outbreak considerably.

Another potentially helpful subtyping tool readily available from the laboratory is the pattern of biochemical reactions seen with the epidemic strain. If unusual, this pattern, known as the biotype, may be as helpful as the antibiogram. If one of the commercially available microtubule bacterial identification systems is used in the laboratory, a distinctive biotype may be recognized and manifested as a distinctive identification code number for the epidemic strain.

Finally, the laboratory should assist in determining what further culturing of patients (or of personnel and environment, if necessary) need to be performed, and by whom, and when, and how much and what kinds of media need to be used. Clearly, some of these activities belong more properly in the category of the more detailed, indepth investigation rather than of a "quick and dirty" one, but the line between the two is entirely arbitrary, and the situation at hand dictates how far the investigation should be carried in any area. The division in the outline is primarily to make the explanation of the various aspects of the investigation easier.

The parts of the basic data base relating to patients should be organized along certain specified lines as well in order to clarify further the epidemiology of the outbreak. Further chart reviewing or interviews with personnel in affected areas may uncover additional cases not detected in the microbiology records review. A line listing of cases should be made, consisting of a list of names of all suspect cases with appropriate associated data which might help solve the outbreak. These data should include such basic information as hospital number; age; sex; dates of admission, discharge, or death; hospital service and areas where the patient stayed; underlying illnesses; types and dates of instrumentation; risk factors present; and all culture results with antibiogram and biotypes if applicable. From these data can be calculated the attack rate, defined as the number of cases of infection divided by the number of persons at risk of becoming infected. A low attack rate may suggest an organism of low virulence or that conditions favorable for acquiring infections occur infrequently, while a high attack rate may indicate the opposite.

The rough time limits of the outbreak should be determined, beginning with the first recognized case of the epidemic and ending with the last, or the most recent if the outbreak is still ongoing. An epidemic curve should be constructed, with cases plotted on a graph by date of onset of infection. A clustering of cases in a narrow range of dates suggests an oubreak due to a common source which infected patients only over a brief time period. Spreading out of cases over a long time period suggests a continuing source of infection or infection propagated from patient to patient or both.

It is also necessary to examine the geographic limits of the outbreak to see if transmission of infection is related to location of cases. Outbreaks of hospital acquired pneumonia are frequently confined to an intensive care unit or a single ward, and determining that that is the the case may allow the investigation to focus on events in that one area. Drawing a floor plan of the area and plotting the location of cases on it may help determine if a particular location on a ward or unit is of singularly high risk. Alternatively, an outbreak may be so diffuse that drawing a floor plan is pointless. This also may be a useful clue, suggesting the possible presence of some unusual factor in the outbreak, different from the more common, patient-to-patient-via-hands-of-personnel type of spread of infection.

During the collection and organization of these preceding data, a hypothesis — or, occasionally, hypotheses — as to the cause of the outbreak usually emerge. Analysis of the accumulated data is performed to test the strength of the hypothesis, and if it seems likely, appropriate control measures are instituted. If the outbreak ceases, the hypothesis is confirmed, the workup is complete, and a final report may be prepared.

Although institution of control measures is placed at the end of this preliminary chain of investigation, in actual fact any appropriate control measure should be instituted as soon as the need for it appears during the investigation. For example, if it appeared that in the initial line listing, all of the cases had had fiberoptic bronchoscopy before contracting pneumonia, the hypothesis immediately suggested would be that bronchoscopy was causing the pulmonary infections. The immediate control measure to institute would be to stop performing bronchoscopies pending investigation of the apparatus. If the geographic analysis implicated no special high-risk ward or unit in the hospital and if the epidemic curve by chance indicated no cases occurring in proximity to a time when the bronchoscope was being repaired and was therefore not in use, the circumstantial evidence would strengthen the case against the instrument. In this hypothetical example, if the epidemic organism were isolated from the bronchoscope and improved disinfection methods eliminated the contamination and curtailed the outbreak, the hypothesis would be confirmed and the investigation would be complete. The initial control measure — cessation of use of the instrument — would be the first step in terminating the outbreak, and the final control measure — elimination of contamination — would finally terminate the outbreak.

In some outbreaks, the need for more data becomes obvious or the necessity for broadening the scope of the investigation becomes apparent when initial control measures prove partially or completely ineffective. An example of this situation might be in an outbreak in an intensive care unit, where the first thought would be to tighten up on sterile technique used on patients by personnel. If this measure had little or no effect on the infection rate, the necessity for a more intensive investigation would become obvious.

First of all, the basic data base might be revised and expanded. Case definitions could be expanded to include three categories: (1) pneumonia, defined as new pulmonary infiltrates on chest X-ray associated with fever and purulent sputum growing the epidemic organism, (2) tracheobronchitis, defined as fever and purulent sputum growing the epidemic organism without any pulmonary infiltrates, and (3) colonization, defined as isolation of the epidemic organism from sputum without evidence of infection. These expanded definitions would cause the inclusion of new cases and lead to review of their charts. Performing a point prevalence culture survey of the respiratory tract of all patients in the suspect area might well lead to the discovery of further unsuspected cases, especially colonizations. This would lead to enlargement of the line listing, its data base could well be enlarged, and the attack rate would have to be recalculated.

This additional information would lead to a refinement of the time limits of the outbreak period and a new, expanded epidemic curve. The geographic limits of the outbreak might well be expanded with preparation of new or additional floor plans. Figure 2 shows the sort of time-bed occupancy chart that might be prepared for patients occupying a single suspect area. A patient's stay is plotted as a linear line stretching from day of entry into the area to day of departure. All positive cultures of infections and colonizations can be plotted on it for each patient, and the resulting pattern may indicate whether or not patient-to-patient spread is conceivable. As this refinement of the previous data base is being carried out, previous lines of communication with other interested parties should be maintained or expanded, and new ones should be opened as necessary.

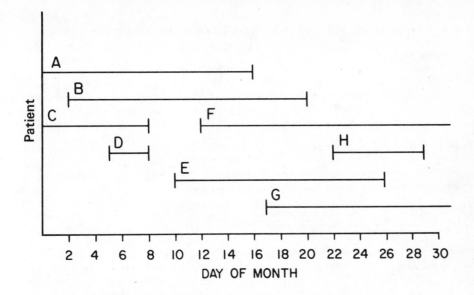

FIGURE 2. Time-bed occupancy chart of a hypothetical four-bed patient unit, showing the overlap of stay of the eight patients (A through H) who occupied beds in it during the month illustrated. From two to four patients occupy the unit on any given day.

The scope of the epidemic investigation should also be broadened which would allow the refinement of previous hypotheses and the development of new ones. Selection of a control group of patients who were admitted at the same time as cases, but who did not become colonized or infected, or selection of a control group of patients carefully matched with cases for certain criteria such as age, sex, and underlying diagnoses, might add an indispensable dimension to the investigation of an outbreak. Careful statistical comparison of differences between cases and controls for various risk factors might reveal the critical one which, when present, led to acquisition of respiratory tract colonization or infection.

Additional cultures of multiple sites in patients, as outlined in Table 1 or of various sites in personnel and the environment, as outlined in Tables 2 and 3, might be obtained. These tables are not all-inclusive, but do offer a guide to sites that might be considered for culture to determine possible reservoirs of epidemic strains or the kinetics of acquisition of these strains by patients. The method of culture and media used for it depend on the source of the culture and growth requirements of the organism. Dry swabs may be used for moist surfaces. Dry surfaces may be cultured with sterile swabs moistened in sterile saline or broth, then planted on or into appropriate culture media. When samples cultured in broth may contain residual disinfectant, the broth should contain 0.07% lecithin and 0.5% polysorbate-80 as neutralizers.[81] Letheen broth used for liquid soap or hand lotion already contains such neutralizers. Other liquids may be cultured by filtration and culture of the filter on agar or in broth, or by adding double-strength broth to a sample of liquid. Air can be cultured by settling plates or by commercial air samplers. Selective media containing appropriate antibiotics or other inhibiting substances may be used to inhibit growth of contaminating organisms, thereby selecting for the epidemic strain.

Staffing levels in appropriate areas should be reviewed. Mayhall et al.[42] have documented the temporal relationship between sharp falls in staffing levels and increases in breaks in sterile technique and concomitant increases in infection rates in a burn unit. Review of turnover in personnel may yield clues as to personnel morale and their

Table 1
SUGGESTED SITES FOR CULTURES FROM PATIENTS

Site	Method	Comments
Nares	Sterile swabs for bacteria Phosphate buffered saline (PBS) wash for viruses	Swab anterior one third of both nares Rinse and withdraw 3 mℓ of PBS from each nostril using a small bulb syringe; culture by the method of Hall and Douglas[9]
Pharynx	Sterile swabs	Plating first, then dropping swab tip into broth for enrichment culture adds considerable sensitivity[19]
Endotracheal tubes	Suction sputum with sterile catheter into trap	
Stool or rectal	Standard procedure for collection of stool specimens; sterile swab for rectal culture	Rectal culture is much easier and probably as good; swab may be moistened with sterile saline
Stomach	Aspirate from nasogastric tube	Perform only if paralytic ileus present
Hands	Sterile swabs	Swab palmar surfaces of both hands, fingertips; moisten swabs with sterile saline or broth
	Large (150 × 15 mm) agar plates	Press palmar surface of each hand lightly to surface of agar; a difficult method as subjects may crush agar or push it out of plate
	Broth rinse	Rub hands together in broth contained in sterile plastic bag or pan; this may be done semiquantitatively[30]
Umbilicus; wounds	Sterile swabs	Umbilicus cultures useful in newborn infants only; moisten swabs with sterile saline if necessary (broth should probably not be applied to wounds or mucosal surfaces)

overall level of experience. Review of aseptic techniques as written in protocols and as actually practiced should be carried out with upgrading of both as necessary. Antibiotic susceptibility tests should be performed on all isolates of epidemic strains not previously tested if the antibiogram appears to be a useful epidemiologic marker.

Better epidemiologic markers are provided by determination of phage types, serotypes, or bacteriocin types if appropriate and available for the epidemic species. It may be necessary to turn to research laboratories or to local, state, or national reference laboratories for these tests or such tests as electron capture gas chromatography,[85] or isolation and restriction endonuclease analysis of plasmids contained in epidemic strains.[107,108] Special studies involving multiple cultures and intensive observation may be necessary to confirm suspected reservoirs of infection and modes of spread.

Finally, all of the above data should be analyzed and the hypotheses should be tested. Hopefully, if the investigation has been thorough and painstaking enough, it should then be possible to complete previous control measures or design new ones and terminate the outbreak. The final report should then be prepared and the findings disseminated to all appropriate parties, not the least of whom are those personnel who are primarily responsible for implementing the control measures and on whose shoulders rest the responsibility of preventing a recurrence of the problem.

PREVENTION OF HOSPITAL ACQUIRED PNEUMONIA

It is impossible to achieve the complete prevention of hospital acquired pneumonia.

Table 2
SUGGESTED SITES FOR CULTURES FROM PERSONNEL

Site	Method	Comments
Hair	Rodac plates	
Nares	Sterile swabs for bacteria	Swab anterior one third of both nares
	Phosphate buffered saline (PBS) wash for viruses	Rinse and withdraw 3 ml of PBS from each nostril using a small bulb syringe; culture by the method of Hall and Douglas[9]
Pharynx	Sterile swabs	Plating first, then dropping swab tip into broth for enrichment culture adds considerable sensitivity[19]
Vagina	Sterile swabs	
Stool or rectal	Standard procedure for collection of stool specimens; sterile swab for rectal culture	Rectal culture is much easier and probably as good; personnel may obtain their own rectal cultures; swab may be moistened with sterile saline
Hands	Sterile swabs	Swab palmar surfaces of both hands, fingertips; moisten swabs with sterile saline or broth
	Large (150 × 15 mm) agar plates	Press palmar surface of each hand lightly to surface of agar; a difficult method as subjects may crush agar or push it out of plate
	Broth rinse	Rub hands together in broth contained in sterile plastic bag or pan; this may be done semiquantitatively[30]

Nevertheless, a number of recommendations may be made which can help to decrease its incidence. A review of the equipment used in anesthesia and respiratory therapy has led to a number of specific recommendations involving such apparatus.[59] The most general statement that can be made in this area is that, while there is no firm evidence to suggest that sterilization of equipment offers a greater margin of safety than disinfection, prudence would favor sterilization.

There is no need to filter air or gas entering respirators or anesthesia equipment[59] nor does there appear to be a need to change the soda lime canisters in the carbon dioxide trap on anesthesia equipment between each case.[68] Changing these canisters after use with a known infected patient is commendable, although it may not be necessary; changing them only as they wear out probably suffices. Sterilization of the inside of anesthesia machines between patients appears to be unnecessary,[68] and the same is true for ventilators,[59,71] although the practice cannot be criticized. Disinfection of the external surfaces of these machines is not clearly necessary but may help prevent secondary hard-borne spread of infection.[71] A somewhat stronger case can be made for filtering exhaust air from ventilators or IPPB machines, especially to prevent environmental contamination[70] and secondary spread of infection.

Equipment such as tubing, face masks, etc., which comes into direct contact with patients should be replaced every 24 hr with fresh sterile or thoroughly disinfected items for each patient and should always be sterilized or thoroughly disinfected before use on another patient.[59] Sterilization is clearly preferable to disinfection in this case. Disposable equipment should never be resterilized after use for reuse as a money-saving maneuver.

All respiratory therapy equipment should be carefully handled, with strict attention paid to sterile technique where required. Fluids and medications used in this equipment should be sterile, preferably of small volume, and for individual use only. Humidifiers

Table 3

SUGGESTED SITES FOR CULTURES FROM THE ENVIRONMENT

Site	Method	Comments

Around patients' beds
  Bedside tables
  Bedrails
  Bed linen
  Cubicle curtains
  Sphygmomanometers
  Stethoscopes
  I.V. poles
  Urinals
  Bedpans
	Sterile swabs	Moisten swabs with sterile saline or broth

Other areas (excluding sinks)
  Door handles
  Bed scales
  Wheelchairs
  Stretchers
  Counter tops
	Sterile swabs	Moisten swabs with sterile saline or broth

Sink areas
  Faucet handles
  Basins
  Drains
	Sterile swabs	Moisten swabs with sterile saline or broth

Faucet aerators	Drop discs in broth	Remove discs from aerator with sterile forceps
Respiratory therapy equipment	Culture respirator output on agar plates	Ryan and Mihalyi[82] have described a simple technique; Lareau et al.[83] recommend the method of Edmondson and Sanford[84] for lower flow rate pediatric ventilators
	Culture water from nebulizers and humidifiers in broth or by filtration	Add water to equal volume of double strength broth or filter water and culture filters on agar or in broth

Liquids
  Saline for irrigation;
  stock solutions for
  respiratory therapy
	Broth or filtration	

Soap from dispensers	Inoculate sample into Letheen Broth (normal strength)	Mix well with broth
Hand lotion	Inoculate sample into Letheen Broth (normal strength)	Mix well with broth; for quantitative cultures an aliquot of broth may be added to pour plates prior to incubation
Air	Settling plates or one of a variety of commercially available air samplers	

are safe and require only cleaning and sterilization between patients, although daily replacement with a fresh sterile unit cannot be criticized. Careful aseptic technique should be observed in refilling their reservoirs, and remaining fluid should be discarded before new fluid is added.

Neither spinning disc[65] nor ultrasonic[32] nebulizers can easily be disinfected; their use should be abandoned in favor of a large-volume mainstream Venturi nebulizer or a Cascade nebulizer if nebulizers are required. In the past, regular disinfection of the large-volume mainstream nebulizers has been tried by nebulizing 0.25% acetic acid through them daily; this method has been consistently effective in the hands of only one group.[64] Placing copper sponges in the reservoirs has maintained sterility of the fluid in the hands of some groups,[70,86] but contamination of the aerosol with copper is a theoretic problem and may be harmful. In addition, normal saline placed in the reservoir may neutralize the effect of the copper for reasons that are unknown.[86] The safest method of handling these units is replacement with a fresh sterile one daily. The same precautions that apply to replenishing humidifier reservoir fluid apply even more forcefully here. The Venturi medication nebulizers should be filled only with sterile medications from small-volume bottles and should be allowed to dry thoroughly between each use.

Probably little can be done to decrease pharyngeal colonization of patients with aerobic Gram-negative bacilli, although such research should be encouraged. One method that should not be used is aerosolization of antibiotics into the pharynx; this favors the emergency of antibiotic-resistant bacteria and may thereby lead to increased mortality from hospital acquired pneumonia.[40,87,88] A vaccine is now commercially available for the 14 most prevalent pneumococcal serotypes; it will have more impact on the prevention of community acquired pneumonia than of hospital acquired pneumonia. However, development of vaccines for certain aerobic Gram-negative rods, especially *P. aeruginosa* and *K. pneumoniae* might help.[7]

General measures such as proper handwashing techniques,[89] sufficient space and personnel for each hospitalized patient, and isolation of selected ill or high-risk patients remain extremely important in the control of hospital acquired pneumonia and of all nosocomial infections. The keystone remains an effective nosocomial infection surveillance program to determine endemic infection rates and to allow identification of outbreaks or high-risk areas or procedures so that they may be dealt with appropriately.

REFERENCES

1. Center for Disease Control, National Nosocomial Infections Study Report, Annual Summary 1976, Center for Disease Control, Atlanta, February 1978.
2. Hemming, V. G., Overall, J. C., Jr., and Britt, M. R., Nosocomial infections in a newborn intensive-care unit: results of forty-one months of surveillance, *N. Engl. J. Med.*, 294, 1310, 1976.
3. Johanson, W. G., Jr., Pierce, A. K., Sanford, J. P., and Thomas, G. D., Nosocomial respiratory infections with gram-negative bacilli: the significance of colonization of the respiratory tract, *Ann. Intern. Med.*, 77, 701, 1972.
4. Stevens, R. M., Teres, D., Skillman, J. J., and Feingold, D. S., Pneumonia in an intensive care unit: a 30-month experience, *Arch. Intern. Med.*, 134, 106, 1974.
5. Hall, C. B., Douglas, R. G., Jr., Geiman, J. M., and Messner, M. K., Nosocomial respiratory syncytial virus infections, *N. Engl. J. Med.*, 293, 1343, 1975.
6. Valdivieso, M., Gil-Extremera, B., Zornoza, J., Rodriguez, V., and Bodey, G. P., Gram-negative bacillary pneumonia in the compromised host, *Medicine (Baltimore)*, 56, 241, 1977.
7. Stamm, W. E., Martin, S. M., and Bennett, J. V., Epidemiology of nosocomial infections due to gram-negative bacilli: aspects relevant to development and use of vaccines, *J. Infect. Dis.*, 136 (suppl.), S151, 1977.
8. Graybill, J. R., Marshall, L. W., Charache, P., Wallace, C. K., and Melvin, V. B., Nosocomial pneumonia: a continuing major problem, *Am. Rev. Respir. Dis.*, 108, 1130, 1973.
9. Hall, C. B. and Douglas, R. G., Jr., Nosocomial influenza infection as a cause of intercurrent fevers in infants, *Pediatrics*, 55, 673, 1975.
10. Wenzel, R. P., Deal, E. C., and Hendley, J. O., Hospital-acquired viral respiratory illness on a pediatric ward, *Pediatrics*, 60, 367, 1977.
11. Gardner, P. S., Court, S. D. M., Brocklebank, J. T., Downham, M. A. P. S., and Weightman, D., Virus cross-infection in paediatric wards, *Br. Med. J.*, 2, 571, 1973.

12. O'Keefe, J. P., Bartlett, J. G., Tally, F. P., and Gorbach, S. L., An heuristic approach to hospital-acquired pneumonia, *Clin. Res.*, 23, 589A, 1975.

13. Lorber, B. and Swenson, R. M., Bacteriology of aspiration pneumonia: a prospective study of community- and hospital-acquired cases, *Ann. Intern. Med.*, 81, 329, 1974.

14. Williams, D. M., Krick, J. A., and Remington, J. S., Pulmonary infection in the compromised host. I, *Am. Rev. Respir. Dis.*, 114, 359, 1976.

15. Williams, D. M., Krick, J. A., and Remington, J. S., Pulmonary infection in the compromised host. II, *Am. Rev. Respir. Dis.*, 114, 593, 1976.

16. Tillotson, J. R. and Lerner, A. M., Characteristics of pneumonias caused by *Escherichia coli*, *N. Engl. J. Med.*, 277, 115, 1967.

17. Teplitz, C., Pathogenesis of *Pseudomonas* vasculitis and septic lesions, *Arch. Pathol.*, 80, 297, 1965.

18. Johanson, W. G., Pierce, A. K., and Sanford, J. P., Changing pharyngeal bacterial flora of hospitalized patients: emergence of gram-negative bacilli, *N. Engl. J. Med.*, 281, 1137, 1969.

19. Rosenthal, S. and Tager, I. B., Prevalence of gram-negative rods in the normal pharyngeal flora, *Ann. Intern. Med.*, 83, 355, 1975.

20. Mackowiak, P. A., Martin, R. M., Jones, S. R., and Smith, J. W., Pharyngeal colonization by gram-negative bacilli in aspiration-prone persons, *Arch. Intern. Med.*, 138, 1224, 1978.

21. Valenti, W. M., Trudell, R. G., and Bentley, D. W., Factors predisposing to oropharyngeal colonization with gram-negative bacilli in the aged, *N. Engl. J. Med.*, 298, 1108, 1978.

22. Pierce, A. K. and Sanford, J. P., Aerobic gram-negative bacillary pneumonias, *Am. Rev. Respir. Dis.*, 110, 647, 1974.

23. Selden, R., Lee, S., Wang, W. L. L., Bennett, J. V., and Eickhoff, T. C., Nosocomial *Klebsiella* infections: intestinal colonization as a reservoir, *Ann. Intern. Med.*, 74, 657, 1971.

24. Schwartz, S. N., Dowling, J. N., Benkovic, C., DeQuittner-Buchanan, M., Prostko, T., and Yee, R. B., Sources of gram-negative bacilli colonizing the tracheae of intubated patients, *J. Infect. Dis.*, 138, 227, 1978.

25. Atherton, S. T. and White, D. J., Stomach as source of bacteria colonising respiratory tract during artificial ventilation, *Lancet*, 2, 968, 1978.

26. Rosendorf, L. L., Diacoff, G., and Baer, H., Sources of gram-negative infection after open-heart surgery, *J. Thorac. Cardiovasc. Surg.*, 67, 195, 1974.

27. Lowbury, E. J. L., Thom, B. T., Lilly, H. A., Babb, J. R., and Whittall, K., Sources of infection with *Pseudomonas aeruginosa* in patients with tracheostomy, *J. Med. Microbiol.*, 3, 39, 1970.

28. Sanders, C. V., Jr., Luby, J. P., Johanson, W. G., Jr., Barnett, J. A., and Sanford, J. P., *Serratia marcescens* infections from inhalation therapy medications: nosocomial outbreak, *Ann. Intern. Med.*, 73, 15, 1970.

29. Buxton, A. E., Anderson, R. L., Werdegar, D., and Atlas, E., Nosocomial respiratory tract infection and colonization with *Acinetobacter calcoaceticus*: epidemiologic characteristics, *Am. J. Med.*, 65, 507, 1978.

30. Stamm, W. E., Feeley, J. C., and Facklam, R. R., Wound infections due to group A *Streptococcus* traced to a vaginal carrier, *J. Infect. Dis.*, 138, 287, 1978.

31. Fierer, J., Taylor, P. M., and Gezon, H. M., *Pseudomonas aeruginosa* epidemic traced to delivery-room resuscitators, *N. Engl. J. Med.*, 276, 991, 1967.

32. Ringrose, R. E., McKown, B., Felton, F. G., Barclay, B. O., Muchmore, H. G., and Rhoades, E. R., A hospital outbreak of *Serratia marcescens* associated with ultrasonic nebulizers, *Ann. Intern. Med.*, 69, 719, 1968.

33. Mertz, J. J., Scharer, L., and McClement, J. H., A hospital outbreak of *Klebsiella* pneumonia from inhalation therapy with contaminated aerosol solutions, *Am. Rev. Respir. Dis.*, 94, 454, 1966.

34. Phillips, I. and Spencer, G., *Pseudomonas aeruginosa* cross-infection due to contaminated respiratory apparatus, *Lancet*, 2, 1325, 1965.

35. Salzman, T. C., Clark, J. J., and Klemm, L., Hand contamination of personnel as a mechanism of cross-infection in nosocomial infections with antibiotic-resistant *Escherichia coli* and *Klebsiella-Aerobacter*, *Antimicrob. Agents Chemother.*, 7, 97, 1967.

36. Knittle, M. A., Eitzman, D. V., and Baer, H., Role of hand contamination of personnel in the epidemiology of gram-negative nosocomial infections, *J. Pediatr.*, 86, 433, 1975.

37. Hendley, J. O., Wenzel, R. P., and Gwaltney, J. M., Jr., Transmission of rhinovirus colds by self-inoculation, *N. Engl. J. Med.*, 288, 1361, 1973.

38. Rubbo, S. D., Gardner, J. F., and Franklin, J. C., Source of *Pseudomonas aeruginosa* infection in premature infants, *J. Hyg. Camb.*, 64, 121, 1966.

39. Teres, D., Schweers, P., Bushnell, L. S., Hedley-Whyte, J., and Feingold, D. S., Sources of *Pseudomonas aeruginosa* infection in a respiratory/surgical intensive-therapy unit, *Lancet*, 1, 415, 1973.

40. Feeley, T. W., du Moulin, G. C., Hedley-Whyte, J., Bushnell, L. S., Gilbert, J. P., and Feingold, D. S., Aerosol polymyxin and pneumonia in seriously ill patients, *N. Engl. J. Med.*, 293, 471, 1975.

41. Ayliffe, G. A. J., Babb, J. R., Collins, B. J., Lowbury, E. J. L., and Newsom, S. W. B., *Pseudomonas aeruginosa* in hospital sinks, *Lancet*, 2, 578, 1974.
42. Mayhall, C. G., Lamb, V. A., Gayle, W. E., Jr., and Haynes, B. W., Jr., *Enterobacter cloacae* septicemia in a burn center: epidemiology and control of an outbreak, *J. Infect. Dis.*, 139, 166, 1979.
43. Mayhall, C. G., personal communication, 1979.
44. Aisner, J., Schimpff, S. C., Bennett, J. E., Young, V. M., and Wiernik, P. H., *Aspergillus* infections in cancer patients: association with fireproofing materials in a new hospital, *J.A.M.A.*, 235, 411, 1976.
45. Arnow, P. M., Andersen, R. L., Mainous, P. D., and Smith, E. J., Pulmonary aspergillosis during hospital renovation, *Am. Rev. Respir. Dis.*, 118, 49, 1978.
46. Green, V. M., Vesley, D., Bond R. G., and Michaelsen, G. S., Microbiological contamination of hospital air. I. Quantitative studies, *Appl. Microbiol.*, 10, 561, 1962.
47. Wenzel, R. P., Hunting, K. J., Osterman, C. A., and Sande, M. A., *Providencia stuartii*, a hospital pathogen: potential factors for its emergence and transmission, *Am. J. Epidemiol.*, 104, 170, 1976.
48. Veazey, J. M., Jr., Sande, M. A., Miller, L. S., Townsend, T. R., Brokopp, C. D., and Wenzel, R. P., Transmission of Gentamicin-Resistant *Klebsiella pneumoniae* and *Pseudomonas aeruginosa* in a Burn Unit, presented at the 17th Interscience Conference on Antimicrobial Agents and Chemotherapy, New York, October 12 to 14, 1977, 427.
49. Mortimer, E. A., Jr., Wolinsky, E., Gonzaga, A. J., and Rammelkamp, C. H., Jr., Role of airborne transmission in Staphylococcal infections, *Br. Med. J.*, 1, 319, 1966.
50. Grieble, H. G., Bird, T. J., Nidea, H. M., and Miller, C. A., Chute-hydropulping waste disposal system: a reservoir of enteric bacilli and *Pseudomonas* in a modern hospital, *J. Infect. Dis.*, 130, 602, 1974.
51. Bynum, L. J. and Pierce, A. K., Pulmonary aspiration of gastric contents, *Am. Rev. Respir. Dis.*, 114, 1129, 1976.
52. Agger, W. A. and Maki, D. G., Mucormycosis: a complication of critical care, *Arch. Intern. Med.*, 138, 925, 1978.
53. Singer, C., Armstrong, D., Rosen, P. P., and Schottenfeld, D., *Pneumocystis carinii* pneumonia: a cluster of eleven cases, *Ann. Intern. Med.*, 82, 772, 1975.
54. Ruebush, T. K., II, Weinstein, R. A., Baehner, R. L., Wolff, D., Bartlett, M., Gonzales-Crussi, F., Sulzer, A. J., and Schultz, M. G., An outbreak of Pneumocystis pneumonia in children with acute lymphocytic leukemia, *Am. J. Dis. Child.*, 132, 143, 1978.
55. Webb, S. F. and Vall-Spinosa, A., Outbreak of *Serratia marcescens* associated with the flexible fiberbronchoscope, *Chest*, 68, 703, 1975.
56. Pereira, W., Kovnat, D. M., Khan, M. A., Iacovino, J. R., Spivack, M. L., and Snider, G. L., Fever and pneumonia after flexible fiberoptic bronchoscopy, *Am. Rev. Respir. Dis.*, 112, 59, 1975.
57. Suratt, P. M., Gruber, B., Wellons, H. A., and Wenzel, R. P., Absence of clinical pneumonia following bronchoscopy with contaminated and clean bronchofiberscopes, *Chest*, 71, 52, 1977.
58. Kellerhals, S., A pseudo-outbreak of *Serratia marcescens* from a contaminated fiberbronchoscope, *Assoc. Pract. Infect. Control J.*, 6, 5, 1978.
59. Wenzel, R. P., Veazey, J. M., Jr., and Townsend, T. R., Role of the inanimate environment in hospital-acquired infections, in *Infection Control in Health Care Facilities: Microbiological Surveillance*, Cundy, K. R. and Ball, W., Eds., University Park Press, Baltimore, 1977, 71.
60. Hoffman, M. A. and Finberg, L., *Pseudomonas* infections in infants associated with high-humidity environments, *J. Pediatr.*, 46, 626, 1955.
61. Klick, J. M. and du Moulin, G. C., An oxygen analyzer as a source of *Pseudomonas*, *Anesthesiology*, 49, 293, 1978.
62. Becker, A. H., Infection due to *Proteus mirabilis* in newborn nursery, *Am. J. Dis. Child.*, 104, 69, 1962.
63. Moffet, H. L. and Allan, D., Colonization of infants exposed to bacterially contaminated mists, *Am. J. Dis. Child.*, 114, 21, 1967.
64. Pierce, A. K., Sanford, J. P., Thomas, G. D., and Leonard, J. S., Long-term evaluation of decontamination of inhalation-therapy equipment and the occurrence of necrotizing pneumonia, *N. Engl. J. Med.*, 282, 528, 1970.
65. Grieble, H. G., Colton, F. R., Bird, T. J., Toigo, A., and Griffith, L. G., Fine-particle humidifiers: source of *Pseudomonas aeruginosa* infections in a respiratory-disease unit, *N. Engl. J. Med.*, 282, 531, 1970.
66. Macpherson, C. R., Oxygen therapy: an unsuspected source of hospital infections?, *J.A.M.A.*, 167, 1083, 1958.
67. Moffet, H. L., Allan, D., and Williams, T., Survival and dissemination of bacteria in nebulizers and incubators, *Am. J. Dis. Child.*, 114, 13, 1967.
68. du Moulin, G. C. and Saubermann, A. J., The anesthesia machine and circle system are not likely to be sources of bacterial contamination, *Anesthesiology*, 47, 353, 1977.

69. **Reinarz, J. A., Pierce, A. K., Mays, B. B., and Sanford, J. P.,** The potential role of inhalation therapy equipment in nosocomial pulmonary infection, *J. Clin. Invest.,* 44, 831, 1965.
70. **Deane, R. S., Mills, E. L., and Hamel, A. J.,** Antibacterial action of copper in respiratory therapy apparatus, *Chest,* 58, 373, 1970.
71. Center for Disease Control, Recommendations for the Decontamination and Maintenance of Inhalation Therapy Equipment, for Training Purposes, Hospital Infections Branch, Bacterial Diseases Division, Bureau of Epidemiology, Center for Disease Control, Atlanta, June 1975.
72. **Meeks, C. H., Pembleton, W. E., and Hench, M. E.,** Sterilization of anesthesia apparatus, *J.A.M.A.,* 199, 276, 1967.
73. **Edmondson, E. B., Reinarz, J. A., Pierce, A. K., and Sanford, J. P.,** Nebulization equipment: a potential source of infection in gram-negative pneumonias, *Am. J. Dis. Child.,* 111, 357, 1966.
74. **Schulze, T., Edmondson, E. B., Pierce, A. K., and Sanford, J. P.,** Studies of a new humidifying device as a potential source of bacterial aerosols, *Am. Rev. Respir. Dis.,* 96, 517, 1967.
75. **Pierce, A. K. and Sanford, J. P.,** Bacterial contamination of aerosols, *Arch. Int. Med.,* 131, 156, 1973.
76. **Veazey, J. M., Jr. and Wenzel, R. P.,** Nosocomial Pneumonia, in *Principles and Practice of Infectious Diseases,* 1st ed., Mandell, G. L., Douglas, R. G., Jr., and Bennett, J. E., Eds., John Wiley & Sons, New York, 1979.
77. Center for Disease Control, Outline for surveillance and control of nosocomial infections, Hospital Infections Branch, Bacterial Diseases Division, Bureau of Epidemiology, Center for Disease Control, Atlanta, revised June 1972, reprinted November 1976.
78. **Wenzel, R. P., Osterman, C. A., Hunting, K. J., and Gwaltney, J. M., Jr.,** Hospital-acquired infections. I. Surveillance in a university hospital, *Am. J. Epidemiol.,* 103, 251, 1976.
79. **Weinstein, R. A. and Stamm, W. E.,** Pseudoepidemics in hospital, *Lancet,* 2, 862, 1977.
80. **Castle, M. and Mallison, G. F.,** Effective investigations of nosocomial outbreaks, *Assoc. Pract. Infect. Control J.,* 5, 13, 1977.
81. **Weinstein, R. A. and Mallison, G. F.,** The role of the microbiology laboratory in surveillance and control of nosocomial infections, *Am. J. Clin. Pathol.,* 69, 130, 1978.
82. **Ryan, K. J. and Mihalyi, S. F.,** Evaluation of a simple device for bacteriological sampling of respirator-generated aerosols, *J. Clin. Microbiol.,* 5, 178, 1977.
83. **Lareau, S. C., Ryan, K. J., and Diener, C. F.,** The relationship between frequency of ventilator circuit changes and infectious hazard, *Am. Rev. Respir. Dis.,* 118, 493, 1978.
84. **Edmondson, E. B. and Sanford, J. P.,** Simple methods of bacteriologic sampling of nebulization equipment, *Am. Rev. Respir. Dis.,* 94, 450, 1966.
85. **Brooks, J. B., Kellogg, D. S., Alley, C. C., Short, H. B., Handsfield, H. H., and Huff, B.,** Gas chromatography as a potential means of diagnosing arthritis. I. Differentiation betwen Staphylococcal, Streptococcal, Gonococcal, and traumatic arthritis, *J. Infect. Dis.,* 129, 660, 1974.
86. **Hughes, R. L., Piergies, M., and Landau, W.,** The effects of copper in heated nebulizers, *Chest,* 69, 500, 1976.
87. **Greenfield, S., Teres, D., Bushnell, L. S., Hedley-Whyte, J., and Feingold, D. S.,** Prevention of gram-negative bacillary pneumonia using aerosol polymyxin as a prophylaxis. I. Effect on the colonization pattern of the upper respiratory tract of seriously ill patients, *J. Clin. Invest.,* 52, 2935, 1973.
88. **Klick, J. M., du Moulin, G. C., Hedley-Whyte, J., Teres, D., Bushnell, L. S., and Feingold, D. S.,** Prevention of gram-negative bacillary pneumonia using polymyxin aerosol as prophylaxis. II. Effect on the incidence of pneumonia in seriously ill patients, *J. Clin. Invest.,* 55, 514, 1975.
89. **Steere, A. C. and Mallison, G. F.,** Handwashing practices for the prevention of nosocomial infections, *Ann. Intern. Med.,* 83, 683, 1975.
90. **Fraser, D. W., Tsai, T. R., Orenstein, W., Parkin, W. E., Beecham, H. J., Sharrar, R. G., Harris, J., Mallison, G. F., Martin, S. M., McDade, J. E., Shepard, C. C., Brachman, P. S., and the Field Investigation Team,** Legionnaires' disease: description of an epidemic of pneumonia, *N. Engl. J. Med.,* 297, 1189, 1977.
91. **McDade, J. E., Shepard, C. C., Fraser, D. W., Tsai, T. R., Redus, M. A., Dowdle, W. R., and the Laboratory Investigation Team,** Legionnaires' disease: isolation of a bacterium and demonstration of its role in other respiratory disease, *N. Engl. J. Med.,* 297, 1197, 1977.
92. **Thacker, S. B., Bennett, J. V., Tsai, T. F., Fraser, D. W., McDade, J. E., Shepard, C. C., Williams, K. H., Jr., Stuart, W. H., Dull, H. B., and Eickhoff, T. C.,** An outbreak in 1965 of severe respiratory illness caused by the Legionnaires' disease bacterium, *J. Infect. Dis.,* 138, 512, 1978.
93. **Saravolatz, L. D., Burch, K. H., Fisher, E., Madhavan, T., Kiani, D., Neblett, T., and Quinn, E. L.,** The compromised host and Legionnaires' disease, *Ann. Intern. Med.,* 90, 533, 1979.
94. **Marks, J. S., Tsai, T. F., Martone, W. J., Baron, R. C., Kennicott, J., Holtzhauer, F. J., Baird, I., Fay, D., Feeley, J. C., Mallison, G. F., Fraser, D. W., and Halpin, T. J.,** Nosocomial Legionnaires' disease in Columbus, Ohio, *Ann. Intern. Med.,* 90, 565, 1979.

95. Haley, C. E., Cohen, M. L., Halter, J., and Meyer, R. D., Nosocomial Legionnaires' disease: a continuing common-source epidemic at Wadsworth Medical Center, *Ann. Intern. Med.*, 90, 583, 1979.

96. Kirby, B. D., Snyder, K. M., Meyer, R. D., and Finegold, S. M., Legionnaires' disease: report of sixty-five nosocomially acquired cases and review of the literature, *Medicine*, 59, 188, 1980.

97. Dondero, T. J., Jr., Rendtorff, R. C., Mallison, G. F., Weeks, R. M., Levy, J. S., Wong, E. W., and Schaffner, W., An outbreak of Legionnaires' disease associated with a contaminated air-conditioning cooling tower, *N. Engl. J. Med.*, 302, 365, 1980.

98. Tobin, J. O'H., Beare, J., Dunnill, M. S., Fisher-Hoch, S., French, M., Mitchell, R. G., Morris, P. J., and Muers, M. F., Legionnaires' disease in a transplant unit: isolation of the causative agent from shower baths, *Lancet*, 2, 118, 1980.

99. Pasculle, A. W., Myerowitz, R. L., and Rinaldo, C. R., Jr., New bacterial agent of pneumonia isolated from renal-transplant recipients, *Lancet*, 2, 58, 1979.

100. Myerowitz, R. L., Pasculle, A. W., Dowling, J. N., Pazin, G. J., Puerzer, M., Yee, R. B., Rinaldo, C. R., Jr., and Hakala, T. R., Opportunistic lung infection due to "Pittsburgh Pneumonia Agent", *N. Engl. J. Med.*, 301, 953, 1979.

101. Rogers, B. H., Donowitz, G. R., Walker, G. K., Harding, S. A., and Sande, M. E., Opportunistic pneumonia: a clinicopathological study of five cases caused by an unidentified acid-fast bacterium, *N. Engl. J. Med.*, 301, 959, 1979.

102. Johanson, W. G., Jr., Woods, D. E., and Chaudhuri, T., Association of respiratory tract colonization with adherence of gram-negative bacilli to epithelial cells, *J. Infect. Dis.*, 139, 667, 1979.

103. Johanson, W. G., Jr., Higuchi, J. H., Chaudhuri, T. R., and Woods, D. E., Bacterial adherence to epithelial cells in bacillary colonization of the respiratory tract, *Am. Rev. Respir. Dis.*, 121, 55, 1980.

104. Hall, C. B. and Douglas, R. G., Jr., Modes of spread of respiratory syncytial virus (RSV), *Pediatr. Res.*, 14, 558, 1980.

105. Tillotson, J. R. and Finland, M., Bacterial colonization and clinical superinfection of the respiratory tract complicating antibiotic treatment of pneumonia, *J. Infect. Dis.*, 119, 597, 1969.

106. Garibaldi, R. A. and Britt, M. R., Risk Factors for Postoperative Pneumonias, presented at the 2nd Int. Conf. on Nosocomial Infections, Atllanta, August 5 to 8, 1980.

107. Markowitz, S. M., Veazey, J. M., Jr., Macrina, F. L., Mayhall, C. G., and Lamb, V. A., Sequential outbreaks of infection due to *Klebsiella pneumoniae* in a neonatal intensive care unit: implication of a conjugative R plasmid, *J. Infect. Dis.*, 142, 106, 1980.

108. Goldmann, D. A. and Macone, A. B., A microbiologic approach to the investigation of bacterial nosocomial infection outbreaks, *Infect. Control*, 1, 391, 1980.

EPIDEMIC NOSOCOMIAL BACTEREMIAS

Dennis G. Maki

As for man, his days are as grass;
as a flower of the field, so he flourisheth;
the wind passeth over it, and it is gone.
Psalm 103:15,16

No infection, with the possible exception of meningitis, evokes greater awe and respect than bacteremia — in the lay jargon, "blood poisoning". Life-threatening bacterial infections of all types typically express themselves early with invasion of the bloodstream. Despite major advances in almost every aspect of therapeutic medicine and the availability of an ever-expanding armamentarium of potent antimicrobial drugs effective against nearly every nosocomial bacterial and fungal pathogen, nearly one half of patients developing bacteremia in the hospital die as a direct or indirect consequence of the infection. A case of bacteremia constitutes a clinical emergency — a cluster of nosocomial cases, an even greater emergency epidemiologically.

Because the diagnosis of bacteremia requires laboratory confirmation that microorganisms are present in the bloodstream, data on bacteremic infections are, as a rule, highly reliable epidemiologically and provide one of our most accurate measures of the present-day problem with nosocomial infection as a whole. Over 100 outbreaks of bacteremic nosocomial infection have been reported in the past two decades; while they are being identified and reported in ever-increasing numbers, the actual occurrence of epidemics of nosocomial bacteremia is probably also truly rising. Recent outbreaks have involved multiple hospitals and assumed national scope.

The goals of this chapter are the following: (1) to define and characterize the problem of nosocomial bacteremia, particularly occurring in epidemic proportions, and (2) to provide a rational, step-by-step approach to the evaluation of a suspected outbreak.

BASIC CONCEPTS AND DEFINITIONS

Bacteremia is defined classically as the presence of bacteria in the bloodstream, as documented by culture or by histopathologic examination. The term bacteremia is often used more broadly (and will be used in this chapter) to also include fungemia, the presence of fungi in the blood.

Whereas it is clear that bacteremia, especially when it is transient, such as when it arises from a dental extraction, is often clinically asymptomatic, in the hospital setting bacteremia is usually associated with clinical signs and symptoms (e.g., fever, chills, or hypotension) or laboratory evidence (e.g., leukocytosis or acid-base abnormalities) suggestive of bloodstream infection; clinically symptomatic bacteremia is referred to as septicemia. In this chapter, the two terms will be used interchangeably. *Sepsis* is a less precise term which refers to a constellation of clinical signs and symptoms suggesting systemic infection, vis-a-vis bacteremia.

Not all blood cultures showing growth of microorganisms represent true bacteremia, the presence of those same microorganisms in the patient's bloodstream. Approximately 5% of positive blood cultures in most hospitals are ultimately judged to be contaminated — by microorganisms introduced during the drawing of the blood culture or during its processing in the laboratory. In most of these cases, only one of multiple blood cultures is positive, usually with a skin commensal such as *Staphylococ-*

cus epidermidis, Bacillus species, or a diphtheroid, in which instance it is easily recognized as a contaminant. If, on the other hand, multiple blood cultures from the same patient are positive, the relevance of the positive cultures must be established on clinical and epidemiologic grounds, and such judgments can sometimes be difficult. Clusters of contaminated blood cultures have given rise to the appellation *epidemic pseudobacteremias.*

The National Nosocomial Infection Surveillance Study of the Center for Disease Control (CDC) subdivides nosocomial bacteremias into two categories, *primary bacteremias* and *secondary bacteremias.*[1] Primary bacteremias are culture-documented bacteremias occurring in the absence of a recognized infection with the responsible pathogen at another (local anatomic) site, such as the urinary tract or a surgical wound; cases of bacteremia thought to be related to infusion therapy, in the absence of purulent (suppurative) thrombophlebitis, are considered as primary. Conversely, culture-documented bacteremia originating from an identifiable infection at a local anatomic site (e.g., the urinary tract) is regarded as a secondary bacteremia; bacteremias deriving from culture-proved purulent thrombophlebitis are also considered as secondary bacteremias. This categorization is admittedly arbitrary, but necessary under the constrictions of the data submitted on many cases reported to the CDC. Whereas bacteremia occurring in severely compromised patients is often cryptogenic, such as those with leukemia and profound granulocytopenia, it is usually possible in most nosocomial cases to identify a local infection which gave rise to the bacteremia. Failure to obtain complete cultures or simply to report the originating source routinely obviously does not imply that a local source for a bacteremia does not exist.

Local infections involving vascular endothelium or the endocardium, usually associated wtih bacteremia, are termed *endovascular infections.* Many bacteremias originate from endovascular foci of infection (e.g., vascular cannulas) or subsequently produce endovascular infection (e.g., suppurative phlebitis or endocarditis). Endocarditis is a local infection of the inside of the heart, usually — but not inevitably — involving one or more heart valves and characterized histopathologically by aggregates of bacteria, platelets, and fibrin known as vegetations; untreated, it is uniformly lethal, death most often ensuing from destruction of vital intracardiac structures, the effects of systemic embolization or, simply, uncontrolled systemic infection. Similarly, infection of a vein segment, documented histopathologically, is called *septic* (or *suppurative) phlebitis* and of an artery, *septic endarteritis.*

Nosocomial infections are those infections that develop in the hospital that were not incubating at the time of admission or are caused by microorganisms that were acquired during a hospitalization.*[2]

Nosocomial infection in a population of patients is quantitated by the *rate* of infection, usually expressed as the number of cases per 100 individuals at risk (see chapter entitled "Surveillance and Reporting of Hospital Acquired Infections"). Nosocomial bacteremias, because they often occur at a lower frequency, are usually expressed as cases per 1000 (or 10,000) hospitalized patients. Based on analysis of data collected over an extended period of observation, nosocomial bacteremias can be shown to occur at a baseline or *endemic* rate (generally between 1 and 6 cases per 1000 patients hospitalized). Although the rate of nosocomial bacteremia typically fluctuates considerably from month to month, it should rarely exceed an "upper limit of normal" — the highest "acceptable" rate which can be determined statistically (e.g., the monthly mean + two standard deviations). A substantial increase in the rate above this level,

---

*   McGowan, Barnes, and Finland[3] have shown that the designation of all bacteremias as nosocomial in which the first positive blood culture was obtained on or after the third hospital day was 98.5% accurate.

especially if it is sustained, is defined as an *epidemic* (or an outbreak) and in the hospital usually indicates an epidemiologically relevant event or events, such as exposure of patients to a common source of contamination or lapses in aseptic technique, causing an increase in the rate of bacteremic infection; it is usually, but not inevitably, associated with a single (epidemic) microbial species. It may not be necessary to know the endemic rate of bacteremic infection accurately in order to detect a large epidemic or one caused by a single unusual species, but if an epidemic is small* or is caused by a common pathogen (e.g., *E. coli*) or multiple pathogens, or cases occur sporadically over a prolonged period of time, or occur in patients in widely separate areas of the hospital, an epidemic can easily remain unrecognized for prolonged periods without reliable baseline (endemic) data. The greatest potential benefit that theoretically derives from continuous surveillance of all nosocomial infections is the greater likelihood that epidemics, especially small ones, will be detected more rapidly. In a large outbreak in this country in 1970 to 1971 traced to the intrinsically contaminated infusion products of one manufacturer, affected hospitals experienced a rise in *Enterobacter* septicemias from approximately 2 per 1000 patients to nearly 20 per 1000 patients during the epidemic period, but because their laboratories did not speciate *Enterobacter* or carry out surveillance of bacteremic infections, some hospitals were unaware of major intrahospital outbreaks that were identified only in retrospect.[4]

Many endemic nosocomial infections and most hospital epidemics stem from exposure of susceptible patients to a source of microbial contamination in the hospital, for instance, a foodstuff, a medication, an infusion product, a ventilator, a dialysis machine, or a physician's hands, to name but a few of the innumerable potential hospital reservoirs of nosocomial pathogens. Contaminants of hospital origin are are referred to as *extrinsic contaminants*.[5] It is now abundantly clear that contamination may be present in a product or device when it arrives at the hospital; introduction of microorganisms during the commercial manufacturing process is termed *intrinsic contamination*.[5]

CLINICAL SYNDROMES AND MANAGEMENT

Clinical Syndromes of Bacteremia

The clinical manifestations of bacteremia range widely, from no symptoms whatsoever or evanescent fever only to fulminant shock, anuria, respiratory failure, and profound metabolic acidosis with death occurring within hours (Table 1). In general with most nosocomial bacteremias — the major exceptions being cases originating from vascular access devices or deep intra-abdominal abscesses — the signs and symptoms of the local infection giving rise to the bacteremia, such as pyelonephritis, peritonitis, or pneumonia, usually predominate. Fever, associated with chills or even shaking rigors and with diaphoresis, is almost universal at the outset, and temperatures exceeding 40°C are common.[6-9] Hypothermia, on the other hand, is rare; seen primarily in newborns, the elderly, or in severely compromised patients, it carries a grave prognosis.[6-9] Most septic patients hyperventilate because of the effects of bacteremia on the medullary respiratory center. Most also show varying degrees of hypotension (systolic arterial pressure less than 90 torr) but are not in shock. Shock, a state of inadequate tissue perfusion, associated with decreased oxygen consumption, oliguria, and metabolic (lactic) acidosis,[10-13] usually reflects a collection of pus under pressure (e.g., an abscess, obstructive cholangitis), untreated endovascular infection (e.g., continued infusion of contaminated intravenous fluid), or simply a severely compromised host. It occurs in

* A nosocomial epidemic can be as small as two cases if the infections are of a type not previously encountered in that hospital or in a specific subpopulation of patients in that hospital.

Table 1

CLINICAL SIGNS AND SYMPTOMS AND LABORATORY ABNORMALITIES
SUGGESTING BACTEREMIC INFECTION

Clinical	Laboratory
Fever (or rarely, hypothermia)	Leukocytosis (>10,000/mm³) or neutropenia,[a] especially with:
Chills or shaking rigors	
Diaphoresis	"Shift to the left" (many immature granulocytes)
Hypotension — frank shock[a]	Vacuolated neutrophils
Hyperventilation	Döhle bodies
Clouded mentation	Thrombocytopenia
Confusion	Sp. Microangiopathic changes in erythrocytes
Delerium	Coagulation abnormalities of disseminated intravascular coagulation (DIC)
Obtundation	
Nonspecific gastrointestinal symptoms	Hypoprothrombinemia (>15 sec)
Abdominal pain	Hypofibrinogenemia (<150 mg/dℓ)
Vomiting	Thrombocytopenia (<100,000/mm³)
Diarrhea	Increased titers of fibrinogen degradation products
Oliguria[a]	
Cutaneous lesions	Hypoxemia
Petechiae, echymosis, mucosal bleeding	Respiratory alkalosis (early) or metabolic acidosis with lactemia[a] (late)
Pustules	
Ecthyma gangrenosum[a]	Azotemia[a]
Osler nodes, Janeway lesions	Hypophosphatemia

[a]   Ominous prognostic signs (mortality increased two- to threefold).

9.7 to 36% of cases,[14-17] and when present, invariably connotes greatly increased mortality. Nonspecific gastrointestinal symptoms such as pain, vomiting, or diarrhea, and nonlocalizing neurologic symptoms such as confusion, delirium, or obtundation, are also frequently encountered in symptomatic bacteremia.

Nosocomial bacteremias more often than community acquired cases exhibit cutaneous signs of systemic infection, including pustules or metastatic skin abscesses, seen most often with *S. aureus* bacteremia.[18] Black necrotic ulcers or palpules with surrounding erythema (echthyma gangrenosum) occur most frequently in leukemic patients with *Pseudomonas aeruginosa* sepsis[19,20] but also can be seen with other Gram-negative bacillemic infections; blood cultures may be negative, but the presence of this lesion, a septic vasculitis with cutaneous infarction, should be regarded as indicative of systemic infection. Distinguishing features of anaerobic bacteremia include frequent jaundice (10 to 40% of cases), septic thrombophlebitis (5 to 12% of cases), and distant metastatic suppurative complications (10 to 28% of cases).[21] While the origin of septicemia in patients with severe granulocytopenia (<500 neutrophils per μℓ) is often initially obscure, careful repeated examinations may disclose indolent perianal cellulitis, most often associated with *P. aeruginosa* bacteremia.[22] A maculonodular rash[23] or exquisitely tender, inflamed maculopapular lesions with underlying myositis[24,25] have been found to be a manifestation of *Candida* sepsis. Petechiae, echymoses, or cutaneous hemorrhaging signal associated coagulation defects, isolated Thrombocytopenia or disseminated intravascular coagulation (DIC)[26-32]

Deep *Candida* sepsis — systemic candidiasis — which, in contradistinction to bacterial septicemia, is frequently associated with negative blood cultures,[33-39] may produce an acute retinitis characterized by multiple paravascular cotton-wool spots.[40-43]

Hematologic and biochemical aberrations commonly encountered in bacteremic infection are also shown in Table 1. Although leukocytosis, often exceeding 20,000/mm³, is relatively common, morphologic abnormalities of granulocytes in the peripheral blood smear are considerably more specific diagnostically: a marked "shift to the left" with many immature neutrophils, vacuolization of neutrophils, and intraneutrophilic Döehle bodies strongly suggest microbial invasion of the bloodstream.[44-50] Hypoprothrombinemia, hypofibrinogenemia, thrombocytopenia, and high titers of fibrin degradation products can be documented in many patients with proven bacteremia;[27-32] these abnormalities denote DIC but rarely pose clinical problems unless refractory shock is present.[32] Early in the course of bacteremia, almost all patients show respiratory alkalosis because of hyperventilation, but if hypotension is prolonged or overt shock develops, metabolic acidosis with hyperlactemia rapidly supervenes.[10-12] Hypoxemia due to pulmonary arteriovenous shunting, which is present in many patients, may culminate in an adult respiratory destress (or "shock-lung") syndrome and severe respiratory failure, again, especially if shock cannot be quickly reversed.[52-55] Oliguria and azotemia usually accompany shock and have ominous portents prognostically.

In their classic 1962 monograph on Gram-negative bacteremia, McCabe and Jackson[6] described a simple system for classifying the severity of patients' underlying diseases. By this system, patients not expected to survive in excess of 1 year under any circumstances (mainly those with acute leukemia) were classified as having a "rapidly fatal disease"; patients whose underlying disease was of such severity that it would likely prove fatal during the next 4 years (e.g., metastatic carcinoma, lymphoma, cirrhosis with bleeding varicies) were classified as having an ultimately fatal disease; patients with diseases not expected to prove fatal during the next 4 years were classified as having nonfatal diseases. Applying this categorization to their cases, McCabe and Jackson showed (and many other investigators have subsequently confirmed[7-9,14-17,56-62]) that the nature and severity of a bacteremic patient's underlying condition is a highly reliable prognostic index: in their patients with rapidly fatal diseases, the mortality was 84%; in patients with ultimately fatal diseases, 48%; and in patients with nonfatal diseases, 16%.[6]

Overall, in patients with bacteremia, advanced age, nosocomial acquisition, septicemia occurring in the setting of granulocytopenia or a fatal underlying disease, hypothermia, shock, acidosis with lactemia, azotemia, polymicrobial bacteremia, *P. aeruginosa* bacteremia in any host, and inappropriate antimicrobial therapy directed at the bacteremia in patients with nonfatal underlying diseases, each connotes a two- to threefold increased mortality (Table 1).[6-9,14-17,56-62]

Systemic signs of bloodstream infection are often masked in neonates, in the elderly, and in immunologically compromised patients receiving corticosteroids or other immunosuppressive therapy.[6-9,14] Most important to an early diagnosis of nosocomial bacteremia is maintaining a high index of suspicion, especially in patients with altered host defenses and in patients in a vulnerable setting, especially those requiring intensive care unit support. Fever alone and mental clouding — especially associated with unexplained tachypnea or hypotension (Table 1) — should prompt an immediate and vigorous search for evidence of nosocomial infection, which should always include blood cultures to identify bacteremia.

Management of Bacteremia

It is beyond the scope of this chapter to discuss the clinical management of nosocomial bactermia in detail, particularly the optimal selection and use of systemic antimicrobial therapy — which should always be administered in maximal doses parenterally,[63] preferably by intravenous injection — and the vital measures necessary to support the failing circulation.[64-69] However, two key facets of management bear emphasis.

In an individual case, *every effort must be made to identify the source of bacteremia* *and, if possible, to extirpate that source* by surgically draining an abscess, decompressing an obstructed ureter or common bile duct, or closing an intestinal perforation; removing an infected intravascular catheter, possibly even resecting a suppurative vein segment; discontinuing an infusion that may contain contaminants; or removing a heavily contaminated ventilator or hemodialysis machine. Such measures are crucial to patient survival and in many instances, such as sepsis from a contaminated infusion[4,70] far supersede antimicrobial therapy in therapeutic importance.* Harris and Cobbs[71] described 20 patients with Gram-negative rod bacteremia and sepsis persisting for 7 days or longer; in every case, bacteremia refractory to antimicrobial therapy originated from a deep abscess or abscesses or an endovascular focus of infection.

By helping to identify the source of the bacteremia accurately — assuring that complete cultures are obtained, including cultures of vascular access devices and infusate in patients without other obvious sources of infection — the infection-control practitioner can make a vital contribution to the management of an individual case. With a cluster of bacteremias that may represent a nosocomial epidemic, the reliable identification of the portal of the bacteremic infections is one of the first and most important steps in defining the outbreak epidemiologically and instituting effective control measures.

It is important to follow patients who develop nosocomial bacteremia or fungemia carefully, even if there is a clear cut favorable response to initial therapy. Latent foci of deep infection — endocarditis,[71-79] an infective aneurysm[79] or endophthalmitis[39-43,78,80] — can be established by even the most transient bloodstream invasion, especially by *S. aureus,* enterococcus, *Salmonella,* or *Candida.* For instance, while the degree of risk is currently a subject of dispute, *S. aureus* bacteremia deriving from a vascular cannula can clearly produce endocarditis; its frequency has been reported as low as 0% by Iannini and Crossley[81] to as high as 40% by Watanakunakorn.[77] Similarly, there are documented cases of *Candida* endocarditis and endophthalmitis not manifesting clinically until 14 months[76] and 2 months,[40] respectively, after a seemingly "self-limiting" cannula-related fungemia. A prospective study by Montgomerie and Edwards[43] found that 5 of 23 patients receiving intravenous hyperalimentation developed *Candida* retinitis, which was usually silent; only 3 patients had positive blood cultures.

LABORATORY DIAGNOSIS OF BACTEREMIA

Cultural Methods

Whereas a patient's clinical picture may strongly suggest bacteremic infection, laboratory confirmation of bacteremia and complete microbiologic characterization of the blood pathogen are imperative for optimal clinical management and, especially, for epidemiologic purposes. Laboratory methods for diagnosis of bacteremia by conventional cultural methods have been thoroughly reviewed in several excellent monographs;[82-85] the scholarly review by Washington and co-workers at the Mayo Clinic is outstanding.** Salient points of the laboratory diagnosis of bacteremia, including both

---

*   During an outbreak of septicemia due to intrinsic contamination of one manufacturer's infusion product in 1970 and 1971, 17 of 19 patients in one hospital treated with gentamicin (to which the epidemic organisms were sensitive) remained clinically septic, continued to have positive blood cultures after 24 hr or more of gentamicin therapy, and did not show improvement until their infusions were fortuitously or intentionally removed[70] (see Figure 9).

**   See review by Washington, J. A., Ed., *The Detection of Septicemia,* CRC Press, Boca Raton, Fla., 1978, 1—155.

conventional culture methods and more recently developed noncultural techniques for detecting the presence of microorganisms in the bloodstream, will be reviewed briefly (see chapter entitled "Optimal Use of the Laboratory for Infection Control").

Drawing Blood Cultures

In general, except for the early phase of brucellosis[86] and typhoid fever, and endo-vascular infections such as infective endocarditis[87,88,92] or infusion-related sepsis[70,71] which produce continuous bacteremia, most bacteremias are intermittent in nature.[88] Thus, except in the aforementioned states, where the timing of blood cultures is prob-ably immaterial, with most infections blood cultures should be drawn at the first clin-ical indication of sepsis — ideally, during a chill or rigor and before the pyrexic episode has begun to abate. In general, the patient's clinical condition will dictate the intervals between cultures; i.e., if septic shock is already present or the patient shows signs of acute infective endocarditis, blood cultures should be drawn immediately and antimi-crobial therapy started without delay.

The fact that a patient may be receiving systemic antimicrobial therapy should never preclude obtaining blood cultures when clinical signs and symptoms suggest bacere-mia;[63] however, in this circumstance, blood cultures obtained immediately before a dose of antibiotics is due to be administered, when the blood antibiotic level will be lowest, may produce a higher yield. There is little evidence that adding beta-lactamase to the media materially improves the yield of blood cultures in patients receiving anti-biotics; conversely, penicillinase readily becomes contaminated, and several outbreaks of pseudobacteremia have been traced to such contamination.[89,90] If penicillinase is to be used, control cultures of (uninoculated) penicillinase-containing media are strongly recommended.[84]

There rarely is any necessity to obtain more than three blood cultures in any 24-hr period. Unless the patient has recently received or is receiving antimicrobial therapy, with bona fide bacteremia, whether due to infective endocarditis or originating from a local infection, one or more of the blood cultures drawn will be positive 90% or more of the time[82,84,91-93] (Figure 1). More than three blood cultures may be indicated in patients who have received antibiotics or who have prosthetic heart valves or other implanted devices, or when there is a clinical picture suggesting occult infection but initial blood cultures are inexplicably negative.

Ideally, when blood cultures are performed, each set should be obtained by separate venipuncture. Half of each specimen should be inoculated into a nonvented (anaero-bic) bottle and the remainder into a vented (aerobic) bottle.[83-85] Determining whether the bottle giving growth represents bona fide, clinically significant bacteremia or con-tamination is greatly aided by performing a separate venipuncture for each set of blood cultures drawn. Moreover, using a dual (anaerobic-aerobic) system should produce the highest yields: between 6% and 8% of bacteremias are caused by anaerobic bacteria;[21,85] conversely, recovery of *P. aeruginosa*[85,94-98] and *Candida*[85,96-100] are con-siderably enhanced when blood culture bottles are transiently vented.

Before drawing blood cultures, the skin must first be disinfected: iodine-containing agents such as tincture of iodine (1 to 2% iodine in 70% alcohol) or an iodophor are most effective,[101-104] but 70% alcohol is an acceptable alternative if it is left on for at least 30 sec before performing the venipuncture.[104-107] Quaternary ammonium antisep-tics such as aqueous benzalkonium should never be used; these agents are notoriously prone to becoming contaminated by Gram-negative bacilli such as *P. aeruginosa* or *Enterobacter* species, and epidemics of both true bacteremia[108,109] and of pseudobac-teremia[110] have derived from such contamination (see chapter entitled "Choosing the Best Antiseptic, Disinfectant, Sterilization Method, and Waste Disposal and Laundry System").

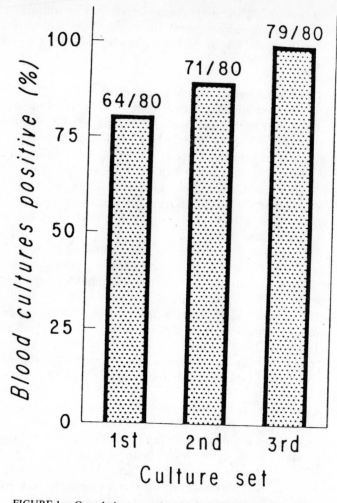

FIGURE 1.   Cumulative rates of positivity in three sets of blood cultures from 80 patients with bacteremia. (From Washington, J. A., II, *Mayo Clin. Proc.*, 50, 91, 1975. With permission.)

Bone marrow cultures may enhance the recovery of *Brucella*[86] *Salmonella typhosa*[111] and *Histoplasma capsulatum* in disseminated disease,[112] but probably confer no advantages in other types of bloodstream infection except possibly in children with leukemia, where Hughes[113] has reported that routinely culturing an aliquot of bone marrow whenever a bone marrow examination is performed may permit earlier diagnosis of opportunistic deep fungal infections. Greene and co-workers[114] however, did not find the practice useful in adult patients with cancer. Roberts and Washington[115] have shown that using biphasic media (the Castaneda system), incorporating both a liquid and solid phase in the same tube, and incubating aerobically at 30°C, considerably enhances the yield of *Candida* and other fungi from blood cultures.

Based on the results of novel animal studies, Stone and co-workers[116] have stated that rapid clearance of blood-borne *Candida* organisms by the liver accounts for the notoriously low yield of venous blood cultures in systemic candidiasis. They provide clinical data to suggest that culturing arterial blood can augment laboratory confirmation of *Candida* sepsis: in a series of 58 patients with histopathologically proven disseminated candidiasis, cultures of arterial blood specimens were positive in 15 of

15 cases, whereas venous blood cultures were positive in only 33 (57%) of the 58 patients. This important finding has not yet been confirmed in other centers.

In a related study of 1197 patients treated in an intensive care unit. Kobza and associates[117] identified nine patients with blood cultures positive for *Candida* during life. All cultures had been drawn through central venous catheters, and, overall, 84% of catheter-drawn cultures in these nine patients yielded *Candida*. Five of these patients died and were autopsied; disseminated candidiasis was confirmed in three. The two without autopsy evidence of candidiasis had received antifungal therapy, as did the three survivors. Only two additional cases of disseminated candidiasis were found in 86 autopsies done on the 91 patients dying during the study; neither had had blood cultures performed during life.

The unresolved issue in both of these intriguing studies is whether the catheters themselves gave rise to candidiasis in patients with positive catheter-drawn cultures (i.e., primary catheter-related septicemias) or whether intravascular catheters "trap" blood-borne organisms originating from other sites, accounting for such a high rate of positive cultures. Neither report provides microbiological data on catheters. It is clear that prolonged vascular cannulation is indeed a major cause of systemic candidiasis,[33,39,76,78,118] and several investigators have demonstrated *Candida* forms in smears of blood drawn through central venous catheters;[119] moreover, catheters have been documented histopathologically to have been the source of *Candida* sepsis.[120] However, vascular catheters can become hematogenously colonized from distant peripheral sites of infection.[71,121-124] The value of arterial or central venous blood cultures in the diagnosis of *Candida* sepsis and the pathophysiologic interpretation of positive specimens cannot be resolved until comparative studies are done with freshly inserted catheters; or, if done with in-use catheters, catheters are also carefully studied on removal, both histologically and microbiologically.

It is common practice in many intensive care units to draw blood cultures through central venous or arterial catheters, or in neonates, through umbilical catheters. The several small studies that have prospectively evaluated this practice found that blood cultures obtained through central venous or arterial catheters in adults show reasonably good concordance with cultures drawn by conventional venipuncture but that rates of false-positive (contaminated) cultures are slightly higher with catheter-drawn specimens.[125,126] In contrast, most studies with umbilical catheters have shown that blood cultures drawn through these catheters are contaminated up to 45% of the time,[127,128] but a recent small study by Cowett and co-workers[129] found that blood cultures drawn through umbilical catheters immediately after they were inserted had no higher rate of false-positivity than concomitant cultures obtained by peripheral venipuncture.

The practice of drawing blood cultures through indwelling vascular catheters ought not to be encouraged because of the risk of introducing contamination into the infusion with added manipulations. If, however, to preserve dwindling superficial veins it is considered necessary to use a vascular catheter to obtain blood cultures, an attempt should be made to use recently inserted catheters and to draw every other specimen by conventional percutaneous venipuncture.

Hall et al.,[130] Tenney et al.,[131] and Washington[85] have shown the importance of obtaining an adequate volume of blood with each culture, to maximize the yield. In infants, where the concentration of organisms in bacteremia is usually considerably higher than in adults (frequently over 10^2 organisms per milliliter[132-134], 1 to 3-ml specimens are probably adequate in most cases.[132,135,136] In a comparative study of a micro-blood culture technique in neonates, Mangurten and LeBeau[137] found that a 0.02-ml capillary blood specimen was positive for the same organism isolated from peripheral venous blood cultures in 8 (73%) of 11 septicemias. Franciosi and Favero[136] have furnished data to suggest that in neonates with sepsis, a single culture will be diagnostic.

In adults a considerably larger volume is needed to maximize the yield; obtaining at least 20 ml, ideally 30 ml, per drawing, each specimen consisting of 10 ml inoculated into a 50 ml, or better, a 100-ml bottle, significantly improves the yield as compared with obtaining only 5-ml aliquots at each drawing and culturing a small total volume.[85,130,131]

Only closed blood culture systems — plugged bottles entered with a needle — should ever be used clinically.[85,138] The specimen may be drawn with a syringe and inoculated directly into the bottle or a transfer set may be used, or the specimen may be drawn directly into an evacuated tube containing the media (Vacutainer® system). This latter system, however, is vulnerable to backflow of tube contents into the bloodstream.[139] Nonsterile evacuated tubes used to collect blood specimens for nonmicrobiologic tests have produced bacteremias,[140,141] and when blood cultures were performed through the same tube holder after drawing nonmicrobiologic specimens, pseudo-bacteremias.[141,142] Contamination of Vacutainer® tube holders was implicated in another outbreak of pseudobacteremia.[143]

Quantitative blood cultures have been evaluated in several studies, using pour-plate techniques.[8,58,132-134] In general, pour-plate cultures proved less sensitive (probably reflecting the smaller volume of blood cultured) than conventional techniques but permitted slightly earlier detection of bacteremia.[132-134] Bacterial counts in bacteremic children, particularly neonates, were found on the average to be higher (50% of cases > 50 organisms per milliliter[132-134], than in adults (80% < 10 organisms per milliliter[8,58]; counts exceeding 10^3 organisms per milliliter in children signaled a 90% likelihood of meningitis.[132,133] In both children and adults, counts correlated inversely with survival.[8,58,132,133] MacGregor and Beatty[144] found that quantitative blood cultures helped discriminate between bacteremia and contaminated cultures: pour-plate cultures were positive in 68% of true bacteremias but only 5.8% of false-positive cultures. Pazin and associates[145] have described an innovative application of quantitative blood cultures: by sampling through cardiac catheters at various points on both sides of the heart, they were able to determine the precise location of endocarditis in two patients.

Up to 25% of all blood cultures in some hospitals are positive with microorganisms subsequently determined to be contaminants.[82,85] It is clear that the experience of the person obtaining the blood cultures heavily influences the rate of contamination. Studies have shown that blood cultures obtained by venipuncture teams have two- to five-fold lower rates of contamination than cultures obtained by medical students and house officers.[85,144]

Processing Blood Cultures

It is beyond the scope of this chapter to discuss laboratory methods of processing blood cultures and the merits of the various blood culture media that are available. This area has also been thoroughly reviewed by Washington and others.[83-85] Several points, however, are extremely important *epidemiologically:*

1. All blood isolates should be identified at least through species, especially Gram-negative bacilli. Failure of hospital laboratories to do so in 1970 and 1971 resulted in large outbreaks of infusion-related *Enterobacter cloacae* and *E. agglomerans* septicemia in several hospitals, which failed to recognize the outbreaks at the time;[4] their epidemics were identified only in retrospect on reviewing laboratory records of positive blood cultures.

2. Similarly, complete antimicrobial susceptibility testing using standardized methods should be performed routinely on all blood isolates. The susceptibility pattern (antibiogram) is often of considerable value as an epidemiologic marker.[4,146,147]

3. An isolate from each clinically relevent bacteremia should be routinely saved for at least 12 to 24 months, ideally, frozen at −70°C for future study, should an epidemic of bacteremias be suspected. This is done routinely in most university and other teaching hospitals and has aided immeasurably in the epidemiologic evaluation of many nosocomial outbreaks of bacteremia reported in the literature.

4. Because many outbreaks of nosocomial bacteremia have derived from contamination of infusion equipment, especially infusate, or from contaminated fluid-filled equipment (such as ventilators and hemodialysis machines) that comes into contact with patients, laboratory personnel should know how to culture infusion fluid, medications, and cannulas,*[123,147,148] specimens from hemodialysis machines,[149] ventilators and other inhalation therapy apparatus,[150-152] and any other environmental specimens[147] that may be epidemiologically important in an epidemic of bacteremias.

5. Similarly, laboratory personnel should be apprised of the concepts of using colonial characteristics and patterns of biochemical reactions (biotype) and antimicrobial susceptibility patterns (antibiogram) for presumptively subtyping epidemiologically relevant isolates.[146-148] They should be aware of reference laboratories such as their own state public health laboratory or the CDC where isolates can be forwarded for further evaluation and complete subtyping by available techniques.**[148]

6. Infection-control personnel should maintain close and continuous dialogue with laboratory personnel. A cluster of isolates of one species from cultures of any site as well as blood, should be immediately reported to infection-control personnel and the isolates retained for possible further analysis.

Interpretation of Positive Blood Cultures

Between 6 and 15% of blood cultures in most hospitals will be positive, representing true bacteremia approximately one half of the time and contaminants introduced during drawing or processing the culture in the rest.[82,85] Multiple blood cultures positive for one species from a given patient, occurring with a clinical picture consistent with bloodstream infection (Table 1), especially if the same species is also isolated from an identifiable local infection such as of the urinary tract, nearly always represents true bacteremia. The increasing frequency of the phenomenon of epidemic pseudobacteremia,[153] which is reviewed in detail in a latter section, bears reminding, however.

Based on a 6-month prospective study of 1707 blood cultures from 857 patients, McGregor and Beatty[144] developed microbiologic criteria to help discriminate between true bacteremia and contaminated blood cultures; isolation of *Streptococcus pneumoniae*, Group A streptococci, *Hemophilus influenzae*, *Neisseria meningitidis* or *N. gonorrhea*, or *Candida* almost always denotes true bacteremia; recovery of *Staphylococcus aureus* or enteric Gram-negative bacilli usually does as well; *S. epidermidis*, *Bacillus* species, and *Proprionibacterium acnes* (diphtheroids) are almost always contaminants*** (especially when recovered from only one of many blood cultures); and isolates of alpha-hemolytic streptococci, enterococci, *Pseudomonas aeruginosa*, or more than one organism from a blood culture represent true bacteremia and contamination about equally. Results and conclusions of MacGregor and Beatty are remarkably similar to those of a similar study done by Kotin[154] 20 years earlier.

---

* Also see the section later in this chapter entitled "Infusion-Related Sepsis".

** Also see section entitled "Approach to an Epidemic", and Table 24.

***Even skin commensals with scant intrinsic pathogenicity such as *S. epidermidis*, *Bacillus* species or diphtheroids demand critical scrutiny when recovered from blood cultures of patients with prosthetic heart valves or other prosthetic implants.[158-162]

Hermans and Washington[155] have reported that at the Mayo Clinic, polymicrobial bacteremia occurs in 6% of cases of bona fide bacteremia and most commonly originates from an intra-abdominal infection. Other studies from teaching hospitals have shown 6 to 8% of bacteremias are polymicrobial.[156,157]

Noncultural Techniques

The clinical gravity of bacteremia and the importance therapeutically of making the earliest diagnosis possible have stimulated intensive efforts to develop methods for diagnosing bacteremia more rapidly by use of noncultural techniques. Anhalt[163] of the Mayo Clinic recently contributed an informative review of progress in this field.

Examining Gram-stained smears of peripheral blood has been the simplest and earliest technique studied. Whereas microorganisms can be seen on a direct smear of venous blood or a buffy coat preparation in occasional cases of staphylococcal septicemia,[164] meningococcemia,[165] or *Candida* sepsis,[119,120,166,167] the few prospective studies indicate that Gram-staining blood is a relative insensitive test that is rarely positive with Gram-negative rod bacteremia.[168-170] In the largest study, by Smith,[168] 17 (30%) of 56 patients with culture-documented bacteremia had microorganisms identified on a Gram stain of peripheral venous blood; invariably, organisms were found within polymorphonuclear leukocytes. Two thirds of positive smears came from patients with staphylococcal or meningococcal septicemia. Powers and Mandell[170] examined leukocyte monolayers from peripheral blood of 16 patients suspected of having infective endocarditis. Intraleukocytic Gram-positive cocci were detected in six of ten patients ultimately determined to have endocarditis, including eight of the nine with positive blood cultures.

Feingold and associates[171-173] and other investigators[174-177] have developed and refined techniques to concentrate microorganisms in blood cultures and remove inhibitory substances by lysing the red cells followed by filtration or centrifugation; concentrated microorganisms are cultured on membrane filters or directly on solid media. Based on parallel trials,[171-177] this approach shows sensitivity at least comparable to conventional culture methods (superior when antibiotics are present) and provides slightly more rapid detection of positive cultures, but is cumbersome and thus far has not received wide application. Komorowski and Farmer[178] found that a lysis-filtration technique doubled the yield of *Candida* isolates (29 vs. 17) and greatly shortened the time for detection of candidemia (1 to 2 days) in a large comparative study with trypticase soy broth with 0.1% agar added. However, the standard culture system was not vented.

Many hospitals now employ a radiometric technique for processing blood cultures which relies on detecting radioactive $^{14}CO_2$ produced by bacterial metabolism of ^{14}C-labeled substrate incorporated in the media. The putative advantage of the technique (the BACTEC® system; Johnston Laboratories, Cockeysville, Md.) is more rapid diagnosis. This system has undergone comparative study in a number of institutions.[179-185] It affords a modest reduction in the time for identification of positive cultures, but its major logistic advantage may be in work-saving, reducing the number of blind subcultures that are necessary. The BACTEC® system appears to be comparably sensitive to conventional culture methods if at least one blind subculture is done. It can be regarded as a significant technological advance in laboratory diagnosis of bacteremia and provides satisfactory results in the many hospitals that now use it routinely.[185]

In 1968, Levin and Bang[186] reported that a lysate of amoebocytes of the horseshoe crab *Limulus polyphemus* gels in the presence of infinitesimal concentrations of Gram-negative lipopolysaccharide — endotoxin. The report immediately raised hopes that a reliable test would shortly be available for rapid diagnosis of Gram-negative bacteremia. Levin and co-workers[187,188] in accounts of their early clinical experiences with the test stated that 53 to 67% of patients with culture-proved Gram-negative rod bacteremia showed a positive *Limulus* lysate assay; most patients with a positive test but without Gram-negative bacteremia had an identifiable local Gram-negative infection which these investigators interpreted as indicating endotoxemia can occur without bacteremia. Further evaluations of the test in a number of other centers, however, have yielded conflicting and mostly less promising results;[189-194] while most trials confirmed that approximately one half of patients with Gram-negative bacteremia have a positive assay, up to 30% of patients without Gram-negative infections in one study did as well.[191] Elin and Wolff[195] have described a number of substances unrelated to endotoxin that produce gelation of the lysate. Although the test is highly sensitive in vitro (0.1 to 1.0 ng of endotoxin per milliliter), approximately 10^2 to 10^3 Gram-negative organisms per milliliter are required to produce a positive test.[196] Except in neonates and infants,[132-134] concentrations of organisms in Gram-negative bacteremia uncommonly exceed 10 to 50 organisms per milliliter[8,58] Thus, at the present time, the *Limulus* assay, which requires considerable technologic expertise, has not yet been sufficiently refined to be of practical utility clinically for diagnosing Gram-negative bacteremia. It has yielded excellent results, however (sensitivity and specificity both > 90%), in Gram-negative meningitis.[197,198]

Gas-liquid chromatography has been successfully applied to detect compounds elaborated by microbial cells or constituents of microorganisms in clinical specimens. The technique forms the basis for characterization of anaerobic isolates in most diagnostic laboratories. Preliminary trials applying gas-liquid chromatography directly to clinical specimens by Mitruka and co-workers[199,200] have shown excellent sensitivity and specificity for the rapid diagnosis of pneumococcal bacteremia (90% accuracy) and bloodstream infections caused by a variety of other Gram-negative organisms and streptococci. Davis and McPherson[201] detected *Candida* sepsis by chromatographic analyses of serum specimens in 13 of 13 cases. This technique holds considerable promise and is currently undergoing clinical study in a number of centers.

Methods for detection of soluble capsular antigens by immunologic techniques, primarily by using counterimmunoelectrophoresis (CIE), are well developed and have been extensively studied clinically with the major agents of bacterial meningitis, *Streptococcus pneumoniae*, *N. meningitidis*, and *H. influenzae* type b.[202-204] Antigenemia can be demonstrated by CIE in approximately one half of patients with bacteremia caused by *H. influenzae* or *S. pneumoniae*;[205-210] antigenemia without bacteremia almost always denotes deep infection caused by the organism, often pneumonia or meningitis. When CIE is performed on cerebrospinal fluid, serum, and urine, over 90% of cases of meningitis caused by *H. influenzae* type b can be reliably detected within 2 to 4 hr.[210] Antigenemia is detectable in only about 25% of patients with meningococcemia.[211-214] With all three organisms, a high level of antigenemia augers a poorer prognosis. Detection of Group B streptococcal[215] and *E. coli* K1[216] capsular antigens in clinical specimens also appears to be feasible by immunologic methods. Studies of the application of CIE to detecting circulating antigens of *Staphylococcus aureus*,[217] *P. aeruginosa*,[205] and *Klebsiella*[218] in bacteremic infections also show promise. Application of other immunodiagnostic techniques, such as latex particle agglutination,[219] radioimmunoassay,[220] and enzyme-linked immunosorbent assay (ELISA)[221] also show considerable clinical promise with certain encapsulated bacteria such as *H. influenzae*, and possibly even *Candida*.[222,223] The extraordinary antigenic heterogeneity of the Enterobacteriaceae has precluded successful application of immunodiagnostic techniques for diagnosing bacteremia caused by enteric Gram-negative bacilli.

Applications of other noncultural methods, such as bioluminescence, microcalorimetry, or electrical impedance changes, to signal the presence of microorganisms in blood, are in considerably more preliminary stages of development at the present time.[163]

PATTERNS OF NOSOCOMIAL BACTEREMIA

Sources of Nosocomial Bacteremia
Endemic Bacteremias

Bacteremia represents the most extreme form of nosocomial infection and occurs in one of three clinical settings: (1) localized infection no longer can be contained and overwhelms the host defenses of an immunologically competent patient; in this setting, the sheer volume of local infection is usually large (e.g., peritonitis) or the infection occurs in association with pus under pressure (e.g., an abscess or an obstructed ureter) when bacteremia develops; (2) bacteremia ensues from a seemingly insignificant local infection (e.g., a small area of cellulitis) or occurs in the absence of any identifiable local infection whatsoever ("cryptogenic bacteremia") in an immunosuppressed host (e.g., a leukemic) or a neonate; or (3) microorganisms are introduced directly into the bloodstream — bypassing local host defenses — through an invasive vascular device.

As shown in Figure 2, the majority of endemic nosocomial bacteremias develop secondarily, as a complication of an identifiable local infection: suppurative surgical wounds or intra-abdominal infections that occasionally develop *de novo* but most often following surgery; infections of the instrumented urinary tract; pneumonias that also commonly occur after instrumentation or anesthesia; or skin and soft tissue infections— especially infected burn wounds. Primary bacteremias, comprised mainly of intravenous cannula-related sepsis and bacteremias of unknown origin, account for only one fourth of all endemic bloodstream infections.*

The risk of acquiring an endemic nosocomial bacteremia is two to four times higher in elderly patients (>60 years of age).[3,57,225] Moreover, patients of any age with a fatal underlying disease, who are as a rule immunocompromised because of their disease or its treatment, develop hospital acquired bacteremia 10 to 15 times more frequently than patients without a fatal underlying disease.[16,227] Patients with leukemia and renal and bone marrow transplants particularly experience very high rates of bacteremic infection, ranging up to 500 cases per 1000;[17,228-232] most of these bacteremias are hospital related. While compromised patients are clearly highly susceptible to infections from invasive devices of all types,[235] most of their bacteremias fall into the first or second aforementioned categories pathophysiologically.[17]

Critical analyses by McGowan et al.[225] and Spengler et al.[234] suggest that at best, only about one fourth of endemic nosocomial bacteremias are putatively preventable by more consistent application of known control measures with regard to devices. Developing effective means to eradicate hospital reservoirs of nosocomial pathogens and preventing, or at least delaying, colonization by hospital organisms would seem of highest priority to reduce the incidence of endemic bacteremia.[235]

---

*   Data from the National Nosocomial Infection Study of the CDC[224] might suggest that one half or more of endemic nosocomial bacteremias are primary bacteremias because a culture-proved local infection is not reported. However, prospective studies of nosocomial infection indicate that the anatomic portal of an individual nosocomial bacteremia should be identifiable much more frequently. In 97 epidemics occurring between 1965 and 1978 and reported in the English literature, the source was identifiable 81% of the time (Figure 2). Thus, to provide a more accurate profile of endemic nosocomial bacteremia and sharpen the comparison between endemic and epidemic cases with respect to sources, pooled data on endemic bacteremias from three prospective studies[16,225,226] are used rather than the otherwise excellent data of the National Study. (It is reasonable to surmise [and data supporting this view will be presented in a later section] that the vast majority of nosocomial bacteremias occurring in hospitals are endemic infections.)

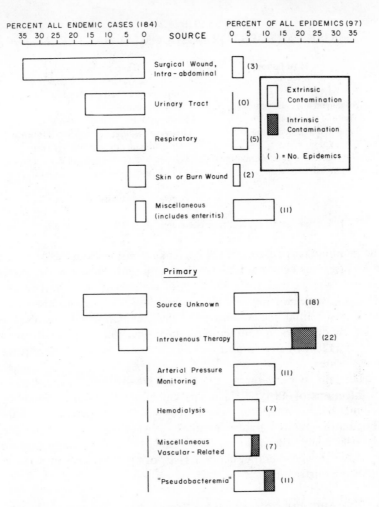

FIGURE 2. Sources of nosocomial bacteremias. (Data on 184 endemic cases from published experiences in three U.S. hospitals: a teaching-community hospital (St. Mary's, Madison, Wis.[16]), a university hospital (Johns Hopkins, Baltimore, Md.[226]), and municipal hospital (Grady Memorial, Atlanta[225]). Data on 97 epidemics occurring between 1965 and 1978 compiled from reports in English world literature in which bacteremias constituted 25% or more of epidemic infections).

Epidemic Bacteremias

Nosocomial bacteremias occurring in epidemics contrast sharply. Fully 78% of all epidemics involve primary bacteremias (Figure 2). Over one third of the 97 outbreaks occurring between 1965 and 1978 stemmed from some aspect of infusion therapy, and in only 19% did the anatomic portal of bacteremia and epidemiologic mechanisms elude detection.* Outbreaks in hemodialysis units accounted for 7% of epidemics — and miscellaneous primary bacteremias, for another 7%. It is noteworthy that in 12% of the outbreaks, the putative epidemic infections were ultimately shown to be pseudobacteremias. An outbreak of local infections at one site giving rise to secondary bacteremias accounted for only 21 (21%) of the 97 tabulated epidemics.

Two thirds of the outbreaks occurred in a closed patient population, usually involv-

---

* Fifteen of the eighteen cryptogenic epidemics took place in a newborn nursery.

Table 2
RISK FACTORS FOR NOSOCOMIAL BACTEREMIA

Host factors	Therapeutic factors
Newborn	*Confinement in an intensive care unit or*
Advanced age (>60 years)	*newborn nursery* [a]
Multiple trauma or burns	Systemic antimicrobial therapy
Fatal underlying disease	*Invasive vascular device* (especially an ar-
Granulocytopenia	terial pressure monitoring system)
Corticosteroid or other immuno-	*Receipt of large volumes of parenteral*
suppressive therapy	*fluids or blood products*
	Hemodialysis
	Nonvascular invasive device

[a]   Prime risk factors for epidemic bacteremias in italics.

ing adults in an intensive care unit (24 epidemics) or a hemodialysis center (7) or new-borns in a nursery or neonatal intensive care unit (26). Furthermore, except for those epidemics involving neonates, the majority of patients affected in the 86 outbreaks of true bacteremia were not intrinsically immunologically compromised. In the largest epidemic of nosocomial bacteremias on record, the nationwide outbreak in 1970 and 1971 caused by one U.S. manufacturer's intrinsically contaminated parenteral prod-ucts,[4] only 29 (12%) of 242 carefully scrutinized cases occurred in patients with fatal underlying diseases.

Whereas certain host and therapeutic factors greatly increase the risk of serious no-socomial infections of all types including endemic bacteremia, (Table 2), epidemics of nosocomial bacteremia occur in large measure irrespective of the character of the patient population, related almost singularly to what has been done to patients thera-peutically after admission to the hospital (Table 2): segregation in a special care unit or exposure to infusion therapy, hemodialysis, or other invasive procedures or devices involving the bloodstream.

Invasive Procedures and Nosocomial Bacteremia

One of the most conspicuous aspects of modern-day medicine is the vast number of invasive procedures to which patients are subjected, primarily for therapeutic purposes but also for monitoring the effects of complex therapies or simply aiding in diagnosis. Every hospitalized patient has countless venipunctures performed to obtain blood spec-imens for analysis; most receive infusion therapy of one or more diverse forms; general anesthesia is synonymous with endotracheal intubation and tracheal suctioning; major surgery and critical care unit support, with urethral catheterization. Intracranial pres-sure monitoring with epidural transducers or indwelling ventricular catheters is consid-ered essential for optimal neurosurgical management, and many centers routinely use internal fetal monitoring in high-risk deliveries. Endoscopic examination through every body orifice — laryngoscopy, bronchoscopy esophagogastroscopy, endoscopic retro-grade cholangiopancreatography (ERCP), proctosigmoidoscopy and colonoscopy, peritoneoscopy, panendoscopy and cystoscopy—angiography of every major organ system, and cardiac catheterization have tremendously enhanced the rapidity and ac-curacy of medical diagnosis.

While each of these procedures provides obvious and often invaluable benefits, it also creates a portal for the entrance of infection. The risk of iatrogenic harm is greatly increased by inexperienced operators and by inadequate attention to aseptic technique. It is to medicine's credit that the cost-benefit of many procedures — such as internal fetal monitoring[236,237] — is increasingly receiving critical scrutiny; studies are attempting to quantify the risks of iatrogenic infection and identify predisposing factors. Guidelines for reducing the hazard of infection with these procedures are now available.

It is very clear that *protracted* exposure to an invasive device or procedure greatly increases the risks of iatrogenic infection, particularly bacteremia. Infections associated with indwelling vascular cannulas, urethral (Foley) catheters, surgery, and prolonged intubation and ventilatory support are covered elsewhere in this book (see chapters entitled "Surveillance and Reporting of Hospital Acquired Infections", "Postoperative Wound Infections", and "Hospital Acquired Pneumonia").

Without discussing methodologic problems that have limited many studies, it also is clear that many short-term invasive procedures commonly produce bacteremia, the incidence of which ranges widely by the type of procedure[238-283] (Table 3). However, except for urologic manipulations which often produce acute septicemia[263-265] (especially if the patient has pre-existent bacteriuria) and manipulations of burn wounds,[273,274] with most short-term procedures, even though demonstrable bacteremia may be relatively frequent (e.g., with dental extractions[238-240] or suction abortion[272]), it is almost always transient — typically lasting for no more than 15 min — and asymptomatic, rarely producing clinical sequelae. However, even an evanescent bacteremia can pose a threat to an immunosuppressed individual or a person with a scarred heart valve, cardiac prosthesis, or some other implanted foreign material (e.g., a prosthetic joint or a ventriculosystemic shunt). Thus, antimicrobial prophylaxis is clearly indicated for susceptible patients undergoing some of the procedures contained in Table 3.[284]

Most bacteremias deriving from brief invasive procedures are endemic bacteremias, caused by the patient's own flora at the site manipulated. However, breaks in technique, improper decontamination of reusable devices and equipment (such as cardiac catheters), or contamination of a disinfectant can result in cross-infection or exposure of multiple patients to a common source of contamination.

Microbiologic Profile of Nosocomial Bacteremia*

Over the past three decades, Gram-negative bacilli have greatly overshadowed Gram-positive organisms as causative agents of nosocomial bacteremia, endemically and especially, in epidemics. Whereas the microbiologic profiles of endemic and epidemic bacteremias have general similarities, a number of important differences bear careful scrutiny. To provide a large, representative base of data on endemic cases occurring in U.S. hospitals for comparison with cases in the 97 epidemics reported between 1965 and 1978, microbiologic data on 4532 bacteremias reported to the CDC's National Nosocomial Infection Study in 1976[224] are displayed in Figure 3, together with data from the 97 outbreaks.

In most hospitals, staphylococci, primarily coagulase-positive *S. aureus*, have continued as major bacteremic pathogens, accounting for approximately 20% of all endemic hospital acquired cases. Nosocomial epidemics of *S. aureus* (6) and *S. epidermidis* (2) bacteremia, however, made up only 8% of reported outbreaks.

---

* CDC[288] recently proposed changes in the taxomony and nomenclature of certain numbers of the Enterobacteriaceae (Table 4). However, because the new designations have not yet received wide currency and because virtually all of the literature cited in this review uses the original nomenclature, the old designations will be used.

  The *Mima-Herellea* were recently designated by an international committee[289] as a new single genus and species, *Acinetobacter calceaceticus*, with two subspecies, *A. calcoaceticus*, var. *anitratus* and *A. calcoaceticus*, var. *lwoffi*. These new designations are now used consistently in the medical literature and will also be used in this review.

Table 3

FREQUENCY AND PROFILE OF BACTEREMIA ASSOCIATED WITH VARIOUS SHORT-TERM INVASIVE PROCEDURES

Anatomic area	Procedure[a]	Reported frequency[a] (%)	Predominant microorganisms	Clinical sequelae	Ref.
Dental	Irrigation	27	Anaerobes, streptococci	Asymptomatic	238
	Extractions	54—92		Rarely symptomatic but clear-cut source endocarditis	239, 240
Respiratory	Fiberoptic bronchoscopy	0	—	Fever, pneumonia—frequent; sepsis—rare	241
	Orotracheal intubation	0	—		242
	Nasal packing (epistaxis)	9		Rare septicemia	243
	Nasotracheal intubation	12—16	Anaerobes, streptococci, rarely Gram-negative bacilli		242
	Tracheal suctioning	16			244
	Tonsillectomy	28		Usually asymptomatic	245
	Peritoneoscopy	0	—		246
GI	Esophagogastroscopy	2—8	Anaerobes, streptococci, rarely Gram-negative bacilli	Rarely symptomatic	247—249
	Rectal exam	4	Anaerobes, Gram-negative bacilli		250
	Sigmoidoscopy	0—11			251—253
	Colonoscopy	0—27			249, 254—258
	ERCP[b]	8	Gram-negative bacilli	0.8% Incidence cholangitis with septicemia	259,260
	Liver biopsy	6—13		Symptomatic septicemia in up to 2%	261,262
Urologic[c]	Insertion of a urethral catheter	2—8	Enterococci, Gram-negative bacilli	Bacteriuric patients, often become clinically septic; risk of bacteremia lower in children	263—267
	Cystoscopy	15—17			
	Urethral dilation	24—40			
	Transurethral prostatectomy	31—67			
	Prostatic massage	67			

Category	Procedure	Risk of bacteremia (%)[a]	Organisms	Comments	Ref.
Gynecologic	Cervical biopsy	0	—		268
	Vaginal delivery	2—11	Anaerobes, streptococci	Rarely symptomatic, but source of endocarditis	269—271
Soft tissue	Suction abortion	85	Anaerobes		272
	Manipulation of boil	34	Staphylococci	Some symptomatic	266
	Incision and drainage of abscess	45			88
	Debride, dress burn wound	21—46	Gram-negative bacilli	Often symptomatic with overt sepsis	273, 274
Vascular	Venipuncture	Unknown	Gram-negative bacilli, staphylococci	Bacteremia very rare but documented	
	Angiography	0	Staphylococci, skin commensals, rarely Gram-negative bacilli	Pyrexic episodes common but usually unrelated to positive blood cultures, most of which may be contaminants	275
	Cardiac catheterization	0—17			276—279
	Hemodialysis	0.03—0.06[d]	Staphylococci, Gram-negative bacilli	Risk of bacteremia, 0.15—0.30 cases per dialysis-year	280—283

Note: From selected published studies; in general, where multiple studies are available, the best controlled and largest are cited.

[a] Risk of bacteremia with single exposure to procedure.
[b] ERCP, endoscopic retrograde cholangiopancreatography.
[c] Preexistent bacteriuria increases risk of bacteremia (and sepsis) up to tenfold.
[d] Assuming dialysis three times per week.
[e] Procedures that have given rise to epidemics of nosocomial bacteremia are italicized.

Table 4
RECENT CHANGES IN TAXONOMY AND NOMENCLATURE OF CERTAIN NOSOCOMIAL GRAM-NEGATIVE BACILLI

Previous designation	New designation
Klebsiella pneumoniae, indole positive	*Klebsiella oxytoca*
Enterobacter cloacae, yellow pigment	*Enterobacter sakazakii* sp.
	Enterobacter gergoviae [a]
Enterobacter hafniae	*Hafnia alvei*
—	*Citrobacter amalonaticus* [a]
Proteus rettgeri, Biogroup 5	*Providencia stuartii,* urea positive
Providencia alcalifaciens, Biogroup 4	*P. stuartii,* Biogroup 4
Proteus rettgeri, Biogroups 1—4	*Providencia rettgeri*
Proteus morganii	*Morganella morganii* sp.
Mima polymorpha	*Acinetobacter calcoaceticus* var. *lwoffii* sp.
Herellea vaginicola	*A. calcoaceticus* var. *anitratus*

[a]   New species based on DNA-homology studies and substantial biochemical differences from other species in the genus.

From Brenner, D. J., Farmer, J. J., III, Hickman, F. W., Asbury, M. A., and Steigerwalt, A. G., *Taxonomic and Nomenclature Changes in Enterobacteriaceae,* H.E.W. Publication No. (CDC) 79-8356, Center for Disease Control, Atlanta, 1977, 15; and Lessel, E. R., *Int. J. Syst. Bacteriol.,* 21, 213, 1971.

Streptococcus pneumoniae, Group A streptococci and the alpha-hemolytic strains of *Streptococcus* now cause relatively few hospital acquired bacteremias. In contrast, Group D streptococci — primarily the enterococci — have become increasingly important nosocomial pathogens in the past two decades[285-287] (Figure 3) Most enterococcal bacteremias stem from silent urinary tract infections related to genitourinary manipulations or from postsurgical polymicrobial intra-abdominal infections; respiratory tract infection with enterococcus is inexplicably rare.[287] In spite of its rising importance as a nosocomial pathogen, epidemics of enterococcal infection have not been identified.

Group B *Streptococcus* has become the predominant agent of neonatal sepsis in many centers during the past two decades. Clusters of cases thought to represent cross-infection have recently been reported.

In 1977 and 1978, multiple hospitals in Durbin and Johannesburg, South Africa, were struck by epidemics of serious pneumococcal disease caused by strains exhibiting resistance to penicillin of a degree previously never encountered.[290-295] These organisms have not yet been detected in significant numbers outside of South Africa.

E. coli remains preeminent in endemic Gram-negative septicemia; in contrast, it has been implicated in relatively few hospital outbreaks of bacteremia (Figure 3); most occurred in newborns.

The Klebsielleae, *Klebsiella, Enterobacter,* and *Serratia,* as a group cause many more endemic bacteremias than *E. coli.* All three members are important epidemic pathogens, particularly in outbreaks linked to infusion therapy or occurring in newborn intensive care units. Of the eight outbreaks caused by *Enterobacter,* seven involved *Enterobacter cloacae* or *E. agglomerans* and only one *E. aerogenes.*

In the past decade, *Serratia marcescans* has also been in sharp ascent, both as an

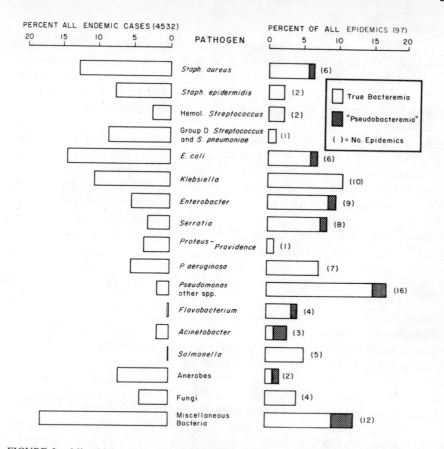

FIGURE 3. Microbial pathogens associated with endemic nosocomial bacteremias and responsible for 97 epidemics occurring between 1965 and 1978. Epidemic pathogens in miscellaneous bacteria: *Citrobacter* (4 epidemics), *Listeria (2), Bacillus* (2), *M. chelonei* (1), *N. meningitidis* (1), *H. influenzae* (1), and *Moraxella* (1). (Data on 4532 endemic bacteremias from 83 U.S. hospitals submitting data on 46,821 nosocomial infections occurring in 1976 to the National Nosocomial Infections Study of the CDC.[224] Data on epidemics compiled from published reports in English world literature in which bacteremias constituted 25% or more of epidemic infections).

endemic and epidemic bacteremic pathogen; 8% of all epidemics since 1965 were caused by *Serratia.*

Proteus-Providence species cause occasional endemic bacteremias and have been responsible for many outbreaks of urinary tract or burn wound infection, but outbreaks of bacteremia caused by these organisms have been rare.

Pseudomonas, particularly *P. aeruginosa,* has become an increasingly important cause of both endemic and epidemic hospital acquired bacteremia. On the other hand, sporadic blood stream infections with the nonaeruginosa species of *Pseudomonas* are infrequent in most hospitals (1.7% of all cases in the National Study, Figure 3). Yet *P. cepacia* has become the preeminent pathogen in epidemics of nosocomial bacteremia. In the past 10 years, 14 *P. cepacia* outbreaks were recorded, more than with any other microorganism (Figure 3).* Every outbreak stemmed from infusion therapy or hemodialysis.

It is now clear that a significant proportion of endemic nosocomial bacteremias (6% of all reported cases in the National Study's hospitals in 1976, Figure 3) are caused by

---

* One outbreak each was caused by *P. acidivorans* and *P. maltophilia.*

Bacteroides fragilis and *Clostridium* species. Epidemics of anaerobic bacteremia, on the other hand, have been exceedingly rare; between 1965 and 1978, clostridia were implicated in one genuine outbreak and in one cluster of pseudobacteremias.

Whereas *Salmonella* has auspicious capacity to produce nosocomial disease of epidemic proportions, it has been a relatively infrequent bloodstream pathogen in the National Study hospitals; in contrast, 5% of reported outbreaks since 1975 were caused by *Salmonella.*

Candida species are now responsible for approximately 3% of all systemic infections, virtually all hospital derived; they have also been implicated in an equivalent percentage of nosocomial outbreaks. A number of miscellaneous organisms, including *Acinetobacter, Flavobacterium, Citrobacter, Listeria, Neisseria meningitidis, H. influenzae,* and the true fungi, that caused only an occasional sporadic nosocomial septicemia in most hospitals or that may even be encountered only very rarely as hospital pathogens, have each been implicated in at least one outbreak of hospital-related bloodstream infection over the past 15 years.

MAGNITUDE OF THE PROBLEM

Endemic Nosocomial Bacteremia

Bacteremic infections have long been a subject of intense interest, both clinically and investigatively, owing in large measure to their gravity clinically and also to the almost mystical aura surrounding infection of the human bloodstream. Over a hundred papers have been published in the past 20 years alone, reporting morbidity and case-fatality rates associated with bacteremic infections in individual institutions.

It is clear from studies in a number of centers[3,6,8,15,16,57,60,61,224,225,296-305] (Table 5), the most comprehensive (longitudinally) being those of Finland and his co-workers at the Boston City Hospital covering the period 1935 to 1972[3,296,297] that the incidence of nosocomial bactermia, particularly Gram-negative rod bacteremia (Figure 4), has risen progressively over the past four decades. Although rates of bacteremia vary considerably from hospital to hospital, it can be seen in Table 4 that between 1 and 14 patients per 1000 hospital admissions develop a nosocomial bacteremia. Rates are lowest in community hospitals (approximately 1 to 2 cases per 1000) and considerably higher in university and municipal institutions (from 4 to 14 cases per 1000).

There has been considerable controversy as to the true magnitude of the problem, particularly with Gram-negative bacteremia, on a national scale.[306,307] The most recent and probably most representative projections,[305] based on data on 1.3 million patients hospitalized in the 83 hospitals submitting data to the National Nosocomial Infections Surveillance Study in 1976,[224] suggest that on the average there are approximately five nosocomial bacteremias per 1000 patients hospitalized in American hospitals. Applying this rate to the approximately 38 million persons hospitalized in this country yearly yields an informed estimate of approximately 185,000 hospital acquired bacteremias each year nationally (Table 6).

It is often very difficult in an individual case of bacteremia that has its onset shortly before the patient dies to determine the exact contribution of the bacteremic infection to a fatal outcome, especially if the patient already had a fatal underlying disease. However, recent careful case-control studies by Rose et al.[301] and Spengler et al. [302] (Table 6) have shown that the risk of a patient's dying is increased 3.8 to 14 times if nosocomial bacteremia is present, compared with fatality ratios of nonbacteremic patients of similar age and with comparable underlying diseases. Thus, it seems reasonable to surmise that nosocomial bacteremia is associated causally with substantial mortality. Mortality is highest in patients with fatal underlying diseases and

Table 5

INCIDENCE (CASES PER 1000 HOSPITALIZED PATIENTS) AND MORTALITY OF ENDEMIC NOSOCOMIAL BACTEREMIA

Hospital, location	Years inclusive	Type of hospital			All types	Case-fatality ratio (%)	Ref.
		Municipal or federal	University	Community			
Boston City, Boston	1935	4.6				57	3
	1947	4.3				40	
	1957	6.3				55	
	1965	8.2				50	
	1972	13.4				39	
Grady Memorial, Atlanta	1975	4.8				NS[a]	225
Bellevue, New York	1975	13.8				17	298
Illinois Research and Development, Chicago	1951—1958		2.8[b]			49	6
University of Minnesota, Minneapolis	1958—1966		4.9[b]			54	8
Stanford University, Palo Alto	1959—1966		1.9[b]			36	15
Royal Free, London	1960—1967		2.5			NS	299
Peter Bent Brigham, Boston	1968—1969		7.7[b]			32	57
Childrens Hospital Medical Center, Boston	1970—1971		6.3			NS	300
Copenhagen City, Copenhagen	1973		3.6			33	60
Johns Hopkins, Baltimore	1968—1974		4.1			37	302
University of Virginia, Charlottesville	1972—1975		5.2			38	301
University of Wisconsin, Madison	1979		7.5			40	303
St. Mary's, Madison, Wis.	1970—1973			1.2		20	16
Riverside Methodist, Columbus, Ohio	1974			1.0[b]		45	304
Hackensack, Hackensack, N.J.	1974—1975			2.4		32	61
80 NNIS[c] hospitals, U.S.	1976	6.9	5.8	1.9	3.1	NS	224
Projections for all U.S. hospitals	1976				5.2	NS	305

Note: From published series providing incidence data and differentiating nosocomial and community acquired cases.

[a] NS, not stated.
[b] Gram-negative cases only.
[c] National Nosocomial Surveillance Study of the Center for Disease Control (CDC).

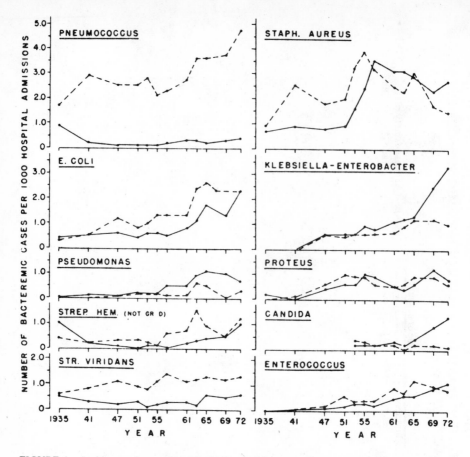

FIGURE 4.   Incidence of nosocomial (solid lines) and community acquired (broken lines) bacteremias at Boston City Hospital with various pathogens in each of 12 selected years between 1935 and 1972. (From McGowan, J. E., Barnes, M. W., and Finland, M., *J. Infect. Dis.*, 132, 316, 1975. With permission University of Chicago Press.)

commensurately lower in patients who do not have fatal diseases.[6-9,15,16,56-62,227] The character of the blood pathogen does not appear to greatly influence mortality, even when it is *Staphylococcus aureus* or a Gram-negative bacillus — except for two organisms, *P. aeruginosa* and *Candida* (Table 7); case-fatality ratios in endemic septicemia caused by these organisms exceed 60% in most centers.

In his scholarly analysis on the impact of infectious diseases nationally, Dixon[305] does not provide mortality data nor, understandably, attempt to make national projections with respect to mortality, presumably because of incomplete reporting from the National Study's hospitals on this subject. However, excellent data on case-fatality rates are available from a number of highly reputable institutions (Table 5). Similar to its incidence, the mortality associated with endemic nosocomial bacteremia has also ranged widely, and appears to be most heavily influenced by the type of patients served by the hospital; in general, muncipal and university hospitals have reported considerably higher case-fatality ratios than community hospitals. On the average, 20 to 40% of patients acquiring a nosocomial bacteremia do not survive. Applying the 4 per 1000 rate of nosocomial bacteremia derived by Dixon and representative of rates found in most prospective studies (Table 5), it can be projected that each year in this country upwards of 75,000 patients die with a hospital acquired bacteremia (Table 6).

The case-control studies of Rose et al.[301] and Spengler et al.[302] have also sought to

Table 6

CASE-FATALITY AND ECONOMIC COSTS OF NOSOCOMIAL BACTEREMIA — NATIONAL PROJECTIONS

Data	Investigator			
	McGowan et al.[3]	Rose et al.[301]	Spengler et al.[302]	Dixon (CDC)[305]
Source of data	Boston City Hospital	University of Virginia Hospital	Johns Hopkins Hospital	83 NNIS[a] hospitals
Dates inclusive	1972	Dec. 1973—Aug. 1974	1968—1974	1976
Number of patients studied	2133	32,073	229,917	1,306,183
Number of nosocomial bacteremias	280	102	435	194,000 (adjusted)[b]
Rate (per 1000 patients)	13.2	5.2	4.1	5.2[b]
Case-fatality rate	39.3%	38%	37.1%	NR[c]
Excess fatality ratio[d]	7.9	3.8[c]	14[c]	NR
Prolongation of hospitalization in patients with nosocomial bacteremia	NR	19 days[e]	14 days[e]	7 days (estimate)
Excess costs associated with nosocomial bacteremia	NR	$4370[e]	$3600[e]	$1225 (estimate)
Projections nationally (per year)				
Number of cases nosocomial bacteremia	—	194,000	156,000	194,000
Number of deaths	—	75,000	58,000	—
Excess costs	—	$863,000,000	$561,000,000	$241,000,000

a   National Nosocomial Infection Study of the CDC.
b   Adjusted for underreporting.
c   NR, not reported.
d   Ratio of case-fatalities of patients with nosocomial bacteremia and hospitalized patients without bacteremia.
e   Case-control analyses; cases matched with control patients cases by age and sex, dates of hospitaization, service, and primary diagnoses.

Table 7

CASE-FATALITY IN ENDEMIC AND EPIDEMIC NOSOCOMIAL BACTEREMIAS

Category	Endemic[a]		Epidemics[b]		
	Number of cases	Case-fatality (per 100 cases)	Number of cases	Number (epidemics[c])	Case-fatality (per 100 cases)
Overall	935	37.1	901	(81)	25.3
Pathogen[c]					
Streptococcus pneumoniae	22	59.1	48	(1)	50.0
Staphylococcus aureus	85	30.6	43	(5)	16.0
Escherichia coli	127	38.6	27	(5[a])	52.0
Klebsiella	233	31.8	63	(10[a])	36.5
Enterobacter	67	35.8	307	(8)	20.2
Serratia	37	32.4	52	(4[a])	42.3
Pseudomonas	74	68.9	33	(7)	39.4 P. aeruginosa
			87	(12)	5.8 other pseudomonads
Candida	56	60.7	22	(1)	0
Miscellaneous	234	27.4	219	(27[a])	25.8
Pyrogens	—	—	163	(10)	0
Origin of bacteremia					
Urinary tract	146	27.4	—	—	—
Surgical or burn wound	111	34.2	42	(4)	50.0
Respiratory tract	99	67.7	60	(5)	48.3
GI	56	45.5	115	(10)	35.7
Vascular access device	118	19.5	527	(36)	13.1
I.V.			397	(21)	14.1
intra-arterial			85	(8)	15.3
hemodialysis			45	(7)	0
Age group					
Newborns	23	26.1	153	(24)	54.3
Adults and children	914	38.5	748	(57)	19.4

[a] From data reported in Spengler, R. F., Grennough, W. B., III, and Stolley, P. O., Johns Hopkins Med. J., 142, 77, 1978.

b   Epidemics reported in world English literature, occurring between 1965 and 1978. Epidemics in which case-fatality data not provided and epidemics of pseudobacteremia and of pyrogenic reactions not included in summary tabulations.

c   Only pathogens for which sufficient data on both endemic and epidemic bacteremias available are analyzed individually.

d   Outbreaks in newborns constituted one half or more of the reported epidemices.

e   *Salmonella* (5 outbreaks), *Citrobacter* (4), *Flavobacterium* (3), *Staphylococcus epidermidis* (2), hemolytic streptococci (2), *Listeria* (2), *Bacillus cereus* (1), *Proteus* (1), *Acinetobacter* (1), *Neisseria meningitidis* (1), *Hemophilus influenzae*(1), *Clostridium sordelli*(1), *Mycobacterium chelonei*(1), *Aspergillus*(1), and *Penicillium*(1).

ascertain the economic impact of nosocomial bacteremia. Their independently derived data are remarkably in agreement (Table 6) and indicate that, in their university hospitals, developing a nosocomial bacteremia portends 14 to 19 days of additional hospitalization and $3600 to $4370 in excess hospital costs, compared with the hospitalizations of (matched) similar patients who do not acquire a bacteremia. Dixon[305] has made similar but uncontrolled projections based on estimates pertinent to the broad spectrum of hospitals contained in the National Nosocomial Infections Study; his figures suggest a somewhat lesser impact economically. Overall, these three studies provide the best data on which to make national estimates: it appears that nosocomial bacteremias account for $280 to $863 million in excess hospital costs each year.

Epidemic Nosocomial Bacteremias

As shown in Figure 5, the frequency of reported epidemics of nosocomial bacteremia has also increased greatly over the past 15 years, especially since 1970.* The rise beginning in 1970 is very likely real and undoubtedly represents major changes in the population of patients hospitalized with respect to age and underlying diseases; in types of surgical operations being performed; in the use of infusion therapy, hemodialysis, and invasive vascular devices of all types; and in the use of systemic antibiotics within hospitals. It also reflects increasing awareness of nosocomial infection as a major health care problem, especially bacteremias related to infusion therapy.

Over 80% of the epidemics tabulated in this review were reported from university centers or other teaching hospitals which comprise but a minute fraction of the 7000-plus hospitals serving 38 million patients each year in this country. While the actual frequency of outbreaks of nosocomial infection of all types, but especially bacteremia, almost certainly is indeed higher in these centers (Table 5), it is also likely that epidemics of bacteremia are being underreported, and that many small outbreaks are never even detected. As previously noted, epidemics due to a common pathogen or multiple pathogens or occurring over a prolonged period of time can easily go unrecognized,[4] especially if a hospital does not fully characterize all blood isolates microbiologically (i.e., through species) or has no central mechanism — vis-a-vis a surveillance program — for routinely classifying every bacteremia as nosocomial or community acquired and for sensing subtle changes in the rate or profile of hospital acquired cases. Further data supporting the notion that outbreaks are being underreported are computer analyses of information from hospitals in the CDC's National Study showing that approximately 5% of all nosocomial infections occur in clusters of five to six cases caused by one strain, suggesting a small outbreak.[309] Further, based on his careful studies in a medium-sized community hospital, Scheckler[310] has reported that approximately 2% of nosocomial infections in his institution occur in significant clusters. Yet, the 97 outbreaks of culture-docmented bacteremia involving approximately 1000 patients that occurred between 1965 and 1978, mostly in hospitals in the U.S., represent less than 0.1% of the estimated million or more nosocomial bacteremias** that occurred in American hospitals over this 14-year period.

The case-fatality ratios of nosocomial bacteremia in epidemics (mean for 86 outbreaks of bona fide bacteremia, 25.3%, Table 7) is also considerably lower on the average than those reported from most centers for endemic bacteremias (Table 5). Except for outbreaks involving neonates that have been associated with an exception-

---

* The apparent decline in 1976 may reflect the usual 2- to 4-year lag between making a biomedical scientific observation and its eventual publication,[308] but could also represent greater general awareness of nosocomial hazards and important progress on a national scale in prevention of device-related infections.

** This estimate is in all likelihood a conservative figure, and is based on extrapolations using rates of nosocomial bacteremia reported during this period (Table 5).

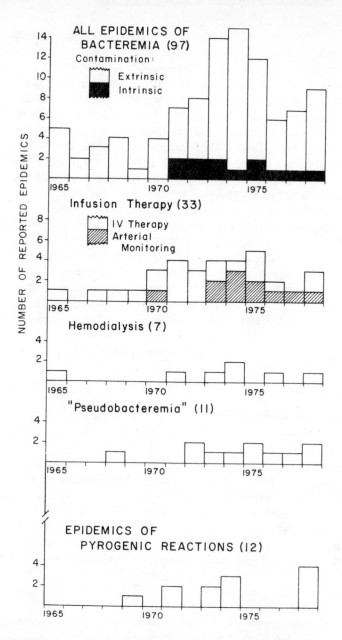

FIGURE 5. Epidemics of nosocomial bacteremia and pyrogenic reactions each year, 1965 to 1978. (From published reports in English world literature; for epidemics of bacteremia, bacteremias constituted at least 25% of epidemic infections).

ally high mortality (mean for 24 outbreaks, 54.3%), this differential mortality obtains for most pathogens, including *P. aeruginosa* and *Candida* (Table 7). Two important observations account for the disparate mortalities: (1) differing populations of patients affected in epidemics and developing bacteremia endemically, and (2) striking contrasts in sources of bacteremia in the two epidemiologic settings (Figure 2).

As previously noted, patients becoming bacteremic in an epidemic tend to be younger and are less likely to have a fatal underlying disease than patients with endemic nosocomial bacteremia. Also, in contrast to endemic bacteremias, most of which are secondary to a local infection (Figure 2), the vast majority of epidemic cases are primary bacteremias; nearly two thirds of the time the source is external to the patient (e.g., a hemodialysis machine, an intravenous infusion) and thus can be immediately and totally extirpated — if identified. The critical importance of this last observation is underscored by noting that even when septicemia due to a vascular cannula occurs endemically, the case-fatality ratio (19.5%, Table 7) is much lower than when bacteremia originates from a natural local infection (mean for all other sites in Table 7, 39.7%, p < 0.001). In the 1970 to 1971 nationwide epidemic due to one manufacturer's contaminated products, the case-fatality of *Enterobacter* septicemia in 258 analyzed cases, 13.4%, was considerably lower than the 35.8% mortality for *Enterobacter* septicemias in the Johns Hopkins Hospital between 1968 and 1974 (Table 7).

The full economic impact of epidemic bacteremias is unknown. The direct consequences in terms of added health care costs are certainly considerably less than the projected costs of endemic bacteremias (Table 6). The aftermath of adverse publicity and litigious action in epidemics may well be much greater. Except for their lamentable sequelae in terms of human suffering, epidemics have indirectly yielded very important gains for preventing hospital related bacteremia: our knowledge of the epidemiology of nosocomial infection, particularly bacteremias related to invasive devices, has been greatly expanded, and epidemics have enhanced general awareness that nosocomial infection — again, particularly nosocomial bacteremia — is a very real risk of modern hospital care, but a risk that may be greatly ameliorable.

EPIDEMIOLOGY OF NOSOCOMIAL BACTEREMIAS

Three points are fundamental to a discussion of the epidemiology of nosocomial bacteremia — particularly epidemic bacteremias — and its application to prevention:

1. While patients with fatal underlying diseases are clearly much more susceptible to hospital related infections of all types,[16,227,310] most nosocomial infections, especially epidemic bacteremias, occur in patients not intrinsically and irreversibly immunosuppressed. Nearly three fourths of the cases in the 84 epidemics of true bacteremia tabulated in this review occurred in patients who did have fatal underlying diseases. This point is even further underscored on reviewing the extraordinarily high rate of nosocomial bacteremia reported to occur in patients in intensive care units[311-314] (Table 8), patients who are not as a rule intrinsically immunologically compromised, but who are subjected to multiple invasive procedures after surgery or trauma.
2. While hepatitis has been a problem in hemodialysis and other multiple-transfused patients, and infections caused by cytomegalovirus, *Candida*, and *Aspergillus*, in severely immunocompromised patients, the vast majority of nosocomial infections of all types, but especially epidemic septicemias (Figure 3), are caused by aerobic bacteremia, primarily Gram-negative bacilli.
3. Many nosocomial infections and the vast majority of epidemic bacteremias (Figure 2) are causally related to transgression of normal host barriers by surgery or invasive devices, such as vascular cannulas used for infusion therapy or hemodialysis. In 41 (48%) of the 84 epidemics of true bacteremia, it was demonstrated that the epidemic pathogens gained direct entry into patients' bloodstreams through a device used for vascular access.

General Concepts

A hospital constitutes an almost unique milieu conducive to the development and

Table 8
INCIDENCE OF NOSOCOMIAL BACTEREMIA IN INTENSIVE CARE UNITS

Hospital	Type of patients	Year(s) of study	Number of patients at risk	Number of bacteremias	Incidence (per 1000 patients)	Ref.
University of Utah	Newborns	1970—1974	904	31	34.3	311
University of Maryland	Trauma and thoracic surgery	1970	135	44	325.9[a]	312
University of Maryland	Trauma	1971	62	7	112.9	313
University of Wisconsin	Medical and surgical	1976	73	16	219.5[a]	314

[a] Analysis restricted to patients confined in unit for more than 2 days.

spread of infection: the most susceptible individuals, many already infected by contagious microorganisms, are confined in close quarters, the most ill closest of all, in intensive care units. Common personnel provide care for large numbers of these patients, affording an almost unique opportunity for cross-infection. In modern medical care, patients are subjected to numerous invasive procedures and are continuously exposed to other infected patients and numerous potential reservoirs of pathogenic microorganisms in the hospital.

Most of our knowledge of the epidemiology of nosocomial infection — the hospital reservoirs of nosocomial pathogens and their mode(s) of transmission to patients — derives from investigations of epidemics. While studies of epidemics have been invaluable in identifying potential reservoirs and modes of transmission, it is less clear how applicable they are to endemic nosocomial infections, which comprise the majority of nosocomial infections in most hospitals.

Figure 6 depicts the major sources and modes of transmission of nosocomial pathogens in the hospital. In this conceptualization, patients' own (community-acquired) flora, the inanimate environment, medical personnel, and colonized or infected patients, all comprise potential reservoirs of nosocomial pathogens. Transmission occurs primarily by contact spread, to a much lesser extent by the airborne route. Antimicrobial therapy greatly modulates the profile of colonizing microorganisms. Pharyngeal aspiration, the presence of surgical wounds and, especially, exposure to invasive devices enormously amplify transmission and susceptibility to infection by all routes. It must be emphasized that while the technology of prevention of infection with regard to devices is far from optimal, employment of basic infection control procedures will assure relative freedom from infection wth limited exposures. In theory, many nosocomial infections, especially epidemic nosocomial bacteremias, are preventable.

Staphylococcus aureus and Hemolytic Streptococci

Although *S. aureus* and Group A streptococci have been greatly overshadowed by Gram-negative bacilli as agents of nosocomial infection in recent years, Gram-positive cocci of all types, primarily *S. aureus* and aerobic streptococci, account for approximately 30% of all endemic hospital acquired bacteremias (Figure 3), especially those occurring in newborns or those deriving from surgical wounds following clean surgery or from vascular access devices.[18,225,285,301,302,315-318] In some hospitals, it has been found that one half of all nosocomial staphylococcal septicemias originate from vascular cannulas.[315]

Group A *Streptococcus*, the scourge of obstetric units and nurseries in the last century ("puerperal fever") and an important cause of nosocomial bacteremia up to the 1940s, is responsible for only a small fraction of hospital acquired bacteremias at the present time.[225,285,286,301,302] Patients with cancer or those otherwise immunosuppressed have been most prone to develop nosocomial Group A streptococcemia.[285,319-321] Although there have continued to be occasional nursery outbreaks[322,323] and epidemics of postoperative surgical wound infection[324-329] caused by Group A streptococci, most epidemic infections have been nonbacteremic.

The majority of *S. aureus* and Group A streptococcal infections are local and involve the skin and soft tissues or the respiratory tract; bacteremia occurs in fewer than 10% of cases, even in epidemics. Nosocomial infections caused by these organisms derive almost solely from human reservoirs:[321-333] either patients' own cutaneous, respiratory, gastrointestinal, or genitourinary strains or organisms acquired through contact with medical personnel who themselves are colonized, harbor low-grade infection, or simply carry the organisms on their hands as a consequence of contacts with colonized or other infected patients. Spread of *S. aureus* and Group A *Streptococcus* on the hands

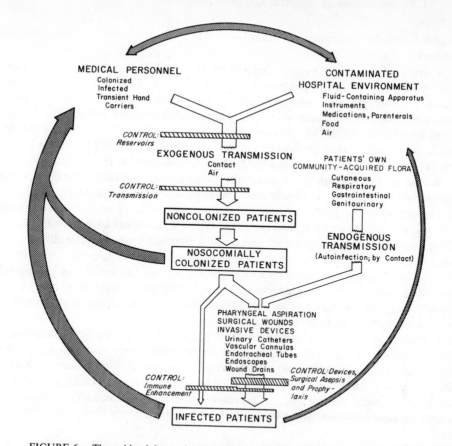

FIGURE 6. The epidemiology of nosocomial infection. Transmission occurs mainly by contact spread, to a much lesser extent by the airborne route. Antimicrobial therapy greatly modulates the profile of colonizing microorganisms. Aspiration, surgical wounds, and especially exposure to invasive medical devices amplify transmission, colonization, and susceptibility to infection by all routes. (From Maki, D. G., *Ann. Intern. Med.*, 89 (Part 2), 77, 1978. With permission).

of medical personnel has been implicated in the genesis of many hospital outbreaks, including most where bacteremias were prodominant (Table 8) — mainly in surgery[334-336] or hemodialysis patients.[337,338] Epidemic infections caused by a single strain of *S. aureus* or Group A *Streptoccus* almost always signifies a medical person who is a chronic carrier, either in the nasopharynx[339,340] or, in the case of Group A *Streptococcus*, the anus[324-328] or vagina[329] and who is also a heavy "shedder".

Two of the five outbreaks with *S. aureus* bacteremia tabulated in this review were caused by strains resistant to methicillin[334,335] — potentially harbingers of the future. Within several years after the introduction of methicillin in 1959, resistant strains of staphylococci, virtually all hospital related, appeared in British, French, Swiss, and Scandinavian hospitals[341-344] and over the next decade became important nosocomial pathogens in these countries. Although comparable antibiotic pressures conducive to selection of resistant strains seemed operative in the U.S., these strains, almost inexplicably, did not pose problems in the U.S. hospitals until quite recently. Since 1975, over a dozen nosocomial outbreaks caused by methicillin-resistant strains have been reported from U.S. hospitals,[345,346] most involving surgical or burn patients. The two outbreaks included in this review underscore the gravity of methicillin-resistance of hospital staphylococci. Klimek and co-workers[334] reported a small epidemic involving ten patients over a 12-month period; the outbreak was perpetuated by cross-infection and could only be controlled by identifying and excluding carriers among hospital personnel.

In a very sobering report by Crossley and co-workers,[335] 108 patients in a large midwestern city-county hospital contracted serious infections caused by strains resistant to methicillin and multiple aminoglycosides. One third of those infected developed bacteremia. The outbreak originated in the hospital's burn unit and coincided with a marked upsurge in the use of antistaphylococcal antibiotics in burn patients for prophylaxis. It rapidly spread outside of the unit to ultimately involve a total of 201 patients over a 2½ year period and had not been fully controlled at the time of the report. The mechanisms of spread of the epidemic strains in this outbreak were not satisfactorily elucidated, but evidence points towards contamination of inanimate objects and airborne spread in the burn unit and carriage on the hands of noncolonized medical personnel in other areas. Four discrete phage-types of *S. aureus* were identified in this outbreak indicating that "epidemic spread of a plasmid" mediating multiple resistances had probably occurred as well as spread of the epidemic organisms.

In both of the aforementioned outbreaks, heavy exposure to antibiotics predisposed to infection with resistant staphylococci. Multiply-resistant strains of *S. aureus*, with resistance to gentamicin as well as methicillin, have now caused outbreaks in Europe as well as in other hospitals in the U.S.[347,348]

The relative importance of endogenous infection by patients' autochthonous strains of *S. aureus* remains unclear. A number of studies have shown that prolonged hospitalization increases the likelihood of nosocomial colonization.[330,333] Moreover, Rifkind and co-workers[349] and others[330,333,350] have stated that nasal carriers undergoing elective surgery are at much greater risk of developing postoperative wound infections with the same strains; however, other studies have not uniformly confirmed these observations.

Although as many as 60% of hospital personnel are nasal carriers of *S. aureus* at some time, only 20% are permanent carriers, and of these, but a fraction are shedders of virulent organisms, capable of causing epidemic disease.[330,333,351,352] Obviously, persons with suppurative lesions, usually caused by *S. aureus* or Group A streptococci,[329] or with clinical pharyngitis[353] that may be streptococcal, pose a hazard to susceptible patients and must be excluded from patient contact. However, in the absence of an identified hospital problem with *S. aureus* or Group A *Streptococcus*, there would appear to be little, if any, epidemiologic value in performing routine culture surveillance of hospital personnel or to exclude those asymptomatic carriers so identified.

The work of Rammelkamp and co-workers,[332] Burke,[354] and others[330,333] suggests that airborne transmission of organisms is relatively unimportant (as compared to contact) in the spread of *S. aureus* and Group A streptococcal infections endemically; but airborne spread may become very important in a burn center[335,919] or when a heavy shedder works within an operating room[329,339,340,353] or laboratory, (*S. aureus* pseudo-bacteremias have stemmed from a shedder laboratory technician who processed blood cultures[708]). Similarly, there is little evidence to suggest that either staphylococci or streptococci are normally spread to any great extent by fomites,[331,355] except possibly within a burn unit.[335]

Isolating colonized and infected patients — in nurseries, instituting cohort nursing — and using hexachlorophene for handwashing by medical personnel and for washing patients, have been the most effective measures for reducing colonization and curtailing spread of *S. aureus* infection endemically and in an epidemic setting.[330,333,356-358] Because of concern regarding possible neurotoxicity, use of hexachlorophene for routine bathing of infants was discontinued in this country in 1972. This was followed by a marked upsurge in the incidence of endemic staphylococcal disease[357] and in outbreaks of staphylococcal infection in newborn nurseries.[358] Cruse and Foord[359] have reported that hexachlorophene showers prior to elective clean surgery can reduce the rate of postoperative wound infection twofold.

Group B *Streptococcus* (*Streptococcus agalactiae*) has become the leading pathogen in sepsis of the newborn in the developed countries where it has had an incidence of 1 to 5 cases per 1000 live births and a mortality of 40 to 50%.[360-366]Bacteremia occurs in over one half of cases, often in association with meningitis. As first delineated by Franciosi,[361] Baker,[362] and their co-workers, disease presents in two forms (which probably also differ epidemiologically): " early infection", occurring in the first hours to days after birth and associated with overwhelming sepsis, respiratory distress, and a mortality of approximately 55%; "late infection", often presenting after the child has been taken home, but much less severe clinically (mortality, approximately 23%) and usually manifesting as isolated meningitis. Early disease appears to be maternally acquired and may even begin *in utero*. Studies by Davis and co-workers[367] suggest that intrauterine fetal monitoring may promote colonization. Most cases of Group B streptococcal sepsis are sporadic, but recently clusters of late-appearing cases have been identified.[368,369] Studies by Steere,[369] Aber,[370] and their CDC co-workers, and by Paredes and associates,[371] have shown that nosocomial colonization of newborns is frequent and often occurs horizontally (i.e., infant-to-infant) rather than vertically (i.e., mother-to-infant). Also, many female nursery personnel are commonly genital or rectal carriers. Following a small cluster of three cases of Group B sepsis in one nursery over a 6-day period in 1974, Steere and co-workers[369] instituted cohort nursing and other measures to prevent contact spread; nosocomial colonization of infants by type IIIB strains in that nursery fell from 31% to 2%, and no further infections occurred.

Hemolytic streptococci of Lancefield's Group C, G, and lower groups also cause occasional nosocomial bacteremias, mainly in compromised patients. But clinical studies by Duma,[285] Armstrong,[372] Broome,[373] and their co-workers indicate that these groups are not important hospital pathogens, particularly when compared with Group A or Group D streptococci. Epidemics caused by these organisms have been rare, but when encountered, resemble outbreaks with Group A *Streptococcus* epidemiologically.[374]

Staphylococcus epidermidis

Coagulase-negative *Staphylococcus epidermidis* (formerly *Staphylococcus albus*) is one of the most frequent isolates from positive blood cultures but turns out to be a contaminant in the vast majority of cases,[82-85,144] reflecting its role as the most common aerobic constituent of the cutaneous microflora.[922] The species possesses much less intrinsic capacity for invasiveness than *S. aureus*, and most *S. epidermidis* infections — folliculitis, skin pustules, "stitch abscesses" of surgical incisions, and community acquired urinary tract infections[923,924] (mainly in females) — are characterized clinically by indolence.

Medical advances of the past two decades, however, have elevated the organism to a position of considerable nosocomial importance. It is now clear that: (1) *S. epidermidis* has a unique predilection to produce infection in association with prosthetic implants of all types, including vascular cannulas,[716,722] ventriculo-atrial shunts,[160,925] prosthetic joints,[926,927] and, especially, prosthetic heart valves;[158,159,875-878] and (2) the species is intrinsically more resistant to antibiotics than *S. aureus* — up to one third of naturally occurring strains are resistant to methicillin.[928] While most *S. epidermidis* infections occurring on implanted prostheses also tend to be indolent clinically, they are characteristically extremely refractory to treatment. In most cases the infected device must be removed to control the infection.

Most nosocomial infections with *S. epidermidis* are considered to derive from the patients' autochthonous strains. However, studies showing a strong correlation between positive intraoperative cultures and subsequent prosthetic valve endocarditis suggest that some of these serious deep infections may originate from extrinsic sources of intra-operative contamination of the surgical wound, the device itself, or the bloodstream.[880,882] *S. epidermidis* is a very common contaminant of ambient air,[431,881,882,926] presumably related to the continuous shedding of skin organisms by individuals in the immediate environment. Counts of airborne organisms in operating rooms are directly proportional to the number of persons present in the room.[881]

Two outbreaks of prosthetic valve endocarditis caused by methicillin-resistant *S. epidermidis* appear to have been of operative origin.[929,930] Perioperative prophylaxis with both isoxazyl penicillins and aminoglycosides may have selected for the more resistant strains. Zaky and co-workers[929] reported a small outbreak involving six postoperative patients over an unstated period. A significantly greater proportion of operating room and surgical intensive care unit personnel was found to carry the epidemic biotype in their noses, compared with laboratory personnel, but the exact mechanism of transmission of infection was not established, and the outbreak ceased spontaneously before control measures were instituted.

Hammond and Stiver[930] describe an outbreak of nine cases of methicillin-resistant prosthetic valve endocarditis in a Canadian hospital; eight of the patients had been operated on over a 9-month period, and baseline rates indicate that the marked upsurge in cases clearly constituted an epidemic. Data were not provided, however, to establish whether the infecting organisms were a common strain or whether surgical personnel were frequent carriers of the resistant strain, but an intraoperative origin of infection is suggested by positive cultures of pump blood in three of the cases. Limiting the number of personnel and traffic in cardiac operating rooms terminated the outbreak.

Whereas the majority of wound infections in clean operations derive from microorganisms of endogenous or exogenous origin introduced into the wound at the time of surgery,[905-907] prosthetic materials can also become infected at any time following surgery by bacteremic seeding. Up to 60% of infections originating from vascular cannulas are caused by *S. epidermidis*.[716,722] It is very conceivable that unrecognized cannula-related infections may be responsible for a significant number of early-appearing infections of prosthetic devices.

Streptococcus pneumoniae

Streptococcus pneumoniae — the pneumococcus — remains the preeminent agent of community acquired bacterial pneumonia throughout the world; approximately 25% of cases are complicated by bacteremia or meningitis. Until very recently, pneumococcal strains were uniformly highly sensitive to benzylpenicillin, and susceptibility testing of clinical isolates was considered unnecessary.[375-377]

Up to the early 1940s, the organism was also an important nosocomial pathogen, and clusters of hospital acquired pneumococcal pneumonia were well known.[378] In the Boston City Hospital in 1935, *S. pneumoniae* was responsible for 22% of all nosocomial bacteremias (34 of 147, Figure 4) and 40% of all bacteremic deaths.[3] With the introduction of penicillin, however, its importance rapidly waned (Figure 4), and hospital outbreaks became very rare. Although transmission of pneumococcal infection occurs almost singularly by droplet spread, the communicability of *S. pneumoniae* infection has been considered so minimal that isolation of infected patients in the hospital has generally been considered unnecessary.

In 1977,[290-293] six children hospitalized in two South African hospitals 300 miles apart developed bacteremic pneumonia or meningitis caused by multiply-resistant pneumococci with greatly reduced susceptibility to penicillin (minimal inhibitory concentrations, 2 to 8 mcg/ml) and resistance to multiple other antibiotics, frequently chloramphenicol, tetracycline, and erythromycin. As recounted by Ward,[294] Koornhoff,[295] and co-workers, the strains, all type 6A or 19A, rapidly spread to other patients, to hospital personnel, and to other South African hospitals. Between January 1977 and August 1978, penicillin-resistant pneumococci were isolated from the blood or cerebrospinal fluid of 48 children, 44% of whom died despite treatment with the usual regimens of high dosage aqueous penicillin or a variety of other antibiotics. Infections with these strains were almost exclusively hospital acquired and occurred most frequently in children previously exposed to antibiotics.

Beginning in August 1977, programs were initiated in some of the involved hospitals aimed at eradicating carriage of these strains and preventing their spread.[295] Efforts were made to reduce unnecessary use of antibiotics and to identify all carriers on an ongoing basis by culture surveillance. Carriers identified were placed in respiratory isolation, and attempts were made to eradicate carriage by treatment with rifampin, fusidic acid, tetracycline, or vancomycin. Although occasional sporadic infections caused by the multiply-resistant strains have continued to occur, these strains have been essentially eliminated from the involved hospitals, and the incidence of systemic infection has declined substantially.

This sobering report indicates that naturally occurring strains of pneumococci also have the potential to develop and express significant resistance to penicillin and multiple other antibiotics, while retaining virulence and communicability. Although a bacteremic infection in a Minnesota child in 1977 was found to have been caused by a similarly resistant strain,[379] recent culture surveys of large numbers of pneumoccal isolates in the U.S. indicate that these strains are not yet prevalent in this country.[380,381] However, if one views the relationship of the South African problem to heavy use of antibiotics, it can be anticipated that their appearance as major nosocomial pathogens in this country may not be far off. The recently released polyvalent pneumococcal vaccine[382-384] would seem most timely in view of the events in South Africa, but it must be pointed out that all infected South African patients were children less than 2 years of age, an age group in which the vaccine has been least immunogenic.

Gram-Negative Bacilli: An Epidemiologic Overview

The extraordinary increase in the past three decades of nosocomial bacteremia caused by Gram-negative bacilli, especially multiply-resistant Enterobacteriaceae such as *Klebsiella-Enterobacter*, *Serratia*, and *Proteus*, and the pseudomonads (Figure 4), directly parallels ever-increasing use of antibiotics in hospitals.[3,296,297,375] Many of these organisms normally colonize the human intestine. Moreover it is clear that hospitalization alone, augmented by inanition, advanced age, and severe underlying disease but independent of exposure to antibiotics, is associated with nosocomial gastrointestinal colonization by these more resistant hospital organisms[385-387] and with Gram-negative colonization of the oropharynx[386,388-392] and skin.[393,394] This affords an opportunity for endogenous infection of the catheterized urinary tract, surgical wounds, the lower respiratory tract, or vascular access sites by these hospital-acquired organisms. Exposure to antibiotics greatly enhances Gram-negative colonization and increases the risk of related infection and superinfection.[396-400]

While many endemic Gram-negative nosocomial infections are thought to derive from patients' own strains, except for a few selective studies of specific organisms such as *Klebsiella* in a hyperendemic setting[401] and *Pseudomonas aeruginosa* in patients with leukemia,[402] comprehensive studies to ascertain the true importance of nosocomial enteric colonization in the genesis of endemic nosocomial infection have not been undertaken. The few epidemics of nosocomial bacteremia linked to enteric colonization caused by organisms other than *Salmonella* occurred mainly in newborns (four outbreaks[403-406]) and once in adults with leukemia.[407]

Gram-negative bacilli differ from Gram-positive cocci by their extraordinary abilities not only to subsist, but also to proliferate, in the countless aqueous environs of the hospital. Pseudomonads in their naturally occurring state, particularly *P. aeruginosa* and *P. cepacia*, attain concentrations of 10^6-10^7 organisms per milliliter in distilled water[408-410] (Figure 7); members of the tribe Klebsielleae — *Klebsiella, Enterobacter*, and *Serratia* — grow luxuriously in various dextrose-containing parenteral solutions.[411,412] A rapidly increasing number of hospital epidemics and the majority of outbreaks of nosocomial Gram-negative bacteremia have been traced to contamination of common source vehicles such as medications, hand lotions, disinfectants, blood products, large-volume parenterals, hemodialysis machines, and ventilators and other respiratory therapy equipment (Table 9). At least 11 outbreaks of true bacteremia and 3 of pseudobacteremia were traced to contaminated disinfectant solutions used for cutaneous antisepsis or for disinfection of apparatus used in patient care. Exposure of susceptible patients to these reservoirs, usually by contact, leads to colonization (Figure 6). If a patient is highly susceptible or the inoculum is large, e.g., 10,000 organisms per cubic foot of effluent from a contaminated inhalation therapy machine,[408] or the organisms are infused directly into the bloodstream, infection becomes almost inevitable. These outbreaks point up the importance of reliable techniques for disinfection of any fluid-containing apparatus which comes into direct contact with patients, especially in association with an invasive device such as a vascular cannula or an endotracheal tube.

The many outbreaks of nosocomial Gram-negative bacteremia originating from environmental reservoirs raise an important question: what areas of the hospital, what products or apparatus should be monitored microbiologically on a routine basis? With the exception of regularly monitoring respiratory therapy equipment, hydrotherapy tanks, hemodialysis machines, and sterilization procedures, in the absence of an identified endemic or epidemic nosocomial problem, the benefits of routine microbiologic surveillance are unclear.

Eight of the epidemics of nosocomial Gram-negative bacteremia were traced to intrinsically contaminated commercial products, primarily large-volume parenterals.[4,140,413-419] The author believes quality assurance is an industry responsibility, and that in the absence of a suspected problem, culture surveillance of presumptively sterile commercial products on a routine basis at the hospital level is not worthwhile.

The endemic rate of nosocomial bacteremia in newborn and adult intensive care units (Table 8) has been extremely high, ranging from 34.3 to 325.9 cases per 1000.[311-314] Not unexpectedly, many epidemics of nosocomial bacteremia, particularly outbreaks caused by Gram-negative bacilli, developed in the closed setting of an intensive care unit or hemodialysis center (21 of 65 epidemics of nosocomial Gram-negative rod bacteremia) or newborn nursery (24 outbreaks). Heavy use of broad-spectrum antibiotics, often for prophylaxis, was considered a central factor in the genesis and propagation of these infections (12 outbreaks). Only by curtailing antimicrobial therapy could epidemic Gram-negative infections be controlled in a number of outbreaks of nonbacteremic infection reported in the literature[397,398] (Figure 8). Nowhere is the hospital does indiscriminate antimicrobial therapy have such far-reaching consequences as in the geographically confined populations of the intensive care, dialysis and burn units, and newborn nursery, where emergence of microbial resistance is combined with unique opportunities for its spread and perpetuation.

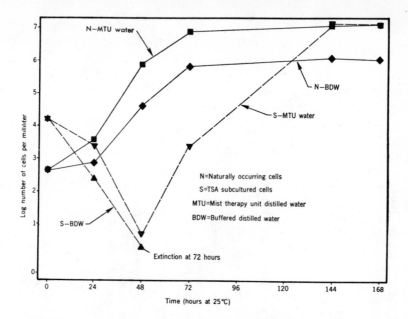

FIGURE 7. Growth of *Pseudomonas aeruginosa* in distilled water at 25°C. Naturally occurring strains grow superiorly to laboratory-adapted subcultures. (From Favero, M. S., Carson, L. A., Bond, W. W., Petersen, N. J., *Science*, 173, 836, copyright 1971 by the American Association for the Advancement of Science. With Permission.

Over 100 studies have implicated carriage of Gram-negative pathogens on the hands of medical personnel in the spread of nosocomial infections, including 12 epidemics of bacteremia occurring in intensive care units and newborn nurseries. Studies by Salzman,[420] Bruun,[421] Petersen,[422], Knittle,[423] and the author[235] and their co-workers have shown that approximately 50% of medical personnel randomly sampled at any one time carry Gram-negative bacilli on their hands, predominantly organisms of the *Klebsiella-Enterobacter* group. In a 4-month study by the author and co-workers[235] (Table 10), all 25 personnel in a neurosurgical unit cultured three times weekly were found to carry Gram-negative bacilli and 64%, *S. aureus*, at some time. Culturing subjects serially showed considerable variation in individual carriage patterns, suggesting major differences in persons' cutaneous microbiologic milieus or in hand-washing practices. Carriage of Gram-negative bacilli and *S. aureus* typically was transient, often reflecting the presence of patients infected by the same species on the ward; *S. aureus* or the same Gram-negative species could be recovered in the next culture only 16% of the time, and prolonged carriage of a single Gram-negative species was uncommon. Whereas several outbreaks have recently been traced to a medical person being permanently colonized by one Gram-negative species, and accordingly a chronic hand carrier,[424,426] the phenomenom appears to be rare.

Except possibly in burn units[427] and in other unusual environmental circumstances,[428-430] there is little evidence that hospital air is a major source of nosocomial infection caused by Gram-negative bacilli. Sampling studies have shown that ambient hospital air normally contains only very small numbers of these organisms ($<1/ft^3$).[431] However, one unusual experience bears mention: a high incidence of endemic nosocomial Gram-negative bacteremia in a new hospital, particularly with *P. aeruginosa*, was linked epidemiologically by Grieble and co-workers[430] to a chute-hydropulping system for solid waste disposal. The system was found to be generating aerosols containing massive numbers of Gram-negative bacilli, exceeding 150 organisms per cubic

Table 9

EPIDEMIOLOGIC MECHANISMS AND PATHOGENS IDENTIFIED IN 86
REPORTED EPIDEMICS OF TRUE NOSOCOMIAL BACTEREMIA, 11 OUTBREAKS
OF PSEUDOBACTEREMIA, AND 12 OUTBREAKS OF PYROGENIC REACTIONS

Epidemiologic mechanisms[a]	Number of epidemics	Epidemic pathogens (number of epidemics)[b]
Medical personnel		
Transient hand carriage	16	*Klebsiella* (5), *S. aureus* (3), *Serratia* (2), *P. aeruginosa* (2), *Citrobacter* (2), *Enterobacter*[d] (1), Gr. B *Streptococcus* (1)
Chronically colonized[c]	4	*Citrobacter* (2), Gr. A *Streptococcus* (1), *Proteus* (1)
Infusion therapy		
Intrinsically contaminated fluid	7	*Enterobacter* (3), *P. cepacia* (3), *Citrobacter* (1), *S. cholerae-suis* (1)
Contaminated intravenous medication	3	*Flavobacterium* (1), *P. cepacia* (1), *Serratia* (1)
Pharmacy-derived contamination	2	*E. aerogenes* (1), *C. parapsilosis* (1)
Extrinsically contaminated fluid, Source indeterminate	4	*P. cepacia* (2), *Klebsiella* (1), *Enterobacter* (1), *E. coli* (1), *Serratia* (1)
Contaminated blood product	6	*P. cepacia* (2), *S. cholerae-suis* (1), *Enterobacter* (1), Pyrogens (2)
Contamination of arterial pressure-monitoring system	10	*P. cepacia* (3), *Serratia* (3), *Enterobacter* (2), *P. aeruginosa* (1), *Flavobacterium* (1), *Candida* (1)
Contaminated disinfectant	11	*P. cepacia* (6), *P. aeruginosa* (4), *Enterobacter* (1)
Hyperalimentation	1	*C. parapsilosis* (1)
Inadequate cutaneous antisepsis	1	*S. aureus* (1)
Intra-arterial cancer chemotherapy	1	*S. aureus* (1)
Hemodialysis		
Contaminated machines, dialyzers	11	Pyrogens (6), *P. aeruginosa* (3), *P. cepacia* (1), *Bacillus cereus* (1)
Cross-infection of access sites	2	*S. aureus* (2)
Evacuated blood collection tubes	2	*Serratia* (2)
Cardiac surgery		
Contaminated porcine heart valves	1	*Mycobacterium chelonei* (1)

Airborne contamination of heart blood in operating room	2	*Aspergillus* (1), *Penicillium* (1)
Cardiac catheterization	4	Pyrogens (4)
Contaminated respiratory nebulizer solution	1	*Klebsiella* (1)
Airborne spread of respiratory infection	3	*N. meningitis* (1), *H. influenzae* (1), *S. pneumoniae* (1)
GI colonization	8[e]	*Salmonella* (4), *P. aeruginosa* (2), *Klebsiella* (1), *E. coli* (1), *Clostridium* (1)
Primary bacteremias, reservoirs of epidemic pathogen and modes of transmission never elucidated	18[f]	*Klebsiella* (5), *E. coli* (3), *Serratia* (2), *Citrobacter* (2), *Listeria* (2), *P. aeruginosa* (1), *Acinetobacter* (1), *Flavobacterium* (1), *Clostridium* (1)
Pseudobacteremia[g]	11	*Acinetobacter* (2), *P. cepacia* (1), *P. maltophilia* (1), *Enterobacter* (1), *Serratia* (1), *E. coli* (1), *Flavobacterium* (1), *S. aureus* (1), *Moraxella* (1), *Bacillus* spp. (1), *Clostridium* (1)

[a] More than one mechanism was often operative in a given epidemic; hence the total of all categories exceeds the number of epidemics tabulated.

[b] For citations to individual epidemics and further details, see text.

[c] Also shown to be an important mechanism in hospital epidemics of *S. aureus* infection and in one outbreak of nonbacteremic *Acinetobacter* infection.[426]

[d] In every outbreak except one specifically noted, *E. cloacae* or *E. agglomerans* was the epidemic pathogen.

[e] All outbreaks with organisms other than *Salmonella* occurred in neonates.

[f] Fifteen (83%) of the 18 occurred in newborn nurseries or neonatal intensive care units.

[g] For further details on epidemiologic mechanisms, see Table 13.

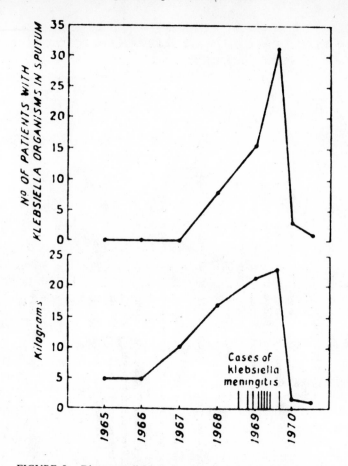

FIGURE 8. Direct parallel between kilograms of antibiotics used and nosocomial colonization and infection with multiply-resistant *Klebsiella* in a neurosurgical intensive care unit, 1965 to 1970. Only by severely restricting use of antibiotics — mainly by curtailing use for prophylaxis — could the epidemic be controlled. (From Price, D. J. E. and Sleigh, J. D., *Lancet*, 2, 1213, 1970. With permission).

Table 10
MICROORGANISMS CARRIED ON THE HANDS OF NURSES AND PHYSICIANS IN A NEUROSURGICAL UNIT

	All microorganisms	Gram-negative bacilli	*Staphylococcus aureus*
Mean $\log_{10}$ CFU recovered from persons' hands	4.59	1.04	0.44
(range individual means)[a]	(3.31—5.76)	(0.29—1.93)	(0—1.45)
Percent all cultures positive[b]	100.0	44.5	11.2
Percent all individuals positive at least once[a]	100	100	64

[a]   Six to 34 cultures were obtained at random from each of 25 medical personnel over a 4-month period.

[b]   Total number of cultures, 348.

From Maki, D. G., *Ann. Intern. Med.*, 89 (Part 2), 77, 1978. With permission.

Table 11
EFFECT OF CLOSING A CHUTE-HYDROPULPING DISPOSAL SYSTEM ON LEVELS OF AIRBORNE ORGANISMS AND NOSOCOMIAL SEPTICEMIA IN A NEW VETERANS HOSPITAL

		Rates of septicemia (per 1000 discharges)	
Period (each, 19 months)	Mean air counts (per ft.³)	Enterobacteriaceae	Pseudomonas aeruginosa
Before closure	>150 (many Gram-negative bacilli)	5.4	0.9
After closure	40 (no Gram-negative bacilli)[a]	1.9[b]	0.3[b]

[a] Five months after closure.
[b] p < 0.0005.

Adapted from Grieble, H. G., Bird, T. J., Nidea, H. M., and Miller, C. A., *J. Infect. Dis.,* 130, 602, 1974.

foot; closure of the disposal system was followed by a marked fall in counts of airborne Gram-negative organisms and a commensurate decline in rates of nosocomial Gram-negative bacteremia (Table 11).

Escherichia coli

E. coli is the most important Gram-negative hospital pathogen on an absolute numbers basis (Figure 3) accounting for 20% of all endemic nosocomial bacteremias, most originating from the urinary tract, infected surgical wounds, or pneumonias. Moreover, E. coli is one of the leading causes of neonatal sepsis and meningitis;[432-435] as reported by Robbins and collaborators,[436] 84% of cases of neonatal meningitis with or without bacteremia, and 39% of cases of bacteremia without meningitis, are caused by strains with the K1 capsular antigen, which confers increased virulence.[437] However, except for nursery outbreaks caused by enterotoxigenic strains which rarely produce invasive disease,[438-440] nosocomial epidemics of E. coli infection — including bacteremia — have been rare, especially in adults.

Three of the five tabulated outbreaks occurring between 1965 and 1978 involved newborns and one involved young children undergoing cardiovascular surgery. In 1966, two children who had had surgical repair of ventricular septal defects on the same day in a Los Angeles hospital developed E. coli 078:H18 septicemia with endocarditis in the early postoperative period; the source of E. coli, however, eluded detection.[441] In 1973, a nursery outbreak of necrotizing enterocolitis in neonates, which had an 88% mortality, was found by Speer and co-workers[403] to be associated with peritonitis and bacteremia caused by one nonenteropathogenic strain of E. coli. Colonization of 41 infants by the epidemic strain over a 2-month period was observed, yet the reservoirs and mode of transmission of the organism in that nursery were never delineated.

Headings and Overall[442] recently reported a cluster of three neonates who developed fulminant E. coli 07:K1:H- meningitis and septicemia over a 9-day period; all three infants died. The outbreak was suspected by the unusual bacteriologic characteristics (nonmotile and ornithine-negative) of the spinal fluid isolates from the three cases. Eight other infants were shown to be colonized, but the mechanisms of spread of E. coli also were not elucidated.

A recent, extraordinary outbreak, reported by Horwitz and Bennett,[443] took place in a small community hospital in 1974 when nine newborns developed pneumoperitoneum with peritonitis and sepsis over a 4-month period; three infants died. Nonenterotoxigenic *E. coli* of differing serotypes were recovered from blood or peritoneal exudate of all infants. Exploratory laparotomy done in several cases failed to reveal sites of intestinal perforation. An in-depth investigation, the basis of which was a series of meticulous case-control analyses, identified a highly significant association between illness and exposure to one of 11 nursing personnel working in the nursery. Further studies showed that this individual routinely inserted rectal thermometers in a manner very likely to produce rectal perforation. After she was removed from the nursery and axillary temperature-taking replaced measurements per rectum, the epidemic ceased. Although by strict definition this was a common-source outbreak, the epidemiologic picture and epidemic curve were atypical for this mechanism of transmission. Only an outstanding clinical-epidemiologic investigation, applying methods to be discussed in detail later in this review, unraveled an extraordinary outbreak.

The single epidemic of nosocomial *E. coli* bacteremia in adult patients derived from infusion therapy; *E. coli* was responsible for two of the four total cases in a small outbreak caused by contaminated intravenous fluid.[444]

Nonenterotoxigenic strains of *E. coli* are the major aerobic constituents of the gastrointestinal flora and are responsible for most endemic *E. coli* infections.[436,445] Epidemiologic studies suggest that most hospital acquired infections are autogenous, caused by patients' own strains,[446] or in the case of neonates, by maternally acquired strains;[447,448] nosocomial gastrointestinal colonization may occasionally derive from contaminated hospital foods.[449]

The sheer number of patients with *E. coli* infections, however, comprises an enormous hospital reservoir of the organism, and it is tempting to speculate that the seeming rarity of epidemic *E. coli* infection, including bacteremia, may be more apparent than real: (1) it is very conceivable that many small common-source outbreaks are concealed in the vast number of endemic infections; (2) except in outbreaks of diarrheal disease in newborns and unusual clusters of infection such as those described above, serotyping of nosocomial isolates is rarely pursued; and (3) while it is not recovered from the hands of medical personnel nearly so frequently as is *Klebsiella* or *Enterobacter*, *E. coli* is commonly present.[235,420-423] Conversely, *E. coli* does not survive in commercial parenteral solutions such as 5% dextrose-in-water,[411] is susceptible to most disinfectants, and is infrequently recovered from cultures of aqueous environments in the hospital. These properties may explain the veritable absence of outbreaks of *E. coli* infection traced to a common vehicle, such as a medication, a disinfectant, or a large-volume parenteral, as have occurred so frequently with pseudomonads, the Klebsielleae, and other more hardy Gram-negative pathogens.

Klebsiella-Enterobacter

These two major groups of organisms in the Enterobacteraceae individually rank second only to *E. coli* in overall frequency as Gram-negative hospital pathogens. Their almost meteoric rise to nosocomial prominence, along with *Serratia* and the pseudomonads (Figure 4), is the unwanted legacy of three decades of unrestricted use of antibiotics in hospitals. Prior to 1960, *Klebsiella-Enterobacter* organisms were relatively infrequent hospital pathogens, including blood[3,296,297] (Figure 4). Together, they now rank first as agents of nosocomial bacteremia, both endemically and especially in epidemics[3,298,302,450-454] (Figure 3, Table 7).

Most endemic nosocomial infections with *Klebsiella* and *Enterobacter* involve postoperative surgical wounds or the instrumented urinary or respiratory tracts of patients who have undergone surgery and received prolonged antimicrobial therapy. *Klebsiella* and *Enterobacter* have also become increasingly important causes of neonatal sepsis. The majority of endemic bacteremias originate from urinary or respiratory tract infections or from vascular catheters.

Klebsiella and *Enterobacter* have minor biochemical differences, but *Klebsiella* is motile and encapsulated and is probably more virulent. It causes two to four times as many endemic nosocomial infections as *Enterobacter,* including bacteremia[298,450-452] (Figure 3, Table 7), and has been implicated in many more hospital outbreaks of non-bacteremic infection. In many outbreaks, the epidemic *Klebsiella* strain was resistant to multiple antibiotics — ascribed to intensive use of broad-spectrum therapy in the population at risk;[397,398,455-463] when studied, resistance was inevitably shown to be plasmid-mediated. Control of epidemic infections with multiply-resistant strains was not achieved in some hospitals until the use of antibiotics was substantially restricted[397,398,455,456,463] (Figure 8). In most outbreaks, the organism was transmitted between patients on the hands of medical personnel.

In contradistinction, few hospital outbreaks of nonbacteremic *Enterobacter* infection have been reported. In most *Enterobacter* outbreaks, whether of localized infection[465] or bacteremia,[4,109,415,416,466-471] the epidemic strain retained its original pattern of antimicrobial susceptibilities. These differences between *Klebsiella* and *Enterobacter* with regard to antimicrobial resistance patterns in an epidemic setting may well reflect the greater propensity for *Klebseilla* to receive and exchange R-factors mediating antibiotic resistance.[394,472]

A small common-source outbreak of overwhelming *Klebsiella* pneumonia, associated twice with bacteremia, was traced by Mertz et al.[464] to a contaminated epinephrine solution used in respiratory nebulizers. Morse and co-workers[473] linked a contaminated container of hand cream to six cases of intravenous catheter-related *Klebsiella* septicemia in an intensive care unit.

Eight epidemics of *Klebsiella* sepsis occurred in newborns.[404,474-480] In four of these outbreaks, the epidemic infections were primary bacteremias, and in three outbreaks, the portal of entry and mode of spread of *Klebsiella* remained obscure.[474,475,477] Nine *Klebsiella* septicemias were traced to intravenous therapy in an outbreak reported by Ross and associates;[479] organisms were spread between infants on the hands of nursery personnel and appear to have infected scalp-vein needle sites. In four nursery epidemics, multiple sites were colonized or infected;[404,476,478,480] in three of these outbreaks, microbiologic studies also suggest that *Klebsiella* was transmitted between infants by organisms carried on the hands of medical personnel.[404,476,478]

Despite its lesser role as an endemic nosocomial pathogen, *Enterobacter* has been a cause of epidemics of hospital acquired bacteremia almost as frequently as *Klebsiella* (Figure 3). In seven of the eight outbreaks with *Enterobacter*, epidemic septicemias were produced by contaminated infusate given parenterally (platelet packs,[466] intravenous fluid,[4,413,415,467-469] or in-line transducer domes used for hemodynamic monitoring[470]). The single outbreak of secondary bacteremias took place in a burn center; Mayhall and co-workers[471] ascribed 15 cases of *Enterobacter cloacae* septicemia originating from infected burn wounds to cross-contamination of burn wounds by organisms carried on the hands of the units' personnel or present in hydrotherapy tanks. Mortality was 87%.

These epidemiologic contrasts between *Klebsiella* and *Enterobacter* may be explained by differences in abilities to subsist in various aspects of the hospital environment; Pollack and co-workers[394] found *Klebsiella* to be the Gram-negative species recovered most frequently from the hands of patients randomly surveyed. *Enterobacter,* especially *E. cloacae* and *E. agglomerans* (formerly *Erwinia, Herbicola-Lathyri* group), survives and even proliferates in aqueous hospital environments, such as parenteral solutions more successfully than *Klebsiella*[411,412] and may be more resistant to certain chemical disinfectants such as those of the quarternary ammonium group. (Outbreaks of true bacteremia[109] and of pseudobacteremia[110] have originated from quaternaries contaminated by *Enterobacter*.)

Serratia marcescens

While it is a fermentative Gram-negative rod and a member of the Enterobacteriaceae, *Serratia* clinically and epidemiologically more closely resembles *P. aeruginosa* in its intrinsic resistance to most antibiotics and ability to subsist in water-containing reservoirs throughout the hospital, and in its propensity to cause nosocomial disease almost singularly. Similar to *Klebsiella* and *Enterobacter*, most infections with *Serratia* involve the manipulated urinary or respiratory tract, surgical wounds, or vascular catheter sites, and occur in premature infants or adults who have undergone surgery or sustained major trauma. In the past decade, *Serratia* has become a major Gram-negative blood stream pathogen in many teaching hospitals and other referral institutions, rivaling *P. aeruginosa*.[481-486] Mortality of *Serratia* bacteremia in most of these centers has exceeded 35%.

Over 50 reported nosocomial outbreaks since 1965 alone attest to *Serratia's* growing importance as a hospital pathogen. Most epidemics have occurred in adults and involved catheter-associated urinary tract infections[487-490] or pneumonias affecting patients receiving ventilatory assistance or some other form of inhalation therapy.[491-494] Exposure to broad-spectrum antibiotics proved to be an almost universal risk factor predisposing to infection. In most outbreaks, if a sufficient number of strains were serotyped, a single epidemic strain or, at most, several strains predominated. Environmental sources of *Serratia*, primarily contaminated solutions used in respiratory therapy equipment or the equipment itself, were implicated in most outbreaks of respiratory infection. In contrast, with epidemics of *Serratia* urinary tract infection, epidemic organisms were transmitted between susceptible patients — most of whom were receiving broad-spectrum antibiotics — and even between hospitals[490] on the hands of uninfected hospital personnel. Confinement in an intensive care unit or nursery or other clustering geographically greatly promoted epidemic spread[488] (Table 12).

Seven intrahospital epidemics of nosocomial *Serratia* bacteremia were reported between 1965 and 1978. Six involved newborns or adults confined to an intensive care unit, and in every outbreak, the bacteremias were primary. Also, when examined, a single epidemic serotype of *Serratia* prevailed. Two devastating outbreaks in newborns[495,496] had an 84 and 100% mortality, but the portal of entry of *Serratia*, its sources in the nursery and modes of spread, were never identified; each outbreak was terminated by greater attention to handwashing and local asepsis. In the other five epidemics, *Serratia* bacteremias stemmed from some aspect of infusion therapy (four outbreaks)[497-500] — or in one epidemic involving multiple hospitals, contaminated blood-collection tubes.[140] *Serratia's* ability to proliferate in parenteral solutions, shared with *Klebsiella* and *Enterobacter*, probably accounts for its preponderance in outbreaks of infusion-related sepsis.[411,412]

Epidemic *Klebsiella*, *Enterobacter*, or *Serratia* bacteremias in a hospital, especially if caused by *E. cloacae* or *E. agglomerans*, should lead to an immediate search for an infusion-related source. Of 33 tabulated outbreaks of infusion-related bacteremia, 16 (48%) were caused by members of the tribe Klebsielleae.

Proteus-Providence

Also members of the Enterobacteriaceae, *Proteus-Providence* are common agents of nosocomial infection, especially of the catheterized urinary tract and surgical wounds; they cause approximately 3% of all bacteremias (Figures 3 and 4). Whereas most endemic infections are caused by indole-negative *Proteus mirabilis*,[501-504] which is susceptible to ampicillin, most hospital outbreaks with this group of Gram-negative organisms have been caused by indole-positive strains, *P. morgagni*, *P. vulgaris*, and *P. rettgeri*, and *Providence* species, which are intrinsically resistant to most antibiotics,

Table 12

RISK OF *SERRATIA* URINARY TRACT INFECTION AMONG CATHETERIZED PATIENTS AS RELATED TO EXPOSURE TO INFECTED CATHETERIZED ROOMMATES

	Shared room with infected catheterized roommate	
Group	Negative	Yes (1 or more days)
Number of catheterized patients at risk (initially uninfected)	12	13
Number of (%) becoming infected with *Serratia* (urine culture > 10^5 per m*l*)	2(17%)	8(62%)[a]

[a] p = 0.029.

Adapted from Maki, D. G., Hennekens, C. G., Phillips, C. W., Shaw, W. V., and Bennett, J. V., *J. Infect. Dis.*, 128, 579, 1973.

including ampicillin. Epidemics of catheter-related urinary tract infection,[505-510] especially in urology wards and neurology units, and of burn units,[427,511] have recently been reported, almost uniformly caused by multiply-resistant strains of indole-negative *Proteus* and *Providence*. As might be expected, exposure of patients to systemic or topical antibiotics has been a major risk factor predisposing to epidemic infection. Plausible environmental reservoirs of the epidemic strains were not consistently identified, however; similar to the many outbreaks caused by *Klebsiella* and *Serratia*, transmission seemed to occur mainly by carriage of organisms on the hands of medical personnel.

Only one epidemic of nosocomial *Proteus* bacteremia has been reported, but it was an extraordinary outbreak epidemiologically. Eleven full-term newborn infants in a hospital nursery developed primary *P. mirabilis* bacteremia over a 4-year period; four infants died. An outstanding investigation by Burke and co-workers[424] traced these infections to one nurse who was shown to be colonized rectally and vaginally by the epidemic strain. She also carried the organism on her hands chronically. Clinical and microbiologic data pointed towards infants' umbilici as the portal of entry of *Proteus*. Removal of the nurse from the nursery terminated the outbreak. (It is sobering to contemplate that if the epidemic organism in this outbreak had been *E. coli*, it is dubious the outbreak would ever have been detected.)

Pseudomonas

Perhaps no organisms are more closely linked to the hospital and nosocomial disease than the pseudomonads, *Pseudomonas aeruginosa* and the nonaeruginosa species, primarily *P. cepacia* and *P. maltophilia*. Innately resistant to most systemic antibiotics and possessed of enormous genetic capacity to develop additional resistance in the setting of heavy antimicrobial pressures,[512-523] these nonfermentative Gram-negative rods proliferate in the innumerable aqueous environs of the hospital. They rarely are encountered environmentally[524] or produce infection outside of the hospital. Like the Klebsielleae, *Pseudomonas* is truly a stepchild of the antibiotic era, and infection with *Pseudomonas* can be considered the prototype disease of medical progress. McGowan et al.[3] and Finland and his co-workers,[296,297] in their unprecedented studies of bacteremia in the Boston City Hospital which began in 1935, encountered blood stream infections with *P. aeruginosa* only rarely before 1957 (Figure 4). Before 1970, infections of any kind caused by *P. cepacia* or other nonaeruginosa species were so uncommon as to almost be reportable;[525-528] in the past 9 years there have been at least 13 epidemics of bacteremia caused by *P. cepacia* alone (Figure 3, Table 9).

Pseudomonas aeruginosa is now a common nosocomial pathogen in most hospitals, causing all types of local infection in immunologically competent hosts — usually in association with instrumentation or prior antibiotic therapy — and producing overwhelming sepsis in immunologically compromised patients, especially patients with inadequate numbers of circulating granulocytes.[530-533] Approximately 5% of hospital acquired bacteremias are caused by *P. aeruginosa* (Figure 3); the mortality of *P. aeruginosa* bacteremia, 60 to 90%, exceeds that of any other bloodstream pathogen[3,530-533] (Table 7). *Pseudomonas aeruginosa* is not normally part of the human gastrointestinal or cutaneous flora and most hospital acquired infections are preceded by nosocomial colonization. Schimpff and co-workers[402] have shown that in patients with leukemia, colonization of any site with *P. aeruginosa*, even enteric colonization alone, connotes a high risk of subsequent bacteremia caused by the colonizing strains. Similar studies by Bodey[534] and Moody,[535] Bruun[536] and their co-workers affirm the importance of colonization as a prelude to nosocomial infection. Hospital foods contaminated by pseudomonads may be a significant source of nosocomial acquisition of the organism.[537]

Countless outbreaks of local infection with *P. aeruginosa* have been traced to contaminated urinals, Foley collection bags, urine measuring containers or urometers,[538-540] cystoscopes,[541] bed pans,[538,539] medications and solutions,[542-544] disinfectants,[545] and particularly, nebulizers and other respiratory therapy equipment.[546-557] *Pseudomonas* in faucet aerators,[558] sink drains[559] or contaminating a plaster bucket,[560] a shaving brush,[561] or a breast pump[562] has been reported to have produced epidemic disease. Carriage of *P. aeruginosa* on the hands of medical personnel has been postulated as the predominant mode of transmission in burn units[563,564] and in most nursery outbreaks,[565,566] including two where bacteremic infections predominated.[405,567]

Four of the five hospital outbreaks of *P. aeruginosa* bacteremia in adults stemmed from contaminated transducers used for hemodynamic monitoring[568,569] or contaminated hemodialysis systems.[570-573] The fifth outbreak, reported by Greene and associates,[407] involved three patients with acute leukemia in the Baltimore Cancer Center who developed fatal *P. aeruginosa* mediastinitis and septicemia following esophagoscopy; microbiologic studies suggest strongly that these patients were cross-colonized and infected by inadequately decontaminated endoscopes. In each of these five epidemics, failure of disinfection by chemical means resulted in an epidemic.

The nonaeruginosa species of *Pseudomonas* probably possess less intrinsic capacity for producing disease than do *P. aeruginosa* and many other Gram-negative bacilli (case fatality in 13 outbreaks caused by *P. cepacia*, 5.8%, Table 7), and have been infrequent endemic nosocomial pathogens, especially of blood (only 1.7% of all nosocomial bacteremias) (Figure 3). In contrast, these organisms, mainly *P. cepacia*, have in the past decade literally soared into prominence as epidemic hospital pathogens. Thirteen outbreaks of nosocomial *P. cepacia* bacteremia[413,417,419,574-583] and one with *P. acidivorans* and *E. cloacae*,[568,569] comprising 16% of the 86 tabulated outbreaks of true bacteremia, have been reported, all since 1971. In every report, the epidemic infections were primary bacteremias and in 13 of the 14 outbreaks, derived from infusion therapy (Table 8) — conventional intravenous therapy,[413,419,575-578,580] intra-arterial infusions for hemodynamic monitoring,[568,569,574,579] or a contaminated blood product.[417,581] In one epidemic, septicemias were caused by contaminated hemodialysis coils,[582] and in a small nursery outbreak reported by Rapkin,[583] the portal of *P. cepacia* bacteremia could not be identified. In all 14 epidemics, an aqueous reservoir was identified: a medication administered parenterally, parenteral solutions of a blood product, a chemical disinfectant used for cutaneous antisepsis, or contamination of in-line transducer domes or hemodialysis coils.

P. cepacia has an almost unique ability to proliferate in distilled water[410] and most large-volume parenterals[412] — and is, in addition, highly resistant to many chemical disinfectants. As with *P. aeruginosa*, many outbreaks of nonbacteremic infection caused by *P. cepacia* or *P. maltophilia* have been traced to contaminated disinfectant solutions.[584-590] In 1969, patients in hospitals across the U.S. developed urinary tract infections with a *P. cepacia*-like organism found to be an intrinsic contaminant of the disinfectant contained in a commercial urinary catheterization tray.[587,588] These properties connote vast potential for producing epidemic nosocomial disease and pseudodisease; *P. cepacia* and *P. maltophilia* were the agents in 2 of the 11 reported outbreaks of pseudobacteremia.[110,141]

While *P. cepacia* has rapidly become a very important nosocomial pathogen, especially in epidemics, it is likely that the organism has been causing hospital acquired infections of epidemic proportions for many years.[108] Until quite recently, many hospital laboratories did not routinely speciate pseudomonads and few could reliably identify *P. cepacia*; in a 1974 proficiency survey carried out by CDC, 34% of 504 participating laboratories were unable to correctly identify a *P. cepacia* isolate.*

Flavobacterium

This slow-growing nonfermentative Gram-negative rod is found in soil, water, and many areas of the natural environment,[591,592] and is resistant to most antibiotics. However, it has been a rare cause of endemic nosocomial infection, including bacteremia. *Flavobacterium* accounted for less than 0.2% of all nosocomial bacteremias reported to the National Nosocomial Infection Study in 1976 (Figure 3). Occasional hospital outbreaks of local *Flavobacterium* infection have been reported, most involving newborns in whom it often also produced meningitis.[593-596] In most outbreaks, environmental sources of *Flavobacterium*, mainly water-containing equipment, were linked to epidemic infections.

A small outbreak of seven cases of primary neonatal septicemia with meningitis caused by *Flavobacterium* was reported from a Brazilian hospital in 1970;[596] all cases were fatal. The source of the organism in the nursery was not identified. Two epidemics of nosocomial *Flavobacterium* bacteremia occurring in adults were both recently traced to infusion therapy; in one, *Flavobacterium* was found in many multidose vials of medications used in operating rooms;[597,598] in the other outbreak, arterial catheter-related bacteremias were linked to contaminated ice used to chill syringes for drawing blood specimens from radial artery catheters.[599]

Like *Pseudomonas* and *Enterobacter*, *Flavobacterium* is resistant to many disinfectants used in hospitals. Six *Flavobacterium* bacteremias occurring in a British hospital over a 2-year period (1973-75), all inexplicably mild clinically, were shown in retrospect to have probably been pseudobacteremias, related to wide scale contamination of aqueous chlorhexidine in that hospital.[600]

Acinetobacter

Acinetobacter (formerly *Mima-Herelleae* group) is also a nonfermentative Gram-negative rod that is characteristically resistant to many antimicrobials. It can be cul-

---

* Personal communication, Dr. Charles Griffin, Chief, Microbiology Section, Licensure and Proficiency Testing Division, Bureau of Laboratories, Center for Disease Control, Atlanta, Ga.

tured from the skin of 17 to 20% of healthy adult males.[601] In most hospitals it has been a relatively infrequent pathogen in endemic nosocomial infection, including bacteremia (<0.2% of the bacteremias reported to the National Study in 1976 [Figure 3]). Most cultures positive for *Acinetobacter* represent colonization or contamination rather than infection.[602,603] Although *Acinetobacter calcoaceticus* var. *lwoffi* (formerly *Mima polymorpha*) is a well-known cause of sporadic cases of meningitis,[604] (it "mimics" *Neisseria meningitidis* on Gram stain), the vast majority of *Acinetobacter* infections are nosocomial and involve the lower respiratory tract, less frequently surgical wounds or the catheterized urinary tract.[606-612] Daly,[605] Green,[610] and Glew[602] and their co-workers have pointed up the frequency with which *Acinetobacter*, especially *A. anitratus*, is implicated in septicemias originating from vascular catheters.

A number of investigators have commented upon a marked seasonal pattern with nosocomial *Acinetobacter* infection; the incidence doubles in summer months.[609,611,612]

The frequency of *Acinetobacter* infection appears to be increasing,[602,611,612] and the organism has become a prominent pathogen (including in bacteremic infections) in some large university hospitals,[602,611] probably related to heavy antimicrobial pressures and a proponderance of elderly and critically ill patients subjected to invasive procedures.

Nosocomial epidemics of *Acinetobacter* infection have mainly involved the respiratory tract and were linked to environmental sources, primarily contaminated inhalation therapy equipment;[426,613] but in an outbreak investigated by Buxton and co-workers,[426] one third of medical personnel carried the organism on their hands intermittently, and one respiratory therapist was found to be a chronic carrier. An outbreak of peritonitis in patients undergoing peritoneal dialysis was traced by Abrutyn and associates[614] to a contaminated water bath used to heat bottles of dialysate.

Two outbreaks of *Acinetobacter* pseudobacteremia have been reported, the etiologic mechanisms attesting to the organism's propensity to subsist in the hospital's inanimate environment. In 1970, 24 *M. polymorpha* (*A. lwoffii*) bacteremias occurred in a large university hospital over a 10-month period. The cluster was ultimately traced by Faris and Sparling[90] to contaminated penicillinase in that hospital's laboratory. In the second incident, an outstanding epidemiologic investigation by Snydman and co-workers[615] showed that large numbers of *Acinetobacter* aerosolized into pediatric mist tents were contaminating blood cultures drawn from children in the tents. Shawker et al.[275] identified three asymptomatic transient bacteremias with *A. lwoffi* in a prospective study of bacteremia during angiography; angiography catheters were apparently contaminated by the organism.

One epidemic of putatively bona fide *Acinetobacter* bacteremias was reported by Smith and Massanari[616] involving 24 patients in a university hospital over a 4-year period. Heavy contamination of unheated humidifiers at patients' bedsides was postulated as the source of these infections; however, little evidence was adduced for respiratory tract colonization of infection, and vascular catheters were hypothesized as the "probable portal of entry" for *Acinetobacter*. Although 20 of the 24 patients were described as significantly compromised, only 3 died. It might reasonably be questioned whether this was an unrecognized outbreak of pseudobacteremia with the same mechanism of contamination of blood cultures as found in the Snydman[615] investigation.

Salmonella

The unique "epidemic geometry" of hospitals undoubtedly accounts for the myriad epidemics of hospital salmonellosis that have been reported in the past two decades. Schroeder,[617] Baine,[618] and their CDC colleagues recorded 112 institutional outbreaks occurring in the U.S. alone between 1963 and 1972, and over 20 more appear in the medical literature during this period. One extraordinary interhospital outbreak of *Sal-*

monella derby infection, linked initially to contaminated cracked eggs by a large CDC investigative team, ultimately involved over 3000 patients and employees in Eastern U.S. hospitals between 1963 and 1965;[619-621] the epidemic was perpetuated by cross-infection between patients and between hospitals. In 1965, intrinsic contamination of a commercial food supplement resulted in cases of epidemic gastroenteritis in nine states, caused by multiple serotypes of *Salmonella,* in 22 institutions for the mentally retarded.[622] In 1966, another interhospital outbreak involved patients in multiple hospitals in the U.S. and Great Britain; the epidemic organism, *Salmonella cubana,* was discovered by Lang and CDC collaborators[623,624] to be a natural contaminant of carmine dye being widely used at the time as a marker in studies of gastrointestinal transit.

Most nosocomial salmonellosis, especially in adults and older children, consists of uncomplicated self-limiting gastroenteritis without bacteremia and can be traced to a common vehicle such as a food or medication. However, cross-contamination on the hands of medical personnel has been thought or shown to be the mode of transmission in many outbreaks,[617,618,625] including virtually all occurring in newborns where bacteremia often accompanies gastrointestinal infection.[626] Besides neonates, patients with impaired gastrointestinal function (e.g., achlorhydria or postgastrectomy), with sickle cell disease or other chronic hemolytic states, as well as immunologically compromised patients — particularly those with reticuloendothelial malignancy — are also highly prone to developing bacteremic infection with *Salmonella.*[627-630]

Over the 14-year period tabulated in this review, five epidemics of nosocomial *Salmonella* bacteremia were reported, each comprising 5 to 56 patients.[414,631-634] In four outbreaks, bacteremia originated from nosocomial gastrointestinal infection with *Salmonella.* Three epidemics involved immunocompromised adults:[414,632,633] one, post-surgical patients;[631] another, 56 infants and children in a large Puerto Rican hospital.[634] Cross-infection was implicated in three of the outbreaks[632-634] — in one, mediated by an inadequately decontaminated endoscope.[633]

One small outbreak of *Salmonella typhimurium* gastroenteritis and bacteremia in the early postoperative period involved four patients who had had a cholecystectomy performed by one surgeon.[631] A case-control study by CDC investigators linked illness epidemiologically to routine use of Gomco gastric suction by that surgeon. It was further found that the hospital had no consistent policy for cleaning and replacing Gomco apparatus used in the operating rooms. Although the epidemic organism was eventually cultured from tubing connecting to nasogastric tubes, the original source of *S. typhimurium* giving rise to this probable common-source outbreak remains obscure.

The last epidemic, discussed in greater detail in a later section, involved seven patients with lymphoproliferative malignancy hospitalized in the Clinical Center of the National Institutes of Health who developed cryptogenic *S. cholerae-suis* bacteremia over a 6-month period in 1970 to 1971.[414] Epidemiologic investigations ultimately traced these infections to contaminated platelet packs obtained from a single donor.

Fungi

A greatly increased incidence of systemic infections caused by fungi such as *Candida* (Figure 3) and closely related *Torulopsis, Aspergillus,* and *Mucorales* has also paralleled the increased use of broad-spectrum antibiotics in hospitals.[33-39,76,78,635-639] Most of these infections are hospital related; the majority prove fatal. Reservoirs and modes of spread of nosocomial fungal pathogens have not been well defined, but autoinfection, originating from strains carried in the gastrointestinal or respiratory tract and greatly enhanced by antimicrobial therapy and corticosteroids or other immunosuppressive therapy, has been thought to account for most deep *Candida* and *Torulopsis* infections; documented outbreaks have been rare.

Recent studies suggest that many — possibly the majority — of nosocomial septicemias with *Candida* and *Torulopsis* originate from vascular catheters;[36,78,635,636] the infrequency with which catheters are cultured in most hospitals probably accounts for the "cryptogenic" nature of most sporadic cases. Both of the two well-documented epidemics of *Candida* septicemia were associated with infusion therapy. In the first outbreak, four infants developed *Candida* sepsis over a 4-week period traced ultimately to contamination of in-line transducer-domes used for arterial pressure monitoring.[569] The second outbreak occurred in one hospital where 22 patients receiving parenteral hyperalimentation developed *Candida parapsilosis* septicemia from contaminated solutions compounded in the hospital's pharmacy.[640]

Aspergillosis is a relatively rare but usually lethal deep fungal infection presumed in most sporadic cases to be acquired by the airborne route; most affected patients are severely immunosuppressed.[35,638] Between 1966 and 1975, five small outbreaks of aspergillosis[641-645] and two of prosthetic valve endocarditis caused by *Aspergillus*[646] and by *Penicillium* species[647] (an exceedingly rare human pathogen) were traced to common-source exposures to airborne fungi. In five epidemics of aspergillosis, immunosuppressed transplant or cancer patients were affected; in the two clusters of endocarditis, immunologically competent patients undergoing open heart surgery were affected. In each outbreak, the epidemic species was recovered from air samples taken in the patients' rooms or in the cardiovascular operating rooms. A plausible source of the fungus was identified in every outbreak: pigeon droppings near an air inlet,[642,646] an inadequate[641] or contaminated[644,647] ventilation system, renovations producing contaminated dust[645] or contaminated fireproofing materials.[643] Improvements in ventilation terminated each outbreak.

Bennett's[648] observations with regard to prevention of hospital acquired systemic mycoses cannot be stated more succinctly or cogently: "Prevention of candidiasis rests upon avoiding therapeutic maneuvers which lead first to enhanced *Candida* colonization of the patient and then to breaks in tissue barriers. Prevention of aspergillosis rests upon protecting the severely immunosuppressed patient from airborne spores."

Anaerobes

Anaerobic bacteria, primarily *Bacteroides fragilis* and clostridia, are recovered from 8 to 11% of positive blood cultures,[21,85] frequently with aerobic bacteria (polymicrobial bacteremia), in large centers with the laboratory expertise to isolate and identify these fastidious microorganisms. In most cases of anaerobic bacteremia, a local infection such as peritonitis or an intra-abdominal abscess can be identified.[21,649-655] Anaerobic bacteria vastly outnumber aerobes in the microflora of the gastrointestinal, female genital, and respiratory tract; with the possible exception of some clostridia infections following major trauma, most infections caused by anaerobes are thought to derive from autochthonous strains.[21] While most anaerobic bacteremias are indeed hospital related and occur following surgery or childbirth, and rare cases of postoperative clostridial infections[107] and an outbreak of pseudobacteremias[656] have been traced to disinfectant solutions contaminated by clostridial spores, clusters of cases that might suggest cross-infection or acquisition of infection from a common hospital source have not been reported in the large published experiences with anaerobic bacteremia.

Howard and co-workers[406] recently described 12 infants in a British hospital's newborn nursery who developed necrotizing enterocolitis over a 6-week period in 1977; all survived. Nine of the ten babies examined showed evidence of *Clostridium butyricum* bacteremia.

Necrotizing enterocolitis is a grave condition of unknown cause affecting newborns, especially low birth weight infants. It has been recognized with increasing frequency since it was first described in 1963.[658-661] A clearcut etiologic agent has not been identified, but other clusters of cases have been reported,[404,661-666] some in association with frequent gastrointestinal colonization — and even bacteremia with C. perfringens[662] or aerobic Gram-negative bacilli such as *P. aeruginosa,*[663] *E. coli,*[403] *Klebsiella*[404,658] or *Salmonella.*[664] It is unclear whether these organisms or the *C. butyricum* in the aforementioned report were etiologic agents or simply secondary invaders. In support of infectious etiology, intensified control measures in several institutions to prevent cross-infection during an apparent outbreak have been associated with a significantly reduced incidence of the disease.[403,404,665]

Listeria

Listeria monocytogenes is a small nonsporulating Gram-positive rod which has an extraordinarily wide host range, producing disease in a large variety of fish, birds, and mammals, as well as man. Best known as an occasional cause of sepsis of the newborn, often with meningitis,[667] it has been encountered increasingly in recent years as an opportunistic pathogen of immunologically compromised adults.[668-670] *Listeria* has been a rare cause of nosocomial infection, however, accounting for less than 0.1% of reported cases, including those with bacteremia.

Occasional reports in the past have suggested that *Listeria* can spread within a nursery.[671] Between 1969 and 1978, four clusters of neonatal listeriosis, each consisting of 7 to 13 cases, occurred in hospitals in New Zealand,[672] South Carolina,[673] Sweden,[674] and South Africa.[675] In three of these experiences, *Listeria* septicemia seemed clinically to represent acquisition *in utero* prior to admission. However, in one Swedish hospital,[675] five secondary cases — one with meningitis, the others with mild enterocolitis or asymptomatic colonization only — appeared to have been acquired nosocomially.

Two recent clusters of unequivocally hospital acquired *Listeria* septicemia in immunocompromised adults, reported by Gantz and co-workers[676] and by Green and Macaulay,[677] indicate that *Listeria* must now be regarded as a potential nosocomial pathogen with clear-cut capacity to produce epidemic disease. Although a hospital source of *Listeria* or mode of spread was not delineated in either outbreak, Green and MaCaulay present convincing circumstantial evidence suggesting case-to-case transmission.

Atypical Mycobacteria

Mycobacteria species other than *Mycobacterium hominis* — the anomalous or "atypical" strains — are common saprophytes of soil, dust, and water, but produce human disease only infrequently and systemic infection but very rarely.[678] In most series, virtually all cases have been thought to be community acquired and involved the lung; documented nosocomial acquisition of atypical mycobacterial infection has been very rare.[679,680] Those rare cases of systemic infection with bacteremia or disseminated granulomatous disease have almost exclusively involved patients with primary myeloproliferative disorders or other conditions of compromised immunity.[678-680]

Recent reports now indicate that these organisms may be more important hospital pathogens than previously thought, owing in part to greater opportunities for nosocomial acquisition and also to improved abilities on the part of diagnostic laboratories to isolate and identify atypical mycobacteria. In 1976, 19 patients in a North Carolina hospital and five in a Colorado hospital who had all undergone open heart surgery developed suppurative infection of their sternotomy wounds caused by organisms of the *Mycobacterium fortuitum* complex, *M. chelonei;*[681,682] two cases progressed to systemic disease, and four patients died of uncontrollable infection by these strains that are resistant to most antituberculous drugs. Risk factors associated with infection or sources of *M. chelonei* in the two hospitals could not be identified. A 1974 outbreak in Spain of 24 surgical infections with *M. chelonei* following vein stripping was traced by Foz and associates[683] to merbromin, a weak mercurial disinfectant used for cutaneous antisepsis; the solution was found to be contaminated with *M. chelonei*. In the past year, contaminated water in peritoneal dialysis machines was shown by Band and Fraser[684] to be the source of an epidemic of *M. chelonei* peritonitis. Most recently, organisms of the *M. fortuitum* complex have been etiologically implicated in late-appearing, indolent infections following augmentation mamoplasty with silicone implants.[685]

These rapid-growing mycobacteriae are widely distributed in nature and possess a high degree of resistance to most chemical disinfectants. Carson and co-workers[686] found that naturally occurring strains of *M. chelonei* multiplied in distilled water at 25°C, losing little viability for periods of up to 1 year. Moreover, the strains were not killed by 24 hr of exposure to 2% aqueous formaldehyde and survived exposure to 0.3 to 0.7 mcg/mℓ of free chlorine for 1 hr and 0.2% alkaline glutaraldehyde for at least 4 days. Only 2% alkaline glutaraldehyde provided reliable bactericidal activity.

Between 1975 and 1977, 25 patients in ten U.S. centers received porcine heterograft prosthetic valves subsequently shown to be intrinsically contaminated by *M. chelonei*.[687-690] The valves were shipped and stored in 0.2% alkaline glutaraldehyde. To date two patients have developed clinical endocarditis.[688,689] It is now strongly recommended that whenever a porcine heart valve prosthesis is used, a tissue remnant or an aliquot of the glutaraldehyde solution be routinely cultured.[690]

The true scope of endemic nosocomial disease caused by these heretofore exceedingly rare (recognized) nosocomial pathogens should become much clearer within the next decade.

Miscellaneous Bacteria

Aerobic Gram-negative bacilli infrequently encountered as pathogens in most hospitals — *Achromobacter* and *Citrobacter* species — have been implicated in a number of small outbreaks of serious nosocomial disease, primarily in newborns.[425,691-695] These organisms probably have minimal intrinsic pathogenicity; most sporadic infections identified in adults have involved debilitated or immunologically compromised individuals.[696]

Between 1970 and 1978, five clusters of devastating neonatal sepsis with meningitis caused by *Citrobacter* species were reported; in four incidents, infections were clearly hospital related and constituted epidemics.[425,693,694] A nursery source of *Citrobacter* could not be identified in any of the investigations, but studies in 1978 by CDC personnel in two small outbreaks in Connecticut and Florida revealed carriage of *Citrobacter* on nurses' hands, in several cases, chronically. Institution of measures to prevent contact transmission terminated both outbreaks.

Bacteremic infection with organisms often labeled as "opportunistic" bacterial pathogens — *Aeromonas hydrophila*,[697,698] *Corynebacterium* species (or diphtheroids),[161,162,699,700] and *Bacillus* species[701-703] — have been encountered with increasing frequency, mainly in patients with cancer or in those who have received organ transplants. Most of these infections have clearly been hospital related and were associated with prolonged immunosuppression and exposure to antibiotics, mucocutaneous defects, surgery, implanted prostheses such as ventriculo-atrial shunts, or exposure to invasive vascular devices of all types. Except for an outbreak of *Bacillus cereus* bacteremia originating from contaminated dialyzers in a British hospital in 1965,[702] clusters of bacteremia with these organisms have not been reported, and the epidemiology and pathogenesis of sporadic nosocomial infections caused by most opportunists remain poorly understood. Longitudinal studies by Stamm and co-workers[700] in a bone marrow transplantation unit experiencing a high endemic rate of bacteremia caused by a multiply-resistant *Corynebacterium* species demonstrated that although colonization (which preceded most infections) was frequently hospital acquired; many patients were already colonized on admission. Two rare human pathogens, a *Bacillus* species and *Moraxella*, were involved in 2 of the 11 outbreaks of pseudobacteremia.[143,704]

Recently small clusters of nosocomial *Hemophilus influenzae* type b septicemia and meningitis (five cases)[705] and nosocomial Group Y *N. meningitidis* bacteremia (two cases)[706] were reported; airborne spread was postulated. In both outbreaks other asymptomatic patients were shown to be colonized by the epidemic organisms.

All of these recent reports of epidemic nosocomial bacteremias caused by organisms uncommonly — or even very rarely — implicated as hospital pathogens in the past, reaffirm the statement made at the outset of this section: in the closed setting of the hospital (especially the critical care unit or the nursery), which constitutes an "epidemic geometry", with increasing numbers of susceptible patients exposed to antibiotics, invasive procedures, and devices, virtually any microorganism can cause nosocomial disease of epidemic proportions.

EPIDEMICS OF PRIMARY NOSOCOMIAL BACTEREMIA

Nearly 80% of all epidemics of nosocomial bacteremia reported to have occurred between 1965 and 1978 involved primary bacteremias (Figure 2), bloodstream infections that did not originate from an identifiable local infection. When a hospital outbreak includes secondary bacteremias, the epidemiologic considerations are essentially those that would apply in an outbreak of local infections at that site unassociated with bacteremia. This section will deal with reported epidemics of primary nosocomial bacteremia.

"Pseudobacteremia"

> Appearances to the mind are of four kinds.
> Things either are what they appear to be;
> or they are neither are, and do not appear to be;
> or they are, and do not appear to be;
> *or they are not, yet appear to be*
> Rightly to aim in all these cases is the wise man's task.

Discourses
Epictetus

A report of multiple patients with positive blood cultures is invariably the first indication of a possible epidemic of nosocomial bacteremia. Before undertaking logistically demanding and costly epidemiologic studies, one must ascertain the following: (1) the positive cultures represent true, clinically significant infections and not laboratory artifact — "pseudobacteremias", and (2) if indeed bona fide bloodstream infections, that the cluster represents an increased incidence of true epidemic magnitude. Pseudoepidemics and pseudobacteremias are both being encountered with increasing frequency by present-day hospital epidemiologists[153,707] (Figure 5).

A pseudoepidemic of nosocomial infection is a cluster of isolates, usually of one species, that is misconstrued as denoting an epidemic. Recognizing an epidemic is predicated upon knowing the expected or base-line (endemic) rate of nosocomial infection caused by the putative epidemic pathogen. Pseudoepidemics usually derive either from inadequate data or even a total lack of base-line data (i.e., no mechanism for ongoing surveillance of nosocomial infections or even failure to atempt to acquire base-line data retrospectively, which is usually possible — and certainly acceptable — epidemiologically) or from misinterpreting clinical or microbiologic information as representing infection — vis-a-vis, pseudoinfection.

Pseudoepidemics of nosocomial bacteremia — alternatively, epidemics of pseudobacteremia — seem to be another one of our maladies of medical progress. There are 11 well-documented reports of pseudobacteremia in the modern medical literature (Table 13); all took place since 1968; eight, since 1974.

Guidelines for interpreting individual positive blood cultures and discriminating between sporadic contaminants and true bacteremia have been developed, based primarily on the characteristic of the isolate[144,154] and the number of cultures that are positive. Here, however, is the crux: the extreme sensitivity of blood culture systems renders them susceptible not only to occasional sporadic contamination but also, in the right circumstances, to contamination of a large number of cultures, producing a cluster of pseudobacteremias. If such contamination is with a plausible pathogen such as a Gram-negative bacillus (8 of the 11 reported outbreaks, Figure 3), it is easy to see why true infection — and even a true epidemic — is logically assumed.

Pseudobacteremia occurring in epidemic numbers can in theory derive from contamination introduced at any stage (Table 13), from drawing the cultures at the bedside to processing them in the laboratory. Clusters of pseudobacteremia which became pseudoepidemics have been traced to extrinsically contaminated antiseptics (aqueous solutions of benzylkonium[110] or chlorhexidine[600],) used to disinfect patients' skin prior to drawing the cultures; to cross-contamination of blood cultures by microorganisms in nonsterile evacuated blood-collection tubes filled with the same syringe prior to inoculating the blood culture;[141,142] to contaminated holders used with evacuated collection tubes;[143] to heavy environmental contamination, including of patients' skin, caused by massive numbers of airborne microorganisms in pediatric mist tents;[615] to contaminated penicillinase added to blood cultures in the laboratory;[89,90] to intrinsic contamination of a commercial blood culture media;[704] to cross-contamination of blood cultures being processed by automated techniques, because the sampling probe did not self-cauterize properly;[707] to a laboratory technician processing the blood cultures who turned out to be a carrier and presumably a shedder of the epidemic strain of *S. aureus*[708]; and, most recently, to a contaminated Merthiolate® solution used to disinfect the diaphragms of blood culture bottles in the laboratory.[656] Several outbreaks involved intrinsic contamination of a nationally distributed product (blood collection tubes,[141,142] blood culture media[704]), resulting in epidemic pseudobacteremias in multiple hospitals in different states, and thus assumed national scope.

Prompt identification and confirmation of pseudobacteremia is obviously of major importance for obvious reasons: patients may be unnecessarily treated with potentially toxic antibiotics; true bacteremia may be concealed by overgrowth of the contaminating species in the blood culture media; the positive blood culture may prevent or delay further search for the cause of patients' fever and other symptoms that prompted blood culturing in the first place; and the circumstances resulting in pseudobacteremia may also have the potential of causing true iatrogenic bacteremia:[110,140,141] e.g., microorganisms from blood collection tubes refluxing into the patient's blood stream.

Recognizing and establishing rapidly that an increased frequency of positive blood cultures represents contamination on a large scale and thus, epidemic pseudobacteremia can be difficult as exemplified by the fact that, of the 11 reported experiences, the median length of time pseudobacteremias had been occurring in the hospital before they were conclusively identified was 6 months (Table 13); in six instances, it took 6 months to 2 years and the occurrence of up to 79 pseudobacteremias before the situation was clarified and resolved.

Epidemic pseudobacteremia should be strongly suspected in the following circumstances:

1. When a cluster of blood culture isolates is positive for a new or "unusual" blood pathogen, such as *Acinetobacter, Moraxella, Bacillus* species, or a nonaeruginosa strain of *Pseudomonas*
2. When the affected patients do not consistently show signs or symptoms consistent with bloodstream infection (this may require a careful case-control analysis to establish)
3. When the putative bacteremias are primary; i.e., the bloodstream pathogen is not isolated from a plausible site of local infection such as a surgical wound or the urinary tract (but it must also be kept in mind that primary nosocomial bacteremias frequently denote infusion-related sepsis)
4. When bacteremia is inexplicably high-grade (most or all of the blood cultures are positive), usually seen only with endovascular infections such as endocarditis

The heart of an investigation of possible pseudobacteremia — or any potential nosocomial epidemic for that matter — should include an early careful case-control study, as described in a later section. This analysis compares exposures of putative epidemic cases and carefully selected control patients (usually randomly selected patients whose blood cultures — drawn during the same time period as cases — were negative or, alternatively, were positive for other species). It strives to identify relevant differences in host or therapeutic factors and, in the case of possible pseudobacteremias, differences in some aspect of drawing and processing blood cultures that point towards the responsible factor or factors. Microbiologic confirmation of the source of contamination should ideally only confirm what is already strongly suspected based on clinical-epidemiologic analyses. If pseudoinfection is suspected or shown to derive from intrinsic contamination of a commercial product, it becomes a problem of major public health concern, and the local and federal health authorities, the Food and Drug Administration (FDA), and the CDC should be immediately informed. Unmanipulated specimens of the implicated product should be retained for analysis by these agencies.

Epidemic pseudoinfections have not been confined to bacteremias, but in recent years have also included pseudopneumonia,[707] pseudotuberculosis,[709] pseudogastroenteritis,[707] and pseudomeningitis[710-712] — due to nonviable contaminants in spinal fluid collection tubes or encountered during Gram staining, both of which resulted in false-positive Gram-stained smears. Weinstein and Stamm reported that pseudoepidemics of all types comprised 11% of 181 nosocomial epidemics investigated by the CDC between 1965 and 1972.[707]

The importance of stringent quality control measures in clinical laboratories, such as routinely preincubating 10% of each lot of blood culture media[713,714] and, whenever it is used, penicillinase,[84] have fundamental importance beyond satisfying the requirements of accreditation agencies.

Infusion-Related Sepsis

Without question, infusion therapy has become an indispensible therapeutic modality in present-day medicine. It has likely saved more lives than all of the antibiotics ever developed. Over one half of the 40 million patients hospitalized each year in this country receive some form of infusion therapy for administration of fluid and electro-

Table 13
REPORTED EPIDEMICS OF PSEUDOBACTEREMIA

Years inclusive (duration)	Epidemic microorganism(s)	No. patients with positive cultures	Mechanism of contamination	Ref.
1968 (5 days)	Escherichia coli	7	Contaminated penicillinase in multidose vial	89
1970 (10 months)	Mima polymorpha[a]	24	Contaminated penicillinase in multidose vial	90
1973 (16 days)	Moraxella nonliquefaciens	8	Contaminated holders for evacuated blood-culture tubes	143
1974 (2 months)	Bacillus spp.	44[b]	Intrinsically contaminated blood-culture media	704
1971—1972 (12 months)	Pseudomonas cepacia or Enterobacter spp.	79	Contaminated aqueous benzalkonium solution used for skin antisepsis	110
1973—1975 (24 months)	Flavobacterium meningosepticum	6	Contaminated aqueous chlorhexidine solution used for disinfection	600
1976 (6 months)	Serratia marcescens	45[b]	Intrinsically contaminated evacuated blood-collection tubes	142
1975—1977 (17 months)	Pseudomonas maltophilia	25[b]	Intrinsically contaminated evacuated blood-collection tubes	141
1975—1976 (7 months)	Acinetobacter calcoaceticus	11	Heavy environmental contamination in pediatric mist tents	615
1978 (4 days)	Staphyloccus aureus	11	Colonized laboratory technician who processed the positive cultures	708

| 1978 (12 days) | Clostridium sordelli | 11 | 656 | Contaminated Merthiolate® solution used to disinfect diaphragms of blood-culture bottles in laboratory |

a Current nomenclature, Acinetobacter lwoffii.
b Multiple hospitals experienced pseudobacteremias.

From Maki, D. G., Arch. Intern. Med., 140, 26, Copyright 1980, American Medical Association. With permission.

lytes, blood products, drugs, or total parenteral nutrition, or increasingly, for hemodynamic monitoring. Yet, infusion therapy carries a substantial and vastly unappreciated potential for producing iatrogenic harm. The awesome litany of potential noninfective complications ranges from protean infusion phlebitis to lethal massive air embolism.[715] Leading the list of all possible complications of infusion therapy is sepsis, bacteremia deriving from infection of the cannula wound or from contaminated infusate. Infusion-related sepsis, which inexplicably did not become widely recognized as a major complication for nearly 30 years,[716] is probably the most insidious and least recognized nosocomial infection. Yet, prospective studies have shown that in some centers up to one half of hospital acquired bacteremias[315] — and, in others, the majority of candidemias[78] — derive from vascular catheters. Between 1968 and 1974, 20.5% of all nosocomial bacteremias with an identified source occurring in the Johns Hopkins Hospital originated from an intravenous device.[302] It is likely that at least 25,000 hospitalized patients develop cannula-related septicemia alone each year in this country.[717] Many of these infections are never recognized as originating from an infusion because neither the cannula or fluid is cultured.

Nothing underscores infusion therapy's potential for causing serious iatrogenic disease more than its enormous and disproportionate role in epidemic nosocomial bacteremia. Whereas only 8% of endemic nosocomial bacteremias are considered as infusion-related, fully 34% of all hospital epidemics of bacteremia derive from infusion therapy in some form (Figure 2, Table 9).

Before discussing the epidemics that have been reported, the clinical features, epidemiology, and pathogenesis of infusion-related infection will be reviewed briefly.

Clinical Recognition of Infusion-Related Sepsis

Although a stringent program of asepsis will considerably reduce the incidence of infusion-related septicemia, because of human errors, intrinsically contaminated products or simply the undue susceptibility to infection of many patients, sporadic cases — and even epidemics — can be expected to occasionally occur. If affected patients are to survive and an epidemic is to be detected, the causal relationship between infusions and infections must be recognized as early as possible.

The general clinical features of infusion-related septicemia are indistinguishable from bloodstream infection arising from any other site such as the urinary tract or an infected surgical wound.[4,70,716-719] Infusion-related sepsis occurring in an intensive care unit population can be particularly insidious. The bacteremia is often attributed to pneumonia, urinary tract, or surgical wound infection, or is simply accepted as "cryptogenic" and treated empirically.

Several key observations should immediately bring to mind the possibility of sepsis arising from an infusion[717] (Figure 9): (1) the patient is receiving infusion therapy at the outset of septicemia; (2) phlebitis (present in about one half of cases); (3) primary septicemia (i.e., no obvious local infection to account for a picture of sepsis); (4) the patient is an unlikely candidate for septicemia (i.e., young or without underlying predisposing diseases); (5) the precipitous onset of overwhelming sepsis, often with shock (usually indicative of massively contaminated infusate or suppurative phlebitis); and (6) most characteristically (Figure 9), sepsis refractory to appropriate antimicrobial therapy until the culpable infusion is purposely (or fortuitously) removed. Focal retinal lesions — cotton wool patches — are present in up to one third of patients with deep *Candida* infection deriving from hyperalimentation catheters,[43] even in those without positive blood cultures, and careful ophthalmologic examination[40,41] should be a routine part of the evaluation of patients receiving parenteral alimentation who are suspected of having sepsis. Septicemia from arterial catheters is frequently heralded by

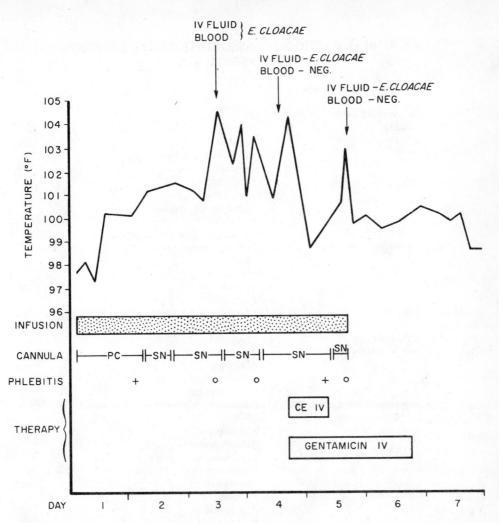

FIGURE 9. Typical case of infusion-related septicemia. A 60-year-old woman hospitalized with un-complicated myocardial infarction had no signs of infection on admission. Low-grade fever appeared on the 2nd hospital day, and on the 3rd hospital day rigors, confusion, and hypotension developed abruptly, and her temperature reached 105°F (39.7°C). Despite administration of gentamicin and cephalothin, and repeated changes of infusion sites through scalp-vein needles, signs of sepsis did not abate. After 3 days of severe illess, results of cultures of blood and I.V. fluid taken at the onset of fever and of infusion fluid on the following 2 days were reported as positive for *E. cloacae.* The entire infusion apparatus was immediately removed, after which the patient defervesced and showed rapid clinical im-provement. (From Maki, D. G., Rhame, F. S., Mackel, D. C., and Bennett, J. V., *Am. J. Med.,* 60, 471, 1976. With permission.)

embolic lesions (Osler's nodes), tender erythematous 5- to 10-mm papules appearing in the distal distribution of the involved artery, usually in the palm or sole.[124,336,720]

The microbiologic profile of septicemia, as outlined in Table 14, can also suggest strongly an infusion-related source. Certain microorganisms are so prevalent in infu-sion-related sepsis — *Staphylococcus aureus* in cannula-related sepsis, *E. cloacae, E. agglomerans,* and *P. cepacia* in sepsis from contaminated infusate, *Candida* in hyper-alimentation — that their recovery from blood cultures, even from only one patient, should prompt an immediate search for an infusion-related etiology. A cluster of cases should mandate a full-scale investigation, which may include culturing of in-use prod-ucts and informing the public health authorities. Such actions in 1973 averted a second

Table 14
MICROBIAL PATHOGENS ASSOCIATED WITH INFUSION-RELATED SEPTICEMIA

Source of septicemia	Major pathogens
Conventional infusion therapy	
Cannula	*Staphylococcus aureus* (>50%)
	S. epidermidis
	Klebsiella-Enterobacter
	Serratia marcescens
	Enterococcus
	Acinetobacter spp.
	Pseudomonas aeruginosa
	P. cepacia
	Corynebacterium spp. (diphtheroids)
Contaminated infusate	Tribe Klebsielleae (90%)
	Klebsiella
	Enterobacter [a]
	Serratia
	P. cepacia [a]
	Citrobacter freundii
	Flavobacterium
Hyperalimentation	*Candida* spp. (30—50%)
(most, catheter-related)	*Torulopsis glabrata*
	S. aureus
	Klebsiella-Enterobacter
	Enterococcus
Contaminated blood products	Pseudomonads other than *P. aeruginosa*
(contaminated infusate)	(>50%) [a]
	S. marcescens
	Achromobacter
	Salmonella cholerae-suis
	Citrobacter
	Flavobacterium
Arterial pressure monitoring	*P. cepacia* [a]
	P. acidivorans
	P. aeruginosa
	Serratia
	Enterobacter
	Flavobacterium
	Candida (rare)
Regional intra-arterial cancer	*S. aureus*
chemotherapy (catheter-related)	

[a] Septicemia caused by *E. cloacae, E. agglomerans,* or *P. cepacia* should especially prompt investigations for contaminated infusate.

Adapted from Maki, D. G., *Microbiologic Hazards of Infusion Therapy*, Phillips, I., Ed., MTP Press, Lancaster, England, 1977, 99.

nationwide U.S. epidemic when, signaled by five unexplained bacteremias in three hospitals, intrinsic contamination of one company's products was identified and a recall put into effect so rapidly that the outbreak was limited to the five initially recognized cases.[416] It must be reemphasized, however, that for surveillance of bacteremias to be maximally effective, all blood isolates must always be characterized completely, i.e., through species (See Laboratory Diagnosis of Bacteremia).

Table 15
RESULTS OF CULTURING INFUSATE AND THE CANNULA IN 790 IN-USE INFUSIONS

Datum	Results on culture	
	Infusion fluid	Cannula
Total number cultured	790	790
Positive culture, number (%)	5 (0.6)	34 (4.3)[a]
Local infection, number (%)	0	29 (3.7)[b]
Related septicemia, number (%)	0	5 (0.6)[c]

[a] p <0.001 by Fischer's exact test.
[b] Positive semiquantitative culture of the cannula.
[c] p = 0.03.

Adapted from Band, J. D., Maki, D. G., *Ann. Intern. Med.*, 91, 173, 1979.

Cannula-Related Infection

There are two potential sources of bacteremic infection associated with administration of a parenteral infusion: infection of the cannula* wound and contaminated infusate. The best available data suggest that cannulas produce endemic nosocomial bacteremia far more frequently than contaminated fluid[717,721] (Table 15).

Expressed as the percentage of cannulas producing sepsis, the incidence of cannula-related bacteremic infection is relatively low, about 1 to 2% with plastic catheters and 0.2% with steel needles.[716,717] These rates are sufficiently low that any single physician is unlikely to encounter and identify more than an occasional case and thus his or her awareness of the problem is likely to be nominal at best. But even a low incidence of infection applied to the approximately 20 million Americans receiving infusion therapy annually in this country supports the author's estimate[717] of at least 25,000 cannula-related septicemias nationwide each year.

Most laboratories culture vascular catheters qualitatively, amputating the tip with a sterile scissors and dropping it into liquid media. A positive culture by this technique is, unfortunately, diagnostically nonspecific. Up to 57% of catheters sampled in some hospitals give growth when cultured in broth.[716] Theoretically, a single bacterium picked up from the skin as the catheter is removed can produce a positive culture.

Considerable evidence indicates that most cannula-related septicemias derive from local infection of the transcutaneous cannula tract or wound.[716,717,722] Thus, quantitative culture of the external surface of the withdrawn cannula should in theory reflect accurately the microbiologic status of the wound and, similar to the use of quantitative urine cultures, distinguish true infection from contamination. The author, Weise, and Sarafin[722] have developed and standardized a semiquantitative method for culturing vascular cannulas on solid media. The technique has been further studied prospectively with vascular catheters from burned patients[123] and with steel ("scalp vein") needles from patients with hematologic malignancy.[233,723]

Before removing a cannula, the skin about the insertion site is first cleansed with an alcohol-impregnated pledget, mainly to remove any residual ointment. After the alcohol dries, the cannula is carefully withdrawn with care to avoid contact with the surrounding skin. If pus can be expressed from the cannula wound, it is always Gram-stained and cultured separately. For short catheters and steel needles, the entire length of the

* Cannula is a general term that encompasses all devices used for temporary vascular access, including steel needles and plastic catheters of all types.

cannula is amputated at the skin junction (Figure 10) with a sterile scissors for plastic catheters and snapping steel needles off with a sterile hemostat. For longer catheters two 2-in segments are cultured: the tip and the intracutaneous segment (Figure 10). Cannula segments are transported to the laboratory in sterile transport tubes (Culturette, Marion Scientific Corporation), first removing and discarding the swab before introducing the segment. Cannulas should be cultured as soon as possible after removal, ideally within 2 hr.

In the laboratory with a flamed forceps, the segment or segments are transferred onto the surface of a 100-mm 5% blood agar plate and, using a sterile forceps (Figure 11), are rolled (or if bent, smeared) back and forth at least four times across the agar surface. Plates are incubated aerobically at 37°C for at least 72 hr before discarding as negative. Each colony type appearing on the semiquantitative plate is enumerated and fully identified and tested for antimicrobial susceptibilities. We do not believe it necessary to routinely culture cannulas anaerobically. Anaerobic bacteria would appear to be rare causes of cannula-related sepsis: in over 30 prospective studies of vascular-cannula-related infection,[716] anaerobes were not identified as bloodstream pathogens deriving from vascular cannulas, even though most of these studies used media and methods for processing blood cultures that would be capable of recovering anaerobes.

Fifteen or more colonies growing on a semiquantitative plate is regarded as a positive culture,[123,722,723] denoting local cannula-related infection, and based on studies with nearly 2000 cannulas, has a 15 to 40% association with concordant bacteremia. With most cannula-related septicemias, growth is confluent (Figure 12). Cannulas positive on semiquantitative culture are strongly associated with local inflammation,[123,722,723] affirming the validity of considering a positive semiquantitative culture ($\geq$15 colonies) as representing infection.

The semiquantitative culture technique shows promise in facilitating the diagnosis of suppurative phlebitis,[123] the most severe form of cannula-related infection, which is often very difficult to diagnose clinically. Compared with the broth method, culturing semiquantitatively also accelerates the microbiologic identification of clinically significant isolates and reduces the cost of culturing cannulas.

Using this culture technique, we use the following stringent criteria for defining an individual nosocomial bacteremia as cannula-related: [123,124,233,721-723] (1) isolation of the same species in significant numbers on semiquantitative culture of the cannula and from blood cultures obtained by separate venipunctures, with a negative culture of the infusate; (2) clinical (or autopsy) and microbiologic data disclosed no other apparent source of septicemia; and (3) clinical features consistent with bloodstream infection.

In reviewing prospective studies of intravascular cannula-related infection[716,717] reported in the literature, [72,77,78,121-124,128,315,336,721-780] several important points can be extracted. Every type of vascular cannula carries some risk of causing bacteremic infection. The degree of risk per cannula varies greatly, depending on the type of cannula and the institution. In general, plastic catheters appear to be considerably more hazardous than small steel needles, long plastic catheters more than short catheters,* catheters inserted into the central circulation more than peripheral venous catheters, and catheters emplaced by surgical cutdown more than catheters inserted by percutaneous puncture. With few exceptions, most studies have found with virtually every type of peripheral venous cannula: the longer the device is left in place, the higher the risk it will cause bacteremia. With reasonable care, few peripheral venous cannulas of any type produce septicemia until they have been in place for at least 48 hr. In most centers, plastic catheters left in place for over 48 to 72 hr have been associated with rates of septicemia ranging between 2 and 5%, but in some hospitals the incidence has been as high as 8%. The lowest rates of infection (consistently less than 1% of all venous catheters) have been reported from institutions with organized intravenous therapy programs that provide a uniform and high level of asepsis at the time of cannula insertion and in maintenance care thereafter, and assure close monitoring of all infusions at least daily.[315,728,731-733,737,742,754]

It must be pointed out that most studies evaluated the older, large polyethylene or

---

* Only if the risk is measured in terms of infections *per 100 catheters* (or %). If *infections per 100 days of cannulation* is used as an index of risk, because they remain in place for much longer periods, central venous catheters inserted directly into the subclavian or internal jugular vein are associated with a considerably *lower* risk of infection than peripheral venous catheters.

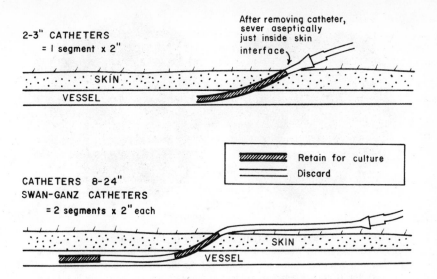

FIGURE 10. Segments of vascular cannulas cultured semiquantitatively. (From Maki, D. G., Jarrett, F., and Sarafin, H. W., *J. Surg. Res.,* 22, 513, 1977. With permission.)

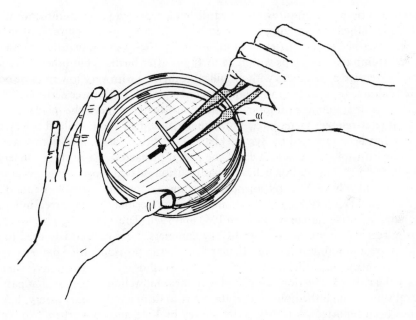

FIGURE 11. Technique for culturing cannula segments semiquantitatively. (From Maki, D. G., Jarrett, F., and Sarafin, H. W., *J. Surg. Res.,* 22, 513, 1977. With permission.)

polyvinyl chloride catheters; the author suspects that the smaller Teflon® catheters now widely used are considerably less hazardous as regards infection, but *controlled comparative* studies of these devices and catheters made of other materials purported to cause less morbidity, such as silastic[754] and steel needles, are needed.

Umbilical catheters are employed almost universally for vascular access in neonates. Prospective studies in a number of centers have documented a high incidence of positive catheter cultures, ranging from 52 to 62%, with rates of concordant bacteremia

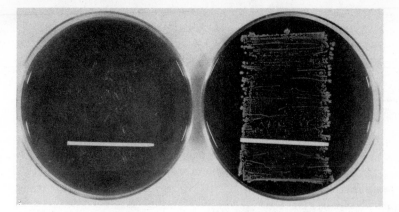

FIGURE 12.   Typical negative (left) and positive (right) semi-quantitative cultures of catheter segments. The two catheters were removed at the same time from a patient with *S. aureus* septicemia originating from the semiquantitative culture-positive catheter. (Catheter segments are left on the plates for perspective only.) (From Maki, D. G., Jarrett, F., and Sarafin, H. W., *J. Surg. Res.*, 22, 513, 1977. With permission.)

— diagnosed by blood cultures obtained through separate venipunctures rather than through the catheter — ranging from 8 to 16%.[128,756,757] These high rates of infection have been ascribed to the difficulty of maintaining asepsis in the luxuriant flora of the umbilical stump that develops within 24 to 48 hr after birth,[758] but other centers have reported extensive experiences with umbilical catheters, with very low rates of positive catheter cultures (6 to 21%) and related bacteremia (0% in all three series).[759-761] Prophylactic use of systemic antibiotics has not consistently reduced the incidence of umbilical catheter-related bacteremia, but catheterization of the umbilical artery rather than vein has been reported by Symanski and Fox[759] to be associated with fewer complications. Infusions were identified as the portal of bacteremia in three nursery outbreaks.[479,498,568,569] The author believes that infusion-related sepsis — unrecognized as such — may also have been responsible for some — possibly many — of the 15 outbreaks of primary, "cryptogenic" Gram-negtive septicemia that occurred in nurseries or neonatal intensive care units between 1965 and 1978 (Table 9).

Flow-directed balloon-tipped Swan-Ganz catheters[762] are now widely used to guide fluid therapy and monitor left ventricular function in post-operative patients and patients with shock or cardiorespiratory failure. Well-designed prospective studies to quantify the risks of infection associated with these indwelling catheters that pass from a central vein through the right side of the heart to lie in a pulmonary artery, however, have not been reported. A retrospective survey by Katz and co-workers[763] of complications encountered with 392 Swan-Ganz catheters identified 17 (4.2%) associated with bacteremia presumably related to the catheter. Retrospective reviews of autopsy records[764,765] have found that 3.4 to 9.3% of monitored patients coming to autopsy show aseptic vegetations in the right side of the heart; related infective endocarditis occurred in 1 of the 54 cases reviewed by Green and co-workers.[764] A small prospective study by Applefield and associates[766] of 57 in-use Swan-Ganz catheters found that catheters in place for more than 72 hr., or that had been repositioned more than three times, were significantly more likely to be associated with positive blood cultures drawn through the catheters, but the clinical relevance of positive catheter-drawn cultures was not ascertained; all blood cultures drawn by percutaneous venipuncture were negative. Unpublished studies by the author indicate that Swan-Ganz catheters produce catheter-related bacteremia at least as frequently as central venous catheters: approximately 3 to 5% of catheters in place for longer than 72 hr. The risk appears to be lower, per day of cannulation, with catheters inserted directly into a subclavian vein than with catheters inserted into a peripheral vein and guided into the central circulation.

The lowest incidence of cannula-related infection has been reported with steel needles, especially the "scalp-vein" or "butterfly" needles widely used in pediatrics. In prospective studies of noncompromised patients given intravenous therapy through steel needles, related septicemia has been rare (<0.2%).[767-771] However, a recent study by Band and the author[233] of steel needles used for intravenous therapy in patients with hematologic malignancy, half of whom had severe granulocytopenia (<1000 granulocytes/mm³), showed that, in this highly susceptible patient population, even steel needles were associated with a significant incidence of septicemia — 1.4% of all needles, affecting 7% of all patients during the study. All septicemias occurred in granulocytopenic patients and with needle placements exceeding 3 days (p = 0.02). Other reports[772-774] also suggest that steel needles pose a significant risk of infection to immunosuppressed patients, especially needles left in place for longer than 3 days.

Tully and co-workers[774a] recently carried out a large, prospective, randomized study which compared the complications associated with small Teflon® catheters and steel needles used for elective intravenous therapy in adult patients. All devices were inserted and cared for by a nurse intravenous therapy team; nearly all of the cannulas in both groups during this study were removed within 3 days. The rate of local and bacteremic device-related infection was extraordinarily low and the same in both groups, although needles infiltrated more frequently and catheters produced significantly more phlebitis. This important study affirms the value of a team approach to the care of intravenous infusions of all types and suggests that if peripheral venous devices receive scrupulous local aseptic care and are removed without fail within 3 days, plastic catheters probably pose no greater risk of bacteremic infection than steel needles. The greater risk of infection associated with plastic catheters in clinical use is most likely due to the reality that catheters are much more likely to be left in place for prolonged periods — often greatly exceeding 3 days — than are steel needles.

In the past decade, providing complete nutritional support by a parenteral route, total parenteral nutrition, or intravenous hyperalimentation, has become a viable therapeutic modality that is often life-saving for patients unable to tolerate oral alimentation or who have insufficient gastrointestinal function to sustain life. Because the solutions used in parenteral alimentation are highly irritating to the vein, the central circulation must be cannulated, usually by percutaneous puncture of the subclavian or internal jugular vein. Catheters routinely remain in the same location for prolonged periods, ranging from weeks to months. Moreover, patients requiring this form of therapy are usually debilitated and malnourished and frequently have peripheral infections.[775] In the early years of this new therapy, from 1969 to 1973, a number of centers reported alarmingly high rates of septicemia complicating hyperalimentation, ranging as high as 27% in several hospitals and averaging 7% in a nationwide survey of major centers.[118] Organisms that commonly cause infections in conventional intravenous therapy, including S. aureus, enterococcus, and Gram-negative bacilli, were often implicated except that approximately 50% of septicemias were caused by Candida species.[118,776] Most sepsis in hyperalimentation originates from the central catheter;[717] despite an outbreak traced to contaminated solutions compounded in one hospital's central pharmacy,[640] there is little evidence that contaminated fluid accounts for many hyperalimentation-related infections. In support of this view, Sanderson,[777] Copeland,[778] Abel,[779] and Myers[780] and their co-workers have shown in the past 5 years that hospitals with special hyperalimentation teams that stress maximal asepsis during catheter insertion and in follow-up care of the catheter, experience very low rates of related sepsis: 2% or less.

A relatively new form of infusion therapy has unique features which predispose to iatrogenic sepsis, especially of epidemic proportions:[568,569,781,782] the use of intra-arterial infusions for hemodynamic monitoring and for obtaining arterial blood specimens. In large centers, most critically ill adults and newborns, and all cardiovascular surgery patients, are monitored routinely; Stamm[783] recently estimated that 76,000 patients are monitored each year nationwide. Long arterial catheters are also being used to deliver antineoplastic drugs directly to an area of unresectable tumor, such as within the liver (regional cancer chemotherapy).[784]

The incidence of endemic bacteremic infection caused by intra-arterial infusions is not as well established as with venous catheters because very few studies of hemodynamic monitoring have specifically addressed the issue of catheter-related infection.[785] Most of the reports of sepsis associated with arterial pressure monitoring involved epidemics related to contamination of the fluid used in these systems[470,497,499,500,568,569,574,579,599] (which are discussed in a later section). A recent prospective study by Band and the author[124] of 130 intra-arterial infusions used for hemodynamic monitoring of critically ill patients identified five catheters that produced septicemia; all had been in place for 5 days or longer (p < 0.001). Catheters placed by cutdown rather than percutaneously had a ninefold increased rate of infection. Because these catheters were used in severely compromised patients, 80% of whom were receiving systemic antibiotics, catheter-related infections were caused primarily by enterococci, Gram-negative bacilli, and *Candida*.

Another study by the author and co-workers[336] prospectively examined the risks of infection with long arterial catheters used for regional cancer chemotherapy. Over a 4-year period, 1.5% of 600 catheters produced septicemia, all with *S. aureus*. Difficult cannulations of the brachial artery, and the need to reposition the catheter, greatly increased the rate of infection (p < 0.01). Requiring patients to shower with hexachlorophene prior to cannulation and periodically applying a topical combination antibiotic ointment to the catheter wound has essentially eliminated these infections in our hospital.

When a plastic catheter is inserted in a vessel, a loosely formed, fibrin sheath develops around the intraluminal portion of the catheter within 24 to 48 hr[786,787] (Figure 13). This sheath forms a nidus within which microorganisms can multiply, shielded from host defenses — and even antibiotics. Thrombogenicity of cannula materials may play an important role in vulnerability to cannula-related infection.[752] Most cannula-produced septicemias begin first as local infections of the intradermal cannula wound.[716,717,722] Aerobic bacteria, especially *S. aureus* (approximately 50% of bacteremias caused by peripheral venous cannulas[716]), enteroccci, and various aerobic Gram-negative bacilli, gain access to the cannula wound (and, ultimately, the fibrin sheath) from external sources at the time the cannula is inserted or afterwards, or colonize the fibrin sheath by hematogenous spread from distant unrelated sites of infection. As previously noted, there is little evidence that anaerobic bacteria are significant pathogens in cannula-related sepsis.

Figure 13 depicts potential sources for contamination and infection of cannula (catheter or needle) wounds. Most cannula-related septicemias derive from the patient's own skin flora or organisms transmitted from the hands of the person inserting the cannula. The presence of preexistent infection, such as an infected surgical wound, connotes an increased risk of infection of the cannula site by the same strains.[121,122,788] The cannula tip and its surrounding fibrin sheath can also become colonized by hematogenous seeding;[71,121-124] the frequency with which this phenomenon occurs is not well defined but central venous and arterial catheters appear to be most prone. In a study of 130 arterial catheters used for hemodynamic monitoring, Band and the author[124] encountered 37 catheters exposed to bacteremias from distant unrelated sites

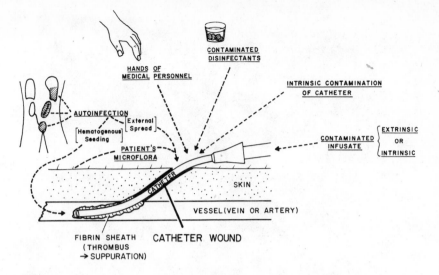

FIGURE 13. Sources of vascular cannula-related infection. (Modified from Maki, D. G., *Microbiological Hazards of Intraveous Therapy,* Phillips, I., Meers, P. O., D'Arcy, P. F., Eds., MTP Press, Lancaster, England, 1977, 106. With permission.)

of infection; 5 appear to have become colonized hematogenously and after a brief latency period, and subsequently perpetuated and amplified the original septicemia. The author and co-workers[123] encountered similar "rebound septicemias" in a prospective study of vascular catheters used in burned patients, and Harris and Cobbs,[71] Henzel and DeWeese,[121] and Morgensen, et al.[122] have identified the phenomenon as well, mainly with central venous catheters. These observations suggest that if a vascular catheter, especially a central venous or arterial catheter or any vascular cannula in a burned patient, is exposed to high grade bacteremia, irrespective of the source of the bacteremia, it may be most prudent to replace it.

In theory, contaminants in the infusate flowing through the cannula (Figure 13) can also colonize the cannula and its fibrin sheath, but recent data suggest this occurs very infrequently. Band and the author[721] found no correlation between organisms recovered from cultures of fluid and the cannula in 790 in-use infusions (Table 15).

The most extreme form of cannula-related infection is septic or suppurative phlebitis; in the central great veins, septic thrombosis. With rare exception, this grave infection derives from plastic catheters that have been left indwelling for more than 48 hr.[123,789-796] In suppurative phlebitis, the vein acts like, and indeed becomes, an intravenous abscess (Figure 14), pouring massive numbers of organisms into the bloodstream. The clinical picture is predictable: refractory and often overwhelming septicemia. When this occurs, few patients survive unless the vein and its affected tributaries are excised surgically.

Suppurative phlebitis has been encountered most often in burn patients whose burn wounds (see chapter entitled "Infections in Burn Patients") commonly harbor 10^5 or more microorganisms per gram of tissue.[123,790,791,794-796] Limited numbers of accessible veins for vascular access, failure to recognize early signs of catheter-induced sepsis because fever is attributed to the burn wound, and an intrinsic hypercoagulable state, combined with the vast number of pathogenic organisms ever near the catheter wound, create a milieu uniquely conducive to this dread infection. Suppurative phlebitis may be most frequent in nonburned patients cannulated through veins of the leg.[789,792]

In the last decade, microorganisms most frequently implicated in suppurative phlebitis have been by and large the same organisms causing uncomplicated cannula-related

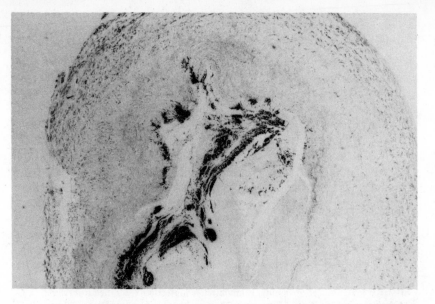

FIGURE 14.   Histopathology of a vein segment associated with suppurative phlebitis (Go-mori-Methenamine Silver × 40). Black masses are *Candida* colonies infiltrating intraluminal thrombus and the vessel wall.

septicemia, coagulase-positive *S. aureus* and, increasingly, resistant strains of *Klebsi-ella-Enterobacter, Pseudomonas, Serratia, Acinetobacter* and *Candida.*

Suppurative phlebitis is characteristically an insidious clinical entity. Local inflammation is present less than half of the time, and the septic picture often does not present until several days after the catheter has been removed. Fever chills, and hypotension are often attributed to infection of the burn wound, the urinary tract, surgical wounds, respiratory tract, or elsewhere. In burned patients, up to two thirds of cases in the past have been identified only at autopsy.[790,791,794,795] Suppuration of the great central veins[793-796] — the vena cavae or subclavian or iliofemoral veins — usually derives from catheters used for hyperalimentation in burn patients and has rarely been diagnosed during life; the patients have typically died of refractory cryptogenic septicemia and septic pulmonary emboli.

Most epidemics of cannula-related septicemia have been caused by Gram-negative bacilli, related to the use of unreliable chemical antiseptics that became heavily contaminated,[108,109,575,580] or derived from cross-contamination of cannula sites,[479,576] often by organisms carried on the hands of medical personnel.[473,498] Although one company's plastic catheters were shown to be intrinsically contaminated in 1973, a clearcut association with clinical disease was not established.[797]

Sepsis from Contaminated Infusate

It took nearly 20 years, after development of the plastic catheter, before intravenous cannulas eventually became recognized as a source of serious iatrogenic infection;[716] but it required 35 years and the occurrence of epidemic bacteremias in hospitals across the country in 1970 to 1971[4] before medicine awakened to the fact that the fluid given in infusions (infusate) also was vulnerable to contamination that could produce serious nosocomial disease. The experience of the past decade (Figures 2 and 5) has shown that nearly one third of all epidemics of nosocomial bacteremia stem from contaminated infusate — organisms introduced during its manufacture (intrinsic contamination) or during its preparation and administration in the hospital (extrinsic contamination).

Table 16
METHOD FOR CULTURING IN-USE INFUSION FLUID IN THE HOSPITAL

1. Record the nature of the fluid and all lot numbers.
2. Cap the administration set with a sterile ensheathed needle and transport the entire delivery system (all bottles or bags and the administration set) promptly to the laboratory in a clean plastic bag. Sampling should be done in a monitored laminar flow hood if possible, at the minimum in a clean, minimally occupied laboratory.
3. Withdraw 10 to 20 ml of fluid from the administration set:
   a. Culture 0.1 ml quantitatively on a surface plate or 1.0 ml in a pour-plate.
   b. Inject remaining fluid into a blood-culture bottle.
   c. If the product is suspected on clinical grounds of having caused illness, a gram-stained smear of the original fluid and of a centrifuged aliquot should always be routinely performed and, if positive, reported immediately to the physician caring for the patient from whom the infusion was obtained.
4. Add an equal volume of double-concentrated brain-heart infusion broth enriched with 0.5% beef extract to remaining fluid in the container — or, if the container is empty, add 50 ml, mix — and incubate the container.
5. Attempt to obtain and culture remaining samples of any other fluids the patient may have received in the preceding 24 to 48 hr.
6. Incubate all containers aerobically at 35 to 37°C for at least 5 to 7 days before discarding.[a]
7. All isolates should be fully identified, through species, and tested for susceptibility to a panel of antimicrobials. All isolates, especially of Gram-negative bacilli, should be retained until the scope of the problem has been fully elucidated.
8. If clinical and epidemiologic data suggest manufacturer-related contamination of a commercial product (intrinsic contamination), the local and federal public health authorities (the Food and Drug Administration and the CDC) should be immediately informed. Remaining unused products in general should probably not be sampled by the hospital, but retained for evaluation by these agencies.

[a] If a blood product is being sampled that may have produced illness, specimens should also be incubated ⁀t 17 to 20°C and anaerobically at 35 to 37°C.

Modified from Center for Disease Control, *National Nosocomial Infections Study,* Quarterly Report, Second Quarter of 1972, Atlanta Ga., U.S. Public Health Service, 1972, 11.

The author uses the following criteria for defining an individual nosocomial bacteremia as caused by contaminated infusate:[124,233,721,723] (1) recovery of the same species from cultures of infusate and from blood cultures obtained by separate venipuncture, with a negative semiquantitative culture of the cannula; (2) no other identifiable source of septicemia; and (3) clinical features consistent with bloodstream infection.

A variety of techniques are available for culturing parenteral admixtures and fluid medications, and have recently been reviewed by the author.[148,412] A relatively simple method, easily adaptable for use in the hospital when in-use fluids or parenteral medications are suspected of harboring contaminants, is outlined in Table 16. There is no evidence that anaerobic bacteria can grow in parenteral admixtures or produce related septicemia; thus, anaerobic culture techniques are not necessary unless a red cell-containing blood product is involved.

An understanding of infection related to infusion fluids must be based on an appreciation of the potential for growth of pathogenic organisms in these fluids. In 1970, the author and Martin[411] evaluated the ability of 105 clinical isolates from human nosocomial infections, representing 9 genera and 13 species, to grow at room temperature (25°C) in 5% dextrose-in-water, the most frequently used commercial large-volume parenteral. Of 51 strains of the tribe Klebsielleae — *Klebsiella, Enterobacter,* and *Serratia* — 50 attained concentrations of 100,000 or more organisms per milliliter in 24 hr , beginning with washed organisms at an initial concentration of one organism per milliliter (Figure 15). In contrast, only 1 of 54 strains of other bacteria, including

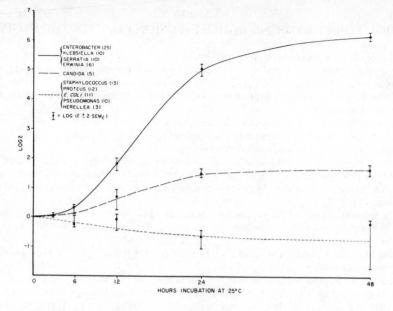

FIGURE 15.   Growth of 106 microbial strains in 5% dextrose-in-water at 25°C. Numbers in parentheses indicate number of strains tested. *Erwinia* = *Enterobacter agglomerans.* c = mean normalized concentration (organisms per milliliter). It is apparent that members of the Klebsielleae *(Klebsiella, Enterobacter, Serratia)* attain counts > 10⁵ organisms per milliliter at room temperature within 24 hr. (From Maki, D. G. and Martin, W. T., *J. Infect. Dis.*, 131, 267, 1975. With permission, University of Chicago Press.)

Staphylococcus, E. coli, P. aeruginosa, Acinetobacter, and *Candida,* displayed any growth abilities in 5% dextrose-in-water. None of 18 strains from 9 genera grew in 0.9% sodium chloride solution over 24 hr, although 3 strains of *Klebsiella* increased 1 log after 48 hr.

The author recently reviewed the growth properties of organisms in various commercial parenteral solutions:[412] rapid multiplication in 5% dextrose-in-water appears to be limited mainly to members of the tribe Klebsielleae and *P. cepacia;* in distilled water, to *P. aeruginosa, P. cepacia, Acinetobacter,* and *Serratia;* and in lactated Ringer's solution to *P. aeruginosa, Enterobacter,* and *Serratia.* Normal (0.9%) sodium chloride solution supports growth of most bacteria and *Candida* rather poorly. *Candida* species grow in the hypertonic glucose solutions used in parenteral hyperalimentation; in the synthetic amino acid-25% glucose solutions now used most frequently, it grows somewhat slowly but considerably better than most bacteria, which are greatly inhibited.[798] But most bacteria as well as *Candida* proliferate rapidly in the casein hydrolysate-25% glucose solutions which are now being used less frequently.

Melly et al.[799] found that most microorganisms were able to grow in commercial 1% lipid emulsion for infusion (Intralipid®). In a similar study by the author,[412] 12 of 13 bacterial species tested and *Candida* multiplied in Intralipid® almost as rapidly as in bacteriologic media. Accordingly, fat emulsions would seem to possess considerable potential for producing epidemic nosocomial disease, but only one sporadic septicemia clearly linked to in-use contamination of the product has been reported.[800] A CDC team[801] encountered frequent contamination of fat emulsion being administered during an outbreak of nosocomial bacteremias in a newborn nursery but was unable to establish a conclusive causal relationship with epidemic infections.

The pathogens implicated in more than 95% of all published reports of septicemia traced to contaminated fluid have been organisms that proliferate rapidly at room temperature in the solution involved;[412] e.g., members of the tribe Klebsielleae in 5% dextrose-in-water. But it should be emphasized that microbial growth in most parenteral solutions — the exception being fat emulsion — is quite selective. Identification of the species isolated from a patient with septicemia can aid greatly in tracing the origin of infection (Table 14). Common nosocomial species such as *E. coli, P. aeruginosa, Acinetobacter, Proteus,* and *Staphylococcus* die in 5% dextrose-in-water. Recovery of these organisms from blood cultures of a patient with sepsis who is receiving parenteral fluids suggests that the infection is unlikely to be due to contaminated infusate. If, however, *Enterobacter* (especially *Enterobacter cloacae* or *E. agglomerans*) or *P. cepacia* is cultured from the blood of a patient receiving infusion therapy, contaminated infusate should be strongly suspected as the possible source.

It should be pointed out that with most organisms, even with counts exceeding 10^6 organisms per milliliter of fluid, visible evidence of microbial growth has usually not been present.[412] Molds, usually introduced into the container through microscopic breaks, may produce cloudiness or filmy precipitates.[802]

The vast majority of nosocomial bacteremias traced to contaminated infusate and reported in the literature occurred in an epidemic setting. However, it is abundantly clear that fluid readily becomes contaminated from extrinsic sources in the hospital, presumably related to the countless manipulations of the infusion in the course of therapy (Figure 16). Culture surveys of intravenous fluids have revealed contamination rates ranging from 0.9 to 38%, with an average of about 5%.[717] Most organisms recovered in positive cultures are common skin commensals that are generally considered of low virulence and grow poorly, if at all, in the fluid. Moreover, the level of contamination is usually very low (< one organism per milliliter), far too low to produce detectable clinical manifestations; but, when contamination occurs with Gram-negative bacilli able to multiply in the fluid, the risk of sepsis increases greatly.

The risk of fluid becoming contaminated during use is related to the duration of uninterrupted infusion through the administration set.[4,70,444,803] Systems in continuous use for periods longer than 48 hr are, in general, more likely to contain contaminants than systems used for less than 48 hr (Table 17). Microorganisms capable of growth in the fluid, once introduced into a running infusion, can perpetuate in the administration set for many days, despite multiple replacements of the bottle or bag and high rates of flow.[716,804] Routinely replacing the entire delivery system (all bottles or bags and the administration set) every 24 to 48 hr and at every change of the cannula, and following the administration of blood products, is one of the most important control measures for reducing the hazard of contaminated infusate.[4,716,717,721,805]

The incidence of endemic nosocomial bacteremia caused by extrinsically contaminated infusate is not accurately known at the present time but appears to be very low, at least tenfold lower than the incidence of endemic cannula-related septicemia. Based on a review of over 20 published studies[717] and his own data[721] (Table 15), the author estimates that there is approximately one case of septicemia from contaminated fluid for every 1000 infusions. Infusate can be identified as a source of septicemia only if it is cultured. This occurs but rarely in most hospitals, and it is likely that the majority of sporadic (endemic) septicemias caused by contaminated fluid are unrecognized or are attributed to the cannula.

From 1 to 6% of blood units have been found to contain bacteria,[466,806-809] yet endemic septicemias deriving from transfusion of contaminated blood products have been rare, most likely because most blood products are routinely refrigerated, contamination is of low level, and because of universal awareness that blood products must be infused promptly after removal from refrigeration. Sepsis traced to contaminated

POTENTIAL SOURCES FOR CONTAMINATION
OF INFUSION FLUID

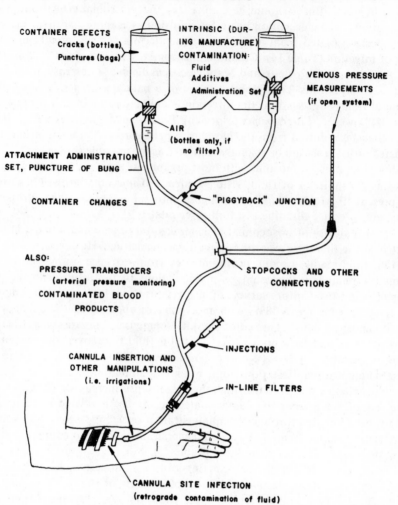

FIGURE 16.   Potential sources for contamination of infusion fluid. (Adapted from Maki, D. G., *Microbiological Hazards of Intravenous Therapy,* Phillips, I., Meers, P. O., D'Arcy, P. F., Eds., MTP Press, Lancaster, England, 1977, 120. With permission.)

Table 17
RELATIONSHIP OF DURATION OF INFUSION THERAPY AND IN-USE CONTAMINATION OF INFUSION FLUID

Duration of continuous infusion therapy	Number of infusions sampled	Number of (%) with contamination
<48 hr	33	1 (3)
≥48 hr	61	9 (15)[a]

[a] $p < 0.05$.

Adapted from Maki, D. G, Anderson, R., and Shulman, J., *Appl. Microbiol.,* 28, 778, 1974.

whole blood has usually been associated with severe shock and high mortality because of the massive numbers of psychrophilic (cold-growing) organisms, most often *Serratia,* pseudomonads other than *P. aeruginosa* or other uncommon nonfermentative Gram-negative bacilli, in the indicted unit.[806,810-812] Bacteria are often visible on a direct gram-stained smear of the product. Recently, outbreaks of pyrogenic reactions[813] and an epidemic of *Pseudomonas* species septicemia[417] were traced to intrinsically contaminated normal serum albumin, and small epidemics of *E. cloacae*[466] and *Salmonella cholerae-suis* septicemia[414] derived from contaminated platelet concentrates (which are maintained at 25°C to enhance viability). Blood products should always be infused promptly after they are removed from refrigeration. Upon completion of the transfusion, the entire delivery system should be replaced. If sepsis is suspected as being related to a contaminated blood product, the entire infusion should be removed; aliquots of the remaining product should be cultured aerobically *and* anaerobically on solid media, and at both 35 to 37°C and 16 to 20°C (Table 14.)

The clinical features of septicemia originating from contaminated infusate are indiscernible from those characterizing cannula-related septicemia; however, shock produced by massive concentrations of viable Gram-negative bacilli or endotoxin in the responsible product, is considerably more frequent.

Prevention of Infusion-Related Sepsis

To accord it due respect, any device for vascular access might best be thought of in very elementary terms, as a direct conduit — almost a funnel — between the external world and its myriad of microorganisms and the patient's bloodstream. All infusion systems, whether for simple intravenous therapy or for hemodynamic monitoring, must be recognized as open portals for the entry of infection. *Vigorous handwashing before inserting — using sterile gloves for high risk cannulas (e.g., for hyperalimentation) and in high-risk patients (e.g., those with leukemia), thoroughly disinfecting the site with a reliable germicide (e.g., 1 to 2% tincture of iodine U.S.P.),* [101-107] *and paying meticulous attention to aseptic technique throughout the insertion, constitute the first line of defense against cannula-related infection.* Thereafter, limiting the duration of placement of peripheral venous cannulas to no longer than 3 days and arterial catheters for hemodynamic monitoring to 4 days, can greatly reduce the risk of cannula-related infection. Maximal care when compounding parenteral admixtures and when handling infusions, and routinely replacing the entire delivery system at least every 48 hr , are pivotal measures for reducing the risk of contaminated infusate. All apparatus used in association with an intravascular infusion, such as pressure transducer components, must be reliably sterile.

Comprehensive published guidelines are now available, dealing with preparation of admixtures,[814,815] administration of infusion therapy[716,717,814,816,817] including total parenteral nutrition,[118,776,817] care of infusions for hemodynamic monitoring[124,568,569,781,782] and arterial catheters used for regional cancer chemotherapy,[336] microbiologic surveillance in infusion therapy,[148,412,818] and for evaluating a possible epidemic of infusion-related sepsis.[819-821]

Epidemics of Infusion-Related Septicemia Traced to Extrinsic Contamination

Even when commercially manufactured products are sterile on arrival in the hospital — as they fortunately almost always are when alleged to be — many circumstances of hospital use can compromise that initial sterility. Most sporadic infections related to infusion therapy, whether due to the cannula or contaminated infusate, are of extrinsic origin. Similarly, most reported epidemics have stemmed from exposure of multiple patients' infusions to a common source of contamination in the hospital (Tables 9 and 18).

One of the earliest reported outbreaks due to extrinsic contamination, reported by Plotkin and Austrian,[108] originated from one hospital's practice of immersing intravenous catheters in aqueous benzalkonium which was also used to disinfect catheter insertion sites. Over a 15-month period in 1955 to 1956, 40 patients developed septicemia with a *Pseudomonas* species. Cultures of an in-use container of the disinfectant showed > 10⁵ organisms per milliliter. Unfortunately, "history forgotten must be history relived". There have been at least ten subsequent outbreaks of infusion-related bacteremia (Table 18) and three of pseudobacteremia (Table 13) due to hospitals' inexplicable proclivity to continue to use unreliable chemical disinfectants such as aqueous benzalkonium in the U.S. and aqueous chlorhexidine in the United Kingdom for preparing cannula sites or, in recent years, for decontaminating transducer components used in hemodynamic monitoring.

In 1970, Sack[467] reported five cases of Gram-negative septicemia with shock occurring in patients who had consecutively received a preoperative infusion from a single bottle of succinycholine in 5% dextrose-in-water, from which *K. pneumoniae* and *E. cloacae* were subsequently cultured. Although the mechanism of contamination was not found in these cases, another case of *Klebsiella-Enterobacter* septicemia in the same hospital was ascribed to a cracked bottle containing contaminated fluid. Entry of organisms through a minute crack was also thought by Robertson[802] to be the cause of two cases of visible contamination of in-use fluid in one hospital in 1970, one with *Trichoderma* species and the other with *Penicillium;* one patient developed transient fungemia.

Preparing medications or solutions for parenteral injection from multidose vials is not dissimilar to the practice of administering the same infusion to more than one patient. Multiple-entered vials or containers are notoriously prone to contamination.[822,823] Three outbreaks of infusion-related septicemia, all caused by Gram-negative bacilli that thrive in aqueous solutions — *Flavobacterium*,[597,598] *P. cepacia*,[578] and *Serratia marcescans*[497] — were traced to contamination of multidose vials used to compound intravenous medications or to flush arterial monitoring systems.

As previously discussed, during their administration infusions readily became contaminated from innumerable hospital sources. Five cases of infusion-related *K. pneumoniae* septicemia in an intensive care unit in 1967 were ascribed by Morse and co-workers[473] to heavily contaminated hand lotions used by nurses. It is unclear whether these were catheter-related infections or microorganisms introduced into in-use fluid. In a very recent outbreak, reported by Rhame and McCullough,[581] contaminated cryoprecipitate caused two cases of *P. cepacia* septicemia in a Minnesota hospital; a water bath used for thawing and warming the product was shown to be heavily contaminated by the epidemic organism.

Investigations in a number of outbreaks have documented contamination of in-use infusate or infection of cannula sites, but the hospital reservoir of the epidemic pathogens — and, often, even the mode of transmission — eluded detection. This was the case in a small outbreak of *E. cloacae* bacteremias traced to contaminated platelet transfusions by Buchholz and associates[466] in 1970. In 1971, Duma and co-workers[444] reported four cases of Gram-negative septicemia with fluid being administered contaminated by organisms identical to those isolated from blood cultures. Manipulations of the delivery system, especially the administration set, were postulated as the probable mode of contamination. Two similar small epidemics of *P. cepacia* septicemia, reported by Meyer[576] and by Thong and Tray,[577] were also ascribed to extrinsic sources of contamination in the hospital. No hospital source of *P. cepacia* could be identified in either outbreak, but in-use contamination of fluid within administration sets was detected in the second outbreak; after adopting a policy of changing delivery sets at

Table 18
EPIDEMICS OF INFUSION-RELATED SEPTICEMIA TRACED TO EXTRINSIC SOURCES OF CONTAMINATION

Years inclusive	Pathogens	Number of cases	Type of infusion[a]	Epidemiology	Ref.
1955—1956	Pseudomonas spp.	40	I.V.	Contaminated aqueous benzalkonium used to disinfect I.V. catheter sites	108[b]
1960	Enterobacter cloacae	11	I.V.	Contaminated aqueous benzalkonium used for cutaneous antisepsis	109[b]
1965	Flavobacterium spp.	8	I.V.	Contaminated multidose vials for intra-operative I.V. injections	597,598
1967	Klebsiella pneumoniae	5	I.V.	Contaminated nurses hand lotions	473
1968	E. cloacae and K. pneumoniae	5	I.V.	Same contaminated infusion containing succinylcholine given to every patient	467
1969	E. cloacae	2	I.V. (blood)	Contaminated platelet transfusions stored at room temperature	466
1970	Pseudomonas cepacia	3	IA	Contaminated reusable pressure transducers used in hemodynamic monitoring; contaminated aqueous benzalkonium used for chemical disinfection of chamber-domes	574
1970	Escherichia coli, Klebsiella, and S. marcescens	4	I.V.	Contaminated in-use fluid, source not identified	444
1970	P. cepacia	5	I.V.	Contaminated aqueous chlorhexidine used for cutaneous antisepsis	575
1971	P. cepacia	4	I.V.	Source and mechanism of contamination not identified	576
1971	P. cepacia	4	I.V.	Contaminated in-use fluid, source not identified	577
1972	P. cepacia	5	I.V.	Contaminated multidose vial of saline for I.V. injections	578
1973	S. marcescens	5	IA	Contaminated multidose vial of heparinized saline used to fill arterial pressure monitors	497

Table 18 (continued)

EPIDEMICS OF INFUSION-RELATED SEPTICEMIA TRACED TO EXTRINSIC SOURCES OF CONTAMINATION

Years inclusive	Pathogens	No. of cases	Type of infusion[a]	Epidemiolgy	Ref.
1973	Flavobacterium spp.	14	IA	Contaminated ice used to chill syringes used for arterial blood specimens	599
1973 — 1974	S. marcescens	6	I.V.	I.V. needle-related septicemias in nursing; Serratia spread on the hands of medical personnel	498
1974	P. cepacia	8	IA	Contaminated aqueous benzalkonium used to disinfect reusable chamber-domes employed in hemodynamic monitoring	579
1975	Candida albicans	4	IA	Contaminated pressure transducers; failure of chemical disinfection of reusable chamber-domes	568, 569
1974	P. aeruginosa	10	IA		
1975	P. acidivorans and E. cloacae	5	IA		
1975	P. cepacia	9	I.V.	Contaminated aqueous benzalkonium used to disinfect cannula sites and I.V. injection ports on administration sets	580
1975	Candida parapsilosis	22	IVH	Contaminated vacuum system used to fill hyperalimentation bottles in hospital's pharmacy	640
1975	K. pneumoniae	9	I.V.	Outbreak in nursery with in-use contamination of I.V. fluid and I.V. needle-related infection; source not identified	479
1975	Staphylococcus aureus	4	IA	Septic endarteritis complicating arterial cannulations used for cancer chemotherapy; outbreak followed discontinuation of preparatory hexachlorophene scrub of catheter sites	336
1976	Enterobacter aerogenes	7	I.V.	Contamination of fluid in hospital pharmacy, using the same syringe to add potassium to multiple bottles of fluid	468, 469

1976	E. cloacae	8	IA	Contaminated transducer heads used with disposable chamber-domes in hemodynamic monitoring	470
1977	S. marcescens	25	IA	Contaminated transducer heads; disposable chamber-domes that were re-used damaged during gas sterilization	499
1978	S. marcescens	17	IA	Contaminated transducer heads used with disposable chamber-domes; fluid thought to have become contaminated by organisms carried on the hands of medical personnel	500
1978	P. cepacia	2	I.V. (blood)	Cryoprecipitate contaminated in water-bath warmer	581

[a] I.V., intravenous; I.V. (blood) intravenous, blood product-related; IA, intra-arterial; IVH, intravenous hyperalimentation.

[b] Provided for completeness, but not included in 1967 to 1978 tabulations (text).

48-hr intervals, no further infusion-related *P. cepacia* bacteremias were identified in that hospital.[577]

Two related outbreaks of infusion-related Gram-negative septicemia occurred in newborn nurseries. In the first outbreak, six *S. marcescens* septicemias originating from winged steel-needle sites were ascribed by Stamm and collaborators[498] to epidemic organisms carried on the hands of nursery personnel. In the second epidemic, Ross and co-workers,[479] linked nine *K. pneumoniae* septicemias to infected winged steel-needle sites and to contaminated fluid; routine use of in-line membrane filters did not prevent sepsis from contaminated infusate. The nursery reservoir of *Klebsiella* was never ascertained, but heightened attention to aseptic practices with respect to infusion therapy curtailed the outbreak.

Compounding of admixtures, whether in the pharmacy or on the patient-care unit, is another important means by which contamination can be introduced. The greatest concern about this mode of contamination, especially if it occurs in a central pharmacy, is that a large number of patients may be exposed. Moreover, the delay between compounding and use provides opportunity for proliferation of introduced organisms. During a 4-month period in 1975, 22 patients in a large university hospital developed *Candida parapsilosis* fungemia traced to contaminated solutions used for intravenous hyperalimentation. The investigators, Plouffe and co-workers,[640] discovered that a vacuum system in the hospital's pharmacy used to evacuate fluid from bottles before introducing additives was heavily contaminated by the epidemic *Candida* strain. Organisms presumably refluxed into bottles during compounding of the admixtures.

In March 1976, seven children in a pediatric hospital developed *E. aerogenes* septicemia traced to contaminated 5% dextrose in 0.2% sodium chloride to which potassium chloride had been added in the hospital's central pharmacy. A CDC team[468,469] found that the pharmacist was using one syringeful of concentrated potassium chloride solution to add potassium to each of eight consecutive units of fluid; after compounding, bottles were permitted to stand at room temperature, before use, for up to 48 hr.

As noted, the use of invasive hemodynamic monitoring systems in critically ill patients has mushroomed in the past decade. While the quantitative hemodynamic data so derived is often of considerable value for the optimal management of these patients, the potential for iatrogenic infective complications is also considerable and, it would appear, has not been adequately explored. Eleven reported outbreaks of bacteremic infection[470,497,499,500,569,574,579,599] or hepatitis[568,569] deriving from intra-arterial monitoring systems (Table 18) — all occurring since 1970 — bears this out. While it is likely that most infections caused by intra-arterial infusions are due to the catheter, these systems have one feature that may increase the risk of sepsis from contaminated infusate — the stagnant column of fluid (Figure 17). In all 11 outbreaks, infections were produced by extrinsically contaminated infusate within the system.

In 1973, Walton and associates[497] traced five cases of *Serratia* septicemia in their hospital to a contaminated heparinized saline solution used to fill manometers and flush arterial catheters. Also in 1973, Stamm and co-workers[599] showed that ice contaminated by *Flavobacterium* species was responsible for 14 cases of *Flavobacterium* septicemia associated with arterial pressure monitoring systems in one hospital's intensive care unit. The organisms are thought to have entered an infusion when a syringe which had been chilled in the ice was used to draw a blood specimen through one of the access ports connected to the arterial catheter (Figure 17). However, the most frequent cause of epidemic septicemias in hemodynamic monitoring has been contamination of the transducer assembly, especially the fluid-filled chamber-dome (Figure 17). Failure of the procedure for disinfecting reusable chamber-domes, employing unreliable chemical agents such as aqueous benzalkonium or chlorhexidine, was impli-

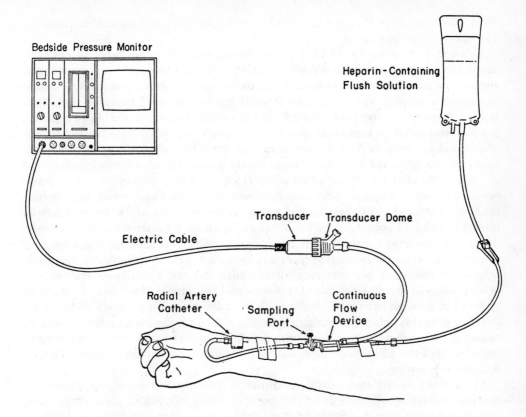

FIGURE 17. Infusion apparatus for arterial pressure monitoring. Besides the catheter wound, the injection port, chamber-dome, and tranducer pose the greatest hazards of in-use contamination.

cated as the cause of contamination in the first outbreak reported by Phillips and co-workers[574] in 1970 and in four outbreaks investigated by the CDC between 1973 and 1976.[568,569,579]

The development and recent availability of disposable chamber-domes seemingly would obviate the problems of resterilization of these critical components by hospitals. However, Buxton and co-workers[470] investigated an outbreak in 1976 of eight cases of *E. cloacae* septicemia in one hospital associated with the use of disposable chamber-domes; the outbreak derived from failure to regularly sterilize the permanent transducer components — specifically the transducer head (Figure 17) — to which disposable domes attach. The mechanism by which organisms on a transducer were transmitted to the isolated fluid circuit (Figure 17), however, could not be determined. Two similar epidemics associated with disposable chamber-domes have now been reported and provide data on possible mechanisms of contamination of fluid. Following an outbreak of 16 *Serratia* septicemias, linked to contaminated transducer-heads, Donowitz and co-workers[500] carried out simulation studies showing that organisms on transducer-heads were readily transmitted to fluid in the (disposable) chamber-dome circuit during manipulations of the system by medical personnel whose hands became contaminated while handling the system. Another potential mechanism of transmission was elucidated by West and associates:[499] they linked 25 *Serratia* septicemias in one hospital to reuse of disposable chamber-domes. Of 25 domes examined after gas sterilization, 8 showed cracks in the membrane that abuts on the transducer. All permanent or reusable transducer components should be cleansed and sterilized with ethylene oxide or glutaraldehyde between use with different patients, and disposable chamber-domes should not be re-used.

Although contamination of fluid within intra-arterial infusions used for hemodynamic monitoring had been implicated in many epidemics of nosocomial bacteremia, virtually no data had been published on *endemic* rates of contamination and related septicemia associated with this unique form of infusion therapy. Recently, the author and Hassemer[823a] prospectively studied 102 intra-arterial infusions used in 56 high-risk patients who required prolonged monitoring. During the study, transducer-chamber-domes and continuous flow devices were used until the infusion was discontinued. Cultures were obtained every 48 hr from the transducer-chamber-dome interface and of fluid in the chamber-dome; 12 infusions (11.8%) showed contamination of chamber-dome fluid, in 8 cases (7.8%) associated with concordant bacteremia. Four bacteremias are considered definitely related and four, possibly related, to the intra-arterial infusion. In all 12 contaminated infusions and with all 8 bacteremias, the chamber-dome had been used for more than 2 days ($p = 0.006$). No concordant contamination of transducer-chamber-dome interfaces was identified. This study indicates that intra-arterial infusions for pressure monitoring cause sporadic septicemias *endemically*. With prolonged monitoring, chamber-domes and continuous flow devices should be replaced at periodic intervals, ideally, with the administration set every 48 hr. After implementing this policy, the authors identified only 3 contaminated infusions and no related septicemias in 53 monitored intra-arterial infusions over 4 months, attesting to the efficacy of this additional simple control measure for preventing infection in hemodynamic monitoring.

All of these reports must further reinforce in the minds of medical personnel the considerable iatrogenic hazards of invasive monitoring. They also demonstrate most convincingly that even if commercial items are sterile when they arrive in the hospital, they can readily become contaminated during clinical use. The use of disposable sterile items must not result in a sense of false security and relaxed attention to good aseptic practices or diminish vigilance for related iatrogenic disease.

With the ever-increasing number of hospital patients who are being exposed to invasive hemodynamic monitoring, the increasing number of reports of infection may well reflect not only an increase in the number of procedures performed and greater general awareness, but a true increase in the incidence of infectious complications. Except during outbreaks, particularly those caused by less common pathogens such as *Flavobacterium* or *P. cepacia,* in many hospitals infusions of any type are rarely considered as a source of nosocomial bacteremia.

One small outbreak of infusion-related septicemia investigated by the author and his colleagues[336] did not involve a common source of contamination. Between January and May 1975, in the University of Wisconsin Hospitals, 4 (5.7%) of 70 patients receiving regional chemotherapy through percutaneously inserted brachial artery catheters developed septic endarteritis with bacteremia caused by *Staphylococcus aureus.* The cluster of infections followed discontinued use of hexachlorophene for scrubbing the patient's arm prior to cannulation; phage-typing suggested the four cases were caused by the patients' own strains of *Staphylococcus.* Reinstituting a policy of using hexachlorophene for the preparatory scrub and routinely applying a topical polyantibiotic (Neosporin) ointment to catheter sites terminated the outbreak. During the next 310 catheterizations, no bacteremic infections occurred ($p < 0.001$).

Epidemics of Infusion-Related Bacteremia Caused by Intrinsic Contamination

Whereas most infection deriving from infusion therapy, whether due to the cannula or contaminated fluid, is of extrinsic origin, since 1970 there have been seven reported epidemics of infusion-related septicemia caused by contaminants of intrinsic origin (Table 19). The occurrence of these outbreaks has greatly abetted wider recognition of the iatrogenic hazards of infusion therapy.

The first and the largest epidemic had its onset in mid-1970,[4,70,824-826] when one U.S. manufacturer of large-volume parenterals began to distribute bottles of fluid with a new elastomer-lined, screw-cap closure. In early December 1970, the first cases of infusion-related septicemia caused by biologically characteristic strains of *E. cloacae* and *E. agglomerans* (formerly designated *Erwinia*) were reported to the CDC although retrospective review subsequently showed that many hospitals had been experiencing epidemic cases for several months (Figure 18). Although it was established very early, virtually at the very outset of investigation, that sepsis was mediated by contaminated fluid, the ultimate source of contamination — intrinsic contamination of the new closures — was not identified conclusively until March 1971. Between July 1970 and March 1971, 25 U.S. hospitals tabulated by the CDC reported nearly 400 cases of infusion-related septicemia.[4] Over 20 microbial species, including *E. cloacae* and *E. agglomerans,* were isolated from closures of previously unopened bottles. Organisms could be shown to gain access to fluid when bottles were handled under conditions duplicating normal in-hospital use.[826] The appearance of epidemic septicemias within individual hospitals and nationally paralleled distribution of the company's product with the new closures (Figure 19). The epidemic was terminated only by a product recall (Figure 18).

Investigations in the company's manufacturing plants[826] showed that the epidemic pathogens were present throughout the environment of the plants and had probably been gaining access to the thread areas and interstices of the screw-cap closure after the autoclaving step for as long as the plants had been in operation. The new closure, which was very similar in design to the old one (Figure 20), however, utilized a synthetic elastomer sealing disk which did not have intrinsic antibacterial activity, whereas the red rubber disk used in the old closure for over 30 years without detectable problems fortuitously possessed antibacterial properties.

An unusual outbreak of *Salmonella cholerae-suis* septicemia in the National Institutes of Health in 1970 to 1971 was ultimately traced to one blood donor whose platelets had been given to every case.[414] This outbreak is discussed in detail in a later section (Approach to an Epidemic).

The third epidemic caused by intrinsically contaminated intravenous products, was reported by Phillips and co-workers.[413] Between April 1971 and January 1972, 40 patients in a London, England hospital developed septicemia, urinary tract infection, or respiratory infection from softened, deionized, distilled water manufactured in the pharmacy and used throughout the hospital. *Pseudomonas cepacia* was recovered from infected patients and the water. When used for cooling bottles of parenteral fluid and other sterilized fluids in the hospital's rapid-cooling autoclave, this water often remained on the rubber stopper beneath a foil seal and entered the bottle when the closure was punctured for clinical use. Water may also have entered some of the bottles directly during the cooling cycle.

In early 1972, seven patients at a Plymouth, England hospital developed profound shock after receiving 5% dextrose-in-water; five patients died. Investigations by Meers and co-workers[415,827] showed that the fluid within approximately one third of 155 bottles cultured from the implicated lot contained viable microorganisms, in some cases up to 10^7 Gram-negative bacilli per milliliter. Contamination was traced to faulty maintenance of autoclaving equipment at the manufacturer's plant.[827]

In both of the aforementioned outbreaks, infusion products with rubber-stopper closures were implicated, emphasizing that no specific design can be assumed to be inherently safe.

Table 19

EPIDEMICS OF INFUSION-RELATED SEPTICEMIA CAUSED BY INTRINSIC CONTAMINATION

Years inclusive	Pathogens	Number of reported cases	Epidemiology	Ref.
1970 — 1971	Enterobacter spp., Enterobacter cloacae and E. agglomerans	378[a]	Contaminated fluid and screwcap closures for I.V. bottles	4, 824, 826
1970 — 1971	Salmonella cholerae-suis	7	Contaminated platelets from one asymptomatic injected donor	414
1971 — 1972	Pseudomonas cepacia	8	Contaminated closures for I.V. bottles	413
1971 — 1972	E. agglomerans	7[a]	Contaminated I.V. fluid	415, 827
1973	Citrobacter freundii, E. cloacae and E. agglomerans	5[a]	Contaminated I.V. fluid	416, 828
1973	P. cepacia	11[a]	Contaminated normal serum albumin	417
1978	P. cepacia	16[a]	Contaminated fentanyl for I.V. injection	418, 419

[a] Epidemic involved multiple hospitals.

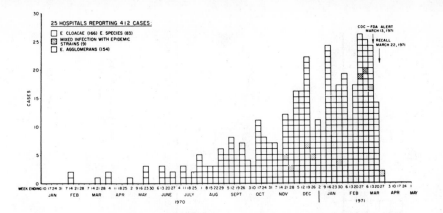

FIGURE 18. Nationwide outbreak of nosocomial bacteremias due to intrinsic contamination of one manufacturer's products; 397 cases of I.V.-associated septicemia in 25 tabulated U.S. hospitals, occurring between July 1, 1970 and April 1, 1971 fulfilled criteria for epidemic cases. The epidemic was curtailed immediately within individual hospitals and nationally by a nationwide recall of the manufacturer's large-volume parenteral products. (From Maki, D. G., Rhame, F. S., Mackel, D. G., and Bennett, J. V., *Am. J. Med.*, 60, 471, 1976. With permission.)

The fifth outbreak — and third in this country — occurred in 1972, when a manufacturer increased pressure in his autoclaves, a move that would be expected to increase their efficiency. Apparently, however, this led to a pressure differential between the outside and the inside of fluid-filled bottles, producing a partial vacuum inside the containers which, in turn, drew contaminated cooling water into the bottles.[828] Between February and March 1973, five patients who received 5% dextrose-in-lactated Ringer's solution developed sepsis;[416] *Citrobacter freundii* was recovered from the blood of three patients; *E. cloacae,* from one patient; and *E. cloacae* and *E. agglomerans,* from one patient. Low-level intrinsic contamination was demonstrated by careful cultures of previously unopened fluid.

The most recently reported outbreak in this country deriving from an intrinsically contaminated product involved 25% normal serum albumin rather than a crystalloid fluid. In 1973, 11 patients at a Maryland hospital developed *Pseudomonas* sp. septicemia, shown by Steere and co-workers[417] to be associated with receipt of 25% normal serum albumin made by a single manufacturer. Cultures of unused units showed contamination with *P. cepacia*. Because the product cannot be autoclaved, it is heated at 60°C for 10 hr and then filtered. Contamination was thought to have been introduced in the manufacturing plant after the heat treatment, most likely during dispensing of the product into individual vials.

In 1978, 16 patients in two European hospitals, one Danish and one Dutch, developed *P. cepacia* bacteremia in the early postoperative period; these infections were fortunately very mild clinically. Investigations by Siboni, Borghans, and associates[418,419] disclosed that all of the affected patients had received intravenous fentanyl intra-operatively, a drug combination used to provide light anesthesia. Two lots of the manufacturer's product, which was not routinely sterilized after preparation and dispensing, were found to be intrinsically contaminated by *P. cepacia*.

All of these epidemics illustrate how subtle and insidious the factors that influence sterility can be. In four outbreaks, there was no documented failure of the sterilization process; instead, seemingly minor alterations in the manufacturing process resulted in contamination of individual units in the manufacturing plant *after* the sterilization stage.

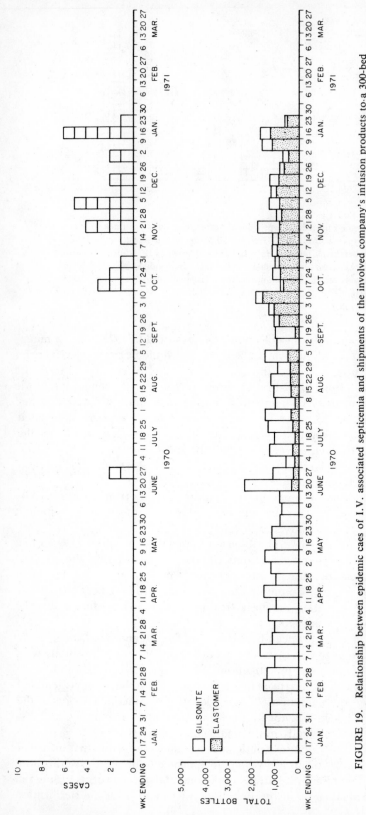

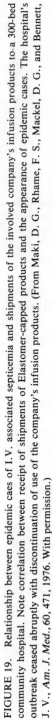

FIGURE 19.   Relationship between epidemic caes of I.V. associated septicemia and shipments of the involved company's infusion products to a 300-bed community hospital. Note correlation between receipt of shipments of Elastomer-capped products and the appearance of epidemic cases. The hospital's outbreak ceased abruptly with discontinuation of use of the company's infusion products. (From Maki, D. G., Rhame, F. S., Mackel, D. G., and Bennett, J. V., *Am. J. Med.,* 60, 471, 1976. With permission.)

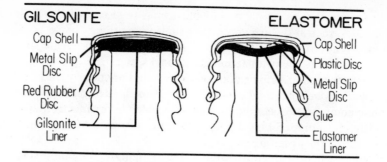

FIGURE 20. The old Gilsonite-lined and new Elastomer-lined screw-cap closures used on bottles of the involved company's parenteral fluids. Micro-organisms were isolated from the threads and lining insert disks of 39.9% of Elastomer-lined closures. The epidemic strain organisms, *E. cloacae* or *E. agglomerans,* were isolated from 8.1% of 1007 of the new closures sampled, but none of 229 Gilsonite-lined closures. (From Maki, D. G., Rhame, F. S., Mackel, D. G., and Bennett, J. V., *Am. J. Med.,* 60, 471, 1976. With permission.)

Intrinsic contamination is fortunately exceedingly rare, but its potential for harm is much greater because numerous hospitals and large numbers of patients may be affected. Also, direct contamination of infusate at the manufacturing level gives contaminants an opportunity to proliferate to very high concentrations. The mortality in outbreaks due to intrinsic contamination (mean, 31.9%; range 0 to 86%) has been considerably higher than in epidemics caused by extrinsic contamination (mean, 8.7%; range 9 to 57%).

The author suspects that intrinsic contamination may well be a continuous, ongoing source of endemic infusion-related sepsis, but of such low magnitude that sporadic septicemias are virtually never identified as being of intrinsic origin, let alone identified as infusion-related. Only when infusion-associated septicemias are encountered in epidemic numbers — especially occurring simultaneously in multiple, widely scattered hospitals — is intrinsic causation likely to be recognized and proved. The key to detection of intrinsic contamination is clinical surveillance: a substantial increase in the incidence of cryptogenic infusion-associated septicemia (i.e., an epidemic) must prompt studies to exclude intrinsic contamination of the cannula, infusate, or some other product used in infusion therapy.

There are no clinical clues to intrinsic contamination. As noted previously, bacteremia deriving from contaminated fluid has the same symptoms and signs as catheter-induced sepsis and other nosocomial septicemias. The few clues to infusion-related bacteremia — such as the lack of an obvious anatomic source of infection, its frequent occurrence in patients without a predilection to systemic infection, and the dramatic clinical response to discontinuation of the infusion — do not differentiate between intrinsic and extrinsic sources of infection.

The author and co-workers[4] have pointed out that the distinction often must be made epidemiologically. Dixon[828] has summarized seven features which strongly suggest intrinsic contamination of an infusion product.

1. Surveillance within the hospital showing a sudden and unexplained rise in blood isolates of one or a few organisms — often with similar sensitivities — vis-a-vis, an epidemic.

2. Establishing that the epidemic organisms have not caused significant disease at other sites, such as the urinary tract — indicating primary bacteremia.

3. An outbreak involving only one or a few species (most endemic infusion-related infections involve many different genera and species).

4. Septicemias with an organism or organisms that are not commonly encountered, such as *E. cloacae, E. agglomerans, C. freundii,* and *P. cepacia*[717] (Table 14).

5. Unlike common nosocomial pathogens, epidemic organisms that are unusually sensitive to antimicrobial drugs, suggesting a source of contamination far removed from the hospital.

6. Epidemiologic investigations which show a highly significant association of epidemic septicemia with infusion therapy.

7. Lastly, similar episodes in multiple hospitals.[4] When only a small proportion of a batch or series of batches of a product is contaminated, the number of infections arising may be too small for a pattern to emerge in a single hospital, but when episodes from several or many hospitals are reported to a central registry — such as the National Nosocomial Infections Study of the CDC — a pattern may evolve that identifies the source, as it did in the outbreak of 1970 to 1971 (Figure 21).[831]

Epidemic Septicemias in Hemodialysis

Technologic advances in the past two decades have made extracorporeal hemodialysis a viable therapeutic modality for the indefinite support of patients with chronic renal failure. Over 38,000 patients were dialyzed in the U.S. in 1978.[571] The necessity of maintaining a stable route for vascular access, however, and the vulnerability of hemodialysis machines to contamination combined with the ability of many Gram-negative "water bacteria" to multiply in dialysis solutions,[832-834] creates a state highly conducive to bacterial sepsis, and in the closed setting of the dialysis unit and sharing of machines, epidemic septicemia. Between 1965 and 1978, six outbreaks of pyrogenic reactions[570,571,835-838] and seven of nosocomial bacteremia[337,338,570-573,582,702] were reported from dialysis centers (Figure 5).

Similar to infusion therapy, dialysis-related infections are of two types: those deriving from the vascular access device and those due to contaminated solutions used in the machine. Three fourths of bacteremias originating from vascular access sites are caused by *S. aureus,* and the rest, by aerobic Gram-negative bacilli.[280-283,839,840] External arteriovenous shunts have been associated with considerably higher rates of infection (approximately 0.3 to 0.6 bacteremias per patient-dialysis-year) than have subcutaneous fistulas (approximately 0.15 bacteremias per patient-year).[280,283,839,840] Septicemia due to an external shunt usually requires that the device be removed to control the infection, whereas sepsis occurring in association with a subcutaneous fistula in most cases can be successfully eradicated with prolonged intravenous antimicrobial therapy (such as by administering weekly doses of vancomycin[280,841,842]). While the case-fatality rate of staphylococcal septicemia deriving from hemodialysis access sites has been much lower (approximately 10%[282,283]) than with other endemic nosocomial bacteremias, septic pulmonary emboli,[282,283,843] endocarditis,[282,283,844,845] and osteomyelitis[282,283,846] are well documented complications.

Frequent staphylococcal infections have plagued many dialysis units, but common-source epidemics or frequent cross-infection caused by one phage-type of *S. aureus* have been surprisingly infrequent. Most staphylococcal infections of access sites appear to be autogenous, produced by patients' own strains;[280,283,839] up to 50% of hemodialysis patients are chronic skin carriers of *S. aureus.*[280,847,848] The relatively few reported "epidemics" of access-site infection with staphylococcal bacteremia involved

Table 20
RELATIONSHIP BETWEEN BACTERIAL COUNTS IN DIALYSIS FLUID AND RATES OF PYROGENIC REACTIONS IN DIALYZED PATIENTS DURING AN OUTBREAK

Concentration Gram-negative bacilli in dialysis fluid (number per ml)	Number of dialyses	Number of pyrogenic reactions	Rate (%)
$<10^2$	25	1	4
$10^2—10^4$	31	4	13
$>10^4$	21	5	24

Adapted from Favero, M. S., Peterson, N. J., Boyer, K. M., Carson, L. A., and Bond, W. W., *Trans. Am. Soc. Artif. Intern. Organs*, (20)A, 175, 1974.

multiple phage-types of *Staphylococcus*; an increased rate of infection was attributed to logistic circumstances resulting in less attention to local asepsis, possibly augmenting cross-infection of indeterminate degree.[337,338] Prevention of access-site infections requires uncompromising commitment to aseptic techniques during dialysis with particular emphasis on rigorous cutaneous antisepsis.

Contaminated dialysate, on the other hand, has been responsible for many outbreaks of pyrogenic reactions[570,571,835-838] or Gram-negative bacteremia,[570-573,582,702] usually with *P. aeruginosa*, in dialysis centers in this country and abroad. Most often illness was linked to high concentrations of Gram-negative bacilli in post-dialysis fluid. During the investigation of an outbreak, Favero and his CDC colleagues[570] identified an almost linear relationship between levels of contamination by Gram-negative bacilli and the appearance of symptomatic illness in dialyzed patients (Table 20); with bacterial counts exceeding 10^4 organisms per milliliter, one fourth of the patients dialyzed developed a pyrogenic reaction. The elegant studies of these investigators[149,570,834,849] have shown that recirculating single-pass and batch-recirculating machines are much more predisposed to heavy contamination than single-pass units and are more difficult to disinfect. Inadequate disinfection of water treatment systems and dialysis machines and suboptimal design and operation of these systems were found to be the major causes of heavy bacterial contamination and epidemic illness in the outbreaks investigated by these workers.[570,571,837]. Institution of proper methods for disinfection and operation of hemodialysis systems and use of water treatment systems that reliably remove endotoxin, such as reverse osmosis,[834] terminated the epidemics.

Reuse of disposable cartridge dialyzer membranes has obvious economic benefits[850,851] but increases the risk of contamination and iatrogenic infecion. Seventeen percent of U.S. dialysis centers surveyed in 1978, 28% of centers performing 100 or more dialyses per week, responded that they practice reuse.[851] Recently, epidemics of *Pseudomonas* bacteremia associated with reuse of disposable dialyzers were reported by Uman, Wagnild, and co-workers[572,573] and by Kuehnel and Lundh.[582] In both outbreaks, one with *P. aeruginosa*[572,573] and the other with *P. cepacia*,[582] contamination was ascribed to gross inadequacy of the disinfecting agent, aqueous benzalkonium, against pseudomonads. Wagnild and associates[573] found that the risk of bacteremia with a given dialyzer coil was directly related to the number of times it was reused; although most coils were contaminated by the second use, bacteremia was not demonstrated until after the fifth use.

Pyrogenic reactions, without demonstrable bacteremia, are very common in many dialysis centers. As noted, most studies — but not all[835,838] — have shown a close relationship between levels of contamination of dialysate and the frequency of reactions. Raij and co-workers[852] reported in 1973 that when present in dialysate, endotoxin readily passes to the blood compartment and shows strong correlation with febrile reactions. In 1974, Hindman and co-workers[838] investigated a large outbreak of pyrogenic reactions in a Washington, D.C. dialysis center occurring despite low levels of bacterial contamination of hemodialysis systems. High concentrations of endotoxin were identified in dialysis fluid and ultimately traced to an increase in endotoxin contamination of the community water supply used to prepare dialysate. Water softeners and deionizers which are commonly used to treat potable water for use in dialysis systems do not remove endotoxin in contrast to reverse osmosis which does.[570,834]

Excellent guidelines for disinfecting hemodialysis systems reliably and for monitoring them bacteriologically have been published by Favero and his co-workers.[149,834] Bacterial counts in water used to prepare dialysis fluids should never exceed 10^2 viable organisms per milliliter, and viable counts in dialysis solutions during use should not exceed 10^3 organisms per milliliter.

Contamination of Evacuated Blood-Collection Tubes

A frightening source of iatrogenic nosocomial bacteremia was brought to light by McLeish and co-workers[140] in 1974 when they identified five patients in two Canadian hospitals who developed *Serratia marcescens* septicemia traced to intrinsically contaminated evacuated blood-collection tubes. One year later, several American hospitals reported clusters of pseudobacteremias, also linked to contaminated blood-collection tubes.[142] Subsequent investigations showed that as many as 38% of tubes in Canadian hospitals contained *Serratia*,[138] and a prospective study by Washington [854] of tubes made by five U.S. manufacturers and obtained from 26 hospital laboratories across the country showed that 11 manufacturers' tubes frequently contained viable contaminants; of 1433 tubes examined, 14% were positive for a variety of microorganisms, including such common hospital pathogens as *P. aeruginosa*, enterococci, *Acinetobacter calcoaceticus,* and *Serratia.*

Virtually all of the over 8000 hospitals in the U.S. and Canada use commercially manufactured blood-collection tubes for obtaining blood samples; over 500 million tubes are sold in North America annually.[139] The obvious question arises: have nosocomial bacteremias due to contaminated blood-collection tubes been occurring on a massive scale, the cause of individual cases always remaining obscure? It is very possible, considering that in 1975 all manufacturers' tubes tested frequently contained contaminants, yet only a comparative handful of hospitals ever identified and reported a problem with either true bacteremias or pseudobacteremias.

Katz and co-workers[139] have studied the mechanisms of backflow and have published detailed guidelines to prevent reflux of tube contents into blood when using evacuated blood-collection tubes. While mandating that all blood-collection tubes must be sterile should obviate the hazards of iatrogenic bacteremia and pseudobacteremia, their precautions still obtain; reflux is always undesirable, because of the potential adverse effects of the liquid or powdered additives (preservatives or anticoagulants) contained in most tubes. All manufacturers now provide sterile tubes.

Epidemic Pyrogenic Reactions

Hospital outbreaks of acute pyrogenic (or pyrexial) reactions have been reported in which bacteremia could not be documented — i.e., blood cultures were consistently negative.[570,571,813,835-838,855-861] Affected patients characteristically had the abrupt onset of high fever, usually associated with rigors, hypotension of varying degrees — even frank shock — and nonlocalizing symptoms such as profound malaise, headache, confusion, and nausea or vomiting. Although two patients in a British hospital in 1961 died shortly after receiving an infusion of an intramurally compounded 5% human albumin solution,[859] the mortality in more recent outbreaks of pyrogenic reactions has been essentially nil; despite severe illness in many of the affected patients, there were no associated deaths in the 12 reported outbreaks occurring since 1965, each involving from 3 to 41 patients (Table 7).

In each outbreak, shortly prior to the onset of illness, each of the affected patients had been exposed to a procedure, such as hemodialysis or cardiac catheterization, or had received a common parenteral product. Investigations showed that the procedure or the administered product introduced nonviable bacterial contaminants — pyrogens — directly into patients' bloodstreams, accounting for a clinical picture indistinguishable from bacteremic sepsis and the characteristic precipitous onset of symptomatic illness. Recent studies using the *Limulus* amoebocyte lysate assay suggest that in most, possibly all, cases, the pyrogenic substance is Gram-negative lipopolysaccharide, endotoxin.[813,837,852,856,857]

All reported outbreaks since 1965 have fallen into one of three categories: (1) dialysate used in hemodialysis machines was found to be heavily contaminated by viable bacteria or endotoxin[570,571,835-838] — concentrations of Gram-negative bacilli exceeding 10^4 per milliliter of dialysate produced pyrogenic reactions in one fourth of exposed patients;[570] (2) pyrogenic reactions followed cardiac catherization with re-used catheters;[855-857] or (3) a blood product linked epidemiologically with pyrogenic reactions, usually normal serum albumin or plasma protein fraction, while sterile, was found to contain pyrogens.[813,860,861]

Febrile reactions associated with, frequently following, cardiac catherization are well known, but are infrequent in most hospitals. Only 0.3% of patients were reported to experience reactions in a large 1967 survey of U.S. centers encompassing 12,367 catheterizations.[277] In 1971, Lee and co-workers[855] traced a cluster of eight pyrogenic reactions to material — thought to be endotoxin — present in the tap water used to clean catheters prior to sterilization with ethylene oxide. Eluents of pyrogen-free distilled water passed through sterilized catheters produced fever in rabbits. Further experiments showed that ethylene oxide sterilization did not inactivate endotoxin placed on catheters. Pyrogenic reactions in patients were curtailed when a 500-mℓ volume of pyrogen-free distilled water (rather than 200 mℓ) was used to rinse each catheter before sterilization.

Three similar outbreaks of pyrogenic reactions associated with cardiac catheterization have recently been reported in the CDC's *Morbidity and Mortality Weekly Report*.[856,857] Each also involved processing of reusable catheters in hospital-distilled water, which was shown to be grossly contaminated with Gram-negative bacteria. Sterilized catheters were shown to contain up to 7.4 ng of endotoxin, as measured by the *Limulus* assay, much of it on the external surface of the catheter.[857]

It is obviously imperative that pyrogen-free distilled water be used for cleaning reusable catheters and that the outer surface, as well as the lumen of the catheter, be copiously rinsed before sterilization. In one center, reactions could not be completely curtailed until switching to disposable catheters.[856]

With regard to the last source of pyrogenic reactions, noncellular blood products such as normal serum albumin or plasma protein fraction are now manufactured commercially; heavy contamination of one lot can result in nosocomial disease involving patients in multiple, widely scattered hospitals. This was recently borne in an outbreak reported by Steere and co-workers.[813] In November, 1974, patients in three U.S. hospitals experienced pyrogenic reactions associated with the infusion of 25% normal serum albumin from the same lot; 65% of 662 vials tested with the *Limulus* lysate assay showed contamination with endotoxin in concentrations ranging from 4 to 64 ng/mℓ.

Sporadic pyrogenic reactions are very common with all types of blood products, cellular and noncellular. It is likely that both normal serum albumin and plasma protein fraction frequently contain small amounts of endotoxin, due to the necessity of sterilizing these solutions by filtration rather than by autoclaving; fortunately the concentrations are usually far too low to produce human illness.

Detection of epidemic pyrogenic reactions due to nosocomial exposures, especially those originating from contamination of a commercial product, is based on awareness of this phenomenon and careful epidemiologic investigations using case-control techniques to be described later in this review.

Pusillanimous Disinfectants and Epidemic Bacteremias

Reliable disinfection and sterilization embrace virtually all measures aimed at prevention of nosocomial infection (see chapter entitled "Choosing the Best Antiseptic, Disinfectant, Sterilization Method, and Waste Disposal and Laundry System").

At least 24 epidemics of nosocomial bacteremia, 6 of pyrogenic reactions, and 3 of pseudobacteremia have stemmed from dismal failure of a chemical germicide utilized in a highly vulnerable setting, such as infusion therapy (Table 18), hemodialysis, or disinfection of porcine heart valves. Aqueous solutions of quaternaries in the U.S., such as benzalkonium chloride or of chlorhexidine in Great Britain, were implicated in most incidents; a cluster of *Clostridium sordelli* pseudobactremias were recently traced to a contaminated Merthiolate® solution used to disinfect the diaphragms of blood culture bottles. Reliance upon these agents for "cold sterilization" of hemodialysis apparatus and transducer components used in hemodynamic monitoring particularly proved disastrous. In many outbreaks, the epidemic organisms were actually cultured from the in-use "working" solution of the agent, usually in concentrations exceeding 10^5 per milliliter, indicating that the organism was multiplying in the "disinfectant".

The unreliable activity of most "quats", the phenolic germicides, and hexachlorophene against many nosocomial Gram-negative pathogens, particularly pseudomonads and *Enterobacter,* has long been known.[862-871] Cork, cotton fibers, and a variety of anionic organic compounds inactivate aqueous benzalkonium;[862,863,866,868,869] and lowering the pH, which occurs when distilled water is used as a diluent, diminishes the activity of chlorhexidine.[586] As aqueous solutions, these agents are likely to become extrinsically contaminated during hospital use. Yet, because they are nonirritating to tissues, they are popular and remain in wide use; related nosocomial outbreaks can be expected to continue to occur.

Iodine-containing solutions, simple tincture of iodine (1 to 2% in 70% alcohol) — which can be compounded inexpensively in a hospital's pharmacy, or commercial iodophors, are most reliable for cutaneous antisepsis.[101-104] Alcohol 70% is an acceptable alternative in the occasional patient unable to tolerate an iodine solution.[104-107]

Any apparatus or device that enters sterile tissues or comes into physical contact with a patient in connection with an invasive device must be sterile. Autoclaving is always preferred, but if the object will not tolerate heat sterilization, gas sterilization with ethylene oxide, or prolonged immersion (for at least 10 hr[872]) in a high-level disinfectant, such as 8% formaldehyde-in-alcohol or 2% glutaraldehyde solution, is acceptable. It is very important that the object always be first vigorously cleansed to remove residual traces of organic matter, such as blood, that can compromise the efficacy of chemical disinfection.

Nosocomial Bacteremias in Cardiovascular Surgery

Patients who have undergone cardiovascular operations experience a high incidence

Table 21
INCIDENCE OF NOSOCOMIAL BACTEREMIA IN CARDIOVASCULAR SURGERY PATIENTS

Hospital	Year(s) of study	Number of patients at risk	Number of bacteremias	Rate (per 1000 patients)	Ref.
New York University	1968—1971	1494	41	27.4	873
University of Florida	1969—1972	466	16	34.3	874
Johns Hopkins	1968—1974	2910	36	12.4	302

of nosocomial bacteremia, ranging from 12.4 to 34.3 cases per 1000[302,873,874] (Table 21), three- to sixfold higher than rates encountered in most general hospital populations at large (Table 5) and exceeded only by the very high rates of nosocomial bacteremia documented in patients requiring prolonged intensive care after trauma or because of multiple organ failure (Table 8). Bacteremia in the early postoperative period is particularly serious in cardiac surgery patients who are often hemodynamically unstable and frequently have fresh vascular grafts or prosthetic heart valves highly vulnerable to becoming seeded and infected. Early prosthetic valve endocarditis (occurring within 60 days after operation) has had a very high mortality, exceeding 60%, in most centers.[875-878]

Most nosocomial bacteremias in this patient population derive from local infections of the surgical wound, pneumonias, or urinary tract infections,[302,873-878] but it is also likely that the multiple vascular cannulas routinely used in the perioperative period give rise to many (cryptogenic) bacteremias. Up to 60% of vascular catheters removed from cardiovascular surgery patients have been reported to be positive on culture.[741,879] Moreover, at least 7 (64%) of the 11 outbreaks of bacteremia from contamination of arterial-pressure monitoring systems involved postcardiac surgery patients.[470,499,500,568,569,574,579]

An additional and unique source of nosocomial bacteremia in this population is the operating room. Ankeney and Parker[880] isolated Staphylococcus epidermidis from 7.5% of 1555 cultures of blood obtained from five different sites of the cardiopulmonary bypass apparatus during 383 open-heart operations; the two sites most frequently positive were the heart-lung machine tubing and the coronary sucker. Three cases of late prosthetic valve endocarditis with S. epidermidis were linked to positive intraoperative cultures. In another careful analysis of intraoperative sources of contamination, Blakemore and associates[881] recovered a variety of organisms, including fungi and Gram-negative bacilli, from 14 (40%) of 35 cultures of blood from the heart-lung machine during open-heart procedures. They further demonstrated a strong concordance between positive cultures and simultaneous cultures of operating room air. In seven instances, the same organism isolated from the extracorporeal apparatus during surgery was later implicated in serious postoperative infection, including three cases of bacteremia. Carey and Hughes[882] and Hammond and Stiver[930] have also reported a correlation between organisms cultured from pump-oxygenator blood and from patients with postoperative endocarditis. These contaminants, many shed by members of the operating room team, are drawn into the extracorporeal apparatus through the coronary sucker which continuously aspirates blood from the surgeon's field. Whereas most are skin commensals and normally would rarely produce disease, S. epidermidis and diphtheroids are leading causes of prosthetic valve endocarditis.[158,159,161,875-878] Blackmore and associates[881] demonstrated that the system particularly constitutes a serious hazard if the ambient operating room air becomes heavily contaminated, especially with more virulent organisms. This point is underscored by the two small outbreaks of fungal prosthetic valve endocarditis caused by *Aspergillus* and *Penicillium,* that proved fatal in five or six cases, traced to an environmental situation producing high counts of fungal pathogens in operating room air.[646,647] In the two outbreaks of *S. epidermidis* prosthetic valve endocarditis described previously,[929,930] the mechanisms of acquisition were not elucidated, but it seems likely that these epidemic infections were also acquired intraoperatively, by the airborne route.

Blood in the heart-lung machine can also become contaminated from improper disinfection of the apparatus after a case. In the early years of open heart surgery, bacteremias caused by Gram-negative water organisms — *Archromobacter* and pseudomonads — were linked to this source of contamination.[691,883,884] This problem has not surfaced (or at least been reported) in recent times.

A last unique source of nosocomial septicemia in the cardiovascular surgery patient is the prosthetic implant itself. To the author's knowledge, there have been no documented cases of bacteremia or endocarditis traced to inadequate sterilization of artificial prosthetic materials; however, as previously discussed, in 1976, *Mycobacterium chelonei* endocarditis developed on two patients' prosthetic porcine heart valves that were already (intrinsically) contaminated at the time of implantation.[687-690] Waterworth and associates[885] have pointed out the difficulties with reliably sterilizing valve homografts by chemical means.

For better perspective, it might be pointed out that the incidence of hospital-related bacteremia in this population (Tables 8 and 21) rivals that reported in patients with acute leukemia.[228] The concern and depth of commitment to aseptic technique that typifies the care given to highly susceptible patients with leukemia[228] and bone marrow transplant patients[231,232] would seem equally fitting for patients undergoing cardiac surgery or requiring prolonged intensive care in any form.

Epidemics of National Scope

We live in an era of unprecendented communication. Products manufactured on one side of a country can be in thousands of homes or hospitals within days or even hours. This has created a potential for the distribution of poisoned or contaminated products on a scale that is almost awesome and which has culminated in at least seven interstate outbreaks of instituitional salmonellesis,[619-623] other nonbacteremic infections,[587,588] or pyrogenic reactions,[813] and six outbreaks of nosocomial bacteremia[4,415-419,687-690] involving multiple hospitals, all of national scope. The largest epidemic of bacteremias occurred in this country when *Enterobacter* septicemias were traced to one company's intrinsically contaminated parenterals in 1970 to 1971[4] (Figure 18). The fact that an outbreak of this magnitude could occur is not surprising; it is very conceivable that an epidemic of similar magnitude and geographic extent could occur in the future.

On a national scale, outbreaks of septicemia arising from intrinsic contamination of nationally distributed products can be exceedingly difficult to recognize if the infections are of low frequency or occur in widely scattered hospitals. Interhospital surveillance networks, such as the CDC's National Nosocomial Infection Study,[829,830] which carries out surveillance of nosocomial infections in a large cross-section of American hospitals, can serve as a sentinel system for the early detection of common source epidemics, as first advocated for bacteremic infections by Martin.[886]

Retrospective review of the data submitted to this program between January 1970 and July 1971 show conclusively that hospitals using the involved company's infusion products experienced a highly significant increase in incidence of *Enterobacter* (especially *E. agglomerans*) bacteremia beginning in June 1970 (Figure 21), even though

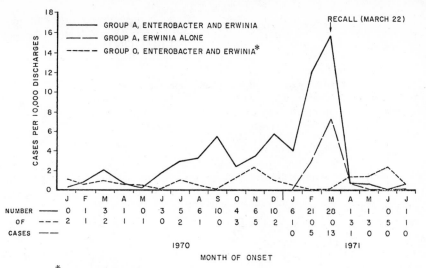

FIGURE 21. Primary bacteremias caused by *Enterobacter* species and by Erwinia *(E. Agglomerans)* reported to the CDC's National Nosocomial Infections Study from 37 U.S. hospitals between January 1970 and June 1971. A, hospitals using the involved manufacturer's products shown to be intrinsically contaminated; O, hospitals using products of other manufacturers. (From Center for Disease Control, *National Nosocomial Infections Study Quarterly Report, Fourth Quarter 1971,* 1972, 14.)

none of these hospitals individually identified the etiology or was even aware of the full scope of the problem nationally before March 1971.[831] No increase in *Enterobacter* bacteremia occurred in hospitals using the infusion products of other companies (p < 0.001). Although this surveillance program (which had its inception only in January 1970) did not detect the outbreak at its outset, the current sophistication with which data submitted by participating hospitals is now processed would almost certainly detect a similar problem in the future.

Outbreaks of national scope have all stemmed from intrinsic contamination of a widely used commercial product. It has been stated previously and will be reiterated once more in this chapter: *any data suggesting iatrogenic contamination of a commercial product, especially if it may have produced human illness or simply has the potential to do so, should be immediately reported to state and federal public health authorities; remaining samples of the product should be quarantined and saved for their analysis.*

APPROACH TO AN EPIDEMIC

Administrative Considerations

If an epidemic is suspected, the epidemiologic approach must be methodical and thorough, yet expeditious. It is directed toward establishing the existence of an epidemic, defining the reservoirs and modes of transmission of the epidemic pathogens and, most importantly, controlling the epidemic — quickly and completely (Table 22).

Knowledge or even suspicion of a possible hospital outbreak, particularly if the infections are as serious as bacteremia, usually spreads rapidly throughout a hospital and even the community, and often gives rise to rumors, panic, and potential for irrational behavior. It is extremely important that a hospital, through its infection

Table 22
EVALUATION OF A POSSIBLE EPIDEMIC
OF NOSOCOMIAL INFECTIONS

Administrative preparedness (Table 23)
Retrieve putative epidemic isolates — *immediately*
Preliminary evaluations
    Identify and characterize individual cases
    Ascertain if situation represents an *epidemic*
    Provisional control measures
    Intensify surveillance
    Review general infection control policies
    Determine need for assistance — especially extramural
Epidemiologic investigations
    Clinical-epidemiologic studies
    Microbiologic studies
Definitive control measures
Report the findings

control program, staff, and administration, be thoroughly prepared to deal with these issues as well as to implement control measures and carry out an effective investigation. Recognizing the vital importance of organization — designating specific responsibilities and maintaining effective communication at all times — the Infection Control Committee of the University of Wisconsin Clinical Sciences Center has developed an administrative protocol for handling suspected outbreaks (Table 23). The Hospital Epidemiologist (or his or her designate) has primary responsibility to direct and coordinate the investigation and to communicate decisions on investigative needs and control measures. The protocol further explicitly defines those persons and departments that must be kept continuously apprised, and provides guidelines for responding to inquiries from patients and their families and the press.

Whether it is the hospital epidemiologist, the nurse epidemiologist, chairman of the infection control committee, chief of the medical staff, or some other respected individual of authority in the hospital with a sound knowledge of applied epidemiology, every hospital should designate *one* person, working closely with the infection control committee, to be in charge of the investigation. It should also draw up contingency plans and administrative policies for dealing with the potentially explosive issues that can arise with an epidemic of nosocomial bacteremia.

Retrieve Putative Epidemic Isolates

One of the first and most important steps to take when any nosocomial outbreak is suspected is to immediately retrieve all available isolates of the putative epidemic pathogens from the laboratory for further testing. The need to move rapidly becomes apparent when it is realized that most hospital laboratories discard cultures as soon as the isolates have been fully characterized. A policy of routinely saving blood isolates, operative in most teaching hospitals, can obviate the frustrating problem of finding that few of the isolates from presumptive cases are yet available.

As noted previously, laboratory personnel should be trained to routinely save clinical isolates of unusual organisms or species that are being encountered in increased numbers, and to immediately inform infection control personnel of the trend and of the availability of the isolates.

If the epidemic organism is a common nosocomial species, such as *S. aureus,* it may be difficult to determine unequivocally that an outbreak is due to a common source, even if there is only a single epidemic species, unless the isolates can be subtyped. If the hospital microbiology department is not equipped to do the required subtyping,

Table 23

ADMINISTRATIVE PROTOCOL FOR INVESTIGATION OF A POSSIBLE EPIDEMIC OF NOSOCOMIAL INFECTIONS[a]

1. The Infection Control Committee shall have ultimate responsibility for investigating epidemics and developing policy aimed at preventing and controlling nosocomial infections in University Hospitals. If an epidemic is suspected, the person designated by the committee to direct the investigation will be the hospital epidemiologist or his/her designate in his/her absence.

2. It will be immediately determined by the hospital epidemiologist (or his/her designate) whether the situation is a probable epidemic that poses a threat to the health of other patients and employees and warrants immediate investigation. The epidemiologist may elect to call an emergency meeting of the entire Infection Control Committee; in most instances, to expedite the investigation, the decision will be made based on one or more meetings of the Executive Committee of the Infection Control Committee (the hospital epidemiologist, the nurse epidemiologists, and the infection control microbiologists), with the director of the Microbiology Laboratory and the representative from Administration of the Infection Control Committee also participating. If the epidemic appears to be large or decisions must be made that have far-reaching implications, an emergency meeting of the entire committee will always be called.

3. Which disciplines and individuals need to be included in immediate planning and action will be determined at the outset; these may include any or all of the following:

   a. All Infection Control Committee members.
   b. Attending staff and house officers caring for the involved patients.
   c. The head nurse of the patient care unit.
   d. Nursing office supervisor.
   e. Employee health director and nurses.
   f. University Hospitals Microbiology Laboratory personnel and possibly State Laboratory of Hygiene personnel.
   g. Student health personnel.
   h. Pharmacy personnel.
   i. Hospital administration.

4. The epidemiologist (or his/her designate) shall call an immediate meeting of such individuals and disciplines in order to:

   a. Clarify the nature and extent of the potential problem.
   b. Discuss proposed investigative steps.
   c. Determine exact criteria for selection of patients and personnel for possible epidemiologic studies.
   d. Determine and assign exact responsibility of each department; determine who will collect and record which data.
   e. Anticipate questions that may arise and develop consistent answers to those questions; in general, certain key individuals will be designated as resource people who will be available to answer queries and keep all personnel informed.

5. Any major decisions involving large numbers of patients or personnel or considerable expense, such as closing a unit to admissions, will be made in conjunction with all investigating personnel, attending staff, and Administration.

   a. If prophylactic or therapeutic medications are required, physicians prescribing the drug should be briefed on potential side effects and therapeutic alternatives if allergies or other contraindications (e.g., pregnancy) to the first-line drug exist. In general, all immunoprophylaxis or medications for employees will be administered through the Employee Health Clinic, at no expense to the employee.
   b. Employees should be informed of the rationale for chemoprophylaxis or immunoprophylaxis and if it is given, all potential side effects.

6. Patient care personnel in general will not be expected to assist with data collection, culturing, or notification of employees. In emergency situations they may reasonably be requested to culture patients or provide a list of involved employees and their phone numbers.

7. The Personnel Office will be appraised in writing of all potentially exposed personnel to avoid any problems with workmen's compensation or hazardous employment.

8. Overreaction or even panic on the part of employees, patients, or families should be anticipated and dealt with by fully informed personnel.

Table 23 (continued)
ADMINISTRATIVE PROTOCOL FOR INVESTIGATION OF A POSSIBLE
EPIDEMIC OF NOSOCOMIAL INFECTIONS[a]

9. Frequent interdisciplinary meetings will be held to review new developments and inform involved personnel of the progress of the investigation and to answer questions.
10. All information released to news media will be cleared with the hospital epidemiologist (or his/her des-
    ignate) and hospital administration.
11. The State Department of Health will always be immediately apprised of the epidemic if it involves a
    reportable disease.
12. At the conclusion of the epidemiologic investigation, after analysis of all data and when the situation is
    fully clarified, a formal written report will be disseminated to the involved departments. Occasionally it
    may be appropriate to distribute interim reports during the investigation, if it is prolonged.

After the investigation is completed, all aspects of the investigation will be critically reviewed by the committee to identify problems which can be averted in the future.

[a]   Policy statement of Infection Control Committee, the Hospital Board, and the Administration, Univer-
     sity of Wisconsin Hospitals, Madison, Wis., 1978 (Authors: Maki, D. G. and McCormick, R. D.).

Table 24
AVAILABLE SYSTEMS FOR SUBTYPING NOSOCOMIAL BACTERIAL
PATHOGENS BESIDES BIOTYPING AND ANTIBIOTIC SUSCEPTIBILITY
PATTERNS (ANTIBIOGRAM)

Microorganism	Subtyping systems
Hemolytic streptococci	(group serologically by Lancefield system; precipitin test)
Group A	*serotyping*[a] (M- and T-type; agglutination)
Group B	*serotyping* (precipitin)
Staphylococcus aureus	*phage typing*, serotyping, *plasmid characterization* by gel electrophoresis
S. epidermidis	*phage typing*, serotyping
Acinetobacter	*serotyping*, bacteriocin typing
Escherichia coli	*serotyping*, bacteriocin (colicin) and phage typing
Flavobacterium spp.	*serotyping* (agglutination)
Klebsiella spp.	*serotyping* (Quellung reaction)
Proteus spp.	*serotyping*, Dienes typing, bacteriocin and phage typing, gas-liquid chromatography
Pseudomonas aeruginosa	*serotyping* (agglutination), *bacteriocin* (pyocin) *typing*, phage typing
Salmonella spp.	*serotyping* (Spicer-Edwards agglutination), phage typing
Serratia marcescens	*serotyping* (agglutination), bacteriocin and phage typing
Shigella spp.	*serotyping*, bacteriocin and phage typing

[a]   Best developed and most widely used systems in italics.

Modified from Bartlett, R. C., Bennett, J. V., Weinstein, R. A., and Mallison, G. F., *Hospital Infections*,
Bennett, J. V. and Brachman, P. S., Eds., Little, Brown, Boston, 1979, 153.

relevant isolates, both from cases and from microbiologic studies such as environmental culture surveys, should be sent to a reference laboratory, usually the state department of health or the CDC, for confirmation of identity and subtyping. Available
methods for subtyping the most common bacterial pathogens are shown in Table 24.
  Even when a reliable subtyping system, such as serologic typing, is unavailable, the
pattern of reactions to large panels of biochemical tests (biotype) and antimicrobial
susceptibilities (antibiogram) can be used to presumptively characterize an epidemic
strain.[4,146,147] For instance, in the 1970 to 1971 nationwide epidemic due to one com-

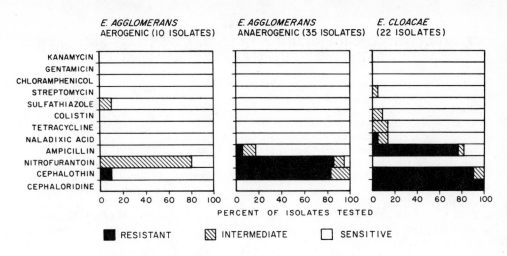

FIGURE 22.   Kirby-Bauer antimicrobial susceptibility patterns of 67 blood isolates from cases of epidemic septicemia due to intrinsic contamination of one manufacturer's infusion products, 1970 to 1971. Note sensitivities of epidemic strains to most antibiotics but resistance of anaerogenic *E. agglomerans* isolates to nitrofurantoin and unusual dissociated susceptibilities to two cephalosporin cogeners. (From Maki, D. G., Rhame, F. S., Mackel, D. G., and Bennett, J. V., *Am. J. Med.*, 60, 471, 1976. With permission.)

pany's intrinsically contaminated intravenous products,[4] the distinctive susceptibility patterns of the epidemic isolates were valuable adjunctive means of identification (Figure 22): *E. cloacae* strains tended to be more susceptible than the usual hospital isolates of this species; anaerogenic isolates of *E. agglomerans* were only intermediately sensitive or more often resistant to nitrofuran and to cephalothin, yet inexplicably were susceptible to cephaloridine.[4]

Preliminary Evaluations

When presented with knowledge of a cluster of nosocomial bacteremias that may denote an epidemic, the epidemiologist or person designated to head a possible investigation must very early make a number of critical decisions. After characterizing the putative epidemic cases, based on the data available, the following questions must be quickly answered: Do the infections represent a true epidemic or not? If so, what provisional control measures need to be instituted immediately? Which direction will the investigation take and what hospital resources and possibly other sources of assistance need to be mobilized? Should extramural consultation or even direct assistance be sought?

Identify and Characterize Individual Cases

Obviously an epidemic of nosocomial bacteremia cannot be characterized unless individual cases are first defined. The clinical features of bacteremia are discussed in detail in the section, "Clinical Syndromes" (cf., Table 1).

In most instances, criteria for defining epidemic cases will be primarily microbiologic: bacteremias caused by the same species or, if characterized sufficiently, by strains of the same biotype with the same or a very similar antibiogram. It is also desirable to require microbiologic concordance in cultures of the local anatomic site of infection giving rise to the bacteremia. In the case of infusion-associated bacteremias, however, cultures from presumptively culpable infusions are usually not available, and in an epidemic setting — i.e., a significant increase in bacteremias, all occurring in association with infusion therapy and caused by one or several distinctive

Table 25
CRITERIA FOR CONSIDERATION AS A CASE OF INFUSION-ASSOCIATED BACTEREMIA IN AN EPIDEMIC SETTING

1. Blood cultures positive for one or more of the epidemic organisms.
2. Cultures of local infections that developed before the onset of septicemia, if obtained, did not yield the bloodstream pathogen.
3. Clinical signs of nosocomial bloodstream infection.
4. Infusion therapy in use at the onset of septicemia.
5. Infusion judged to have been a possible cause of the septicemia.

Adapted from Maki, D. G., Rhame, F. S., Mackel, D. C., and Bennett, J. V., *Am. J. Med.,* 60, 71, 1976.

species — it is acceptable epidemiologically to tabulate individual cases of infusion-associated septicemia as epidemic cases based solely on epidemiologic and clinical criteria (Table 25).

Conversely, because blood culture data are often the first indication of a possible outbreak (e.g., a cluster of patients with blood cultures positive for *P. cepacia)*, the importance of assuring that positive blood cultures represent clinically significant infection (i.e., septicemia) cannot be emphasized too strongly. In other words, before undertaking an in-depth investigation, it must be quickly established that the putative outbreak represents true infection of patients and not laboratory artifact. As discussed, an increasing number of outbreaks of pseudobacteremia have recently been reported (Table 13): clusters of patients with blood cultures positive for one species that were found not to represent bacteremic infections, but rather, contamination introduced during drawing or laboratory processing. This phenomenon must always be suspected when the "epidemic" bacteremias are primary — the epidemic pathogen is not cultured from a clinically plausible site of infection — and, obviously, when affected patients do not consistently show signs of bacteremic infection.

On the other hand, if the clinical picture is that of true sepsis but conventional blood cultures are negative, the possibility of infection caused by more fastidious microorganisms (that might require special media or methods of processing to recover in culture) or of nonviable contaminants (such as endotoxin)* should be entertained.

After developing a working criteria for an epidemic case, the investigator should organize each case by time, place, and person. Particular attention should be paid to the possible origin of the bacteremia. The date and, if identifiable, time of onset, the patient's exact locations in the hospital prior to and up to the onset of bacteremia, and details of underlying medical conditions and other host factors predisposing to infection should be recorded. Exposure to various diagnostic and therapeutic factors should also be carefully tabulated.

These data for each case are best recorded on a horizontal line listing; after data have been entered for all (or a subgroup) of the cases, the group can be quickly scanned for commonality with respect to host conditions or exposures to environmental or therapeutic factors that may be significant epidemiologically; this preliminary review may point up areas for immediate further study microbiologically. For instance, all cases may have received a certain drug by intravenous injection, possibly a drug normally used infrequently; or all of the cases may have been operated on by one surgeon.

Ascertain if the Infections Represent an Epidemic
Many suspected outbreaks are simply fluctuations in the endemic rate of infection

---

* See the section entitled "Epidemic Pyrogenic Reactions".

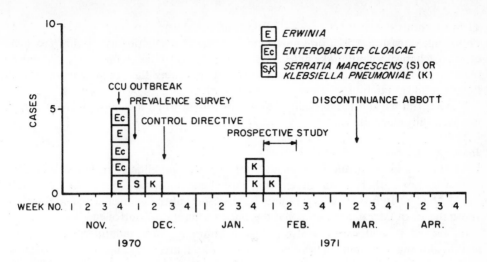

FIGURE 23.   Epidemic curve for infusion-related septicemias occurring in one hospital during nationwide outbreak due to one manufacturer's intrinsically contaminated products, 1970 to 1971. Provisional control measure in mid-December, routinely replacing all I.V. delivery systems (bottles and administration sets) every 24 hr, seemed relatively effective for nearly 3 months despite continued use of the company's parenteral products, pending the results of epidemiologic investigations. When the intrinsic nature of contamination was identified, use of the company's products was discontinued. (From Maki, D. G., Mandell, G. L., Sher, N., and Mackel, D. G., unpublished data.)

and are not actual epidemics. For example, with infections that are normally encountered only two or three times a month on the average, an epidemic may seem likely if three cases occur within one week, especially on a single patient care unit. The rate of bacteremia with the epidemic species should be calculated, not only for the hospital as a whole, but also for the area(s) experiencing epidemic cases, i.e., the population at risk. Careful comparison with base-line rates, which can be done quickly if the hospital has an ongoing surveillance program, makes it possible to determine promptly if the increase or the cluster of infections represents a genuine epidemic and calls, therefore, for immediate epidemiologic investigation. If surveillance data are unavailable, however, it may be necessary to do a retrospective chart survey to ascertain the base-line (endemic) rate of infection. Even if a hospital does not have a formal surveillance program for all nosocomial infections, the base-line rate of nosocomial bacteremia over several years with any species can usually be ascertained relatively quickly by reviewing the laboratory's blood culture records, kept in a separate log in most hospital laboratories. In any event, it usually is possible to ascertain within 24 hr or less whether the apparent increased number of bacteremias represents a bona fide epidemic.

A plot of the number of bacteremias caused by the epidemic species by date of onset (the "epidemic curve", Figure 23) can help to discern a common-source exposure as opposed to intermittent exposures with cross-infection producing secondary cases.

Provisional Control Measures

Preliminary control measures, based on the known ecology and epidemiology of the epidemic pathogen (in a *S. aureus* outbreak, screening personnel for suppurative infection, and initiating the use of hexachlorophene for handwashing) or based on the results of preliminary epidemiologic study of the cases, are usually implemented early, long before the investigation is completed. In the 1970 to 1971 nationwide epidemic caused by one parenteral manufacturer's contaminated products,[4] before the source of contamination was identified as intrinsic but after contaminated fluid was identified as responsible for the infections, it was recommended that hospitals routinely change all intravenous delivery systems — bottles and administration sets — every 24 hr.[824] This simple measure, based on knowledge that organisms getting into fluid (regardless of the mechanism) would take at least 24 hr to multiply to dangerous levels, did indeed reduce epidemic septicemias in several hospitals adopting the policy (Figure 23), although it understandably did not totally prevent them.

More definitive control measures may be instituted when the cause of the outbreak has been fully elucidated.

Intensify Surveillance

As soon as an epidemic is suspected, the existent surveillance program should be intensified (or if there is not an existing surveillance program, one should be established) to identify future cases that may occur, especially subclinical cases, and to provide a means of later determining that the epidemic has been controlled.

Intensified surveillance may also include encouraging or mandating more frequent blood culturing, especially in areas of the hospital that are experiencing epidemic cases. If the tentative hypothesis based on the preliminary case review suggests that the epidemic bacteremias seem to be associated with infection at one site (such as the urinary tract) or exposure to some single factor (such as infusion therapy), routinely culturing urine (or in-use infusions), as well as the blood of patients with fever, may also be considered.

Review General Infection Control Policies

This step also is an early one instituted before undertaking a full-scale epidemiologic investigation. It is an immediate attempt to identify, while the trail is fresh, recent events or changes in medical or nursing procedures that may be responsible for the outbreak. A quick but careful review of all aspects of infusion therapy in the hospital may bring to light recent changes in aseptic practices or a newly introduced product that the next steps in the investigation will show to underlie the outbreak: For instance, are new or different routines in intravenous therapy, either in the pharmacy or on patient-care units, being followed? Are new admixtures or cannulas or different skin disinfectants being used? Are there new personnel on patient-care units where epidemic cases have occurred? Has there been an increased incidence of phlebitis or of positive cannula cultures? Has the pharmacy noted an increase in the frequency of positive quality-control cultures of parenteral admixtures?

Information derived from this early review may identify fruitful areas for immediate microbiologic study before more comprehensive clinical-epidemiologic investigations begin.

Determine Need for Assistance

Once it is clear that a hospital is experiencing (or has experienced) an epidemic of nosocomial bacteremias, contact with local and national health authorities, such as the Hospital Infections Section of the CDC (telephone 404-329-3311) — and if a commercial product may be responsible, the manufacturer — can be helpful. Are these authorities or the manufacturer aware of an ongoing problem, possibly of national scope? Are other hospitals experiencing similar unexplained infections?

Although valuable information and sometimes even epidemiologic assistance may accrue to an individual hospital from early contacts with these sources, the contact conversely furnishes the sources with data that may be of national importance. In the 1970 to 1971 U. S. outbreak, the first indication to the CDC that there might be a problem of national scope derived from inquiries and voluntary reporting by numerous individual hospitals.[4,824]

At this time, it should be determined whether on-site consultation and epidemiologic assistance might be advisable. If preliminary data indicate the epidemic is large or very complex, or if the infections are unduly severe, producing substantial mortality, and always, if intrinsic contamination of a commercial product is suspected, direct assistance from state or federal health authorities should be sought.

Epidemiologic Investigations
Clinical-Epidemiologic Studies

When an epidemic occurs, there is often a strong temptation to immediately begin extensive culturing of the inanimate environment and even of medical personnel. Although early culture surveys based on the probable ecology and epidemiology of the epidemic organisms (Table 9) are often appropriate, it is equally important — in many respects more important — to carry out careful clinical-epidemiologic analyses: (1) The population at greatest risk should be clearly defined by determining the rates of epidemic infection among different populations in the hospital and on the various patient care units. (2) In general, a careful retrospective case-control study should be carried out. The records of epidemic cases and a carefully selected control group should be exhaustively reviewed. Controls are usually randomly selected patients on the same patient-care unit as epidemic cases but who did not develop bacteremia with the epidemic pathogen or, alternatively, hospitalized patients who also had a bacteremia on the same day as an epidemic case but with a different organism. By comparing epidemic cases and control patients who had similar exposures as cases but did not develop bacteremia, an association between epidemic cases and a possible causal factor or factors can often be identified.

In general, the number of control patients chosen should be at least as many as the number of epidemic cases, or if the number of cases is less than 20, there should be at least 20 controls, in order to have large enough numbers for meaningful analysis. The goal is to show that epidemic cases were exposed to one or more factors in a very high frequency (or ideally uniformly), whereas control patients were infrequently exposed. Controls should always be selected randomly.

Besides demographic data, underlying medical conditions, and exact hospital location, information collected and compared on both epidemic cases and controls might include: exposures to antiseptics and invasive devices of all types, to all forms of infusion therapy, to various admixtures and medications given intravenously; all diagnostic and therapeutic procedures performed; diet and oral medications; medical personnel who had direct contact with the patient; inflammation (phlebitis) at infusion sites; the presence of fever and other clinical signs or symptoms suggesting infection; and the results of all cultures done during hospitalization.

Exposure of all (or most) epidemic cases to one (or more) factors (e.g., the same admixture or intravenous drug), combined with little or no exposure of control cases to the factor(s), constitutes strong presumptive evidence implicating that factor or factors in the causation of the outbreak.

Case-control analysis is almost mandatory with epidemic nosocomial bacteremias unless the source is patently obvious at the outset, because the number of risk factors, potential sources of the epidemic pathogen, and portals for its entry is so vast that only by carrying out such a study are the responsible factors likely to be delineated.

Example 1 — Between August 1970 and February 1971, seven patients with hematologic malignancy hospitalized in widely separated areas of the clinical center of the National Institutes of Health developed nosocomial *cholerae-suis* septicemia.[414] All were primary bacteremias; no local anatomic sites in these patients yielded *S. cholerae-suis* on culture. The source of these infections eluded exhaustive clinical studies and

Table 26

**EXPOSURES OF PATIENTS WITH
SALMONELLA CHOLERAE-SUIS
SEPTICEMIA AND CONTROL PATIENTS
TO SELECTED THERAPEUTIC FACTORS**

No. (%) of patients
exposed

Factor	Septicemia patients (n = 5)	Control patients (n = 22)	P-value
I.V. therapy	5 (100)	22 (100)	NS
Allopurinol	4 (80)	12 (55)	NS
Platelet transfusions	4 (80)	8 (36)	0.01
Red cell transfusions	3 (60)	9 (41)	NS
Narcotic	2 (40)	8 (36)	NS
Prednisone	2 (40)	15 (68)	NS

Adapted from Rhame, F. S., Root, R. K., MacLowry, M. D., Dadisman, T. A., and Bennett, J. V., *Ann. Intern. Med.*, 78, 633, 1973.

extensive culture surveys of medications, blood products, medical personnel, and patients, but was strongly suspected after the first five cases, based on an outstanding investigation by Rhame and co-workers.[414] Carrying out a meticulous and extremely comprehensive case-control analysis of all exposures of the first five cases and a randomly selected group of 22 control patients who had been hospitalized on the same services as the five cases (which included exposures to 43 different medications and to numerous diagnostic tests and therapeutic measures), a single factor stood out: platelet transfusions (Table 26). Four (80%) of the first cases had received platelet transfusion in the week prior to the first positive blood culture, whereas only 8 (36%) of the 22 control patients had received platelets in the same period. Further review showed that all five cases had received platelets prior to the onset of sepsis (p < 0.001). A program of routinely culturing an aliquot of every platelet pool given in the National Institutes of Health was established, but all cultures continued to be negative for *S. cholerae-suis*.

After a sixth and seventh case occurred, the epidemiologic lead that alone pointed toward platelet transfusions as being somehow associated with epidemic cases was pursued further. Of the 116 professional donors who had given platelets to one or more of the seven cases, it was found that a single individual had donated to all seven cases (p<0.01). Previous surveillance cultures of his blood products had been negative. Although the donor was asymptomatic, he was immediately excluded from further donations. Six 130-m*l* units of his platelet-rich plasma, obtained in three plasmaphereses over 10 days, were cultured by dividing the entire volume of each unit among 10 separate culture tubes; 4 tubes of the 60 cultured were positive for *S. cholerae-suis*. It was subsequently shown that the donor had an asymptomatic focus of tibial osteomyelitis and presumably was experiencing intermittent, very low-level, asymptomatic bacteremia.

Epidemiologic data alone — Specifically a careful case-control analysis — not the extensive earlier culture studies, identified the cause of this extraordinary outbreak. The epidemic was controlled without the latter positive microbiologic data, which only confirmed the epidemiologic hypothesis.

Table 27

COMPARISON OF EPIDEMIOLOGIC FACTORS: PATIENTS WITH EPIDEMIC BACTERIMIC INFECTION AND UNINFECTED CONTROL PATIENTS IN TWO HOSPITALS

Factor	Patients with Epidemic Infection (n = 28)	Control[a] Subjects (n = 59)
Mean duration:		
Intravenous cannula in place	49 hr	33 hr
Intravenous bottle hung[b]	30 hr	14 hr
Continuous infusion[b]	4.5 days	2.0 days
Percentage with:		
Plastic catheter	75	69
Infusion phlebitis[b]	36	10
Additives to intravenous bottle[b]	89	64
Injections into intravenous line	57	58
Received dextrose-containing solutions	96	94
Underlying serious illness	21	20

[a]   Patients receiving I.V. therapy on the same nursing units as cases but who did not develop septicemia.
[b]   Differences statistically significant, $p < 0.05$.

Adapted from Maki, D. G., Rhame, F. S., Mackel, D. C., and Bennett, J. V., *Am. J. Med.*, 60, 71, 1976.

Example 2 — In the nationwide outbreak in 1970 to 1971 traced to the intrinsically contaminated infusion products of one manufacturer,[4] it was apparent very early in the investigation that *E. cloacae* and *E. agglomerans* septicemias in the involved hospitals were unequivocally infusion-related: simple case-control analyses in several carefully studied hospitals showed that every patient with epidemic *E. cloacae* or *E. agglomerans* septicemia was receiving infusion products of the involved manufacturer at the onset of septicemia and, conversely, no cases of sepsis with the epidemic strains were detected among patients who had not received intravenous fluid therapy. Moreover, in a number of instances, in-use cultures of fluid had been positive for the same (epidemic) species recovered simultaneously from blood cultures; but the source of contamination — even whether it was extrinsic or intrinsic — was not immediately apparent. Early culture surveys of fluid from several hundred freshly opened bottles had been nonrevealing.

Epidemiologic studies within two hospitals which carefully compared exposures of epidemic cases with those of uninfected control patients who had also received intravenous therapy on the same patient-care units as cases delineated several key factors associated with a greater risk of infection (Table 27). The frequency and mean duration of plastic catheter use were comparable in epidemic cases and control subjects; however, the incidence of phlebitis was significantly greater in epidemic cases. Most importantly, the mean length of time the intravenous fluid bottle had been hanging and the mean number of hours the patient had received continous infusion therapy were both considerably greater in epidemic cases ($p < 0.05$). "Keep-open" infusions were also used more frequently in epidemic cases. Although a significantly higher proportion of epidemic cases than control subjects received fluid additives, no single medication was common to all or even a majority of cases. It was clear that prolonged exposure to the involved company's parenteral products, especially through one delivery system, was a major risk factor.

About this time it was learned that the company had developed a new closure for fluid bottles that they had introduced into use the preceding summer, shortly before infections began to appear (Figure 15). Further studies showed that the frequency of epidemic septicemias in individual hospitals closely paralleled the receipt and use of products with the new closures (Figure 19). Cultures of the new closures (Figure 20) subsequently showed frequent contamination by the epidemic strains.

The results of the investigations in two hospitals (Table 27) then became even more clear: the common practice of recapping and shaking a bottle after introducing additives was probably more of a factor than the risk of extrinsic contamination. In laboratory studies,[826] this manipulation produced frequent transfer of organisms from closures to fluid. Patients with epidemic infection had greater mean durations of infusion for intravenous bottles and for continuous use of administration sets than control subjects; in vitro studies showed that small inocula of the epidemic organisms that may have been in fluid or introduced into fluid by uncapping the bottle required 12 to 24 hr to attain concentrations of 100 organisms per milliliter or higher.[411]

It must be emphasized that clinical-epidemiologic studies implicated the company's products and eventually pointed toward the new closures. Microbiologic confirmation of contaminated closures was the final step in a comprehensive epidemiologic investigation.

Intrinsic contamination in this outbreak is suggested epidemiologically even more strongly by a subsequent simple but compelling case-control analysis done on a macroscopic scale[831] (cases: hospitals using the involved company's products; controls: hospitals using other manufacturers' products). Analyzing all primary nosocomial septicemias occurring in hospitals participating in the CDC's National Nosocomial Infection Surveillance Study (Figure 21), only hospitals using the involved manufacturer's products (A) experienced a marked increase in septicemias caused by *Enterobacter*, particularly *E. agglomerans (Erwinia)*, during the epidemic period.

Microbiologic Studies

Armed with specific epidemiologic information that may point toward one (or at most several) product(s) or procedure(s), more specific microbiologic studies of the inanimate environment — or even of medical personnel — can then be undertaken. Empiric wide-scale environmental culturing is expensive and often fruitless; even if the epidemic strain is recovered, the findings may be difficult to interpret. When environmental sampling is directed and complemented by the results of clinical-epidemiologic investigations, however, the source of the outbreak can usually be identified with certainty.

In regard to infusion therapy, it may be elected to culture fluid (and possibly cannulas) from all intravenous systems in use in the hospital at one point in time (a "culture-prevalence survey") to identify unsuspected contamination by the epidemic strains. It may be elected to culture the fluid or cannulas from infusions of patients with fever. It may even be elected to culture unused products which are suspected as contaminated based on the results of epidemiologic studies or the physical appearance of the product.

In general, however, large-scale culturing of unused commercial products in the hospital is not recommended. This is probably better done in state and federal laboratories equipped to handle large volumes of fluids using total-volume sampling techniques under highly controlled conditions of environmental sterility.

Selective environmental culturing should ideally be based on the results of epidemiologic investigations which point to one or more of the items discussed earlier or begin with what is known regarding the usual ecology and epidemioloy of the epidemic organisms (Table 9); e.g., *S. aureus* infections of one phage-type or epidemic Group A streptococcal infection — seeking to identify a medical person who is a nasal, anal, or vaginal carrier of the epidemic strain; with *P. cepacia* septicemias, culturing in-use parenteral fluids, medications, disinfectants, or arterial pressure-monitoring systems.

Definitive Control Measures

With epidemiologic information and possibly even microbiologic data pointing towards a specific reservoir of the epidemic pathogen and a mode or modes of transmission to patients, more specific control measures can then be implemented. These may consist simply of reemphasis or refinement of the earlier control measures that were based on suspected or hypothesized epidemiologic mechanisms. They may be as simple as removing the implicated product from use (Figures 18, 19, and 23). In any event, continued surveillance should be maintained for at least 3 to 6 months to confirm complete control of the epidemic.

If epidemiologic or microbiologic studies suggest or indicate intrinsic contamination of a commercial product, the local and state health authorities, the Food and Drug Administration, the CDC, and the manufacturer should always be immediately informed. Remaining products should always be quarantined and retained for evaluation by these agencies.

Report the Findings

The hospital infection control committee's responsibility does not end with control of the outbreak, but includes the task of preparing and disseminating a final report that summarizes the results of the investigation, with conclusions, and spells out the lessons that have been learned and steps being taken to prevent a similar epidemic from occurring in the future. This report should be distributed to all members of the hospital staff, supervisory personnel, and all involved departments, and, ideally, to other local hospitals and to public health authorities.

PREVENTION OF NOSOCOMIAL BACTEREMIA

Whereas measures to prevent nosocomial bacteremia using novel techniques of immune enhancement, such as vaccines directed against shared antigens of the enteric Gram-negative bacilli or against the prevalent serogroups of *P. aeruginosa*, have attracted great interest,[62, 887-890] immediate benefits would derive from achieving wider and more consistent application of existent knowledge of infection control. Many nosocomial bacteremias occurring endemically do not appear to be preventable with the current state of knowledge,[225,234] especially those occurring in immunologically severely compromised patients; however, greater attention to high-priority aseptic practices could materially reduce the incidence of local nosocomial infection and, in the process, secondary bacteremia. More rapid diagnosis and prompter and more effective treatment of local infections with antimicrobial therapy and, when necessary, surgically, could also prevent many secondary bacteremias that might otherwise develop. However, the potential for prevention would seem greatest with epidemic bacteremias, the majority of which are related to exposure to invasive devices, to heavy levels of environmental contaminants (often a common source), or both.

Infection control guidelines have been published dealing with most of the high-risk areas, devices, or procedures in the hospital where lapses in aseptic practices or contamination often results in bacteremia: isolation procedures;[891,892] handwashing;[893-894] cutaneous antisepsis;[103,716,893] disinfection and sterilization;[872,895] urethral catheters;[896,897] use of evacuated blood-collection tubes;[139] infusion therapy, including hyperalimentation,[148,715-717,816-821,898] hemodynamic arterial pressure monitoring systems,[124,568,569,781,782] and intra-arterial cancer chemotherapy;[336] respiratory therapy;[150-152,899-904] surgery;[905-907] the newborn nursery;[908-910] hemodialysis;[149,834,853] environmental microbiologic surveillance;[895,911] quality control in the laboratory;[147,713,714] prophylaxis for endocarditis with invasive procedures;[284] and utilization of antibiotics.[912-914]

The value and necessity of continuous surveillance of all nosocomial infections as an infection control measure remain unclear at the present time in the current national atmosphere of intense concern with containment of health-care costs.[931,932] However, ongoing surveillance of nosocomial bacteremias, which is considerably simpler and much less expensive than surveillance of all nosocomial infections,[298] would seem likely to be more cost-effective. Besides providing an accurate reflection of a hospital's experience with nosocomial infection in general, it makes available immediately the baseline data necessary to detect significant increases in rates of bacteremia caused by individual pathogens or clusters that may denote an epidemic.

The author[235] believes that a national commitment in the following areas could substantially reduce the incidence of endemic nosocomial bacteremia and reverse the upward trend in hospital epidemics of the past decade:

1.   Studies are needed to better define the epidemiology of endemic nosocomial infections, especially those caused by Gram-negative bacilli, to develop more effective control measures and to derive more rational guidelines for decontamination and microbiologic surveillance of the hospital environment. The significance of microorganisms carried on the hands of medical personnel and of nosocomial enteric colonization should be determined.

    Although many studies show that any colonization by hospital Gram-negative bacilli is associated with a high risk of subsequent infection,[228,386,389,396,398,401,402] these studies have not consistently identified the hospital sources of colonizing pathogens. There should be an intensive effort to identify these sources.

2.   Major resources have been committed to study the efficacy of complex isolation systems for patients with acute leukemia,[915-918] with aplastic anemia, and who have undergone bone marrow transplantation;[231,232] in these patients, extreme degrees of environmental decontamination combined with floral suppression reduce the frequency of infection. However, except for limited studies in burn patients,[919-921] few studies have examined the efficacy of these measures in preventing infection in the vast population of susceptible patients without fatal underlying diseases — neonates, trauma patients, and others confined to intensive care units. A major commitment should be made to evaluate critically the efficacy of various forms of protective isolation of these patients who usually have limited periods of susceptibility.

3.   Improvements in the design of devices and development of new techniques to enhance their safety are of highest priority.

4.   Many physicians are unaware of basic precepts of infection control, and in most hospitals nurses are far better informed and are the most effective force for assuring compliance with infection-control practices. In a survey of recent graduates of 47 American medical schools, the author found only 15 schools (or 33%) that offered lectures to medical students on infection control, and only five (10%) that provided any formal clinical training in aseptic technique. Innovative programs to enhance awareness of nosocomial disease and to communicate knowl-

edge of infection control — especially with regard to the use of devices and antibiotics — are greatly needed.

> When old age shall this generation waste,
> Thou shalt remain, in midst of other woe
> Than ours, a friend to man, to whom thou sayst,
> "Beauty is truth, truth beauty," — that is all
> Ye know on earth and all ye need to know.

Ode on a Grecian Urn
John Keats

ACKNOWLEDGMENTS

I am deeply appreciative to my family for their forbearance and support during the period of writing this review, to my wife Gail, Mrs. Cheryl Beckett, Ms. Donna Davis, and Ms. Patricia Schaul for excellent secretarial support, and to Mr. Scott Wesley for generous assistance in carrying out computer literature searches. I also wish to acknowledge my co-workers in those collaborative investigations cited.

Portions of the sections "Infusion-Related Sepsis" and "Approach to an Epidemic" are excerpted, with modification, from three recent monographs[148,817,819] I contributed to *Modern IV Practices* (1979), by permission of Medical Directions Inc., Chicago, Ill. Portions of the section "Pseudobacteremia" are excerpted in part from an editorial written for the *Archives of Internal Medicine*,[153] by permission of the American Medical Association.

REFERENCES

1. Center for Disease Control, Definitions used by the *National Nosocomial Infections Study, Quarterly Report*, Second Quarter 1972, 1973, 26.
2. Brachman, P. S., Introduction, in *Hospital Infections,* Bennett, J. V. and Brachman, P.S., Eds., Little, Brown, Boston, 1979, 3.
3. McGowan, J. E., Jr., Barnes, M. W., and Finland, M., Bacteremia at Boston City Hospital: occurrence and mortality during 12 selected years (1935-1972), with special reference to hospital-acquired cases, *J. Infect. Dis.,* 132, 3, 1975.
4. Maki, D. G., Rhame, F. S., Mackel, D. C., and Bennett, J. V., Nationwide epidemic of septicemia caused by contaminated intravenous products. I. Epidemiologic and clinical features, *Am. J. Med.,* 60, 471, 1976.
5. Maki, D. G., Rhame, F. S., Mackel, D. C., and Bennett, J. V., A national epidemic of septicemias consequent to contaminated infusion fluid, Abstract of the Annual Meeting of the American Society for Microbiology, Minneapolis, May 1971.
6. McCabe, W. R. and Jackson, G. G., Gram-negative bacteremia. I. Etiology and Ecology. II. Clinical, laboratory, and therapeutic observations, *Arch. Intern. Med.,* 110, 83, 1962.
7. Hodgin, U. G. and Sanford, J. P., Gram-negative rod bacteremia: an analysis of 100 patients, *Am. J. Med.,* 39, 952, 1965.
8. DuPont, H. L. and Spink, W. W., Infections due to gram-negative organisms: an analysis of 860 patients with bacteremia at the University of Minnesota Medical Center, 1958-1966, *Medicine,* 48, 307, 1969.
9. Bryant, R. F., Hood, A. F., Hood, C. E., and Koenig, M. G., Factors affecting mortality of gram-negative rod bacteremia, *Arch. Intern. Med.,* 127, 120, 1971.

10. Nishijima, H., Weil, M. H., Shubin, H., and Cavanilles, J., Hemodynamic and metabolic studies on shock associated with gram-negative bacteremia, *Medicine (Baltimore),* 52, 287, 1973.
11. Winslow, E. J., Loeb, H. S., Rahimtoola, S. H., Kamath, S., and Gunnar, R. M., Hemodynamic studies and results of therapy in 50 patients with bateremic shock, *Am. J. Med.,* 54, 421, 1973.
12. Gunnar, R. M., Lock, H. S., Winslow, E. J., Blain, C., and Robinson, J., Hemodynamic measurements in bacteremia and septic shock in man, *J. Infect. Dis.,* 128, S295, 1973.
13. Weil, M. H. and Nishijima, H., Cardiac output in bacterial shock, *Am. J. Med.,* 64, 920, 1978.
14. Weil, M. H., Shubin, H., and Biddle, M., Shock caused by gram-negative microorganisms: analysis of 169 cases, *Ann. Intern. Med.,* 60, 384, 1964.
15. Freid, M. A. and Vosti, K. L., The importance of underlying disease in patients with gram-negative bacteremia, *Arch. Intern. Med.,* 121, 418, 1968.
16. Scheckler, W. E., Septicemia in a community hospital, 1970-1973, *J.A.M.A.,* 237, 1938, 1977.
17. Singer, C., Kaplan, M. H., and Armstrong, D., Bacteremia and fungemia complicating neoplastic disease: a study of 364 cases, *Am. J. Med.,* 62, 731, 1977.
18. Nolan, C. M. and Beaty, H. N., Staphylococcus aureus bacteremia: current clinical patterns, *Am. J. Med.,* 60, 495, 1976.
19. Teplitz, C., Pathogenesis of *Pseudomonas* vasculitis and septic lesions, *Arch. Pathol.,* 80, 297, 1965.
20. Dorff, G. J., Geimer, N. F., Rosenthal, D. R., and Rytel, M. W., *Pseudomonas* septicemia, *Arch. Intern. Med.,* 128, 591, 1971.
21. Gorbach, S. L. and Bartlett, J. G., Anaerobic infections, *N. Engl. J. Med.,* 290, 1177, 1974.
22. Schimpff, S. C., Wiernik, P. H., and Block, J. B., Rectal abscesses in cancer patients, *Lancet,* 2, 844, 1972.
23. Balandran, L., Rothschild, H., Pugh, N., and Seabury, J., A cutaneous manifestation of systemic candidiasis, *Ann. Intern. Med.,* 78, 400, 1973.
24. Kressel, B., Szewczyk, C., and Tuazon, C. U., Early clinical recognition of disseminated candidiasis by muscle and skin biopsy, *Arch. Intern. Med.,* 138, 429, 1978.
25. Jarowski, C. I., Fialk, M. A., Murray, H. W., Gottlieb, G. J., Coleman, M., Steinberg, C. R., and Silver, R. T., Fever, rash, and muscle tenderness: a distinctive clinical presentation of disseminated candidiasis, *Arch. Intern. Med.,* 138, 544, 1978.
26. Cohen, P. and Gardner, F. H., Thrombocytopemia as a laboratory sign and complication of gram-negative bacteremic infection, *Arch. Intern. Med.,* 117, 113, 1966.
27. Corrigan, J. J., Jr., Ray, W. L., and May, N., Changes in blood coagulation system associated with septicemia, *N. Engl. J. Med.,* 279, 851, 1968.
28. Colman, R. W., Robboy, S. J., and Minna, J. D., Disseminated intravascular coagulation: an approach, *Am. J. Med.,* 52, 679, 1972.
29. Beller, F. K. and Douglas, G. W., Thrombocytopenia indicating gram-negative infection and endotoxemia, *Obstet. Gynecol.,* 41, 521, 1973.
30. Corrigan, J. J., Jr., Thrombocytopenia: a laboratory sign of septicemia in infants and children, *J. Pediatr.,* 85, 219, 1974.
31. Kim, H. S., Suzuki, M., Lie, J. T., and Titus, J. L., Clinically unsuspected disseminated intravascular coagulation (DIC): an autopsy survey, *Am. J. Clin. Pathol.,* 60, 31, 1976.
32. Corrigan, J. J., Jr., Medical progress: heparin therapy in bacterial septicemia, *J. Pediatr.,* 91, 695, 1977.
33. Andriole, V. T., Kravetz, H. M., Roerts, W. C., and Utz, J. P., *Candida* endocarditis: clinical and pathologic studies, *Am. J. Med.,* 32, 251, 1962.
34. Louria, D. B., Stiff, D. P., and Bennett, B., Disseminated moniliasis in the adult, *Medicine (Baltimore),* 41, 307, 1962.
35. Hart, P. D., Russel, E., Jr., and Remington, J. S., The compromised host and infection. III. Deep fungal infection, *J. Infect. Dis.,* 120, 169, 1969.
36. MacMillan, B. G., Law, E. J., and Holder, I. A., Experience with *Candida* infections in the burn patient, *Arch. Surg. (Chicago),* 104, 509, 1972.
37. Seelig, M. S., Speth, C. P., Kozinn, P. J., Taschdjian, C. L., Toni, E. F., and Goldberg, P., Patterns of *Candida* endocarditis following cardiac surgery: importance of early diagnosis and therapy (an analysis of 91 cases), *Prog. Cardiovas. Dis.,* 17, 125, 1974.
38. Myerowitz, R. L., Pazin, G. J., and Allen, C. M., Disseminated candidiasis: changes in incidence, underlying diseases, and pathology, *Am. J. Clin. Pathol.,* 68, 29, 1977.
39. Lehrer, R. I., Stiehm, E. R., Fischer, T. J., Young, L. S., Severe candidal infections: Clinical perspective, immune defense mechanisms, and current concepts of therapy, UCLA Conference, *Ann. Intern. Med.,* 89, 91, 1978.
40. Fishman, L. S., Griffin, J. R., Sapic, F. L., and Hecht, R., Hematogenous candida endophthalmitis: a complication of candidemia, *N. Engl. J. Med.,* 286, 675, 1972.

41. Edwards, J. E., Jr., Foos, R. Y., Montgomerie, J. Z., and Guze, L. B., Ocular manifestations of candida septicemia: review of seventy-six cases of hematogenous candida endophthalmitis, *Medicine (Baltimore)*, 53, 47, 1974.

42. Weinstein, A. J., Johnson, E. H., and Moellering, R. C., Jr., *Candida* endophthalmitis: a complication of candidemia, *Arch. Intern. Med.*, 132, 749, 1973.

43. Montgomerie, J. Z. and Edwards, J. E., Jr., Association of infection due to *Candida albicans* with intravenous hyperalimentation, *J. Infect. Dis.*, 137, 197, 1978.

44. Zieve, P. D., Haghshenass, M., Blanks, M., and Krevans, J. R., Vacuolization of the neutrophil: an aid in the diagnosis of septicemia, *Arch. Intern. Med.*, 118, 356, 1966.

45. Emerson, W. A., Zieve, P. D., and Krevans, J. R., Hematologic changes in septicemia, *Johns Hopkins Med. J.*, 126, 69, 1970.

46. Riedler, G. F., Platelet count, white blood cell differential count, and inorganic phosphate: 3 useful laboratory signs in septicemia, *Schweiz. Med. Wochenschr.*, 102, 497, 1972.

47. Steigbigel, R. T., Johnson, P. K., and Remington, J. S. The nitroblue tetrazolium reduction test versus conventional hematology in the diagnosis of bacterial infection, *New Engl. J. Med.*, 290, 235, 1974.

48. Todd, J. K., Childhood Infections, *Am. J. Dis. Child*, 127, 810, 1974.

49. Zipursky, A., Palko, J., Milner, R., and Akenzua, G. I., The hematology of bacterial infections in premature infants, *Pediatrics*, 57, 839, 1976.

50. Boyle, R. J., Chandler, B. D., Stonestreet, B. X., and Oh, W., Early identification of sepsis in infants with respiratory distress, *Pediatrics*, 62, 744, 1978.

51. Duff, J. H., Groves, A. C., McLean, A. P. H., LaPointe, R., and MacLean, L. D., Defective oxygen consumption in septic shock *Surg. Gynecol. Obstet.*, 1051, 1969.

52. Burke, J. F., Pontoppidan, H., and Welch, C. E., High output respiratory failure: an important cause of death ascribed to peritonitis or ileus, *Ann. Surg.*, 158, 581, 1963.

53. Clowes, G. H. A., Jr., Zuschneid, W., Turner, M., Blackburn, G., Rubin, J., Toala, P., and Green, G., Observations on the pathogenesis of the pneumonitis associated with severe infections in other parts of the body, *Ann. Surg.*, 167, 630, 1965.

54. Riordan, J. F. and Walters, G., Pulmonary oedema in bacterial shock, *Lancet*, 719, 1968.

55. Vito, L., Dennis, R. C., Weisel, R. D., and Hectman, H. B., Respiratory failure can signal sepsis, *Surg. Gynecol. Obstet.*, 138, 896, 1974.

56. Altemeier, W. A., Todd, J. C., and Inge, W. W., Gram-negative septicemia: a growing threat, *Ann. Surg.*, 166, 228, 1967.

57. Myerowitz, R. L., Medeiros, A. A., and O'Brien, T. F., Recent experience with bacillemia due to gram-negative organisms, *J. Infect. Dis.*, 124, 239, 1971.

58. Kluge, R. M. and DuPont, H. L., Factors affecting mortality of patients with bacteremia, *Surg. Gynecol. Obstet.*, 137, 267, 1973.

59. McHenry, M. C., Gavan, T. L., Hawk, W. A., Ma, C., and Berrettoni, J. N., Gram-negative bacteremia: variable clinical course and useful prognostic factors, *Cleveland Clin. Q.*, 42, 15, 1975.

60. Jepsen, O. B. and Korner, B., Bacteremia in a general hospital: a prospective study of 102 consecutive cases, *Scand. J. Infect. Dis.*, 7, 179, 1975.

61. Setia, U. and Gross, P. A., Bacteremia in a community hospital: spectrum and mortality, *Arch. Intern. Med.*, 137, 1698, 1977.

62. Martin, W. J., Meyer, R. D., Weinstein, R. J., and Anderson, E. T., Gram-negative rod bacteremia: microbiologic, immunologic, and therapeutic considerations, UCLA Conference, *Ann. Intern. Med.*, 86, 456, 1977.

63. Anderson, E. T., Young, L. S., Hewitt, W. L., Simultaneous antibiotic levels in "breakthrough" gram-negative rod bacteremia, *Am. J. Med.*, 61, 493, 1976.

64. Hardaway, R. M., James, P. M., Jr., Anderson, R. W., Bredenberg, C. E., and West, R. L., Intensive study and treatment of shock in man, *J.A.M.A.*, 199, 115, 1967.

65. Tarazi, R. C., Sympathomimetic agents in the treatment of shock, *Ann. Intern. Med.*, 81, 364, 1974.

66. Weil, M. H., Shubin, H., and Carlson, R., Treatment of circulatory shock: use of sympathomimetic and related vasoactive agents, *J.A.M.A.*, 231, 1280, 1975.

67. Schumer, W., Steroids in the treatment of clinical septic shock, *Ann. Surg.*, 333, 1976.

68. Shubin, H., Weil, M. H., and Carlson, R. W., Bacterial Shock, *Am. Heart J.*, 94, 112, 1977.

69. Ledingham, I. M. and McArdle, C. S., Prospective study of the treatment of septic shock, *Lancet*, 1194, 1978.

70. Fisher, E. J., Maki, D. G., Eisses, J., Neblett, T. R., and Quinn, E. L., Epidemic septicemias due to intrinsically contaminated infusion products, Abstracts of the Eleventh Interscience Conf. on Antimicrobial Agents and Chemotherapy, Atlantic City, October 20, 1971.

71. Harris, J. A. and Cobbs, C. G., Persistent gram-negative bacteremia: observations in twenty patients, *Am. J. Surg.*, 125, 705, 1973.

72. **Smits, H. and Freedman, L. R.,** Prolonged venous catheterization as a cause of sepsis, *N. Engl. J. Med.,* 276, 1229, 1967.

73. **Quintiliani, R. and Gifford, R. H.,** Endocarditis from *Serratia marcescens, J.A.M.A.,* 208, 2055, 1969.

74. **Darrell, J. H. and Garrod, L. P.,** Secondary septicemia from intravenous cannulae, *Br. Med. J.,* 2, 481, 1969.

75. **Mandell, G. L., Kaye, D., Levison, M. E., and Hook, E. W.,** Enterococcal Endocarditis: an analysis of 38 patients observed at the New York Hospital-Cornell Medical Center, *Arch. Intern. Med.,* 125, 258, 1970.

76. **Rubinstein, E., Noriega, E. R., Simberkoff, M. S., Holzman, R., and Rahal, J. J., Jr.,** Fungal endocarditis: analysis of 24 cases and review of the literature, *Medicine (Baltimore),* 54, 331, 1975.

77. **Watanakunakorn, C. and Baird, I. M.,** *Staphylococcus aureus* bacteremia and endocarditis associated with a removable infected intravenous device, *Am. J. Med.,* 63, 253, 1977.

78. **Rose, H. D.,** Venous catheter-associated candidemia, *Am. J. Med. Sci.,* 275, 265, 1978.

79. **Cohen, P. S., O'Brien, T. F., Schoenbaum, S. C., and Medeiros, A. A.,** The risk of endothelial infection in adults with salmonella bacteremia, *Ann. Intern. Med.,* 89, 931, 1978.

80. **Bloomfield, S. E., David, D. S., Cheigh, J. S., Kim, Y., White, R. P., Stenzel, K. H., and Rubin, A. L.,** Endophthalmitis following staphylococcal sepsis in renal failure patients, *Arch. Intern. Med.,* 138, 706, 1978.

81. **Iannini, P. B. and Crossley, K.,** Therapy of *Staphylococcus aureus* bacteremia associated with a removable focus of infection, *Ann. Intern. Med.,* 84, 558, 1976.

82. **Bartlett, R. C.,** Contemporary blood culture practices, in *Bacteremia: Laboratory and Clinical Aspects,* Sonnenwirth, A. C., Ed., Charles C Thomas, Springfield, Ill., 1973, 15.

83. **Bartlett, R. C., Ellner, P. D., and Washington, J. A., II,** in *Blood Cultures,* Sherris, J. C., Ed., Cumitech 1, American Society for Microbiology, Washington, D.C., 1974.

84. **Washington, J. A., II,** Blood cultures: principles and techniques, *Mayo Clin. Proc.,* 50, 91, 1975.

85. **Washington, J.A., II,** Conventional approaches to blood culture, in *The Detection of Septicemia,* Washington, J. A., II, Ed., CRC Press, West Palm Beach, Fla., 1978, 41.

86. **Spink, W. W.,** *The Nature of Brucellosis,* University of Minnesota Press, Minneapolis, 1956.

87. **Beeson, P. B., Brannon, E. S., and Warren, J. V.,** Observations on the sites of removal of bacteria from the blood in patients with bacterial endocarditis, *J. Exp. Med.,* 81, 9, 1945.

88. **Bennett, I. L., Jr. and Beeson, P. B.,** Bacteremia: a consideration of some experimental and clinical aspects, *Yale J. Biol. Med.,* 26, 241, 1954.

89. **Norden, C. W.,** Pseudosepticemia, *Ann. Intern. Med.,* 71, 789, 1969.

90. **Faris, H. M. and Sparling, F. F.,** *Mima polymorpha* bacteremia: false-positive cultures due to contaminated penicillinase, *J.A.M.A.,* 219, 76, 1972.

91. **Belli, J. and Waisbren, B. A.,** The number of blood cultures necessary to diagnose most cases of bacterial endocarditis, *Am. J. Med. Sci.,* 232, 284, 1956.

92. **Werner, A. S., Cobbs, C. G., Kaye, D., and Hook, E. W.,** Studies on the bacteremia of bacterial endocarditis, *J.A.M.A.,* 202, 199, 1967.

93. **Washington, J. A., II,** Characteristics of bacteremia relevant to its laboratory diagnosis, in *The Detection of Septicemia,* Washington, J. A., II, Ed., CRC Press, West Palm Beach, Fla., 1978, 27.

94. **Slotnick, I. J. and Sacks, H. J.,** The growth of pseudomonas in blood cultures, *Am. J. Clin. Pathol.,* 58, 723, 1972.

95. **Knepper, J. G. and Anthony, B. F.,** Diminished growth of *Pseudomonas aeruginosa* in unvented blood-culture bottles, *Lancet,* 2, 285, 1973.

96. **Blazevic, D. J., Stemper, J. E., and Matsen, J. M.,** Effect of aerobic and anaerobic atmospheres on isolation of organisms from blood cultures, *J. Clin. Microbiol.,* 1, 154, 1975.

97. **Harkness, J. L., Hall, M., Ilstrup, D. M., and Washington, J. A., II,** Effects of atmosphere of incubation and of routine subcultures on detection of bacteremia in vacuum blood culture bottles, *J. Clin. Microbiol.,* 2, 296, 1975.

98. **Braunstein, H. and Tomasulo, M.,** A quantitative study of the multiplication of *Pseudomonas aeruginosa* in vented and unvented blood-culture bottles, *Am. J. Clin. Pathol.,* 66, 80, 1976.

99. **Gantz, N. M., Swain, J. L., Medeiros, A. A., and O'Brien, T. F.,** Vacuum blood-culture bottles inhibiting growth of *Candida* and fostering growth of *Bacteroides, Lancet,* 2, 1174, 1974.

100. **Braunstein, H. and Tomasulo, M.,** A quantitative study of the growth of *Candida albicans* in vented and unvented blood-culture bottles, *Am. J. Clin. Pathol.,* 66, 87, 1976.

101. **King, T. C. and Price, P. B.,** An evaluation of iodophors as skin antiseptics, *Surg. Gynecol. Obstet.,* 105, 361, 1963.

102. **Gershenfeld, L.,** Iodine, in *Disinfection, Sterilization, and Preservation,* Lawrence C. A. and Block, S. S., Eds., Lea & Febiger, Philadelphia, 1968, 329.

103. White, J. J., Wallace, C. K., and Burnett, L. S., Drug letter: skin disinfection, *Johns Hopkins Med. J.*, 126, 169, 1970.

104. Selwyn, S. and Ellis, H., Skin bacteria and skin disinfection reconsidered, *Br. Med. J.*, 1, 136, 1972.

105. Spaulding, E. H., Alcohol as a surgical disinfectant, *Assoc. Oper. Rm. Nurses J.*, 2, 67, 1965.

106. Lee, S., Schoen, I., and Malkin, A., Comparison of use of alcohol with that of iodine for skin antisepsis in obtaining blood cultures, *Am. J. Clin. Pathol.*, 47, 646, 1967.

107. Morton, H. D., Alcohols, in *Disinfection, Sterilization, and Preservation*, Lawrence, C. A. and Black, S. S., Eds., Lea & Febiger, Philadelphia, 1968, 237.

108. Plotkin, S. A. and Austrian, R., Bacteremia caused by *Pseudomonas* sp. following the use of materials stored in solutions of a cationic surface-active agent, *Am. J. Med. Sci.*, 235, 621, 1958.

109. Malizia, W. F., Gangarosa, E. J., and Goley, A. F., Benzalkonium chloride as a source of infection, *N. Engl. J. Med.*, 263, 800, 1960.

110. Kaslow, R. A., Mackel, D. C., and Mallison, G. F., Nosocomial pseudobacteremia: positive blood cultures due to contaminated benzalkonium antiseptic, *J.A.M.A.*, 236, 2407, 1976.

111. Gilman, R. H., Terminel, M., Levine, M. M., Hernandez-Mendoza, P., and Hornick, A. R., Relative efficacy of blood urine, rectal swab, bone marrow, and rose-spot cultures for recovery of *Salmonella typhi* in typhoid fever, *Lancet*, 1, 1211, 1975.

112. Smith, J. W. and Utz, J. P., Progressive disseminated histoplasmosis: a prospective study of 26 patients, *Ann. Intern. Med.*, 76, 557, 1972.

113. Hughes, W. T., Leukemia monitoring with fungal bone marrow cultures, *J.A.M.A.*, 218, 441, 1971.

114. Greene, W. H., Schimpff, S. C., Vermeulen, G. D., et al., The value of routine bone marrow and cerebrospinal fluid cultures in patients with cancer — a negative report, *Am. J. Clin. Pathol.*, 60, 404, 1973.

115. Roberts, G. D. and Washington, J. A., II, Detection of fungi in blood cultures, *J. Clin. Microbiol.*, 1, 309, 1975.

116. Stone, H. H., Kolb, L. D., Currie, C. A., Geheber, C. E., and Cuzzell, J. Z., *Candida* sepsis: pathogenesis and principles of treatment, *Ann. Surg.*, 179, 697, 1974.

117. Kobza, K., Perruchoud, A., Mihatsch, J. M., and Herzog, H., Candidaemia and bacterial infections in patients with lung disease, *Lancet*, 2, 1084, 1976.

118. Goldmann, D. A. and Maki, D. G., Infection control in total parenteral nutrition, *J.A.M.A.*, 223, 1360, 1973.

119. French, G. and Shenoi, V., Disseminated moniliasis with demonstration of organism in blood, *Can. Med. Assoc. J.*, 71, 238, 1954.

120. Portnoy, J., Wolf, P. L., Webb, M., and Remington, J. S., *Candida* blastospores and pseudohyphae in blood smears, *N. Engl. J. Med.*, 285, 1010, 1971.

121. Henzel, J. H. and DeWeese, M. S., Morbid and mortal complications associated with prolonged central venous cannulation, *Am. J. Surg.*, 121, 600, 1971.

122. Morgensen, J. V., Frederiksen, W., Jensen, J. K., Subclavian vein catheterization and infection: a bacteriologic study of 130 catheter insertions, *Scand. J. Infect. Dis.*, 4, 31, 1972.

123. Maki, D. G., Jarrett, F., and Sarafin, H. W., A semiquantitative culture method for identification of catheter-related infection in the burn patient, *J. Surg. Res.*, 22, 513, 1977.

124. Band, J. D. and Maki, D. G., Infections caused by indwelling arterial catheters for hemodynamic monitoring, *Am. J. Med.*, 67, 735, 1979.

125. Tonnesen, A., Peuler, M., and Lockwood, W. R., Cultures of blood drawn by catheters vs. venipuncture, *J.A.M.A.*, 235, 1877, 1976.

126. Felices, F. J., Hernandez, J. L., Ruiz, J., Mesguer, J., Gomez, J. A., and Monlina, E., Use of the central venous pressure catheter to obtain blood cultures, *Crit. Care Med.*, 7, 78, 1979.

127. Nelson, J. D., Richardson, J., and Shelton, S., The significance of bacteremia with exchange transfusions, *J. Pediatr.*, 66, 291, 1965.

128. Anagnostakis, D., Kamba, A., Petrochilou, V., Arseni, A., and Marsaniotis, N., Risk of infection associated with umbilical vein catheterization: a prospective study in 75 newborn infants, *J. Pediatr.*, 86, 759, 1975.

129. Cowett, R. M., Peter, G., Hakanson, D. O., and Oh, W., Reliability of bacterial culture of blood obtained from an umbilical artery catheter, *J. Pediatr.*, 88, 1035, 1976.

130. Hall, M. M., Ilstrup, D. M., and Washington, J. A., II, Effect of volume of blood cultured on detection of bacteremia, *J. Clin. Microbiol.*, 3, 643, 1976.

131. Tenney, J. H., Reller, L. B., Stratton, C. W., and Wang, W-L. L., Controlled evaluation of volume of blood cultured and atmosphere of incubation in detection of bacteremia, Abstr. 16th Interscience Conf. Antimicrobial Agents and Chemotherapy, Chicago, October 1976.

132. Dietzman, D. E., Fischer, G. W., and Schoenknecht, F. D., Neonatal *Escherichia coli* septicemia — bacterial counts in blood, *J. Pediatr.*, 85, 128, 1974.

133. Santosham, M. and Moxon, E. R., Detection and quantitation of bacteremia in childhood, *J. Pediatr.,* 91, 719, 1977.

134. Durbin, W. A., Szymczak, E. G., and Goldman, D. A., Quantitative blood cultures in childhood bacteremia, *J. Pediatr.,* 92, 778, 1978.

135. Minkus, R. and Moffet, H. L., Detection of bacteremia in children with sodium polyanethol sulfonate: a prospective clinical study, *Appl. Microbiol.,* 22, 805, 1971.

136. Franciosi, R. A. and Favero, B. E., A single blood culture for confirmation of the diagnosis of neonatal septicemia, *Am. J. Clin. Pathol.,* 57, 215, 1972.

137. Mangurten, H. H. and LeBeau, L. J., Diagnosis of neonatal bacteremia by a microblood culture technique: a preliminary report, *J. Pediatr.,* 90, 990, 1977.

138. Conner, V. and Mallery, O. T., Blood culture: a clinical laboratory study of two methods, *Am. J. Clin. Pathol.,* 21, 785, 1951.

139. Katz, L., Johnson, D. L., Neufeld, P. D., and Gupta, K. G., Evacuated blood-collection tubes — the backflow hazard, *Can. Med. Assoc. J.,* 113, 210, 1975.

140. McLeish, W. A., Corrigan, E. N., Elder, R. H., and Westwood, J. C. N., Contaminated vacuum tubes (letter to the editor), *Can. Med. Assoc. J.,* 112, 682, 1975.

141. Semel, J. D., Trenholme, G. M. Harris, A. A., Jupa, J. E., and Levin, S., *Pseudomonas* maltophilia pseudosepticemia, *Am. J. Med.,* 64, 403, 1978.

142. Hoffman, P. C., Arnow, P. M., Goldmann, D. A., Parrott, P. L., Stamm, W. E., and McGowan, J. E., Jr., False-positive blood cultures: association with nonsterile blood collection tubes, *J.A.M.A.,* 236, 2073, 1976.

143. DuClos, T. W., Hodges, G. R., and Killian, J. E., Bacterial contamination of blood-drawing equipment: a cause of false positive blood cultures, *Am. J. Med. Sci.,* 266, 459, 1973.

144. MacGregor, R. R. and Beatty, H. N., Evaluation of positive blood cultures: guidelines for early differentiation of contaminated from valid positive cultures, *Arch. Intern. Med.,* 130, 84, 1972.

145. Pazin, G. J., Peterson, K. L., Griff, F. W., Shaver, J. A., and Ho, M., Determination of site of infection in endocarditis, *Ann. Intern. Med.,* 82, 746, 1975.

146. Center for Disease Control, Epidemiologic uses of antimicrobial susceptibility testing, *National Nosocomial Infections Study Quarterly Report, Third & Fourth Quarters 1973,* 1975, 29.

147. Bartlett, R. C., Bennett, J. V., Weinstein, R. A., and Mallison, G. F., The microbiology laboratory: its role in surveillance, investigation, and control, in *Hospital Infections,* Bennett, J. V. and Brachman, P. S., Eds., Little, Brown, Boston, 1979, 147.

148. Maki, D. G., Microbiological surveillance in *Modern IV Practices,* Medical Directions, Chicago, Ill., 1979, 1.

149. Favero, M. S. and Petersen, N. J.: Microbiologic guidelines for hemodialysis systems, *Dialysis Transplant.,* 6, 34, 1977.

150. Edmondson, E. B. and Sanford, J. P., Simple methods of bacteriologic sampling of nebulization equipment, *Am. Rev. Respir. Dis.,* 94, 450, 1966.

151. Nazemi, M. M., Musher, D. M., and Martin, R. R., A practical method for monitoring bacterial contamination of inhalation therapy machines, *Am. Rev. Respir. Dis.,* 106, 920, 1972.

152. Mackel, D. C., Sterilization and disinfection of respiratory therapy equipment, Assoc. Pract. Infect. Control (APIC) Newsletter, 2, 1, 1974.

153. Maki, D. G., Through the glass darkly — nosocomial pseudoepidemics and pseudobacteremias, *Arch. Intern. Med.,* 140, 26 1980.

154. Kotin, P.,Techniques and interpretation of routine blood cultures: observations in five thousand consecutive patients, *J.A.M.A.,* 149, 1273, 1952.

155. Hermans, P. E. and Washington, J. A., II, Polymicrobial bacteremia, *Ann. Intern. Med.,* 73, 387, 1970.

156. Lufkin, E. G., Silverman, M., Callaway, J. J., and Glenchur, H., Mixed septicemias and gastrointestinal disease, *Am. J. Dig. Dis.,* 11, 930, 1966.

157. Hochstein, H. D., Kirkham, W. R., and Young, V. M., Recovery of more than 1 organism in septicemias, *N. Engl. J. Med.,* 273, 468, 1965.

158. Geraci, J. E., Hanson, K. C., and Giuliani, E. R., Endocarditis caused by coagulase-negative staphylococci, *Mayo Clin. Proc.,* 43, 420, 1968.

159. Keys, T. F. and Hewitt, W. L., Endocarditis due to micrococci and *Staphylococcus epidermidis,* *Arch. Intern. Med.,* 132, 216, 1973.

160. Schimke, R. T., Black, P. H., Mark, V. H., and Swartz, M. N., Indolent *Staphylococcus albus* or *aureus* bacteremia after ventriculoatriostomy: role of foreign body in its initiation and perpetuation, *N. Engl. J. Med.,* 264, 264, 1961.

161. Gerry, J. L. and Greenough, W. B., III, Diphtheroid endocarditis. Report of nine cases and review of the literature, *Johns Hopkins Med. J.,* 139, 61, 1976.

162. Beeler, B. A., Crowder, J. G., Smith, J. W., and White, A.,Propionibacterium acnes; pathogen in central nervous system shunt infection. Report of three cases including immune complex glomerulonephritis, *Am. J. Med.,* 61, 935, 1976.

163. Anhalt, J. P., New or experimental approaches to detection of bacteremia, in *The Detection of Septicemia,* Washington, J. A., II, Ed., CRC Press, West Palm Beach, Fl., 1978.

164. McCabe, W. R. and LaPorte, J. J., Intracellular bacteria in the peripheral blood in staphylococcal bacteremia, *Ann. Intern. Med.,* 57, 141, 1962.

165. Humphrey, A. A., Use of the buffy layer in the rapid diagnosis of septicemia, *Am. J. Clin. Pathol.,* 14, 358, 1944.

166. Silverman, E. M., Norman, L. E., Goldman, R. T., and Simmons, J., Diagnosis of systemic candidiasis in smears of venous blood stained with Wright's stain, *Am. J. Clin. Pathol.,* 60, 473, 1973.

167. Kobza, K. and Steenblock, U., Demonstration of candida in blood smears, *Br. Med. J.,* 1, 1640, 1977.

168. Smith, H., Leucocytes containing bacteria in plain blood films from patients with septicaemia, *Australas. Ann. Med.,* 15, 210, 1966.

169. Brooks, G. F., Pribble, A. M., and Beaty, H. N., Early diagnosis of bacteremia by buffy-coat examinations, *Arch. Intern. Med.,* 132, 673, 1973.

170. Powers, D. L. and Mandell, G. L., Intraleukocytic bacteria in endocarditis patients, *J.A.M.A.,* 227, 312, 1974.

171. Finegold, S. M., White, M. L., Ziment, I., and Winn, W. R., Rapid diagnosis of bacteremia, *Appl. Microbiol.,* 18, 458, 1969.

172. Sullivan. N. M., Sutter, V. L., Carter, W. T., Attebery, H. R., and Finegold, S. M., Bacteremia after genitourinary tract manipulation: bacteriological aspects and evaluation of various blood culture systems, *Appl. Microbiol.,* 23, 1101, 1972.

173. Sullivan. N. M., Sutter, V. L., and Finegold, S. M., Practical aerobic membrane filtration blood culture technique: clinical blood culture trial, *J. Clin. Microbiol.,* 1, 37, 1975.

174. Rose, R. E. and Bradley, W. J., Using the membrane filter in clinical microbiology, *Med. Lab.,* 3, 22, 1969.

175. Farmer, S. G. and Komorowsk, R. A., Evaluation of the Sterifil lysis-filtration blood culture system, *Appl. Microbiol.,* 23, 500, 1972.

176. Dorn, G. L., Burson, G. G., and Haynes, J. R., Blood culture technique based on centrifugation: clinical evaluation, *J. Clin. Microbiol.,* 5, 46, 1977.

177. Zierdt, C. H., Kagan, R. L., and MacLowry, J. D., Development of a lysis-filtration blood culture technique, *J. Clin. Microbiol.,* 5, 46, 1977.

178. Komorowski, R. A. and Farmer, S. G., Rapid detection of candidemia, *Am. J. Clin. Pathol.,* 59, 56, 1973.

179. DeBlanc, H. J., Jr., DeLand, F., and Wagner, H. N., Jr., Automated radiometric detection of bacteria in 2,967 blood cultures, *Appl. Microbiol.,* 22, 846, 1971.

180. Renner, E. D., Gatherdige, L. A., and Washington, J. A., II, Evaluation of radiometric system for detecting bacteremia, *Appl. Microbiol.,* 26, 368, 1973.

181. Brooks, K. and Sodeman, T., Rapid detection of bacteremia by a radiometric system, *Am. J. Clin. Pathol.,* 61, 859, 1974.

182. Randall, E. L., Long-term evaluation of a system for radiometric detection of bacteremia, in *Microbiology—1975,* Schlessinger, D., Ed., American Society for Microbiology, Washington, D.C., 1975.

183. Morello, J. A., Automated radiometric detection of bacteremia, in *Automation in Microbiology and Immunology,* Heden, C. G. and Illemi, T., Eds., John Wiley & Sons, New York, 1975.

184. Thiemke, W. A. and Wicher, K., Laboratory experience with a radiometric method for detecting bacteremia, *J. Clin. Microbiol.,* 1, 302, 1975.

185. Randall, E. L., Radiometric techniques in microbiology, in *Modern Methods in Medical Microbiology.* Prier, J. E., Bartola, J. T., and Friedmand, H., Eds., University Park Press, Baltimore, Md., 1976.

186. Levin, J. and Bang, F. B., Clottable protein in Limulus: its localization and kinetics of its coagulation by endotoxin, *Thromb. Diath. Haemorrh.,* 19, 186, 1968.

187. Levin, J., Poore, T. E., Zauber, N. P., and Oser, R. S., Detection of endotoxin in the blood of patients with sepsis due to Gram-negative bacteria, *N. Engl. J. Med.,* 283, 1313, 1970.

188. Levin, J., Poore, T. E., Young, N. S., Margolis, S., Zauber, N. P., Townes, A. S., and Bell, W. R., Gram-negative sepsis: detection of endotoxemia with the limulus test, *Ann. Intern. Med.,* 76, 1, 1972.

189. Caridis, D. T., Reinhold, R. B., Woodruff, P. W. H., and Fine, J., Endotoxaemia in man, *Lancet,* 1, 1381, 1972.

190. **Martinez-G., L. A., Quintiliani, R. and Tilton, R. C.,** Clinical experience on the detection of endotoxemia with the Limulus test, *J. Infect. Dis.,* 127, 102, 1973.

191. **Stumacher, R. J., Kovnat, M. J., and McCabe W. R.,** Limitations of the usefulness of the limulus assay for endotoxin, *N. Engl. J. Med.,* 288, 1261, 1973.

192. **Feldman, S. and Pearson, T. A.,** The *Limulus* test and Gram-negative bacillary sepsis, *Am. J. Dis. Child.,* 128, 172, 1974.

193. **Elin, R. J., Robinson, R. A., Levine, A. S., and Wolff, S. M.,** Lack of clinical usefulness of the limulus test in the diagnosis of endotoxemia, *N. Engl. J. Med.,* 293, 521, 1975.

194. **Young, L. S.,** Opsonizing antibodies, host factors, and the limulus assay for endotoxin, *Infect. Immun.,* 12, 88, 1975.

195. **Elin, R. J. and Wolff, S. M.,** Nonspecificity of the limulus amebocyte lysate test: positive reactions with polynucleotides and proteins, *J. Infect. Dis.,* 128, 349, 1973.

196. **Jorgensen, J. H., Carvajal, H. F., Chipps, B. E., and Smith, R. F.,** Rapid detection of Gram-negative bacteriuria by use of the *Limulus* endotoxin assay, *Appl. Microbiol.,* 26, 38, 1973.

197. **Nachum, R., Lipsey, A., Siegel, S. E.,** Rapid detection of Gram-negative bacterial meningitis by the limulus lysate test, *N. Engl. J. Med.,* 289, 931, 1973.

198. **Ross, S., Rodriguez, W., Controni, G., Korengold, G., Watson, S., and Khan, W.,** Limulus lysate test for Gram-negative bacterial meningitis, *J.A.M.A.,* 233, 1366, 1975.

199. **Mitruka, B. M., Kundargi, R. S., and Jonas, A. M.,** Gas chromatography for rapid differentiation of bacterial infections in man, *Med. Res. Eng.,* 11, 7, 1972.

200. **Mitruka, B. M.,** Rapid automated identification of microorganisms in clinical specimens by gas chromatography, in *New Approaches to the Identification of Microorganisms,* Heden, C. G. and Illeni, T., Eds., John Wiley & Sons, New York, 1975.

201. **Davis, C. E. and McPherson, R. A.,** Rapid diagnosis of septicemia and meningitis by gas-liquid chromatography, in *Microbiology — 1975,* Schlessinger, D., Ed., American Society for Microbiology, Washington, D. C., 1975.

202. **Coonrod, J. D. and Rytel, M. W.,** Determination of aetiology of bacterial meningitis by counterimmunoelectrophoresis, *Lancet,* 1, 1154, 1972.

203. **Rytel, M. W.,** Rapid diagnostic methods in infectious diseases, *Adv. Intern. Med.,* 20, 37, 1975.

204. **Edwards, E. A., Muehl, P. M., and Peckinpaugh, R. O.,** Diagnosis of bacterial meningitis by counterimmunoelectrophoresis, *J. Lab. Clin. Med.,* 80, 449, 1972.

205. **Bartram, C. E., Jr., Crowder, J. G., Beeler, B., and White, A.,** Diagnosis of bacterial diseases by detection of serum antigens by counterimmunoelectrophoresis, sensitivity, and specificity of detecting *Pseudomonas* and pneumococcal antigens, *J. Lab. Clin. Med.,* 83, 591, 1974.

206. **Tugwell, P. and Greenwood, B. M.,** Pneumococcal antigen in lobar pneumonia, *J. Clin. Pathol.,* 28, 118, 1975.

207. **Coonrod, J. D. and Drennan, D. P.,** Pneumococcal pneumonia: capsular polysaccharide antigenemia and antibody responses, *Ann. Intern. Med.,* 84, 254, 1976.

208. **Shackelford, P. G., Campbell, J., and Feigin, R. D.,** Countercurrent immunoelectrophoresis in the evaluation of childhood infections, *J. Pediatr.,* 85, 478, 1974.

209. **Feigin, R. D., Stechenberg, B. W., Chang, M. J., Dunkle, L. M., Wong, M. L., Palkes, H., Dodge, P. R., and Davis, H.,** Prospective evaluation of treatment of *Haemophilus influenzae* meningitis, *J. Pediatr.,* 88, 542, 1976.

210. **Feigin, R. D., Wong, M., Shackelford, P. G., Stechenberg, B. W., Dunkle, L. M., and Kaplan, S.,** Countercurrect immunoelectrophoresis of urine as well as of CSF and blood for diagnosis of bacterial meningitis, *J. Pediatr.,* 89, 773, 1976.

211. **Edwards, E. A.,** Immunologic investigations of meningococcal disease. I. Group-specific *Neisseria meningitidis* antigens present in the serum of patients with fulminant meningococcemia, *J. Immunol.,* 106, 314, 1971.

212. **Greenwood, B. M., Whittle, H. C., and Dominic-Rajkovic, O.,** Countercurrent immunoelectrophoresis in the diagnosis of meningococcal infections, *Lancet,* 2, 519, 1971.

213. **Hoffman, T. A. and Edwards, E. A.,** Group-specific polysaccharide antigen and humoral antibody response in disease due to *Neisseria meningitidis,* *J. Infect. Dis.,* 126, 636, 1972.

214. **Whittle, H. C., Greenwood, B. M., Davidson, N. M., Tomkins, A., Tugwell, P., Warrell, D. A., Zalin, A., Bryceson, A. D. M., Parry, E. H. O., Brueton, M., Duggan, M., Oomen, J. M. V., and Rajkovic, A. D.,** Meningococcal antigen in diagnosis and treatment of group A meningococcal infections, *Am. J. Med.,* 58, 823, 1975.

215. **Edwards, M. S., Kasper, D. L., and Baker, C. J.,** Rapid diagnosis of type III group B streptococcal meningitis by latex particle agglutination, *J. Pediatr.,* 95, 202, 1979.

216. **McCracken, G. H., Jr., Sarff, L. D., Glode, M. P., Mize, S. G., Schiffer, M. S., Robbins, J. B., Gotschlich, E. C., Orskov, I., and Orskov, F.,** Relation between *Escherichia coli* K1 capsular polysaccharide antigen and clinical outcome in neonatal meningitis, *Lancet,* 2, 246, 1974.

217. Jackson, L. J., Aguilar-Torres, F. G., Dorado, A., Rose, H. D., and Ryte, M. W., Detection of staphylococcal teichoic acid antigen in body fluids and tissue, Abstracts of the Annual Meeting of the American Society for Microbiology, 1977.

218. Pollack, M., Significance of circulating capsular antigen in *Klebsiella* infections, *Infect. Immun.*, 13, 1543, 1976.

219. Ward, J. I., Siber, G. R., Scheifele, D. W., and Smith, D. H., Rapid diagnosis of *Hemophilus influenzae* type b infections by latex particle agglutination and counterimmunoelectrophoresis, *J. Pediatr.*, 93, 37, 1978.

220. Kayhty, H., Makela, P. H., Ruoslahti, E., Radioimmunoassay of capsular polysaccharide antigens of group A and C meningococci and *Hemophilus influenzae* type b in cerebrospinal fluid, *J. Clin. Pathol.*, 30, 831, 1977.

221. Drow, D. L., Manning, D. D., Maki, D. G., An indirect sandwich enzyme-linked immunosorbent-assay (ELISA) for the rapid detection of *Hemophilus influenzae* type b infection, *J. Clin. Microbiol.*, 10, 442, 1979.

222. Wiener, M. H., and Yount, W. J., Mannan antigenemia in the diagnosis of invasive *Candida* infections, *J. Clin. Inv.*, 58, 1045, 1976.

223. Warren, R. C., Bartlett, A., Bidwell, D. E., Richardson, M. D., Voller, A., and White, L. O., Diagnosis of invasive candidiasis by enzyme immunoassay of serum antigen, *Br. Med. J.*, 1, 1183, 1977.

224. Center for Disease Control, Reported nosocomial infections, 1976, *National Nosocomial Infections Study Report, Annual Summary 1976*, 1978, 1.

225. McGowan, J. E., Parrott, P. L., and Duty, V. P., Nosocomial bacteremia: potential for prevention of procedure-related cases, *J.A.M.A.*, 237, 2737, 1977.

226. Thoburn, R., Fekety, F. R., Jr., Cluff, L. E., and Melvin, V. B., Infections acquired by hospitalized patients: an analysis of the overall problem. *Arch. Intern. Med.*, 121, 1, 1968.

227. Britt, M. R., Schleupner, C. J., and Matsumiya, S., Severity of underlying disease as a predictor of nosocomial infection: utility in the control of nosocomial infection, *J.A.M.A.*, 239, 1047, 1978.

228. Schimpff, S. C., Young, V. M., Greene, W. H., Vermeulen, G. D., Moody, M. R., and Wiernik, P. H., Origin of infection in acute nonlymphocytic leukemia: significance of hospital acquisition of potential pathogens, *Ann. Intern. Med.*, 77, 707, 1972.

229. Myerowitz, R. L., Medeiros, A. A., and O'Brien, T. F., Bacterial infection in renal homotransplant recipients, *Am. J. Med.*, 53, 308, 1972.

230. Murphy, J. F., McDonald, F. D., Dawson, M., Reite, A., Turcotte, J., and Fekety, F. R., Jr., Factors affecting the frequency of infection in renal transplant recipients, *Arch. Intern. Med.*, 136, 1976.

231. The UCLA Bone Marrow Transplantation Group, Bone marrow trnsplantation with intensive combination chemotherapy/radiation therapy (SCARI) in acute leukemia, *Ann. Intern. Med.*, 86, 155, 1977.

232. Buckner, C. D., Clift, R. A., Sanders, J. E., Meyers, J. D., Counts, G. W., Farewell, V. T., Thomas, E. D., and The Seattle Marrow Transplant Team, Protective environment for marrow transplant recipients: a prospective study, *Ann. Intern. Med.*, 89, 893, 1978.

233. Band, J. D. and Maki, D. G., Morbidity associated with steel needles in patients with hematologic malignancy, *Arch. Intern. Med.*, 140, 31, 1980.

234. Spengler, R. F. and Grenough, W. B., III, Hospital costs and mortality attributed to nosocomial bacteremias, *J.A.M.A.*, 240, 2455, 1978.

235. Maki, D. G., Control of colonization and transmission of pathogenic bacteria in the hospital, *Ann. Intern. Med.*, 89, 77, 1978.

236. Gassner, C. B. and Ledger, W. J., The relationship of hospital-acquired maternal infection to invasive intrapartum monitoring techniques, *Am. J. Obstet. Gynecol.*, 126, 33, 1976.

237. Davis, J. P., Moggio, M. V., Klein, D., Tiosejo, L. L., Welt, S. I., and Wilfert, C. M., Vertical transmission of group B *Streptococcus:* relation to intrauterine fetal monitoring, *J.A.M.A.*, 242, 42, 1979.

238. Berger, S. A., Weitzman, S., Edberg, S. C., and Casey, J. I., Bacteremia after the use of an oral irrigation device: a controlled study in subjects with normal-appearing gingiva: comparison with use of toothbrush, *Ann. Intern. Med.*, 80, 510, 1974.

239. McEntegart, M. G. and Porterfield, J. S., Bacteraemia following dental extractions, *Lancet*, 2, 596, 1949.

240. Crawford, J. J., Sconyers, J. R., Moriarty, J. D., King, R. C., and West, J. F., Bacteremia after tooth extractions studied with the aid of prereduced anaerobically sterilized culture media, *Appl. Microbiol.*, 27, 927, 1974.

241. Kane, R. C., Cohen, M. H., Fossieck, B. E., Jr., and Tvardzik, A. V., Absence of bacteremia after fiberoptic bronchoscopy, *Am. Rev. Respir. Dis.*, 111, 102, 195.

242. Berry, F. A., Blankenbaker, W. L., and Ball, C. G., A comparison of bacteremia occurring with nasotracheal and orotracheal intubation, *Anesth. Analg. (Cleveland)*, 52, 873, 1973.

243. Herzon, F. S., Bacteremia and local infections with nasal packing, *Arch. Otolaryngol.*, 94, 317, 1971.

244. LeFrock, J. L., Klainer, A. S., Wu, W. H., and Turndorf, H., Transient bacteremia associated with nasotracheal suctioning, *J.A.M.A.*, 236, 1610, 1976.

245. Rhoads, P. S., Sibley, J. R., and Billings, C. E., Bacteremia following tonsillectomy: effect of preoperative treatment with antibiotics in postoperative bacteremia and in bacterial content of tonsils, *J.A.M.A.*, 157, 877, 1955.

246. Zwelling, L. A., Mandell, G. L., and Young, R. C., Peritoneoscopy: an invasive procedure without bacteremia, *Ann. Intern. Med.*, 87, 454, 1977.

247. Shull, H. J., Greene, B. M., Allen, S. D., Dunn, G. D., and Schenker, S., Bacteremia with upper gastrointestinal endoscopy, *Ann. Intern. Med.*, 83, 212, 1975.

248. Mellow, M. H. and Lewis, R. J., Endoscopy-related bacteremia, *Arch. Intern. Med.*, 136, 667, 1976.

249. Liebermann, T. R., Bacteremia and fiberoptic endoscopy *Gastrointest. Endosc.*, 23, 36, 1976.

250. Hoffman, Bruce I., Kobasa, W., and Kaye, D., Bacteremia after rectal examination, *Ann. Intern. Med.*, 88, 658, 1978.

251. Unterman, D., Milberg, M. B., and Kranis, M., Evaluation of blood cultures after sigmoidoscopy, *Med. Intel.*, 257, 773, 1957.

252. LeFrock, J. L., Ellis, C. A., Turchik, J. B., and Weinstein, L., Transient bacteremia associated with sigmoidoscopy, *Med. Intel.*, 289, 467, 1973.

253. Engeling, E. R. and Eng, B. F., Bacteremia after sigmoidoscopy: another view, *Ann. Intern. Med.*, 85, 77, 1976.

254. Dickman, M. D., Farrell, R., Higgs, R. H., Wright, L. E., Humphries, T. J., Wojcik, J. D., and Chappelka, R., Colonoscopy associated bacteremia, *Surg. Gynecol. Obstet.*, 142, 173, 1976.

255. Pelican, G., Hentges, D., Butt, J., Haag, T., Rolfe, R., and Hutcheson, D., Bacteremia during colonoscopy, *Gastrointest. Endosc.*, 23, 33, 1976.

256. Norfleet, R. G., Mulholland, D. D., Mitchell, P. D., Philo, J., and Walters, E. W., Does bacteremia follow colonoscopy?, *Gastroenterology*, 70, 20, 1976.

257. Hartong, W. A., Barnes, W. G., and Calkins, W. G., The absence of bacteremia during colonoscopy, *Am. J. Gastroenterol.*, 67, 240, 1977.

258. Coughlin, G. P., Butler, R. N., Alp, M. H., and Grant, A. K., Colonoscopy and bacteraemia, *Gut*, 18, 678, 1977.

259. Lam, S. K., Chan, P. K. W., Wong, K. P., and Ong, G. B., How often does bacteraemia occur following endoscopic retrograde cholangiopancreatography (ERCP)?, *Endoscopy*, 9, 231, 1977.

260. Bilbao, M. K., Dotter, C. T., Lee, T. G., and Katon, R. M., Complications of endoscopic retrograde cholangiopancreatography (ERCP): a study of 10,000 cases, *Gastroenterology*, 70, 314, 1976.

261. McCloskey, R. V., Gold, M., and Weser, E., Bacteremia after liver biopsy, *Arch. Intern. Med.*, 132, 213, 1973.

262. LeFrock, J. L., Ellis, C. A., Turchik, J. B., Zawacki, J. K., and Weinstein, L., Transient bacteremia associated with percutaneous liver biopsy, *J. Infect. Dis.*, 131, S104, 1975.

263. Slade, N., Bacteraemia and septicaemia after urological operations, *Proc. R. Soc. Med.*, 51, 331, 1958.

264. Last, P. M., Harbison, P. A., and Marsh, J. A., Bacteraemia after urological instrumentation, *Lancet*, 1, 74, 1966.

265. Sullivan, N. M., Sutter, V. L., Mims, M. M., Marsh, V. H., and Finegold, S. M., Clinical aspects of bacteremia after manipulation of the genitourinary tract, *J. Infect. Dist.*, 127, 49, 1973.

266. Richards, J. H., Bacteremia following irritation of foci of infection, *J.A.M.A.*, 99, 1496, 1932.

267. Speck, W. T., Dresdale, S. S., Krongrad, E., Gersony, W. M., Absence of bacteremia after instrumentation of the genitourinary tract in children, *J. Pediatr.*, 85, 224, 1974.

268. Regetz, M. J., Starr, S. E., Dowell, V. R., Jr., Balows, A., and Wenger, N. K., Absence of bacteremia after diagnostic biopsy of the cervix: chemoprophylactic implications, *Chest*, 65, 223, 1974.

269. Redleaf, P. D. and Fadell, E. J., Bacteremia during parturition: prevention of subacute bacterial endocarditis, *J.A.M.A.*, 169, 1284, 1959.

270. Baker, T. H., Machikawa, J. A., and Stapleton, J., Asymptomatic puerperal bacteremia, *Am. J. Obstet. Gynecol.*, 94, 903, 1966.

271. Baker, T. H. and Hubbell, R., Reappraisal of asymptomatic puerperal bacteremia, *Am. J. Obstet. Gynecol.*, 97, 575, 1967.

272. Ritvo, R., Monroe, P., and Andriole, V. T., Transient bacteremia due to suction abortion: implications for SBE antibiotic prophylaxis, *Yale J. Biol. Med.*, 50, 471, 1977.

273. Beard, C. H., Ribeiro, C. D., and Jones, D. M., The bacteraemia associated with burns surgery, *Br. J. Surg.*, 62, 638, 1975.

274. Sasaki, T. M., Welch, G. W., Herndon, D. N., Kaplan, J. Z., Lindberg, R. B., and Pruitt, B. A., Jr., Burn wound manipulation-induced bacteremia, *J. Trauma,* 19, 46, 1979.

275. Shawker, T. H., Kluge, R. M., and Ayella, R. J., Bacteremia associated with angiography, *J.A.M.A.,* 229, 1090, 1974.

276. Gould, L. and Lyon, A. F., Penicillin prophylaxis for cardiac catheterization, *J.A.M.A.,* 202, 662, 1967.

277. Cooperative Study on Cardiac Catheterization, Braunwald, E. and Swan, E., Eds., *Circulation,* 37 (Suppl. 3), 1, 1968.

278. Clark, H., An evaluation of antibiotic prophylaxis in cardiac catheterization, *Am. Heart J.,* 77, 767, 1969.

279. Sande, M. A., Levinson, M. E., Lukas, D. S., and Kaye, D., Bacteremia associated with cardiac catheterization, *N. Engl. J. Med.,* 281, 1104, 1969.

280. Ralston, A. J., Harlow, G. R., Jones, D. M., and Davis, P., Infections of Scribner and Brescia arteriovenous shunts, *Br. Med. J.,* 3, 408, 1971.

281. Kaslow, R. A. and Zellner, S. R., Infection in patients on maintenance haemodialysis, *Lancet,* 2, 117, 1972.

282. Keane, W. F., Shapiro, F. L. and Raiji, L., Incidence and type of infections occuring in 445 chronic hemodialysis patients, *Trans. Am. Soc. Artif. Intern. Organs,* 23, 41, 1977.

283. Dobkin, J. F., Miller, M. H., and Steigbiegel, N., Septicemia in patients on chronic hemodialysis, *Ann. Intern. Med.,* 88, 28, 1978.

284. Kaplan, E. L., Anthony, B. F., Bisno, A., Durack, D., Houser, H., Millard, D., Sanford, J., Shulman, S. T., Stillerman, M., Taranta, A., and Wenger, N., Prevention of bacterial endocarditis, *Circulation,* 56, 139A, 1977.

285. Duma, R., Weinberg, A. N., Medrek, T. F., and Kunz, L. J., Streptococcal infections: a bacteriologic and clinical study of streptococcal bacteremia, *Medicine (Baltimore),* 48, 87, 1969.

286. Horstmeier, C. and Washington, J. A., II, Microbiological study of streptococcal bacteremia, *Appl. Microbiol.,* 26, 589, 1973.

287. Maki, D. G., and Agger, W. A., Enterococcal bacteremia: clinical features and risk of endocarditis, Abstracts of the 18th Interscience Conference on Antimicrobial Agents and Chemotherapy, Atlanta, Ga., October 1978.

288. Brenner, D. J., Farmer, J. J., III, Hickman, F. W., Asbury, M. A., and Steigerwalt, A. G., Taxonomic and nomenclature changes in *Enterobacteriaceae,* Publ. No. (CDC) 79-8356, Department of Health, Education and Welfare, 1979.

289. Lessel, E. R., International committee on nomenclature of bacteria, subcommittee on the taxonomy of Moraxella and allied bacteria, *Int. J. Syst. Bacteriol.,* 21, 213, 1971.

290. Applebaum, P. C., Koornhof, H. J., Jacobs, M., Robins-Browne, R., Isaacson, M., Gilliland, J., and Austrian, R., Multiple-antibiotic resistance of pneumococci—South Africa, *Morbid. Mortal, Weekly Rep.,* 26, 285, 1977.

291. Koornhof, H. J., Jacobs, M., Issacson, M., Appelbaum, P., Miller, B., Stevenson, C. M., Freeman, I., Naude, A., Botha, P., Glathaar, E., and Gilliland, J., Follow-up on multiple-antibiotic-resistant pneumococci—South Africa, *Morbid. Mortal. Weekly Rep.,* 27, 1, 1978.

292. Appelbaum, P. C., Bhamjee, A., Scragg, J. N., Bowen, A. J., *Streptococcus pneumoniae* resistant to penicillin and chloramphenicol, *Lancet,* 2, 995, 1977.

293. Jacobs, M. R., Koornhof, H. J., Robins-Browne, R. M. Stevenson, C. M., Vermaak, Z. A., Freiman, I., Miller, G. B., Witcomb, A. A., Isaacson, M., Ward, J. I., and Austrian, R., Emergence of multiply resistant pneumococci, *N. Engl. J. Med.,* 299, 735, 1978.

294. Ward, J. I., Koornhof, H., Jacobs, M., and Appelbaum, P., Clinical and epidemiological features of multiply resistant pneumococci, South Africa, in *Microbiology — 1979,* Schlessinger, Ed., American Society for Microbiology, Washington, D.C., 1979, 283.

295. Koornhof, H. J., Jacobs, M. R., Ward, J. I., Appelbaum, P. C., and Hallet, F. A., Therapy and Control of antibiotic-resistant pneumococcal disease, in *Microbiology — 1979,* American Society for Microbiology, Washington, D.C. 1979, 286.

296. Finland, M., Jones, W. F., Jr., and Barnes, M. W., Occurrence of serious bacterial infections since introduction of antibacterial agents, *J.A.M.A.,* 170, 2188, 1959.

297. Finland, M., Changing ecology of bacterial infections as related to antibacterial therapy, *J. Infect. Dis.,* 122, 419, 1970.

298. Holzman, R. S., Florman, A. L., and Toharsky, B., The clinical usefulness of an ongoing bacteremia surveillance program, *Am. J. Med. Sci.,* 274, 13, 1977.

299. Crowley, N., Some bacteraemias encountered in hospital practice, *J. Clin. Pathol.,* 23, 166, 1969.

300. Gardner, P. and Charles, D. G., Infections acquired in a pediatric hospital, *J. Pediatr.,* 81, 1205, 1972.

301. Rose, R., Hunting, K. J., Townsend, T. R., and Wenzel, R. P., Morbidity/mortality and economics of hospital-acquired blood stream infections: a controlled study, *South. Med. J.,* 70, 1267, 1977.

302. Spengler, R. F., Greenough, W. B., III, and Stolley, P. D., A descriptive study of nosocomial bacteremias at The Johns Hopkins Hospital, 1968-1974, *Johns Hopkins Med. J.,* 142, 77, 1978.

303. Maki, D. G. and Zilz, M. A., (Surveillance of Nosocomial Infections in the University of Wisconsin Hospitals), unpublished data, 1979.

304. File, T. M., Jr. and Vincent, D. J., The pattern of gram-negative-rod bacteremia in a community hospital, *Ohio State Med. J.,* 551, August 1977.

305. Dixon, R. E., Effect of infections on hospital care, *Ann. Intern. Med.,* 89, 749, 1978.

306. Wolff, S. M. and Bennett, J. V., Gram-negative-rod bacteremia, *N. Engl. J. Med.,* 291, 733, 1974.

307. McCabe, W. R., Letter to the editor, *N. Engl. J. Med.,* 292, 111, 1974.

308. Roland C. G. and Kirkpatrick, R. A., Time lapse between hypothesis and publication in the medical sciences, *N. Engl. J. Med.,* 292, 1273, 1975.

309. Bennett, J. V., Incidence and nature of endemic and epidemic nosocomial infections, in *Hospital Infections,* Bennet, J. V. and Brachman, P. S., Eds., Little, Brown, Boston, 1979, 233.

310. Scheckler, W. E., Nosocomial infections in a community hospital — 1972-1976, *Arch. Intern. Med.,* 138, 1792, 1978.

311. Hemming, V. G., Overall, J. C., Jr., Britt, M. R., Nosocomial infections in a newborn intensive-care unit: results of forty-one months of surveillance, *N. Engl. J. Med.,* 294, 1310, 1976.

312. Miller, R. M., Polakavetz, S. H., Hornick, R. B., and Cowley, R. A., Analysis of infections acquired by the severely injured patient, *Surg. Gynecol. Obstet.,* 137, 7, 1973.

313. Schimpff, S. C.; Miller, R. M. Polakvetz, S., and Hornick, R. B., Infection in the severely traumatized patient, *Ann. Surg.,* 179, 352, 1974.

314. Maki, D. G., McCormick, R., Nosocomial Infections in Patients in the Trauma and Life Support Center of the University of Wisconsin Hospitals, unpublished data, presented in part by Maki, D. G., Symposium on the Impact of Infections on Medical Care in the United States: problems and Priorities for future Research, National Institutes of Health, Bethesda, Md., May 1978.

315. Bentley, D. W. and Lepper, M. H., Septicemia related to indwelling venous catheter, *J.A.M.A.,* 206, 1749, 1968.

316. Austin, T. W. and Wallace, J. F., Staphylococcus aureus bacteremia: a critical review of its treatment and association with infective endocarditis, *Infection,* 1, 214, 1973.

317. Musher, D. M. and McKenzie, S. O., Infections due to *Staphylococcus aureus, Medicine (Baltimore),* 56, 383, 1977.

318. Ladisch, S. and Pizzo, P. A., *Staphylococcus aureus* sepsis in children with cancer, *Pediatrics,* 61, 231, 1978.

319. Dudding, B., Humphrey, G. B., and Nesbit, M. E., Beta-hemolytic streptococcal septicemias in childhood leukemia, *Pediatrics,* 43, 359, 1969.

320. Henkel, J. S., Armstrong, D., Blevins, A., and Moody, M. D., Group A β-Hemolytic *Streptococcus* bacteremia in a cancer hospital, *J.A.M.A.,* 211, 983, 1970.

321. Hable, K. A., Horstmeier, C., Wold, A. D., and Washington, J. A., II. Group A β-Hemolytic Streptococcemia: bacteriologic and clinical study of 44 cases, *Mayo Clin. Proc.,* 48, 336, 1973.

322. Geil, C. C., Castle, W. K., and Mortimer, E. A., Jr., Group A streptococcal infections in newborn nurseries, *Pediatrics,* 46, 849, 1970.

323. Nelson, J. D., Dillon, H. C., Jr., and Howard, J. B., A prolonged nursery epidemic associated with a newly recognized type of group A streptococcus, *J. Pediatr.,* 89 792, 1976.

324. McKee, W. M., DiCaprio, J. M., Roberts, C. E., Jr., Sherris, J. C., Anal carriage as the probable source of a streptococcal epidemic, *Lancet,* 2, 1007, 1966.

325. Schaffner, W., Lefkowitz, L. B., Jr., Goodman, J. S., and Koenig, M. G., Hospital outbreak of infections with group A streptococci traced to an asymptomatic anal carrier, *N. Engl. J. Med.,* 280, 1224, 1969.

326. Gryska, P. F. and O'Dea, A. E., Postoperative streptococcal wound infection: the anatomy of an epidemic, *J.A.M.A.,* 213, 1189, 1970.

327. Decker, J., MacArthur, M., Bailey, J., and Fukushima, T., Hospital outbreak of streptococcal wound infection — Utah, *Morbid. Mortal. Weekly Rep.,* 25, 141, 1976.

328. Richman, D. D., Breton, S. J., and Goldmann, D. A., Scarlet fever and group A streptococcal surgical wound infection traced to an anal carrier, *J. Pediatr.,* 90, 387, 1977.

329. Stamm, W. E., Feeley, J. C., and Facklam, R. R., Wound infections due to group A *Streptococcus* traced to a vaginal carrier, *J. Infect. Dis.,* 138, 287, 1978.

330. Nahmias, A. J. and Eickhoff, T. C., Staphylococcal infections in hospitals: recent developments in epidemiologic and laboratory investigation, *N. Engl. J. Med.,* 265, 74, 1961.

331. Howe, C. W. and Marston, A. T., A study on sources of postoperative staphylococcal infection, *Surg. Gynecol.,* 103, 266, 1962.

332. Rammelkamp, C. H., Jr., Mortimer, E. A., Jr., and Wolinsky, E., Transmission of streptococcal and staphylococcal infections, *Ann. Intern. Med.*, 60, 753, 1964.

333. Fekety, F. R., Jr., The epidemiology and prevention of staphylococcal infection, *Medicine (Baltimore)*, 43, 593, 1964.

334. Klimek, J. J., Marsik, F. J., Bartlett, R. C., Weir, B., Shea, P., and Quintiliani, R., Clinical, epidemiologic and bacteriologic observations of an outbreak of methicillin-resistant *Staphylococcus aureus* at a large community hospital, *Am. J. Med.*, 61, 340, 1976.

335. Crossley, K., Loesch, D., Landesman, B., Mead, K., Chern, M., and Strate, R., An outbreak of infections caused by strains of *Staphylococcus aureus* resistant to methicillin and aminoglycosides. I. Clinical Studies. II. Epidemiologic Studies, *J. Infect. Dis.*, 139, 273, 1979.

336. Maki, D. G., McCormick, R., and Wirtenan, G. W., Septic endarteritis due to intra-arterial catheters for cancer chemotherapy. I. Clinical features and management. II. Investigation of an outbreak. III. Risk factors and guidelines for prevention, *Cancer*, 44, 1228, 1979.

337. Gross, P. A., Lyons, R., Flower, M., and Barden, G., Endemicity of multiple staphylococcal phage types: relation to two common source outbreaks, *Nephron*, 16, 462, 1976.

338. Linnemann, C. C., Jr., McKee, E., and Laver, M.C., Staphylococcal infections in a hemodialysis unit, *Am. J. Med. Sci.*, 276, 67, 1978.

339. Payne, R. W., Severe outbreak of surgical sepsis due to *Staphlococcus aureus* of unusual type and origin, *Br. Med. J.*, 4, 17, 1967.

340. Walter, C. W., Kundsin, R. B., and Brubaker, M. M. The incidence of airborne wound infection during operation, *J.A.M.A.*, 186, 122, 1963.

341. Barber, M., Naturally occurring methicillin-resistant staphylococci, *J. Gen. Microbiol.*, 35, 183, 1964.

342. Charbert, Y. A., Baudens, J. G., Agar, J. F., and Gerband, G. R., La resistance naturelle des Staphylocoques a la methicilline et l'oxacilline, *Rev. Fr. Etud. Clin. Biol.*, 10, 495, 1965.

343. Jessen, O., Rosendal, K., Bulow, P., Faber, V., and Eriksen, K. R., Changing staphylococci and staphylococcal infections: a ten-year study of bacteria and cases of bacteremia, *N. Engl. J. Med.*, 281, 627, 1969.

344. Kayser, F. H., Methicillin-resistant staphylococci — 1965-75 *Lancet*, 2, 650, 1975.

345. Seiger, B. E., Long, J. M., Lindberg, R. B., Pruitt, B. A., Jr., McNitt, T. R., Methicillin resistant staphylococci in thermally injured patients: epidemiologic aspects, Abstracts 16th Interscience Conf. on Antimicrobial Agents and Chemotherapy, Washington, D.C., October 1976.

346. Richmond, A. S., Simberkoff, M. S., Schaefler, S., Rahal, J. J., Jr., Reistance of *Staphylococcus aureus* to semi-synthetic penicillins and cephalothin, *J. Infect. Dis.*, 135, 108, 1977.

347. Shanson, D. C., Kensit, J. G., and Duke, R., Outbreak of hospital infection with a strain of *Staphylococcus aureus* resistant to gentamicin and methicillin, *Lancet*, 2, 1347, 1976.

348. Center for Disease Control, Gentamicin-resistant *Staphylococcus aureus* in a Gerogia Hospital, National Nosocomial Infections Study Report, Annual Summary 1975, October 1977.

349. Rifkind, D., Marchioro, T. L., Waddell, W. R., and Starzl, T. E., Infectious disease associated with renal homotransplantation, *J.A.M.A.*, 189, 397, 1964.

350. Calia, F. M., Wolinsky, E., Mortimer, E. A., Jr., Abrams, J. S., and Rammelkamp, C. H., Jr., Importance of the carrier state as a source of *Staphylococcus aureus* in wound sepsis, *J. Hyg. Camb.*, 67, 49, 1969.

351. White, A., Relation between quantitative nasal cultures and dissemination of staphylococci, *J. Lab. Clin. Med.*, 58, 273, 1961.

352. Stokes, E. J., Bradley, J. M., Thompson, R. E. M., Hitchcock, N. M., Parker, M. J., and Walker, J. S., Hospital staphylococci in three London teaching hospitals, *Lancet*, 1, 84, 1972.

353. Rountree, P. M., Streptococcus pyogenes infections in a hospital, *Lancet*, 2, 172, 1955.

354. Burke, J. F., Identification of the sources of staphylococci contaminating the surgical wound during operation, *Ann. Surg.*, 158, 898, 1964.

355. Gonzaga, A. J., Mortimer, E. A., Jr., Wolinsky, E., and Rammelkamp, C. H., Jr., Transmission of staphylococci by fomites, *J.A.M.A.*, 189, 109, 1964.

356. Gezon, H. M., Thompson, D. J., Rogers, K. D., Hatch, T. F., and Taylor, P. M., Hexachlorophene bathing in early infancy: effect on staphylococcal disease and infection, *N. Engl. J. Med.*, 270, 379, 1964.

357. Kaslow, R. A., Dixon, R. E., Martin, S. M., Mallison, G. F., Goldman, D. A., Lindsey, J. D., II, Rhame, F. S., and Bennett, J. V., Staphylococcal disease related to hospital nursery bathing practices — a nationwide epidemiologic investigation, *Pediatrics*, 51, 418, 1973.

358. Dixon, R. E., Kaslow, R. A., Mallison, G. F., Bennett, J. V., Staphylococcal disease outbreaks in hospital nurseries in the United States — December 1971 through March 1972, *Pediatrics*, 51 (Part II), 413, 1973.

359. Cruse, P. J. E. and Foord, R., A five-year prospective study of 23,649 surgical wounds, *Arch. Surg. (Chicago)*, 107, 206, 1973.

360. Eickhoff, T. C., Klein, J. O., Daly, A. K., Ingall, D., and Finland, M., Neonatal sepsis and other infections due to group B Beta-Hemolytic streptococci, *N. Engl. J. Med.*, 271, 1221, 1964.

361. Franciosi, R. A., Knostam, J. D., and Zimmerman, R. A., Group B streptococcal neonatal and infant infections, *J. Pediatr.*, 82, 707, 1973.

362. Baker, C. J., Barrett, F. F., Gordon, R. C., and Yow, M. D., Suppurative meningitis due to streptococci of Lancefield group B: a study of 33 infants, *J. Pediatr.*, 82, 724, 1973.

363. Horn, K. A., Meyer, W. T., Wyrick, B. C., Zimmerman, R. A., Group B streptococcal neonatal infection, *J.A.M.A.*, 230, 1165, 1974.

364. Anthony, B. F. and Okada, D. M., The emergence of group B streptococci in infections of the newborn infant, *Annu. Rev. Med.*, 28, 355, 1977.

365. Parker, M. T., Neonatal streptococcal infections, *Postgrad. Med. J.*, 53, 598, 1977.

366. Embil, J. A., Belgaumkar, T. K., and MacDonald, S. W., Group B Beta-hemolytic streptococci in an intramural neonatal population, *Scand. J. Infect. Dis.*, 10, 50, 1978.

367. Davis, J. P., Gutman, L. T., Higgins, M. V., Katz, S. L., Welt, S. I., and Wilfert, C. M., Nasal colonization of infants with group B *Streptococcus* associated with intrauterine pressure transducers, *J. Infect. Dis.*, 138, 804, 1978.

368. MacKnight, J. F., Ellis, P. J., Jensen, K. A., and Franz, B., Group B streptococci in neonatal deaths, *Appl. Microbiol.*, 17, 926, 1969.

369. Steere, A. C., Aber, R. C., Warford, L. R., Murphy, K. E., Feeley, J. C., Hayes, P. S., Wilinson, H.W., Facklam, R. R., Possible nosocomial transmission of group B streptococci in a newborn nursery, *J. Pediatr.*, 87, 784, 1975.

370. Aber, R. C., Allen, N., Howell, J. T., Wilkenson, H. W., and Facklam, R. R., Nosocomial transmission of group B strepococci, *Pediatrics*, 58, 346, 1976.

371. Paredes, A., Wong, P., Mason, E. O., Jr., Taber, L. H., and Barrett, F. F., Nosocomial transmission of group B streptococci in a newborn nursery, *Pediatrics*, 59, 679, 1977.

372. Armstrong, D., Blevins, A., Louria, D. B., Henkel, J. S., Moody, M. D., and Sukany, M. II. Gram-positive bacteria: Groups B, C, and G streptococcal infections in a cancer hospital, *Ann. N.Y. Acad. Sci.*, 174, 511, 1970.

373. Broome, C. V., Moellering, R. C., Jr., and Watson, B. K., Clinical significance of Lancefield groups L-T streptococci isolated from blood and cerebrospinal fluid, *J. Infect. Dis.*, 133, 382, 1976.

374. Goldmann, D. A. and Breton, S. J., Group C streptococcal surgical wound infections transmitted by an anorectal and nasal carrier, *Pediatrics*, 61, 235, 1978.

375. Finland, M., Changing patterns of susceptibility of common bacterial pathogens to antimicrobial agents., *Ann. Intern. Med.*, 76, 1009, 1971.

376. Finland, M., Increased resistance in the pneumococcus, *N. Engl. J. Med.*, 284, 212, 1971.

377. Performance Standards for Antimicrobial Disc Susceptibility Tests, NCCLS Publ. No. ASM-2, Villanova, Pa., American Society of Microbiology, 1975.

378. Smilie, W. G., Study of an outbreak of Type II pneumococcus pneumonia in Veterans Administration Hospital at Bedford, Mass. *Am. J. Hyg.*, 24, 522, 1936.

379. Blazevic, D. J., Bleeker, E. Z., Gates, K. L., Gerrard, J. M., Giebink, G. S., Lund, M. E., Quie, P. G., and Fifer, E. Z., Penicillin-resistant *Streptococcus pneumoniae* — Minnesota, *Morbid. Mortal. Weekly Rep.*, 26, 345, 1977.

380. Cooksey, R. C., Facklam, P. R., and Thornsberry, C., Antimicrobial susceptibility patterns of *Streptococcus pneumoniae, Antimicrob. Agents Chemother.*, 13, 646, 1978.

381. Maki, D. G., Helstad, A. G., Kimball, J. L., Screening for penicillin-resistant pneumococci, *Am. J. Clin. Pathol.*, 73, 177, 1980.

382. Austrian, R., Vaccines of pneumococcal capsular polysaccharides and the prevention of pneumococcal pneumonia in the role of immunological factors, in *Infectious, Allergic and Autoimmune Process*, Beers, R. F. and Bassett, E. G., Eds., Eighth Miles International Symposium, Raven Press, New York, 1976, 79.

383. Ammann, A. J., Addiego, J., Wara, D. W., Lubin, B., Smith, W. B., and Mentzer, W. C., Polyvalent Pneumococcal-polysaccharide immunization of patients with sickle-cell anemia and patients with splenectomy, *N. Engl. J. Med.*, 297, 897, 1977.

384. Center for Disease Control, Pnemococcal polysaccharide vaccine, *Morbid. Mortal. Weekly Rep.*, 27, 48, 1978.

385. Rose, H. D. and Schreier, J., The effect of hospitalization and antibiotic therapy on gram-negative fecal flora, *Am. J. Med. Sci.*, 255, 288, 1968.

386. Rose, H. D. and Babcock, J. B., Colonization of intensive care unit patients with gram-negative bacilli, *Am. J. Epidemiol.*, 101, 495, 1975.

387. LeFrock, J. L., Ellis, C. A., Weinstein, L., The impact of hospitalization on the aerobic fecal microflora, *Am. J. Med. Sci.,* 277, 269, 1979.

388. Johanson, W. G., Pierce, A. K., and Sanford, J. P., Changing pharyngeal bacterial flora of hospitalized patients, *N. Engl. J. Med.,* 281, 1127, 1969.

389. Johanson, W. G., Jr., Pierce, A. K., Sanford, J. P., and Thomas, G. D., Nosocomial respiratory infections with gram-negative bacilli: the significance of colonization of the respiratory tract, *Ann. Intern. Med.,* 77, 701, 1972.

390. Harris, H., Wirtschafter, D., and Cassady, G., Endotracheal intubation and its relationship to bacterial colonization and systemic infection of newborn infants, *Pediatrics,* 56, 816, 1976.

391. Goodpasture, H. C., Romig, D. A., Voth, D. W., Liu, C., and Brackett, C. E., A prospective study of tracheobronchial bacterial flora in acutely brain-injured patients with and without antibiotic prophylaxis, *J. Neurosurg.,* 47, 228, 1977.

392. LeFrock, J. L., Ellis, C. A., Weinstein, L., The relation between aerobic fecal and oropharyngeal microflora in hospitalized patients, *Am. J. Med. Sci.,* 277, 275, 1979.

393. Stratford, B., Gallus, A. S., Matthiesson, A. M., and Dixson, S., Alteration of superficial bacterial flora in severely ill patients, *Lancet,* 1, 68, 1968.

394. Pollack, M., Charache, P., Nieman, R. E., Jett, M. P., Reinhardt, J. A., Harby, P. H., Jr., Factors influencing colonization and antibiotic-resistance patterns of gram-negative bacteria in hospital patients, *Lancet,* 2, 668, 1972.

395. Weinstein, L., Goldfield, M., and Chang, T. W., Infections occurring during chemotherapy: a study of their frequency, type and predisposing factors, *N. Engl. J. Med.,* 251, 247, 1954.

396. Tillotson, J. R. and Finland, M., Bacterial colonization and clinical superinfection of the respiratory tract complicating antibiotic treatment of pneumonia, *J. Infect. Dis.,* 119, 597, 1969.

397. Price, D. J. E. and Sleigh, J. D., Control of infection due to *Klebsiella aerogenes* in a neurosurgical unit by withdrawal of all antibiotics, *Lancet,* 1, 1213, 1970.

398. Franco, J. A., Eitzman, D. V., and Baer, H., Antibiotic usage and microbial resistance in an intensive care nursery, *Am. J. Dis. Child.,* 126, 318, 1973.

399. Finland, M., Superinfections in the antibiotic era, *Postgrad. Med.,* 54, 175, 1973.

400. Philp, J. R. and Spencer, R. C., Secondary respiratory infection in hospital patients: effect of antimicrobial agents and environment, *Br. Med. J.,* 2, 359, 1974.

401. Selden, R., Lee, S., Want, W. L. L., Bennett, J. V., and Eickhoff, T. C., Nosocomial *Klebsiella* infections: intestinal colonization as a reservoir, *Ann. Intern. Med.,* 72, 657, 1971.

402. Schimpff, S. C., Young, V. M., Greene, W. H., Vermeulen, G. D., Moody, M. R., and Wiernik, P. H., Origin of infection in acute nonlymphocytic leukemia: Significance of hospital acquisition of potential pathogens, *Ann. Intern. Med.,* 77, 707, 1972.

403. Speer, M. E., Taber. L. H., Yow, M. D., Rudolph, A. J., Urteaga, J., and Waller, S., Fulminant neonatal sepsis and necrotizing enterocolitis associated with a "nonenteropathogenic" strain of *Escherichia coli, J. Pediatr.,* 89, 91, 1976.

404. Hill, H. R., Hunt, C. E., and Matsen, J. M., Nosocomial colonization with *Klebsiella,* type 26, in a neonatal intensive-care unit associated with an outbreak of sepsis, meningitis, and necrotizing enterocolitis, *J. Pediatr.,* 85, 415, 1974.

405. Jellard, C. H. and Churcher, G. M., An outbreak of *Pseudomonas aeruginosa* (pyocyanea) infection in a premature baby unit, with observations on the intestinal carriage of *Pseudomonas aeruginosa* in the newborn, *J. Hyg. Camb.,* 65, 219, 1967.

406. Howard, F. M., Flynn, D. M., Bradley, J. M., Noone, P., and Szawatkowski, M., Outbreak of necrotising enterocolitis caused by *Clostridium butyricum, Lancet,* 2, 1099, 1977.

407. Greene, W. H., Moody, M., Hartley, R., Effman, E., Aisner, J., Young, V. M., and Wiernik, P. H., Esophagoscopy as a source of *Pseudomonas aeruginosa* sepsis in patients with acute leukemia: the need for sterilization of endoscopes, *Gastroenterology,* 67, 912, 1974.

408. Reinarz, J. A., Pierce, A. K., Mays, B. B., and Sanford, J. P., The potential role of inhalation therapy equipment in nosocomial pulmonary infection, *J. Clin. Invest.,* 44, 831, 1965.

409. Favero, M. S., Carson, L. A., Bond, W. W., and Petersen, N. J., *Pseudomonas aeruginosa:* growth in distilled water for hospitals, *Science,* 173, 836, 1971.

410. Carson, L. A., Favero, M. S., Bond, W. W., and Petersen, N. J., Morphological, biochemical, and growth characteristics of *Pseudomonas cepacia* from distilled water, *Appl. Microbiol.,* 25, 476, 1973.

411. Maki, D. G. and Martin, W. T., Nationwide epidemic of septicemia caused by contaminated infusion products. IV. Growth of microbial pathogens in fluids for intravenous infusion, *J. Infect. Dis.,* 131, 267, 1975.

412. Maki, D. G., Growth properties of microorganisms in infusion fluid and methods of detection, in *Microbiologic Hazards of Intravenous Therapy,* Phillips, I., Meers, P. D., and D'Arcy, P. F., Eds., MTP Press Ltd., Lancaster, England, 1977, 13.

413. Phillips, I., Eykyn, S., and Laker, M., Outbreak of hospital infection caused by contaminated auto-claved fluids, *Lancet*, 1, 1258, 1972.

414. Rhame, F. S., Root, R. K., MacLowry, J. D., Dadisman, T. A., and Bennett, J. V., Salmonella septicemia from platelet transfusions: study of an outbreak traced to a hematogenous carrier of *Salmonella cholerae-suis, Ann. Intern. Med.*, 78, 633, 1973.

415. Meers, P. D., Calder, M. W., Mazhar, M. M., and Lawrie, G. M., Intravenous infusion of contaminated dextrose solution: the Devonport incident, *Lancet*, 2, 1189, 1973.

416. Center for Disease Control, Septicemias associated with contaminated intravenous fluids — Wisconsin, Ohio, *Morbid. Mortal. Weekly Rep.*, 22; 99, 115, and 124; 1973.

417. Steere, A. C., Tenney, J. H., Mackel, D. C., Snyder, M. J., Polakavetz, S., Dunne, M. E., and Dixon, R. E., *Pseudomonas* species bactermia caused by contaminated normal human serum albumin, *J. Infect. Dis.*, 135, 729, 1977.

418. Siboni, K., Olsen, H., Ravn, E., Søgaard P., Hjorth, A., Nielsen, K. N., Askgaard, K., Secher, B., Borghans, J., Khing-ting, L., Joosten, H., Frederiksen, W., Jensen, K., Mortensen, N., and Sebbesen, O., *Pseudomonas cepacia* in 16 non-fatal cases of postoperative bacteremia derived from intrinsic contamination of the anaesthetic fentanyl, *Scand. J. Infect. Dis.*, 11, 39, 1979.

419. Borghans, J. G. A., Hosli, M. Th. C., Olsen, H., Ravn, E. M., Siboni, K., and Søgaard, P., *Pseudomonas cepacia* bacteraemia due to intrinsic contamination of an anaesthetic, *Acta. Pathol. Microbiol. Scand.*, 87, 15, 1979.

420. Salzman, T. C., Clark, J. J., and Klemm, L., Hand contamination of personnel as a mechanism of cross-infection in nosocomial infections with antibiotic-resistant *Escherichia coli* and *Klebsiella-Aerobacter, Antimicrob. Agents Chemother.*, 97, 1968.

421. Bruun, J. N. and Solberg, C. O., Hand carriage of gram-negative bacilli and *Staphylococcus aureus* among hospital personnel, *Br. Med. J.*, 2, 580, 1973.

422. Petersen, N. J., Collins, D. E., and Marshall, J. H., Evaluation of skin cleansing procedures using the wipe-rinse technique, *Health Lab. Sci.*, 11, 182, 1974.

423. Knittle, M. A., Eitzman, D. V., and Baer, H., Role of hand contamination of personnel in the epidemiology of gram-negative nosocomial infections, *J. Pediatr.*, 86, 433, 1975.

424. Burke, J. P., Ingall, D., Klein, J. O., Gezon, H. M., and Finland, M., *Proteus mirabilis* infections in a hospital nursery traced to a human carrier, *N. Engl. J. Med.*, 284, 115, 1971.

425. Parry, M. F., Hutchinson, J., Gofstein, R. M., Murray, R., Checko, P. J., Bruce, A., Lewis, J. N., Boer, H., Ariel, F. E., and Yeller, R. M., Nosocomial meningitis caused by *Citrobacter diversus* — Connecticut, Florida, *Morbid. Mortal. Weekly Rep.*, 28, 249, 1979.

426. Buxton, A. E., Anderson, R. L., Werdegar, D., and Atlas, E., Nosocomial respiratory tract infection and colonization with *Acinetobacter calcoaceticus:* epidemiologic characteristics, *Am. J. Med.*, 65, 507, 1978.

427. Wenzel, R. P., Hunting, K. J., Osterman, C. A., and Sande, M. A., *Providencia stuartii*, a hospital pathogen: potential factors for its emergence and transmission, *Am. J. Epidemiol.*, 104, 170, 1976.

428. Grieble, H. G., Colton, F. R., and Bird, J. J., Fine particle humidifiers: source of *Pseudomonas aeruginosa* infections in a respiratory disease unit, *N. Engl. J. Med.*, 282, 531, 1970.

429. Kelsen, S. G., McGuckin, M., Kelsen, D. P., and Cherniack, N. S., Airborne contamination of fine-particle nebulizers, *J.A.M.A.*, 237, 2311, 1977.

430. Grieble, H. G., Bird, T. J., Nidea, H. M., and Miller, C. A., Chute-hydropulping waste disposal system: a reservoir of enteric bacilli and *Pseudomonas* in a modern hospital, *J. Infect. Dis.*, 130, 602, 1974.

431. Greene, V. W., Vesley, D., Bond, R. G., and Michaelsen, G. S., Microbiological contamination of hospital air. I. Quantitative studies. II. Qualitative studies, *Appl. Microbiol.*, 10, 561, 1962.

432. Buetow, K. C., Klein, S. W., and Lane, R. B., Septicemia in premature infants: the characteristics, treatment, and prevention of septicemia in premature infants, *Am. J. Dis. Child.*, 110, 29, 1965.

433. Quie, P. G., Neonatal Septicemia, *Antibiot. Chemother. (Basel)*, 21, 128, 1976.

434. Crosson, F. J., Feder, H. M., Jr., Bocchini, J. A., Jr., Hackell, J. M., and Hackell, J. G., Neonatal sepsis at The Johns Hopkins Hospital, 1969-1975: bacterial isolates and clinical correlates, *Johns Hopkins Med. J.*, 140, 37, 1977.

435. Jeffrey, H., Mitchison, R., Wigglesworth, J. S., and Davies, P. A., Early neonatal bacteraemia: comparison of group B streptococcal, other gram-positive and gram-negative infections, *Arch. Dis. Child.*, 52, 683, 1977

436. Robbins, J. B., McCracken, G. H., Jr., Gotschlich, E. C., Ørskov, F., Ørskov, I. and Hanson, L. A., *Escherichia coli* K1 capsular polysaccharide associated with neonatal meningitis, *N. Engl. J. Med.*, 290, 1216, 1974.

437. Weinstein, R. and Young, L. S., Phagocytic resistance of *Escherichia coli* K-1 isolates and relationship to virulence, *J. Clin. Microbiol.*, 8, 748, 1978.

438. South, M. A., Enteropathogenic *Escherichia coli* disease: new developments and perspectives, *J. Pediatr.*, 79, 1, 1971.

439. Behrman, R. E., An outbreak of gastroenteritis due to *E. coli* 0142 in a neonatal nursery, *J. Pediatr.*, 86, 919, 1975.

440. Ryder, R. W., Wachsmuth, I. K., Buxton, A. E., Evans, D. G., DuPont, H. L., Mason, E., and Barrett, F. F., Infantile diarrhea produced by heat-stable enterotoxigenic *Escherichia coli*, *N. Engl. J. Med.*, 295, 849, 1976.

441. Stanton, R. E., Lindesmith, G. G., Meyer, B. W., *Escherichia coli* endocarditis after repair of ventricular septal defects, *N. Engl. J. Med.*, 279, 737, 1968.

442. Headings, D. L. and Overall, J. C., Jr., Outbreak of meningitis in a newborn intensive care unit caused by a single *Escherichia coli* K1 serotype, *J. Pediatr.*, 90, 99, 1977.

443. Horwitz, M. A. and Bennett, J. V., Nursery outbreak of peritonitis with pneumoperitoneum probably caused by thermometer-induced rectal perforation, *Am. J. Epidemiol.*, 104, 632, 1976.

444. Duma, R. J., Warner, J. F., Dalton, H. P., Septicemia from intravenous infusions, *N. Engl. J. Med.*, 284, 257, 1971.

445. Wachsmuth, I. K., Stamm, W. E., and McGowan, J. E., Jr., Prevalence of toxigenic and invasive strains of *Escherichia coli* in a hospital population, *J. Infect. Dis.*, 132, 601, 1975.

446. Shaw, D., Infection associated with modern surgical procedures, *Postgrad. Med. J.*, 48, 330, 1972.

447. Davies, P. A., Bacterial infection in the fetus and newborn, *Arch. Dis. Child.*, 46, 1, 1971.

448. Sarff, L. D., McCracken, G. H., Jr., Schiffer, M. S., Glode, M. P., Robbins, J. B., Ørskov, I. and Ørskov, F., Epidemiology of *Escherichia coli* K1 in healthy and diseased newborns, *Lancet*, 1, 1099, 1975.

449. Shooter, R. A., Crooke, E. M., Faiers, M. C., Breaden, A. L., and O'Farrell, S. M., Isolation of *Escherichia coli*, *Pseudomonas aeruginosa*, and *Klebsiella* from food in hospitals, canteens, and schools, *Lancet*, 2, 390, 1971.

450. Steinhaurer, B. W., Eickhoff, T. C., Kislak, J. W., and Finland, M., The *Klebsiella- Enterobacter-Serratia* division: clinical and epidemiologic characteristics, *Ann. Intern. Med.*, 65, 1180, 1966.

451. Edmondson, E. B. and Sanford, J. P., The *Klebsiella-Enterobacter (Aerobacter)-Serratia* group: a clinical and bacteriological evaluation, *Medicine (Baltimore)*, 46, 323, 1967.

452. Dans, P. E., Barrett, F. F., Casey, J. I., and Finland, M., *Klebsiella-Enterobacter* at Boston City Hospital, 1967, *Arch. Intern. Med.*, 125, 94, 1970.

453. Terman, J. W., Alford, R. H., Bryant, R. E., Hospital-acquired *Klebsiella* bacteremia, *Am. J. Med. Sci.*, 264, 191, 1972.

454. Umsawasdi, T., Middleman, E. A., Luna, M., and Bodey, G. P., *Klebsiella* bacteremia in cancer patients, *Am. J. Med. Sci.*, 265, 473, 1973.

455. Gardner, P. and Smith, D. H., Studies on the epidemiology of resistance (R) factors. I. Analysis of *Klebsiella* isolates in a general hospital. II. A prospective study of R factor transfer in the host, *Ann. Intern. Med.*, 71, 1, 1969.

456. Noriega, E. R., Leibowitz, R. E., Richmond, A. S., Rubinstein, E., Schaefler, S., Simberkoff, M. S., and Rahal, J. H., Jr., Nosocomial infection caused by gentamicin-resistant, streptomycin-sensitive *Klebsiella*, *J. Infect. Dis.*, 131, S45, 1975.

457. Schaberg, D. R., Weinstein, R. A., and Stamm, W. E., Epidemics of nosocomial urinary tract infection caused by multiply resistant gram-negative bacilli: epidemiology and control, *J. Infect. Dis.*, 133, 363, 1976.

458. Rennie, R. P. and Duncan, I. B. R., Emergence of gentamicin-resistant *Klebsiella* in a general hospital, *Antimicrob. Agents Chemother.*, 11, 179, 1977.

459. Thomas, F. E., Jr., Jackson, R. T., Melly, A., and Alford, R. H., Sequential hospitalwide outbreaks of resistant *Serratia* and *Klebsiella* infections, *Arch. Intern. Med.*, 137, 581, 1977.

460. Casewell, M. W., Dalton, M. T., Webster, M., and Phillips, I., Gentamicin-resistant *Klebsiella aerogenes* in a urological ward, *Lancet*, 2, 444, 1977.

461. Holzman, R. S., Florman, A. L., Podrid, P. J., Simberkoff, M. S., and Toharsky, B., Drug-associated diarrhoea as a potential reservoir for hospital infections, *Lancet*, 1, 1195, 1974.

462. Curie, K., Speller, D. C. E., Simpson, R. A., Stephens, M., and Cooke, D. I., A hospital epidemic caused by a gentamicin-resistant *Klebsiella aerogenes*, *J. Hyg. Camb.*, 80, 115, 1978.

463. Forbes, I., Gray, A., Hurse, A., and Pavillard, R., The emergence of gentamicin-resistant *Klebsiellae* in a large general hospital, *Med. J. Aust.*, 1, 14, 1977.

464. Mertz, J. J., Scharer, L., and McClement, J. H., A hospital outbreak of *Klebsiella* pneumonia from inhalation therapy with contaminated aerosol solutions, *Am. Rev. Respir. Dis.*, 95, 454, 1966.

465. Newsom, S. W. B., Hospital infection from contaminated ice, *Lancet*, 2, 620, 1968.

466. Buchholz, D. H., Young, V. M., Friedman, N. R., Reilly, J. A., and Mardiney, M. R., Jr., Bacterial proliferation in platelet products stored at room temperature: transfusion-induced enterobacter sepsis, *N. Engl. J. Med.*, 285, 429, 1971.

467. Sack, R. A., Epidemic of gram-negative organism septicemia subsequent to elective operation, *Am. J. Obstet. Gynecol.,* 107, 394, 1970.

468. Davis, A. T., Nadler, H. L., Brown, M. C., Brolnitsky, O., and Francis, B. J., Primary Bacteremia—Illinois, *Morbid. Mortal. Weekly Rep.,* 25, 110, 1976.

469. Edwards, K. E., Allen, J. R., Miller, M. J., Yogev, R., Hoffman, P. C., Klotz, R., Marubio, S., Burkholder, E., Williams, T., and Davis, A. T., *Enterobacter aerogenes* primary bacteremia in pediatric patients, *Pediatrics,* 62, 304, 1978.

470. Buxton, A. E., Anderson, R. L., Klimek, J., and Quintiliani, R., Failure of disposable domes to prevent septicemia acquired from contaminated pressure transducers, *Chest,* 74, 508, 1978.

471. Mayhall, C. G., Lamb, V. A., Gayle, W. E., Jr., and Haynes, B. W., Jr., *Enterobacer cloacae* septicemia in a burn center: epidemiology and control of an outbreak, *J. Infect. Dis.,* 139, 166, 1979.

472. Allison, M. J., Punch, J. D., and Dalton, H. P., Frequency of transferable drug resistance in clinical isolates of *Klebsiella, Aerobacter,* and *Escherichia, Antimicrob. Agents Chemother.,* 94, 1969.

473. Morse, L. J., Williams, H. L., Grenn, F. P., Jr., Eldridge. E. E., and Rotta, J. R., Septicemia due to *Klebsiella pneumoniae* originating from a handcream dispenser, *N. Engl. J. Med.,* 277, 472, 1967.

474. Weil, A. J., Ramchand, S., and Arias, M. E., Nosocomial infection with *Klebsiella* type 25, *N. Engl. J. Med.,* 275, 17, 1966.

475. Adler, J. L., Shulman, J. A., Terry, P. M., Feldman, D. B., and Skaliy, P., Nosocomial colonization with kanamycin-resistant *Klebsiella pneumoniae,* Types 2 and 11, in a premature nursery, *J. Pediatr.,* 77, 376, 1970.

476. Hable, K. A., Matsen, J. M., Wheeler, D. J., Hunt, C. E., and Quie, P. G., *Klebsiella* type 33 septicemia in an infant intensive care unit, *J. Pediatr.,* 80, 920, 1972.

477. Pierog, S., Nigam, S., Lala, R. V., Crichlow, D. K., and Evans, H. E., Neonatal septicemia due to *Klebsiella pneumoniae* type 60, *N. Y. State J. Med.,* 77, 737, 1977.

478. Cichon, M. J., Craig, C. P., Sargent, J., and Brauner, L., Nosocomial *Klebsiella* infections in an intensive care nursery, *South. Med. J.,* 70, 33, 1977.

479. Ross, B. S., Peter, G., Dempsey, J. M., and Oh, W., *Klebsiella pneumoniae* nosocomial epidemic in an intensive care nursery due to contaminated intravenous fluid, *Am. J. Dis. Child.,* 131, 712, 1977.

480. Eidelman, A. I. and Reynolds, J., Gentamicin-resistant *Klebsiella* infections in a neonatal intensive care unit, *Am. J. Dis. Child.,* 132, 421, 1978.

481. Dodson, W. H., *Serratia marcescens* septicemia, *Arch. Intern. Med.,* 121, 145, 1968.

482. Wilfert, J. N., Barrett, F. F., and Kass, E. H., Bacteremia due to *Serratia marcescens, N. Engl. J. Med.,* 279, 286, 1968.

483. Altemeier, W. A., Culbertson, W. R., Fullen, W. D., and McDonough J. J., *Serratia marcescens* septicemia, *Arch. Surg. (Chicago),* 99, 232, 1969.

484. Davis, J. T., Foltz, E., Blakemore, W. S., *Serratia marcescens:* a pathogen of increasing clinical importance, *J.A.M.A.,* 214, 2190, 1970.

485. Henjyoji, E. Y., Whitson, M. C., Ohashi, D. K., and Allen, B. D., Bacteremia due to *Serratia marcescens, J. Trauma,* 11, 417, 1971.

486. Yu, V. L., Oakes, C. A., Axnick, K. J., and Merigan, T. C., Patient factors contributing to the emergence of gentamicin-resistant *Serratia marcescens, Am. J. Med.,* 66, 468, 1979.

487. Allen, S. D. and Conger, K. B., *Serratia marcescens* infection of the urinary tract: a nosocomial infection, *J. Urol.,* 101, 621, 1969.

488. Maki, D. G., Hennekens, C. G., Phillips, C. W., Shaw, W. V., and Bennett, J. V., Nosocomial urinary tract infection with *Serratia marcescens:* an epidemiologic study, *J. Infect. Dis.,* 128, 579, 1973.

489. Farmer, J. J., III, Davis, B. R., Hickman, F. W., Presley, D. B., Bodey, G. P., Negut, M., and Bobo, R. A., Detection of *Serratia* outbreaks in hospital, *Lancet,* 2, 455, 1976.

490. Schaberg, D. R., Alford, R. H., Anderson, R., Farmer, J. J., III, Melly, M. A., and Schaffner, W., An outbreak of nosocomial infection due to multiply resistant *Serratia marcescens:* evidence of interhospital spread, *J. Infect. Dis.,* 134, 181, 1976.

491. Ringrose, R. E., McKown, B., Felton, F. G., Barclay, B. O., Muchmore, H. G., and Rhoades, E. R., A hospital outbreak of *Serratia marcescens* associated with ultrasonic nebulizers, *Ann. Intern. Med.,* 69, 719, 1968.

492. Cabrera, H. A., An outbreak of *Serratia marcescens,* and its control, *Arch. Intern. Med.,* 123, 650, 1969.

493. Sanders, C. V., Jr., Luby, J. P., Johanson, W. G., Barnett, J. A., and Sanford, J. P., *Serratia marcescens* infections from inhalation therapy medications: nosocomial outbreak, *Ann. Intern. Med.,* 73, 15, 1970.

494. Webb, S. F. and Vall-Spinosa, A., Outbreak of *Serratia marcescens* associated with the flexible fiberbronchoscope, *Chest,* 68, 703, 1975.

495. Stenderup, A., Faergeman, O., and Ingerslev, M., *Serratia marcescens* infections in premature infants, *Acta Pathol. Microbiol. Scand.,* 68, 157, 1966.

496. Cardos, S. F., Florman, A. L., Simberkoff, M. S., and Lanier, L., *Serratia marcescens:* use of detailed characterization of strains to evaluate an increase of isolates in an intensive care unit, *Am. J. Med. Sci.,* 266, 447, 1973.

497. Walton, J. R., Shapiro, B. A., Harrison, R. A., Davison, R., and Reisberg, B. E., *Serratia* bacteremia from mean arterial pressure monitors, *Anesthesiology,* 43, 113, 1975.

498. Stamm, W. E., Kolff, C. A., Dones, E. M., Javariz, R., Anderson, R. L., Farmer, J. J., III, and Rivera de Quinones, H., A nursery outbreak caused by *Serratia marcescens* — scalp-vein needles as a portal of entry, *J. Pediatr.,* 89, 96, 1976.

499. West, C. M., Wayle, B., Touneson, A., et al., Nosocomial *Serratia marcescens* bacteremia associated with reuse of disposable pressure monitoring domes (abstract), 17th Interscience Conf. on Antimicrobial Agents and Chemotherapy, 1977, 429.

500. Donowitz, L. G., Marsik, F. J., Hoyt, J. W., and Wenzel, R. P., Control of nosocomial *Serratia marcescens* bacteremia traced to contaminated pressure transducers, *J.A.M.A.,* 242, 1749, 1979.

501. Lewis, J. and Fekety, F. R., Jr., Proteus bacteremia, *Bull. Johns Hopkins Hosp.,* 116, 151, 1969.

502. Adler, J. L., Burke, J. P., Martin, D. F., and Finland, M., Proteus infections in a general hospital. II. Some clinical and epidemiological characteristics, *Ann. Intern. Med.,* 75, 531, 1971.

503. Lorian, V. and Topf, B., Microbiology of nosocomial infections, *Arch. Intern. Med.,* 130, 104, 1972.

504. Center for Disease Control, *Proteeae, National Nosocomial Infections Study Quarterly Report, Third Quarter 1972,* 1973, 18.

505. Washington, J. A., II. Senjem, D. H., Haldorson, A., Schutt, A. H., and Martin, W. J., Nosocomially acquired bacteriuria due to *Proteus rettgeri* and *Providencia stuartii, Am. J. Clin. Pathol.,* 60, 836, 1973.

506. Edwards, L. D., Cross, A., Levin, S., and Landau, W., Outbreak of a nosocomial infection with a strain of *Proteus rettgeri* resistant to many antimicrobials, *Am. J. Clin. Pathol.,* 61, 41, 1974.

507. Lindsey, J. O., Martin, W. T., Sonnenwirth, A. C., and Bennett, J. V., An outbreak of nosocomial *Proteus rettgeri* urinary tract infection, *Am. J. Epidemiol.,* 103, 261, 1976.

508. Kaslow, R. A., Lindsey, J. O., Bisno, A. L., and Price, A., Nosocomial infection with highly resistant *Proteus rettgeri:* report of an epidemic, *Am. J. Epidemiol.,* 104, 278, 1976.

509. Whiteley, G. R., Penner, J. L., Stewart, I. O., Stokan, P. C., and Hinton, N. A., Nosocomial urinary tract infections caused by two O-serotypes of *Providencia stuartii* in one hospital, *J. Clin. Microbiol.,* 6, 551, 1977.

510. Yoshikawa, T. T., Shibata, S. A., Chow, A. W., and Guze, L. B., Outbreak of multiply drug-resistant *Proteus mirabilis* originating in a surgical intensive care unit: in vitro susceptibility pattern, *Antimicrob. Agents Chemother.,* 13, 177, 1978.

511. Curreri, P. W., Bruck, H. M., Lindberg, R. B., Mason, A. D., and Pruitt, B. A., *Providencia stuartii* sepsis: a new challenge in the treatment of thermal injury, *Ann. Surg. (Chicago),* 177, 133, 1973.

512. Shulman, J. A., Terry, P. M., and Hough, C. E., Colonization with gentamicin-resistant *Pseudomonas aeruginosa,* pyocine type 5, in a burn unit, *J. Infect. Dis.,* 124, S18, 1971.

513. Lowbury, E. J. L., Babb, J. R., and Roe, E., Clearance from a hospital of gram-negative bacilli that transfer carbenicillin-resistance to *Pseudomonas aeruginosa, Lancet,* 2, 941, 1972.

514. Greene, W. H., Moody, M., Schimpff, S., Young, V. M., and Wiernik, P. H., *Pseudomonas aeruginosa* resistant to carbenicillin and gentamicin, *Ann. Intern. Med.,* 79, 684, 1973.

515. Meyer, R. D., Lewis, R. P., Halter, J., and White, M., Gentamicin-resistant *Pseudomonas aeruginosa* and *Serratia marcescens* in a general hospital, *Lancet,* 1, 580, 1976.

516. Gaman, W., Cates, C., Snelling, C. F. T., Lank, B., and Ronald, A. R., Emergence of gentamicin- and carbenicillin-resistant *Pseudomonas aeruginosa* in a hospital environment, *Antimicrob. Agents Chemother.,* 9, 474, 1976.

517. Baird, I. M., Slepack, J. M., Kauffman, C. A., and Phair, J. P., Nosocomial infection with gentamicin-carbenicillin-resistant *Pseudomonas aeruginosa, Antimicrob. Agents Chemother.,* 10, 626, 1976.

518. Guerrant, R. L., Strausbaugh, L. J., Wenzel, R. P., Hamory, B. H., and Sande, M. A., Nosocomial bloodstream infections caused by gentamicin-resistant gram-negative bacilli, *Am. J. Med.,* 62, 894, 1977.

519. Keys, T. F. and Washington, J. A., II, Gentamicin-resistant *Pseudomonas aeruginosa:* Mayo Clinic experience, 1970-1976, *Mayo Clin. Proc.,* 52, 797, 1977.

520. Roberts, N. J., Jr. and Douglas, R. G., Jr., Gentamicin use and *Pseudomonas* and *Serratia* resistance: effect of a surgical prophylaxis regimen, *Antimicrob. Agents Chemother.,* 13, 214, 1978.

521. Block, C. S., Gentamicin-resistant gram-negative bacilli in hospital patients. I. Preliminary epidemiological assessment, *S. Afr. Med. J.,* 53, 391, 1978.

522. Ruben, F. L., Norden, C. W., and Hruska, E., Factors associated with acquisition of *Pseudomonas aeruginosa* resistant to gentamicin, *Am. J. Med. Sci.,* 275, 173, 1978.

523. Kauffman, C. A., Ramundo, N. C., Williams, S. G., Dey, C. R., Phair, J. P., and Watanakunakorn, C., Surveillance of gentamicin-resistant gram-negative bacilli in a general hospital, *Antimicrob. Agents Chemother.*, 13, 918, 1978.

524. Whitby, J. L. and Rampling, A., *Pseudomonas aeruginosa* contamination in domestic and hospital environments, *Lancet*, 1, 15, 1972.

525. Pickett, M. J. and Pedersen, M. M., Nonfermentative bacilli associated with man. II. Detection and identification, *Am. J. Clin. Pathol.*, 54, 164, 1970.

526. Pedersen, M. M., Marso, E., and Pickett, M. J., Nonfermentative bacilli associated with man. III. Pathogenicity and antibiotic susceptibility, *Am. J. Clin. Pathol.*, 54, 178, 1970.

527. Ederer, G. M. and Matsen, J. M., Colonization and infection with *Pseudomonas cepacia*, *J. Infect. Dis.*, 125, 613, 1972.

528. Gilardi, G. L., Infrequently encountered *Pseudomonas* species causing infections in humans, *Ann. Intern. Med.*, 77, 211, 1972.

529. Young, L. S. and Armstrong, D., *Pseudomonas aeruginosa* infections, *CRC Crit. Rev. Clin. Lab. Sci.*, September, 1972, 291.

530. Baltch, A. L. and Griffin, P. E., *Pseudomonas aerugnosa:* pyocine types and clinical experience with infections in a general hospital, *Am. J. Med. Sci.*, 264, 233, 1972.

531. Schimpff, S. C., Green, W. H., Young, V. M., and Wiernik, P. H., *Pseudomonas* septicemia: incidence, epidemiology, prevention and therapy in patients with advanced cancer, *Eur. J. Cancer*, 9, 449, 1973.

532. Levine, A. S., Wood, R. E., Zierdt, C. H., Dale, D. C., and Pennington, J. E., *Pseudomonas aeruginosa* infections: persisting problems and current research to find new therapies, *Ann. Intern. Med.*, 82, 819, 1975.

533. Flick, M. R. and Cluff, L. E., *Pseudomonas* bacteremia: review of 108 cases, *Am. J. Med.*, 60, 501, 1976.

534. Bodey, G. P., Epidemiological studies of *Pseudomonas* species in patients with leukemia, *Am. J. Med. Sci.*, 260, 82, 1970.

535. Moody, M. R., Young, V. M., Kenton, D. M., and Vermeulen, G. D., *Pseudomonas aeruginosa* in a center for cancer research. I. Distribution of intraspecies types from human and environmental sources, *J. Infect. Dis.*, 125, 95, 1972.

536. Bruun, J. N., McGarrity, G. J., Blakemore, W. S., and Coriell, L. L., Epidemiology of *Pseudomonas aeruginosa* infections: determination by pyocin typing, *J. Clin. Microbiol.*, 3, 264, 1976.

537. Kominos, S. D., Copeland, C. E., Grosiak, B., and Postic, B., Introduction of *Pseudomonas aeruginosa* into a hospital via vegetables, *Appl. Microbiol.*, 24, 567, 1972.

538. McLeod, J. W., The hospital urine bottle and bedpan as reservoirs of infection by *Pseudomonas pyocyanea*, *Lancet*, 1, 394, 1958.

539. Falkiner, F. R., Keane, C. T., Dalton, M., Clancy, M. T., and Jacoby, G. A., Cross infection in a surgical ward caused by *Pseudomonas aeruginosa* with transferable resistance to gentamicin and tobramycin, *J. Clin. Pathol.*, 30, 731, 1977.

540. Marrie, T. J., Major, H., Gurwith, M., Ronald, A., Harding, G. K., Forrest, G., and Forsythe, W., Prolonged outbreak of nosocomial urinary tract infection with a single strain of *Pseudomonas aeruginosa*, *Can. Med. Assoc. J.*, 119, 593, 1978.

541. Moore, B. and Forman, A., An outbreak of urinary *Pseudomonas aeruginosa* infection acquired during urological operations, *Lancet*, 2, 929, 1966.

542. Baird, R. M. and Shooter, R. A., *Pseudomonas aeruginosa* infections associated with use of contaminated medicaments, *Br. Med. J.*, 2, 349, 1976.

543. Corbett, J. J. and Rosenstein, B. J., Pseudomonas meningitis related to spinal anesthesia, *Neurology*, 21, 946, 1971.

544. Thomas, E. T., Jones, L. F., Simao, E., Sole-Vernin, C., and Farmer, J. J., III, Epidemiology of *Pseudomonas aeruginosa* in a general hospital: a one-year study, *J. Clin. Microbiol.*, 2, 397, 1975.

545. Shickman, M. D., Guze, L. B., and Pearce, M. L., Bacteremia following cardiac catheterization. Report of a case and studies on the source, *N. Engl. J. Med.*, 260, 1164, 1959.

546. Barrie, D., Incubator-borne *Pseudomonas pyocyanea* infection in a newborn nursery, *Arch. Dis. Child.*, 40, 555, 1965.

547. Sutter, V. L., Hurst, V., Grossman, M., and Calonje, R., Source and significance of *Pseudomonas aeruginosa* in sputum: patients requiring tracheal suction, *J.A.M.A.*, 197, 132, 1966.

548. Rubbo, S. D., Gardner, J. F., and Franklin, J. C., Source of *Pseudomonas aeruginosa* infection in premature infants, *J. Hyg. Camb.*, 64, 121, 1966.

549. McNamara, M. J., Hill, M. C., Balows, A., and Tucker, E. B., A study of the bacteriologic patterns of hospital infections, *Ann. Intern. Med.*, 66, 480, 1967.

550. Fierer, J., Taylor, P. M., and Gezon, H. M., *Pseudomonas aeruginosa* epidemic traced to delivery-room resuscitators, *N. Engl. J. Med.*, 276, 991, 1967.

551. Phillips, I., *Pseudomonas aeruginosa* respiratory tract infections in patients receiving mechanical ventilation, *J. Hyg. Camb.*, 65, 229, 1967.

552. Tinne, J. E., Gordon, A. M., Bain, W. H., and Mackey, W. A., Cross-infection by *Pseudomonas aeruginosa* as a hazard of intensive surgery, *Br. Med. J.*, 4, 313, 1967.

553. Lowbury, E. J. L., Thom, B. T., Lilly, H. A., Babb, J. R., and Whittall, K., Sources of infection with *Pseudomonas aeruginosa* in patients with tracheostomy, *J. Med. Microbiol.*, 3, 39, 1970.

554. Drewett, S. E., Payne, D. J. H., Tuke, W., and Verdon, P. E., Eradication of *Pseudomonas aeruginosa* infection from a special-care nursery, *Lancet*, 1, 946, 1972.

555. Olds, J. W., Kisch, A. L., Eberle, B. J., and Wilson, J. N., *Pseudomonas aeruginosa* respiratory tract infection acquired from a contaminated anesthesia machine, *Am. Rev. Respir. Dis.*, 105, 628, 1972.

556. Bobo, R. A., Newton, E. J., Jones, L. F., Farmer, L. H., and Farmer, J. J., III, Nursery outbreak of *Pseudomonas aeruginosa:* epidemiological conclusions from five different typing methods, *Appl. Microbiol.*, 25, 414, 1973.

557. Tinne, J. E., Persistence of a specific *Pseudomonas* infection in a large general hospital, *Scott. Med. J.*, 22, 16, 1977.

558. Cross, D. F., Benchimol, A., and Dimond, E. G., The faucet aerator — a source of *Pseudomonas* infection, *N. Engl. J. Med.*, 274, 1430, 1966.

559. Teres, D., Schweers, P., Bushnell, L. S., Hedley-Whyte, J., and Feingold, D. S., Sources of *Pseudomonas aeruginosa* infection in a respiratory/surgical intensive-therapy unit, *Lancet*, 1, 415, 1973.

560. Sussman, M. and Stevens, J., *Pseudomonas pyocyanea* wound infection: an outbreak in an orthopaedic unit, *Lancet*, 2, 734, 1960.

561. Ayliffe, G. A. J., Lowbury, E. J. L., Hamilton, J. G., Small, J. M., Asheshov, E. A., and Parker, M. T., Hospital infection with *Pseudomonas aeruginosa* in neurosurgery, *Lancet*, 2, 365, 1965.

562. Thom, A. R., *Pseudomonas aeruginosa* infection in a neonatal nursery, possibly transmitted by a breast-milk pump, *Lancet*, 1, 560, 1970.

563. Lowbury, E. J. L. and Fox, J. The epidemiology of infection with *Pseudomonas pyocyanea* in a burn unit, *J. Hyg. (Camb.)*, 52, 403, 1954.

564. Kominos, S. D., Copeland, C. E., and Grosiak, B., Mode of transmission of *Pseudomonas aeruginosa* in a burn unit and an intensive care unit in a general hospital, *Appl. Microbiol.*, 23, 309, 1972.

565. Knights, H. T., France, D. R., and Harding, S., *Pseudomonas aeruginosa* cross infection in a neonatal unit, *N.Z. Med. J.*, 67, 617, 1968.

566. Brown, D. G. and Baublis, J., Reservoirs of *Pseudomonas* in an intensive care unit for newborn infants: mechanisms of control, *J. Pediatr.*, 90, 453, 1977.

567. Morehead, C. D. and Houck, P. W., Epidemiology of *Pseudomonas* infections in a pediatric intensive care unit, *Am. J. Dis. Child.*, 124, 564, 1972.

568. Weinstein, R. A., Stamm, W. E., Kramer, L., and Corey, L., Pressure monitoring devices: overlooked source of nosocomial infection, *J.A.M.A.*, 236, 936, 1976.

569. Center for Disease Control, The infection hazards of pressure monitoring devices, *National Nosocomial Infections Study Report, Annual Summary 1974*, 1977, 15.

570. Favero, M. S., Petersen, N. J., Boyer, K. M., Carson, L. A., and Bond, W. W., Microbial contamination of renal dialysis systems and associated health risks, *Trans. Am. Soc. Artif. Intern. Organs*, XX-A, 175, 1974.

571. Center for Disease Control, An outbreak of bacteremia and pyrogenic reactions in a dialysis unit — Pennsylvania, *Morbid. Mortal. Weekly Rep.*, 27, 307, 1978.

572. Uman, S. J., Johnson, C. E., Beirne, G. J., and Kunin, C. M., *Pseudomonas aeruginosa* bacteremia in a dialysis unit. I. Recognition of cases, epidemiologic studies and attempts at control, *Am. J. Med.*, 62, 667, 1977.

573. Wagnild, J. P., McDonald, P., Craig, W. A., Johnson, C., Hanley, M., Uman, S. J., Ramgopal, V., and Beirne, G. J., *Pseudomonas aeruginosa* bacteremia in a dialysis unit. II. Relationship to reuse of coils, *Am. J. Med.*, 62, 672, 1977.

574. Phillips, I., Eyken, S., Curtis, M. A., and Snell, J. J. S., *Pseudomonas cepacia* (multivorans) septicaemia in an intensive-care unit, *Lancet*, 1, 375, 1971.

575. Speller, D. C. E., Stephens, M. E., and Viant, A. C., Hospital infection by *Pseudomonas cepacia*, *Lancet*, 1, 798, 1971.

576. Meyer, G. W., *Pseudomonas cepacia* septicemia associated with intravenous therapy, *West. J. Med.*, 119, 15, 1973.

577. Thong, M. L. and Kay, L. K., Septicaemia from prolonged intravenous infusions, *Arch. Dis. Child.*, 50, 886, 1975.

578. Cabrera, H. A. and Drake, M. A., An epidemic in a coronary care unit caused by *Pseudomonas* species, *Am. J. Clin. Pathol.*, 64, 700, 1975.

579. Weinstein, R. A., Emori, T. G., Anderson, R. L., and Stamm, W. E., Pressure transducers as a source of bacteremia after open heart surgery: report of an outbreak and guidelines for prevention, *Chest*, 69, 338, 1976.

580. Frank, M. J. and Schaffner, W., Contaminated aqueous benzalkonium chloride: an unnecessary hospital infection hazard, *J.A.M.A.*, 236, 2418, 1976.

581. Rhame, F. S. and McCullough, J., Nosocomial *Pseudomonas cepacia* infection, *Morbid. Mortal. Weekly Rep.*, 28, 289, 1979.

582. Kuehnel, E. and Lundh, H., Outbreak of *Pseudomonas cepacia* bacteremia related to contaminated reused coils, *Dial. Transplant.*, 5, 44, 1976.

583. Rapkin, R. H., *Pseudomonas cepacia* in an intensive care nursery, *Pediatrics*, 57, 239, 1976.

584. Mitchell, R. G., and Hayward, A. C., Postoperative urinary tract infections caused by contaminated irrigating fluid, *Lancet*, 1, 793, 1966.

585. Burdon, D. W. and Whitby, J. L., Contamination of hospital disinfectant with *Pseudomonas* species, *Br. Med. J.*, 2, 153, 1967.

586. Bassett, D. C. J., Stokes, K. J., and Thomas, W. R. G., Wound infection with *Pseudomonas multivorans*, *Lancet*, 1, 1188, 1970.

587. Hardy, P. C., Ederer, G. M., and Matsen, J. M., Contamination of commercially packaged urinary catheter kits with Pseudomonad EO-1, *N. Engl. J. Med.*, 282, 33, 1970.

588. Mackel, D. C., Contamination of disposal catheter kits with EO-1, *N. Engl. J. Med.*, 282, 752, 1970.

589. Wishart, M. M. and Riley, T. V., Infection with *Pseudomonas maltophilia* hospital outbreak due to contaminated disinfectant, *Med. J. Aust.*, 2, 710, 1976.

590. Dixon, R. E., Kaslow, R. A., Mackel, D. C., Fulkerson, C. C., and Mallison, G. F., Aqueous quarternary ammonium antiseptics and disinfectants, *J.A.M.A.*, 236, 2415, 1976.

591. Center for Disease Control, Laboratory aspects in the control of nosocomial infections, *Flavobacterium sp.*, *National Nosocomial Infections Study Quarterly Report Third & Fourth Quarters 1973*, 1975, 34.

592. Olsen, H., *Flavobacterium meningosepticum* isolated from outside hospital surroundings and during examination of patient specimens, *Acta Pathol. Microbiol. Scand.*, 75, 313, 1969.

593. Cabrera, H. A. and Davis, G. H., Epidemic meningitis of the newborn caused by *Flavobacteria*. I. Epidemiology and bacteriology, *Am. J. Dis. Child.*, 101, 289, 1961.

594. Plotkin, S. A. and McKitrick, J. C., Nosocomial meningitis of the newborn caused by a *Flavobacterium*, *J.A.M.A.*, 198, 194, 1966.

595. Hazuka, B. T., Dajani, A. S., Talbot, K., and Keen, B. M., Two outbreaks of *Flavobacterium meningosepticum* type E in a neonatal intensive care unit, *J. Clin. Microbiol.*, 6, 450, 1977.

596. Madruga, M., Zanon, U., Pereira, G. M. N., and Galvao, A. C., Meningitis caused by *Flavobacterium meningosepticum*. The first epidemic outbreak of meningitis in the newborn in South America, *J. Infect. Dis.*, 121, 328, 1970.

597. Olsen, H., Frederiksen, W. C., and Siboni, K. E., *Flavobacterium meningosepticum* in 8 non-fatal cases of postoperative bacteraemia, *Lancet*, 1, 1294, 1965.

598. Olsen, H., An epidemiological study of hospital infection with *Flavobacterium meningosepticum*, *Dan. Med. Bull.*, 14, 6, 1967.

599. Stamm, W. E., Colella, J. J., Anderson, R. L., and Dixon, R. E., Indwelling arterial catheters as a source of nosocomial bacteremia. An outbreak caused by *Flavobacterium* species, *N. Engl. J. Med.*, 292, 1099, 1975.

600. Coyle-Gilchrist, M. M., Crewe, P. and Roberts, G., *Flavobacterium meningosepticum* in the hospital environment, *J. Clin. Pathol.*, 29, 824, 1976.

601. Taplin, D., Rebell, G., and Zaias, N., The human skin as a source of *Mima-Herellea* infections, *J.A.M.A.*, 186, 952, 1963.

602. Glew, R. H., Moellering, R. C., Jr., and Kunz, L. J., Infections with *Acinetobacter calcoaceticus* (*Herellea-vaginicola*): clinical and laboratory studies, *Medicine (Baltimore)*, 56, 79, 1977.

603. Rosenthal, S. L. and Freundlich, L. F., The clinical significance of *Acinetobacter* species, *Health Lab. Sci.*, 14, 194, 1977.

604. Donald, W. D. and Doak, W. M., Mimeae meningitis and sepsis, *J.A.M.A.*, 200, 111, 1967.

605. Daly, A. K., Postic, B., and Kass, E. H., Infections due to organisms of the genus *Herellea*, *Arch. Intern. Med.*, 110, 580, 1962.

606. Graber, C. D., Rabin, E. R., Mason, A. D., Jr., and Vogel, E. H., Jr., Increasing incidence of nosocomial *Herellea vaginicola* infection in burned patients, *Surg. Gynecol. Obstet.*, 114, 109, 1962.

607. Reynolds, R. C. and Cluff, L. E., Infection of man with *Mimeae*, *Ann. Intern. Med.*, 58, 759, 1963.

608. Robinson, R. G., Garrison, R. G., and Brown, R. W., Evaluation of the clinical significance of the genus *Herellea*, *Ann. Intern. Med.*, 60, 19, 1964.

609. Inclan, A. P., Massey, L. C., Crook, B. G., and Bell, J. S., Organisms of the tribe *Mimeae*: incidence of isolation and clinical correlation at the City of Memphis Hospitals, *South. Med. J.*, 58, 1261, 1965.

610. Green, G. S., Johnson, R. H., Jr., and Shively, J. A., *Mimeae:* opportunistic pathogens, *J.A.M.A.*, 194, 163, 1965.
611. Ramphal, R. and Kluge, R. M., *Acinetobacter calcoaceticus* variety *anitratus:* an increasing nosocomial problem, *Am. J. Med. Sci.*, 277, 57, 1979.
612. Retailliau, H. F., Hightower, A. W., Dixon, R. E., and Allen, J. R., *Acinetobacter calcoaceticus:* a nosocomial pathogen with an unusual seasonal pattern, *J. Infect. Dis.*, 139, 371, 1979.
613. Castle, M., Tenney, J. H., Weinstein, M. P., Eickhoff, T. C., Outbreak of a multiply resistant *Acinetobacter* in a surgical intensive care unit: epidemiology and control, *Heart Lung*, 7, 641, 1978.
614. Abrutyn, E., Goodhart, G. L., Roos, K., Anderson, R., and Buxton, A., *Acinetobacter calcoaceticus* outbreak associated with peritoneal dialysis, *Am. J. Epidemiol.*, 107, 328, 1978.
615. Snydman, D. R., Maloy, M. F., Brock, S. M., Lyons, R. W., and Rubin, S. J., Pseudobacteremia: false-positive blood cultures from mist tent contamination, *Am. J. Epidemiol.*, 106, 154, 1977.
616. Smith, P. W. and Massanari, R. M., Room humidifiers as the source of *Acinetobacter* infections, *J.A.M.A.*, 237, 795, 1977.
617. Schroeder, S. A., Aserkoff, B., and Brachman, P. S., Epidemic salmonellosis in hospitals and institutions: a five-year review, *N. Engl. J. Med.*, 279, 674, 1968.
618. Baine, W. B., Gangarosa, E. J., Bennett, J. V., and Barker, W. H., Jr., Institutional salmonellosis, *J. Infect. Dis.*, 128, 357, 1973.
619. Sanders, E., Sweeney, F. J., Jr., Friedman, E. A., Boring, J. R., Randall, E. L., and Polk, L. D., An outbreak of hospital-associated infections due to *Salmonella derby*, *J.A.M.A.*, 186, 984, 1963.
620. Sweeney, F. J., Jr. and Randall, E. L., Clinical and epidemiological studies of *Salmonella derby* infections in a general hospital, in *Proceedings, National Conference on Salmonellosis, March 11-13, 1964*, (U.S. Public Health Service Publ. No. 1262), Government Printing Office, Washington, D.C., 1965, 130.
621. Sokol, E. M., *Salmonella derby* infections after gastrointestinal surgery, *J. Mt. Sinai Hosp., N.Y.*, 33, 36, 1965.
622. McCall, C. E., Collins, R. N., Jones, D. B., Kaufmann, A. F., and Brachman, P. S., *Am. J. Epidemiol.*, 84, 32, 1966.
623. Lang, D. J., Kunz, L. J., Martin, A. R., Schroeder, S. A., Thomson, L. A., Carmine as a source of nosocomial Salmonellosis, *N. Engl. J. Med.*, 276, 829, 1967.
624. Lang, D. J., Schroeder, S. A., Kunz, L. J., Thompson, L. A., Hobbs, B. C., and Butler, N. J., Salmonella-contaminated carmine dye. Another example of in-plant contamination during processing, *Am. J. Public Health*, 61, 1615, 1971.
625. Steere, A. C., Craven, P. J., Hall, W. J., III, Leotsakis, N., Wells, J. G., Farmer, J. J., III, Gangarosa, E. J., Person-to-person spread of *Salmonella typhimurium* after a hospital common-source outbreak, *Lancet*, 1, 319, 1975.
626. Center for Disease Control, Epidemiologic aspects of nursery Salmonellosis, National Nosocomial Infections Study Report May 1970, 1970, 15.
627. Hook, E. W., Salmonellosis: certain factors influencing the interaction of *Salmonella* and the human host, *Bull. N.Y. Acad. Med.*, 37, 499, 1961.
628. Han, T., Soral, J. E., and Neter, E., Salmonellosis in disseminated malignant diseases: a seven-year review (1959-1965), *N. Engl. J. Med.*, 276, 1045, 1967.
629. Cherubin, C. E., Fodor, T., Denmark, L. I., Master, C. S., Fuerst, H. T., and Winter, J. W., Symptoms, septicemia and death in salmonellosis, *Am. J. Epidemiol.*, 90, 285, 1969.
630. Wolfe, M. S., Armstrong, D., Louria, D. B., and Blevins, A., Salmonellosis in patients with neoplastic disease, *Arch. Intern. Med.*, 128, 546, 1971.
631. Center for Disease Control, Nosocomial Salmonellosis—2 outbreaks, National Nosocomial Infections Study Quarterly Report, First & Second Quarters, 1973, 1974, 13.
632. Lintz, D., Kapila, R., Pilgrim, E., Tecson, F., Dorn, R., and Louria, D., Nosocomial *Salmonella* epidemic, *Arch. Intern. Med.*, 136, 968, 1976.
633. Chmel, H. and Armstrong, D., Salmonella oslo: a focal outbreak in a hospital, *Am. J. Med.*, 60, 203, 1976.
634. Rice, P. A., Craven, P. C., and Wells, J. G., Salmonella heidelberg enteritis and bacteremia, *Am. J. Med.*, 60, 509, 1976.
635. Pankey, G. A. and Daloviso, J. R., Fungemia caused by torulopsis glabrata, *Medicine (Baltimore)*, 52, 395, 1973.
636. Young, R. C., Bennett, J. E., Geelhoed, G. W., and Levine, A. S., Fungemia with compromised host resistance: a study of 70 cases, *Ann. Intern. Med.*, 80, 605, 1974.
637. Meyer, R. D., Rosen, P., and Armstrong, D., Phycomycosis complicating leukemia and lymphoma, *Ann. Intern. Med.*, 77, 871, 1972.
638. Meyer, R. D., Young, L. S., Armstrong, D., and Uy, B., Aspergillosis complicating neoplastic disease, *Am. J. Med.*, 54, 6, 1973.

639. **Agger, W. A. and Maki, D. G.,** Mucormycosis: a complication of critical care, *Arch. Intern. Med.,* 138, 925, 1978.
640. **Plouffe, J. F., Brown, D. G., Silva, J., Jr., Eck, T., Stricof, R. L., and Fekety, R., Jr.,** Nosocomial outbreak of *Candida parapsilosis* fungemia related to intravenous infusions, *Arch. Intern. Med.,* 137, 1686, 1977.
641. **Rose, H. D.,** Mechanical control of hospital ventilation and *Aspergillus* infections, *Am. Rev. Respir. Dis.,* 105, 306, 1972.
642. **Burton, J. R., Zachery, J. B., Bessin, R., Rathbun, H. K., Greenough, W. B., III, Sterioff, S., Wright, J. R., Slavin, R. E., and Williams, G. M.,** Aspergillosis in four renal transplant recipients: diagnosis and effective treatment with amphotericin B, *Ann. Intern. Med.,* 77, 383, 1972.
643. **Aisner, J., Schimpff, S. C., Bennett, J. E., Young, V. M., and Wiernik, P. H.,** *Aspergillus* infections in cancer patients: association with fireproofing materials in a new hospital, *J.A.M.A.,* 235, 411, 1976.
644. **Kyriakides, G. K., Zinneman, H. H., Hall, W. H., Arora, V. K., Lifton, J., DeWolf, W. C., and Miller, J.,** Immunologic monitoring and aspergillosis in renal transplant patients, *Am. J. Surg.,* 131, 246, 1976.
645. **Arnow, P. M., Andersen, R. L., Mainous, P. D., and Smith, E. J.,** Pulmonary aspergillosis during hospital renovation, *Am. Rev. Respir. Dis.,* 118, 49, 1978.
646. **Gage, A. A., Dean, D. C., Schimert, G., Minsley, N.,** *Aspergillus* infection after cardiac surgery, *Arch. Surg. (Chicago),* 101, 384, 1970.
647. **Hall, W. J., III,** Penicillium endocarditis following open heart surgery and prosthetic valve insertion, *Am. Heart J.,* 87, 501, 1974.
648. **Bennett, J. E.,** Prevention of hospital-acquired systemic mycoses, *Prev. Med.,* 3, 515, 1974.
649. **Tynes, B. S. and Utz, J. P.,** Fusobacterium septicemia, *Am. J. Med.,* 30, 879, 1960.
650. **Gelb, A. F. and Seligman, S. J.,** Bacteroidaceae bacteremia: effect of age and focus of infection upon clinical course, *J.A.M.A.,* 212, 1038, 1970.
651. **Bodner, S. J., Koenig, M. G., and Goodman, J. S.,** Bacteremic bacteroides infections, *Ann. Intern. Med.,* 73, 537, 1970.
652. **Felner, J. M. and Dowell, V. R., Jr.,** Anaerobic bacterial endocarditis, *N. Engl. J. Med.,* 283, 1188, 1970.
653. **Kagnoff, M. F., Armstrong, D., and Blevins, A.,** *Bacteroides* bacteremia: experience in a hospital for neoplastic diseases, *Cancer,* 29, 245, 1972.
654. **Chow, A. W. and Guze, L. B.,** *Bacteroidaceae* bacteremia: clinical experience with 112 patients, *Medicine, (Baltimore),* 53, 93, 1974.
655. **Chow, A. W., Leake, R. D., Yamauchi, T., Anthony, B. F., and Guze, L. B.,** The significance of anaerobes in neonatal bacteremia: analysis of 23 cases and review of the literature, *Pediatrics,* 54, 736, 1974.
656. **Lynch, J. M., Anderson, A., Camacho, F. R., Winters, A. K., Hodges, G. R., and Barnes, W. G.,** Pseudobacteremia caused by *Clostridium sordellii, Arch. Intern. Med.,* 1979, in press.
657. **Bradley, J. M., Szawatkowski, M., Noone, P., Howard, F. M., and Flynn, D. M.,** Clostridia in necrotising enterocolitis, *Lancet,* 1, 389, 1978.
658. **Roback, S. A., Foker, J., Frantz, I. V., Hunt, C. E., Engel, R. R., and Leonard, A. S.,** Necrotizing enterocolitis: an emerging entity in the regional infant intensive care facility, *Arch. Surg. (Chicago),* 109, 314, 1974.
659. **Santulli, T. V., Schullinger, J. N., Heird, W. C., Gongaware, R. D., Wigger, J., Barlow, B., Blanc, W. A., and Berdon, W. E.,** Acute necrotizing enterocolitis in infancy: a review of 64 cases, *Pediatrics,* 55, 376, 1975.
660. **Kliegman, R. M.,** Neonatal necrotizing enterocolitis: implications for an infectious disease, *Pediatr. Clin. North Am.,* 26, 327, 1979.
661. **Virnig, N. L. and Reynolds, J. W.,** Epidemiological aspects of neonatal necrotizing enterocolitis, *Am. J. Dis. Child.,* 128, 186, 1974.
662. **Engel, R.,** Report of 68th Ross Conference on Pediatric Research, 1974, 66.
663. **Waldhausen, J. A., Herendeen, T., and King, H.,** Necrotizing colitis of the newborn: common cause of perforation of the colon, *Pediatr. Surg.,* 54, 365, 1963.
664. **Stein, H., Beck, J., Solomon, A., and Schaman, A.,** Gastroenteritis with necrotizing enterocolitis in premature babies, *Br. Med. J.,* 2, 616, 1972.
665. **Book, L. S., Overall, J. C., Jr., Herbst, J. J., Britt, M. R., Epstein, B., and Jung, A. L.,** Clustering of necrotizing enterocolitis; interruption by infection-control measures, *N. Engl. J. Med.,* 297, 984, 1977.
666. **Moomjian, A. S., Packham, G. J., and Fox, W. W.,** Necrotizing enterocolitis-endemic vs. epidemic form, *Pediatr. Res.,* 12, 530, 1978.
667. **Shackelford, P. G. and Feigin, R. D.,** *Listeria* revisited, *Am. J. Dis. Child.,* 131, 391, 1977.

668. Louria, D. B., Hensle, T., Armstrong, D., Collins, H. S., Blevins, A., Krugman, D., and Buse, M., Listeriosis complicating malignant disease, *Ann. Intern. Med.*, 67, 261, 1967.

669. Bojsen-Møller, J., Human listeriosis: diagnostic, eidemiological and clinical studies, *Acta Pathol. Microbiol. Scand. (B)*, suppl. 229, 1972.

670. Isiadinso, O. A., *Listeria* sepsis and meningitis: a complication of renal transplantation, *J.A.M.A.*, 234, 842, 1975.

671. Florman, A. L. and Venkatesan, S., Listeriosis among nursery mates, *Pediatrics*, 41, 784, 1968.

672. Becroft, D. M. O., Farmer, K., Seddon, R. J., Sowden, R., Stewart, J. H., Vines, A., Wattie, D. A., Epidemic listeriosis in the newborn, *Br. Med. J.*, 3, 747, 1971.

673. Filice, G. A., Cantrell, H. F., Smith, A. B., Hayes, P. S., Feeley, J. C., and Fraser, D. W., *Listeria monocytogenes* infection in neonates: investigation of an epidemic, *J. Infect. Dis.*, 138, 17, 1978.

674. Jacobs, M. R., Stein, H., Buqwane, A., Dubb, A., Segal, F., Rabinowitz, L., Ellis, U., Freiman, I., Witcomb, M., and Vallabh, V., Epidemic listeriosis: report of 14 cases detected in 9 months, *S. Afr. Med J.*, 389, 1978.

675. Larsson, S., Cederberg, A., Ivarsson, S., Svanberg, L., Cronberg, S., *Listeria monocytogenes* causing hospital-acquired enterocolitis and meningitis in newborn infants, *Br. Med. J.*, 2, 473, 1978.

676. Gantz, N. M., Myerowitz, R. L., Medeiros, A. A., Carrera, G. F., Wilson, R. E., and O'Brien, T. F., Listeriosis in immunosuppressed patients: a cluster of eight cases, *Am. J. Med.*, 58, 637, 1975.

677. Green, H. T. and Macaulay, M. B., Hospital outbreak of *Listeria monocytogenes* septicaemia: a problem of cross infection?, *Lancet*, 2, 1039, 1978.

678. Wolinsky, E., Nontuberculous mycobacteria and associated diseases, *Am. Rev. Respir. Dis.*, 119, 107, 1979.

679. Katz, M. A. and Hull, A. R., Probable *Mycobacterium fortuitum* septicemia: complication of home dialysis, *Lancet*, 1, 499, 1971.

680. Graybill, J. R., Silva, J., Jr., Fraser, D. W., Lordon, R., and Rogers, E., Disseminated mycobacteriosis due to *Mycobacterium abscessus* in two recipients of renal homografts, *Am. Rev. Respir. Dis.*, 109, 4, 1974.

681. Center for Disease Control, Atypical mycobacteria wound infections—North Carolina, Colorado, National Nosocomial Infections Study Report, Annual Summary 1974, 1977, 12.

682. Robicsek, F., Daugherty, H. K., Cook, J. W., Selle, J. G., Masters, T. N., O'Bar, P. R., Fernandez, C. R., Mauney, C. U., and Calhoun, D. M., *Mycobacterium fortuitum* epidemics after open-heart surgery, *J. Thorac. Cardiovas C. Surg.*, 75, 91, 1978.

683. Foz, A., Roy, C., Jurado, J., Arteaga, E., Ruiz, J. M., and Moragas, A., *Mycobacterium chelonei* iatrogenic infections, *J. Clin. Microbiol.*, 7, 319, 1978.

684. Band, J. D. and Fraser, D. W., Peritonitis caused by a *Mycobacterium chelonei*-like organism (MCLO) associated with chronic peritoneal dialysis. Center for Disease Control, Atlanta, Ga., Abstracts of the Nineteenth Interscience Conference on Antimicrobial Agents and Chemotherapy, Boston, Mass., 1979.

685. Foster, M. T. and Sanders, W. E., Atypical mycobacterial infections complicating mammary implants, Abstracts of the Eighteenth Interscience Conference on Antimicrobial Agents and Chemotherapy, October 1978, Atlanta, Ga., 1978.

686. Carson, L. A., Petersen, N. J., Favero, M. S., Aguero, S. M., Growth characteristics of atypical mycobacteria in water and their comparative resistance to disinfectants, *Appl. Environ. Microbiol.*, 36, 839, 1978.

687. Center for Disease Control, Isolation of mycobacteria species from porcine heart valve prostheses—United States, *Morbid. Mortal. Weekly Rep.*, 26, 42, 1977.

688. Laskowski, L. F., Marr, J. J., Spernoga, J. F., Frank, N. J., Barner, H. B., Kaiser, G., and Tyras, D. H., Fastidious mycobacteria grown from porcine prosthetic-heart-valve cultures, *N. Engl. J. Med.*, 297, 101, 1977.

689. Levy, C., Curtin, J. A., Watkins, A., Marsh, B., Garcia, J., and Mispireta, L., (letter to the editor), *Mycobacterium chelonei* infection of porcine heart valves, *N. Engl. J. Med.*, 297, 667, 1977.

690. Laskowski, L. F., Marr, J. J., Curgin, J. A., Levy, C., Levy, M. E., Cohen, R. L., Field, R., Simon, L. S., Freeman, D., Chin, J., Schwarzmann, S. W., Smith, J. D., Bartlett, R. C., Carrington, G. O., Doyle, K., and McLaughlin, J. C., Follow-up on mycobacterial contamination of porcine heart valve prosthesis—United States, *Morbid. Mortal. Weekly Rep.*, 27, 92, 1978.

691. Linde, L. M. and Heins, H. L., Bacterial endocarditis following surgery for congenital heart disease, *N. Engl. J. Med.*, 263, 65, 1960.

692. Foley, J. F., Gravelle, C. R., Englehard, W. E., and Chin, T. D. Y., Achromobater septicemia—fatalities in prematures, *Am. J. Dis. Child.*, 101, 279, 1961.

693. Gwynn, C. M. and George, R. H., Neonatal *citrobacter* meningitis, *Arch. Dis. Child.*, 48, 455, 1973.

694. Gross, R. J., Rowe, B. and Easton, J. A., Neonatal meningitis caused by *Citrobacter koseri*, *J. Clin. Pathol.*, 26, 138, 1973.

695. Vogel, L. C., Ferguson, L., and Gotoff, S. P., *Citrobacter* infections of the central nervous system in early infancy, *J. Pediatr.*, 93, 86, 1978.

696. Madrazo, A., Geiger, J., and Lauter, C. B., *Citrobacter diversus* at Grace Hospital, Detroit, Mich., *Am. J. Med. Sci.*, 270, 497, 1975.

697. Washington, J. A., II, *Aeromonas hydrophila* in clinical bacteriologic specimens, *Ann. Intern. Med.*, 76, 611, 1972.

698. Ketover, B. P., Young, L. S., and Armstrong, D., Septicemia due to *Aeromonas hydrophila:* clinical and immunologic aspects, *J. Infect. Dis.*, 127, 284, 1973.

699. Pearson, T. A., Braine, H. G., and Rathbun, H. K., *Corynebacterium* sepsis in oncology patients: predisposing factors, diagnosis, and treatment, *J.A.M.A.*, 238, 1737, 1977.

700. Stamm, W. E., Tompkins, L. S., Wagner, K. F., Counts, G. W., Thomas, E. D., and Meyers, J. D., Infection due to *Corynebacterium* species in marrow transplant patients, *Ann. Intern. Med.*, 91, 167, 1979.

701. Farrar, W. E., Jr., Serious infections due to "non-pathogenic" organisms of the genus bacillus: review of their status as pathogens, *Am. J. Med.*, 34, 134, 1963.

702. Curtis, J. R., Wing, A. J., and Coleman, J. C., Bacillus cereus bacteraemia: a complication of intermittent haemodialysis, *Lancet*, 1, 136, 1967.

703. Ihde, D. C. and Armstrong, D., Clinical spectrum of infection due to Bacillus species, *Am. J. Med.*, 55, 839, 1973.

704. Noble, R. C. and Reeves, S. A., *Bacillus* species pseudosepsis caused by contaminated commercial blood culture media, *J.A.M.A.*, 230, 1002, 1974.

705. Glode, M. P., Schiffer, M. S., Robbins, J. B., Khan, W., Battle, C. U., and Armenta, E., An outbreak of *Hemophilus influenzae* type b meningitis in an enclosed hospital population, *J. Pediatr.*, 88, 36, 1976.

706. Cohen, M. S., Steere, A. C., Baltimore, R., von Graevenitz, A., Pantelick, E., Camp, B., and Root, R. K., Possible nosocomial transmission of group y *Neisseria meningitidis* among oncology patients, *Ann. Intern. Med.*, 91, 7, 1979.

707. Weinstein, R. A. and Stamm, W. E., Pseudoepidemics in hospital, *Lancet*, 2, 862, 1977.

708. Dolan, J., Joachim, G. R., Khapra, A., and Greenwald, P., Pseudobacteremia due to *Staphylococcus aureus*—New York, *Morbid. Mortal. Weekly Rep.*, 28, 82, 1979.

709. Weinstein, R. A. and Stamm, W. E., Early detection of false-positive acid-fast smears, *Lancet*, 2, 173, 1975.

710. Musher, D. M. and Schell, D. F., False-positive gram stains of cerebrospinal fluid, *Ann. Intern. Med.*, 79, 603, 1973.

711. Weinstein, R. A., Bauer, R. W., Hoffman, R. D., Tyler, P. G., Anderson, R. L., and Stamm, W. E., Factitious meningitis. Diagnostic error due to nonviable bacteria in commercial lumbar puncture trays, *J.A.M.A.*, 233, 878, 1975.

712. Ericsson, C. D., Carmichael, M., Pickering, L. K., Mussett, R., and Kohl, S., Erroneous diagnosis of meningitis due to false-positive gram stains, *South. Med. J.*, 71, 1524, 1978.

713. Russell, R. L., Quality control in the microbiology laboratory, in *Manual of Clinical Microbiology*, 2nd ed., Lennette, E. H., Spaulding, E. H., and Truant, J. P., Eds., American Society for Microbiology, 1974, 862.

714. Ellis, R. J., Quality control procedures for microbiological laboratories, Center for Disease Control, October 1976.

715. Maki, D. G., Non-infective complications of infusion therapy, *Infusion*, 2, 89, 1978.

716. Maki, D. G., Goldmann, D. A., and Rhame, F. S., Infection control in intravenous therapy, *Ann. Int. Med.*, 79, 867, 1973.

717. Maki, D. G., Sepsis arising from extrinsic contamination of the infusion and measures for control, in *Microbiologic Hazards of Intravenous Therapy*, Phillips, I., Meers, P. D., and D'Arcy, P. F., Eds., MTP Press, Lancaster, England, 1977, 99.

718. Altemeier, W. A., McDonough, J. J., and Fullen, W. D., Third day surgical fever, *Arch. Surg. (Chicago)*, 103, 158, 1971.

719. Freeman, R. and King, B., Recognition of infection associated with intravenous catheters, *Br. J. Surg.*, 62, 404, 1975.

720. Michaelson, E. D. and Walsh, R. E., Osler's node—a complication of prolonged arterial cannulation, *N. Engl. J. Med.*, 283, 472, 1970.

721. Band, J. D. and Maki, D. G., Safety of changing intravenous delivery systems at longer than 24-hour intervals, *Ann. Intern. Med.*, 91, 173, 1979.

722. Maki, D. G., Weise, C. E., and Sarafin, H. W., A semiquantitative culture method for identifying intravenous-catheter-related infection, *N. Engl. J. Med.*, 296, 1305, 1977.

723. Band, J. D., Alvarado, C. J., and Maki, D. G., A semiquantitative culture technique for identifying infection due to steel needles used for intravenous therapy, *Am. J. Clin. Pathol.*, 72, 980, 1979.

724. Druskin, M. S. and Siegel, P. D., Bacterial contamination of indwelling intravenous polyethylene catheters, *J.A.M.A.*, 185, 966, 1963.
725. Cheney F. W., Jr. and Lincoln, J. R., Phlebitis from plastic intravenous catheters, *Anesthesiology*, 25, 650, 1964.
726. Moran, J. M., Atwood, R. P., and Rowe, M. I., A clinical and bacteriologic study of infections associated with venous cutdowns, *N. Engl. J. Med.*, 272, 554, 1965.
727. Collins, R. N., Braun, P. A., Zinner, S. H., and Kass, E. H., Risk of local and systemic infection with polyethylene intravenous catheters: a prospective study of 213 catheterizations, *N. Engl. Med. J.*, 279, 340, 1968.
728. Brereton, R. B., Incidence of complications from indwelling venous catheters, *Del. Med. J.*, 41, 1, 1969.
729. Zinner, S. H., Denny-Brown, B. C., Braun, P., Burke, J. P., Toala, P., and Kass, E. H., Risk of infection with intravenous indwelling catheters: effect of application of antibiotic ointment, *J. Infect. Dis.*, 120, 616, 1969.
730. Norden, C. W., Application of antibiotic ointment to the site of venous catheterization: a controlled trial, *J. Infect, Dis.*, 120, 611, 1969.
731. Corso, J. A., Agostinelli, R., and Brandriss, M. W., Maintenance of venous polyethelene catheters to reduce risk of infection, *J.A.M.A.*, 210, 2075, 1969.
732. Banks, D. C., Yates, D. B., Cawdrey, H. M., Harries, M. G., and Kidner, P. H., Infection from intravenous catheters, *Lancet*, 1, 443, 1970.
733. Bolasny, B. L., Shepard, G. H., and Scott, H. W., Jr., The hazards of intravenous polyethylene catheters in surgical patients, *Surg. Gynecol. Obstet.*, 130, 342, 1970.
734. Levy, R. S., Goldstein, J., and Pressman, R. S., Value of a topical antibiotic ointment in reducing bacterial colonization of percutaneous venous catheters, *J. Albert Einstein Med. Cent.*, 18, 67, 1970.
735. Glover, J. L., O'Byrne, S. A., and Jolly, L., Infusion catheter sepsis: an increasing threat, *Ann. Surg.*, 173, 148, 1971.
736. Bernard, R. W., Stahl, W. M., and Chase, R. M., Jr., Subclavian vein catheterizations: a prospective study. II. Infectious complications, *Ann. Surg.*, 173, 191, 1971.
737. Fuchs, P. C., Indwelling intravenous polyethylene catheters: factors influencing the risk of microbial colonization and sepsis, *J.A.M.A.*, 216, 1447, 1971.
738. Bolasny, B. L., Martin, C. E., and Conkle, D. M., Careful technique with plastic intravenous catheters, *Surg. Gynecol. Obstet.*, 132, 1030, 1971.
739. Crenshaw, C. A., Kelly, L., Turner, R. J., III, and Enas, D., Bacteriologic nature and prevention of contamination to intravenous catheters, *Am. J. Surg.*, 123, 264, 1972.
740. Walters, M. B., Stanger, H. A., and Rotem, C. E., Complications with percutaneous central venous catheters, *J.A.M.A.*, 220, 1445, 1972.
741. Freeman, R. and King, B., Infective complications of indwelling intravenous catheters and the monitoring of infections by the nitrobluetetrazolium test, *Lancet*, 1, 992, 1972.
742. Colvin, M. P., Blogg, C. E., Savege, T. M., Jarvis, J. D., and Strunin, L., A safe long-term infusion technique?, *Lancet*, 2, 317, 1972.
743. Hoshal, V. L., Intravenous catheters and infection, *Surg. Clin. North Am.*, 52, 1407, 1972.
744. Sketch, M. H., Cole M., Mohiuddin, S. M., and Booth, R. W., Use of percutaneously inserted subclavian venous catheters in coronary care units, *Chest*, 6, 684, 1972.
745. Buchsbaum, H. J. and White, A. J., The use of subclavian central venous catheters in gynecology and obstetrics, *Surg. Gynecol. Obstet.*, 136, 561, 173.
746. Irwin, G. R., Jr., Hart, B. J., and Martin, C. M., Pathogenesis and prevention of intravenous catheter infections, *Yale J. Biol. Med.*, 46, 85, 1973.
747. Smith, J. A., Selick, A., and Edelist, G., A clinical and microbiological study of venous catheterization, *Can. Med. Assoc. J.*, 109, 115, 1973.
748. Collin, J., Collin, C., Constable, F. L., and Johnston, I. D. A., Infusion thrombophlebitis and infection with various cannulas, *Lancet*, 2, 150, 1975.
749. Stephen, M., Loewenthal, J., Wong, J., and Benn, R., Complications of intravenous therapy, *Med. J. Aust.*, 557, 1976.
750. Silva, J., Prager, R. L., and Harkema, J., Infections of central venous catheters, *Clin. Res.*, 24 (Abstr.), 546A, 1976.
751. Freeman, R. and King, B., Analysis of results of catheter tip cultures in open-heart surgery patients, *Thorax*, 30, 26, 1975.
752. Stillman, R. M., Soliman, F., Garcia, L., and Sawyer, P. N., Etiology of catheter-associated sepsis: correlation with thrombogenicity, *Arch. Surg. (Chicago)*, 112, 1497, 1977.
753. Herbst, C. A., Jr., Indications, management and complications of percutaneous subclavian catheters: an audit, *Arch. Surg. (Chicago)*, 113, 1421, 1978.

754. Bottino, J., McCredie, K. B., Groschel, D. H. M., and Lawson, M., Long-term intravenous therapy with peripherally inserted silicone elastomer central venous catheters in patients with malignant diseases, *Cancer,* 43, 1937, 1979.

755. Maki, D. G. and Band, J. D., Comparative study of polyantibiotic and iodophor ointments in prevention of vascular catheter-related infection, *Am. J. Med.,* 1981, in press.

756. Balagtas, R. C., Bell, C. E., Edwards, L. D., and Levin, S., Risk of local and systemic infections associated with umbilical vein catheterization: a prospective study in 86 newborn patients, *Pediatrics,* 48, 359, 1971.

757. Hall, R. T. and Rhodes, P. G., Total parenteral alimentation via indwelling umbilical catheters in the newborn period, *Arch. Dis. Child.,* 51, 929, 1976.

758. Fairchild, J. P., Graber, C. D., Vogel, E. H., and Ingersoll, R. L., Flora of the umbilical stump, *J. Pediatr.,* 53, 538, 1958.

759. Symansky, M. R. and Fox, H. A., Umbilical vessel catheterization: indications, management, and evaluation of the technique, *J. Pediatr.,* 80, 820, 1972.

760. Powers, W. F. and Tooley, W. H., (letter to the editor), Contamination of umbilical vessel catheters: encouraging information, *Pediatrics,* 49, 470, 1972.

761. Cowett, R. M., Peter, G., Hakanson, D. O., Stern, L., and Oh, W., Prophylactic antibiotics in neonates with umbilical artery catheter placement: a prospective study of 137 patients, *Yale J. Biol. Med.,* 50, 457, 1977.

762. Swan, H. J. C., Ganz, W., Forrester, J., Marcus, H., Diamond, G., and Chonette, D., Catheterization of the heart in man with the use of a flow-directed balloon-tipped catheter, *N. Engl. J. Med.,* 283, 447, 1970.

763. Katz, J. D., Cronau, L. H., Barash, P. G., and Mandel, S. D., Pulmonary artery flow-guided catheters in the perioperative period, *J.A.M.A.,* 237, 2832, 1977.

764. Greene, J. F., Jr., Fitzwater, J. E., and Clemmer, T. P., Septic endocarditis and indwelling pulmonary artery catheters, *J.A.M.A.,* 233, 891, 1975.

765. Pace, N. L. and Horton, W., Indwelling pulmonary artery catheters: their relationship to aseptic thrombotic endocardial vegetations, *J.A.M.A.,* 233, 893, 1975.

766. Applefeld, J. J., Caruthers, T. E., Reno, D. J., and Civetta, J. M., Assessment of the sterility of long-term cardiac catheterization using the thermodilution Swan-Ganz catheter, *Chest,* 74, 377, 1978.

767. Peter, G., Lloyd-Still, J. D., and Lovejoy, F. H., Jr., Local infection and bacteremia from scalp-vein needles and polyethylene catheters in children, *J. Pediatr.,* 80, 78, 1972.

768. Crossley, K. and Matsen, J. M., The scalp-vein needle: a prospective study of complications, *J.A.M.A.,* 220, 985, 1972.

769. Crenshaw, C. A., Kelly, L., Turner, R. J., and Enas, D., Prevention of infection at scalp-vein sites of needle insertion during intravenous therapy, *Am. J. Surg.,* 124, 43, 1972.

770. Keough, E. J. and Hopkins, B. E, Risk of infection with scalp-vein needles — a prospective study, *Aust. N.Z. J. Med.,* 3, 389, 1973.

771. Ferguson, R. L., Resett, W., Hodges, G. R., and Barnes, W. G., Complications with heparin-lock needles — a prospective evaluation, *Ann. Intern. Med.,* 85, 583, 1976.

772. Harbin, R. L. and Schaffner, W., Septicemia associated with scalp-vein needles, *South. Med. J.,* 66, 638, 1973.

773. Maki, D. G., Drinka, P. J., and Davis, T. E., Suppurative phlebitis of an arm vein from a "scalp-vein needle", *N. Engl. J. Med.,* 202, 1116, 1975.

774. Agger, W. A. and Maki, D. G., Septicemia from heparin-lock needles, *Ann. Intern. Med.,* 86, 657, 1977.

774a. Tully, J. L., Friedland, G. H., and Goldmann, D. A., Complications of intravenous therapy with steel needles and small-bone Teflon® catheters, *Am. J. Med.,* 1981, in press.

775. Dillon, J. D., Schaffner, W., Van Way, C. W., and Meng, H. C., Septicemia and total parenteral nutrition. Distinguishing catheter-related from other septic episodes, *J.A.M.A.,* 223, 1341, 1973.

776. Allen, J. R., The incidence of nosocomial infection in patients receiving total parenteral nutrition, in *Advances in Parenteral Nutrition,* Johnston, I. D. A., Ed., Proc. International Symp., Bermuda, May, 1977, MTP Press, Lancaster, England, 1977, 339

777. Sanderson, I. and Deitel, M., Intravenous hyperalimentation without sepsis, *Surg. Gynecol. Obstet.,* 136, 577, 1973.

778. Copeland, E. M., MacFayden, B. V. McGown, C., and Dudrick, S. J., The use of hyperalimentation in patients with potential sepsis, *Surg. Gynecol. Obstet.,* 137, 377, 1974.

779. Abel, R. M., Fischer, J. E., Buckley, M. J., and Austen, W. G., Hyperalimentation in cardiac surgery: a review of sixty-four patients, *J. Thorac. Cardiovasc. Surg.,* 67, 294, 1974.

780. Myers, R. N., Smink, R. D., and Goldstein, F., Parenteral hyperalimentation—five years' clinical experience, *Am. J. Gastroenterol.,* 62, 313, 1974.

781. Weinstein, R. A., The design of pressure monitoring devices: infection control considerations, *Med. Instrum. (Baltimore),* 10, 287, 1976.

782. Retailliau, H. F., Infection control with invasive pressure monitoring devices, *A.P.I.C.J.*, 110, 597, 1969.

783. Stamm, W. E., Infections related to medical devices, *Ann. Intern. Med.*, 89, 764, 1978.

784. Ansfield, F. J., Ramirez, G., Davis, H. L., Wirtanen, G. W., Johnson, R. O., Bryan, G. T., Manalo, F. B., Borden, E. C., Davis, T. E., and Esmaili, M., Further clinical studies with intrahepatic arterial infusion with 5-fluorouracil, *Cancer*, 36, 2413, 1975.

785. Gardner, R. M., Schwartz, R., Wong, H. C., and Burke, J. P., Percutaneous indwelling radial-artery catheters for monitoring cardiovascular function, *N. Engl. J. Med.*, 290, 1227, 1974.

786. Hoshal, V. L., Ause, R. G., and Hoskins, P. A., Fibrin sleeve formation on indwelling subclavian central venous catheters, *Arch. Surg. (Chicago)*, 102, 353, 1971.

787. Peters, W. R., Bush, W. H., Jr., McIntyre, R. D., and Hill, L. L., The development of fibrin sheath on indwelling venous catheters, *Surg. Gynecol. Obstet.*, 137, 43, 1973.

788. Edwards, L. D., The epidemiology of 2056 remote site infections and 1966 surgical wound infections occurring in 1865 paitents: a four year study of 40,923 operations at Rush-Presbyterian-St. Luke's Hospital, Chicago, *Ann. Surg.*, 184, 758, 1978.

789. Crane, C., Venous interruption for septic thrombophlebitis, *N. Engl. J. Med.*, 262, 947, 1960.

790. Stein, J. M. and Pruitt, B. A., Jr., Suppurative thrombophlebitis: a lethal iatrogenic disease, *N. Engl. J. Med.*, 282, 1452, 1970.

791. Pruitt, B. A., Jr., Stein, J. M., Foley, F. D., Moncrief, J. A., and O'Neill, J. A., Jr., Intravenous therapy in burn patients: suppurative thrombophlebitis and other life-threatening complications, *Arch. Surg. (Chicago)*, 100, 399, 1970.

792. Munster, A. M., Septic thrombophlebitis: a surgical disorder, *J.A.M.A.*, 230, 1010, 1974.

793. Vic-Dupont, J. M., Cormier, M., and Lecompte, Y., Ligation of veins in suppurative thrombophlebitis secondary to venous catheterization, *Chururg*, 99, 285, 1973.

794. Warden, G. D., Wilmore, D. W., and Pruitt, B. A., Central venous thrombosis: a hazard of medical progress, *J. Trauma*, 13, 620, 1973.

795. Popp, M. G., Law, E. J., and MacMillan, B. G., Parenteral nutrition in the burned child: a study of twenty-six patients, *Ann. Surg.*, 179, 219, 1974.

796. Jarrett, F., Maki, D. G., and Chan, C., Septic thrombosis of the inferior vena cava caused by *Candida*, *Arch. Surg. (Chicago)*, 113, 637, 1978.

797. Center for Disease Control, Recall of contaminated intravenous cannulae, *Morbid. Mortal. Weekly Rep.*, 23, 57, 1964.

798. Goldmann, D. A., Martin, W. T., and Worthington, J. W., Growth of bacteria and fungi in total parenteral nutrition solutions, *Am. J. Surg.*, 126, 314, 1973.

799. Melly, M. A., Meng, H. C., and Schaffner, W., Microbial growth in lipid emulsions used in parenteral nutrition, *Arch. Surg. (Chicago)*, 110, 1479, 1975.

800. McKee, K. T., Melly, M. A., Greene, H. L., and Schaffner, W., Gram-negative bacillary sepsis associated with use of lipid emulsion in parenteral nutrition, *Am. J. Dis. Child.*, 133, 649, 1979.

801. West, C. M., Highsmith, A. K., Dixon, R. E., and Bennett, J. V., Nosocomial bacteremia in a neonatal intensive care unit, Georgia, *Epidemic Aid Report*, (78-4-2), Center for Disease Control, Atlanta, Ga.

802. Robertson, M. H., Fungi in fluids—a hazard of intravenous therapy, *J. Med. Microbiol.*, 3, 99, 1970.

803. Maki, D. G., Anderson, R. L., and Shulman, J. A., In-use contamination of intravenous infusion fluid, *Appl. Microbiol.*, 28, 778, 1974.

804. Michaels, L. and Ruebner, B., Growth of bacteria in intravenous infusion fluids, *Lancet*, 1, 722, 1953.

805. Buxton, A. E., Highsmith, A. K., Garner, J. S., West, C. M., Stamm, W. E., Dixon, R. E., and McGowan, J. E., Contamination of intravenous infusion fluid: effects of changing administration sets, *Ann. Intern. Med.*, 90, 764, 1979.

806. Braude, A. I., Sanford, J. P., Bartlett, J. E., and Mallery, O. T., Effects and clinical significance of bacterial contaminants in transfused blood, *J. Lab. Clin. Med.*, 39, 902, 1952.

807. James, J. D., Bacterial contamination of reserved blood, *Vox Sang.*, 4, 177, 1959.

808. Buchholz, D. H., Young, V. M., Friedman, N. R., Reilley J. A., and Mardiney, M. R., Jr., Detection and quantitation of bacteria in platelet products stored at ambient temperature, *Transfusion (Philadelphia)*, 13, 268, 1973.

809. Wrenn, H. E. and Speicher, C. E., Platelet concentrates: sterility of 400 single units stored at room temperature, *Transfusion (Philadelphia)*, 14, 171, 1974.

810. Borden, C. W. and Hall, W. H., Fatal transfusion reactions from massive bacterial contamination of blood, *N. Engl. J. Med.*, 245, 760, 1951.

811. Braude, A. I., Transfusion reactions from contaminated blood: their recognition and treatment, *N. Engl. J. Med.*, 258, 1289, 1958.

812. McEntegart, M. G., Dangerous contaminants in stored blood, *Lancet*, 2, 909, 1956.

813. Steere, A. C., Rifaat, M. K., Seligmann, E. B., Jr., Hochstein, H. D., Friedland, G., Dasse, P., Wustrack, K. O., Axnick, K. J., and Barker, L. F., Pyrogen reactions associated with the infusion of normal serum albumin (human), *Transfusion (Phildelphia)*, 18, 102, 1978.

814. National Coordinating Committee on Large Volume Parenterals, Recommended methods for compounding intravenous admixtures in hospitals, *Am. J. Hosp. Pharm.*, 32, 261, 1975.

815. Garrison, T. J. and Ravin, R., Operating a centralized admixture program: politics & procedures, in *Modern IV Practices*, Medical Directions, Chicago, 1979, 1.

816. Goldmann, D. A., Maki, D. G., Rhame, F. S., Kaiser, A. B., Tenney, J. H., and Bennett, J. V., Guidelines for infection control in intravenous therapy, *Ann. Intern. Med.*, 79, 848, 1973.

817. Maki, D. G., Infectious complications of infusion therapy and their prevention, in *Modern IV Practices*, Medical Directions, Chicago, 1979, 1.

818. National Coordinating Committee on Large Volume Parenterals, Recommended procedures for in-use testing of large volume parenterals suspected of contamination or of producing a reaction in a patient, *Am. J. Hosp. Pharm.*, 35, 678, 1978.

819. Maki, D. G., Evaluation of a suspected epidemic, in *Modern IV Practices*, Medical Directions, Chicago, 1979, 1.

820. National Coordinating Committee on Large Volume Parenterals, Recommended system for surveillance and reporting of problems with large-volume parenterals in hospitals, *Am. J. Hosp. Pharm.*, 32, 1251, 1975.

821. National Coordinating Committee on Large Volume Parenterals, Recommendations to pharmacists for solving problems with large-volume parenterals, *Am. J. Hosp. Pharm.*, 33, 231, 1976.

822. Herman, L. G., A critical evaluation of microbiological hazards associated with the pharmacy and the hospital, *Am. J. Hosp. Pharm.*, 27, 56, 1970.

823a. Maki, D. G. and Hassemer, C. A., Endemic rate of fluid contamination and related septicemia in arterial pressure monitoring, *Am. J. Med.*, 1981, in press.

824. Center for Disease Control, Nosocomial bacteremias associated with intravenous fluid therapy—USA, *Morbid. Mortal. Weekly Rep.*, 20 (Suppl. No. 9), 12 March, 1971.

825. Felts, S. K., Schaffner, W., Melly, M. A., and Koenig, M. G., Sepsis caused by contaminated intravenous fluids: epidemiologic, clinical, and laboratory investigation of an outbreak in one hospital, *Ann. Intern. Med.*, 77, 881, 1972.

826. Mackel, D. C., Maki, D. G., Anderson, R. L., Rhame, F. S., and Bennett, J. V., Nationwide epidemic of septicemia caused by contaminated intravenous products: mechanisms of intrinsic contamination, *J. Clin. Microbiol.*, 2, 486, 1975.

827. Report of the committee appointed to inquire into the circumstances, including the production, which led to the use of contaminated infusion fluids in the Devenport Section of Plymouth General Hospital, London, Her Majesty's Stationery Office, 1972.

828. Dixon, R. E., Intrinsic contamination—the associated infective syndrome, in *Microbiologic Hazards of Intravenous Therapy*, Phillips, I., Ed., MTP Press, Lancaster, England, 1977, 145.

829. Bennett, J. V., Scheckler, W. E., Maki, D. G., and Brachman, P. S., Current national patterns, in *Proc. International Conf. on Nosocomial Infections*, Brachman, P. S. and Eickhoff, T. E., Eds., American Hospital Association, Chicago, 1971, 42.

830. Garner, J. S., Bennett, J. V., Scheckler, W. E., Maki, D. G., and Brachman, P. S., Surveillance of nosocomial infections, in *Proc. of the International Conf. on Nosocomial Infections*, Brachman, P. S. and Eickhoff, T. E., Eds., American Hospital Association, Chicago, 1971, 277.

831. Goldmann, D. A., Fulkerson, C. C., Dixon, R. E., Maki, D. G., and Bennett, J. V., Nationwide epidemic of septicemia caused by contaminated intravenous products. II. Assessment of the problem by a national nosocomial infection surveillance system, *Am. J. Epidemiol.*, 108, 207, 1978.

832. Sherris, J. C., Cole, J. J., and Scribner, B. H., Bacteriology of continuous-flow-hemodialysis, *Trans. Am. Soc. Artif. Intern. Organs*, 7, 37, 1961.

833. Kidd, E. E., Bacterial contamination of dialyzing fluid of artificial kidney, *Br. Med. J.*, 1, 880, 1964.

834. Favero, M. S., Petersen, N. J., Carson, L. A., Bond, W. W., and Hindman, S. H., Gram-negative water bacteria in hemodialysis systems, *Health Lab. Sci.*, 12, 321, 1975.

835. Robinson, P. J. A. and Rosen, S. M., Pyrexial reactions during haemodialysis, *Br. Med. J.*, 1, 528, 1971.

836. Jones, D. M., Tobin, B. M., Harlow, G. R., and Ralston, A. J., Bacteriological studies of the modified Kiil dialyser, *Br. Med. J.*, 3, 135, 1970.

837. Petersen, N. J., Boyer, K. M., Carson, L. A., and Favero, M. S., Pyrogenic reactions from inadequate disinfection of a dialysis fluid distribution system, *Dial. Transplant.*, 7, 52, 1978.

838. Hindman, S. H., Favero, M. S., Carson, L. A., Petersen, N. J., Schonberger, L. B., and Solano, J. T., Pyrogenic reactions during haemodialysis caused by extramural endotoxin, *Lancet*, 2, 732, 1975.

839. Martin, A. M., Clunie, G. J. A., Tonkin, R. W., and Robson, J. S., The aetiology and management of shunt infections in patients on intermittent haemodialysis, dialysis, and renal transplantation, *Proc. Eur. Dial. Transplant Assoc.*, 4, 67, 1967.

840. Ozeran, R. S., Gral, T., Sokol, A., and Gordon, H. E., Long-term experience with arteriovenous shunts for hemodialysis, *Am. Surg.*, 38, 259, 1972.

841. Eykyn, S., Phillips, I., and Evans, J., Vancomycin for staphylococcal shunt site infections in patients on regular haemodialysis, *Br. Med. J.*, 3, 80, 1970.

842. Barcenas, C. G., Fuller, T. J., Elms, J., Cohen, R., and White, M. G., Staphylococcal sepsis in patients on chronic hemodialysis regimens: intravenous treatment with vancomycin given once weekly, *Arch. Intern. Med.*, 136, 1131, 1976.

843. Levi, J., Robson, M., and Rosenfeld, J. B., Septicaemia and pulmonary embolism complicating use of arteriovenous fistula in maintenance of haemodialysis, *Lancet*, 2, 288, 1970.

844. Leonard, A., Raij, L., and Shapiro, F. L., Bacterial endocarditis in regularly dialyzed patients, *Kidney Int.*, 4, 407, 1973.

845. Cross, A. S., Steigbigel, R. T., Infective endocarditis and access site infections in patients on hemodialysis, *Medicine (Baltimore)*, 55, 453, 1976.

846. Leonard, A., Comty, C. N., Shapiro, F. L., and Raij, L., Osteomyelitis in hemodialysis patients, *Ann. Intern. Med.*, 78, 651, 1973.

847. Goldblum, S. E., Reed, W. P., Ulrich, J. A., and Goldman, R. S., Staphylococcal carriage and infections in hemodialysis patients, *Dial. Transplant.*, 7, 1140, 1978.

848. Kirmani, N., Tuazon, C. U., Murray, H. W., Parrish, A. E., and Sheagren, J. N., *Staphylococcus aureus* carriage rate of patients receiving long-term hemodialysis, *Arch. Intern. Med.*, 138, 1657, 1978.

849. Favero, M. S., Carson, L. A., Bond, W. W., and Petersen, N. J., Factors that influence microbial contamination of fluids associated with hemodialysis machines, *Appl. Microbiol.*, 28, 822, 1974.

850. Vercellone, A., Piccoli, G., Alloatti, S., Segoloni, G. P., Stratta, P., Triolo, G., Canavese, C., and Grott, G., Reuse of dialyzers, *Dial. Tranplant.*, 7, 350, 1978.

851. Deane, N., Blagg, C., Bower, J., De Palma, J., Gutch, C., Kanter, A., Ogden, D., Sadler, J., Siemsen, A., Teehan, Br., and Sosin, A., A survey of dialyzer reuse practice in the United States, *Dial. Transplant.*, 7, 1128, 1978.

852. Raij, L., Shapiro, F. L., and Michael, A. F., Endotoxemia in febrile reactions during hemodialysis, *Kidney Int.*, 4, 57, 1973.

853. Cossart, Y. E., Gillespie, E. H., Jones, D. M., Kelsey, J. C., Moore, B., Murray, I. G., Polakoff, S., Turner, G. C., Burbridge, D. H. D., Coleman, J. C., and Stirland, R. M., Infection risks of haemodialysis—some preventive aspects: a report to the public health laboratory service by the working party on haemodialysis units, *Br. Med. J.*, 3, 454, 1968.

854. Washington, J. A., II, The microbiology of evacuated blood collection tubes, *Ann. Intern. Med.*, 86, 186, 1977.

855. Lee, R. V., Drabinsky, M., Wolfson, S., Cohen, L. S., and Atkins, E., Pyrogen reactions from cardiac catheterization, *Chest*, 63, 757, 1973.

856. Brown, W. J., Fowler, N., Friedman, C., Ganguly, S., Gatmaitan, B., Lerner, A. M., Reyes, M. P., Davis, L. R., Herrera, L. F., Kloepfer, J., Leader, I., Tusnell, P., Huggett, D. O., Hayner, N. S., and Weber, J. A., Endotoxic reactions associated with the reuse of cardiac catheters—Michigan, *Morbid. Mortal. Weekly Rep.*, 28, 25, 1979.

857. Bauer, E., Densen, P., Faxon, D., Kloster, C., Melidossian, C., Kundsin, R., Ryan, P., and Fiumara, N., Endotoxic reactions associated with the reuse of cardiac catheters—Massachusetts, *Morbid. Mortal. Weekly Rep.*, 28, 25, 1979.

858. Wichelhausen, R. H., Clark, H. W., Griffing, V. F., and Robinson, L. B., The concealment of heavy bacterial contamination in 25 per cent human serum albumin: its mechanism and clinical significance, *J. Lab. Clin. Med.*, 51, 276, 1958.

859. Dykes, P. W., Fatal pyrogenic reactions in man, *Lancet*, 1, 563, 1962.

860. Bland, J. H. L., Laver, M. B., and Lowenstein, E., Hypotension due to 5 per cent plasma protein fractions, *N. Engl. J. Med.*, 286, 109, 1972.

861. Bland, J. H. L., Laver, M. B., and Lowenstein, E., Vasodilator effect of commercial 5% plasma protein fraction solutions, *J.A.M.A.*, 224, 1721, 1973.

862. Lowbury, E. J. L., Contamination of centrimide and other fluids with *Pseudomonas pyocyanea*, *Br. J. Ind. Med.*, 8, 22, 1951.

863. Kundsin, R. B. and Walter, C. W., Investigation on absorption of benzalkonium chloride U.S.P. by skin, gloves and sponges, *Arch. Surg. (Chicago)*, 75, 1036, 1957.

864. Editorial, Failure of disinfectants to disinfect, *Lancet*, 2, 306, 1958.

865. Editorial, Bacteria in antiseptic solutions, *Br. Med. J.*, 2, 436, 1958.

866. Anderson, K. and Keynes, R., Infected cork closures and the apparent survival of organisms in antiseptic solutions, *Br. Med. J.*, 2, 274, 1958.

867. Anderson, K., The contamination of hexachlorophene soap with *Pseudomonas pryoyanea*, *Med. J. Aust.*, 2, 463, 1962.

868. **Lee, F. C. and Fialkow, P. J.,** Benzalkonium chloride—source of hospital infection with gram-negative bacteria, *J.A.M.A.,* 177, 708, 1961.

869. **Adair, F. W., Geftic, S. G., and Gelzer, J.,** Resistance of *Pseudomonas* to quaternary ammonium compounds. I. Growth in benzalkonium chloride solution, *Appl Microbiol.,* 18, 299, 1969.

870. **Simmons, N. A. and Gardner, D. A.,** Bacterial contamination of a phenolic disinfectant, *Br. Med. J.,* 2, 668, 1969.

871. **Sanford, J. P.,** Disinfectants that don't (editorial), *Ann. Intern. Med.,* 72, 282, 1970.

872. **Spaulding, E. H. and Groschel, D. H. M.,** Hospital Disinfectants and antiseptics in *Manual of Clinical Microbiology, Second Edition,* Lennette, E. H., Spaulding, E. H., and Truant, J. P., Eds., American Society for Microbiology, Washington, D.C., 1974, 852.

873. **Engelman, R. M., Chase, R. M., Jr., Boyd, A. D., and Reed, G. E.,** Lethal postoperative infections following cardiac surgery: review of four years' experience, *Circulation,* 47 and 48 (Suppl. 3), 31, 1973.

874. **Rosendorf, L. L., Daicoff, G., and Baer, H.,** Sources of gram-negative infection after open-heart surgery *J. Thorac. Cardiovasc. Surg.,* 67, 195, 1974.

875. **Wilson, W. R., Jaumin, P. M., Danielson, G. K., Giuliani, E. R., Washington, J. A., II, and Geraci, J. E.,** Prosthetic valve endocarditis, *Ann. Intern. Med.,* 82, 751, 1975.

876. **Kloster, F. E.,** Diagnosis and management of complications of prosthetic heart valves, *Am. J. Cardiol.,* 35, 872, 1975.

877. **Saffle, J. R., Gardner, P., Schoenbaum, S. C., Wild, W.,** Prosthetic valve endocarditis: a case for prompt valve replacement, *J. Thorac. Cardiovasc. Surg.,* 73, 416, 1977.

878. **Quenzer, R. W., Edwards, L. D., and Levin, S.,** A comparative study of 48 host valve and 24 prosthetic valve endocarditis cases, *Am. Heart J.,* 92, 15, 1976.

879. **Kluge, R. M., Calia, F. M., McLaughlin, J. S., Hornick, R. B.,** Sources of contamination in open heart surgery, *J.A.M.A.,* 230, 1415, 1974.

880. **Ankeney, J. F. and Parker, R. F.,** Staphylococcus endocarditis following open-heart surgery related to positive intraoperative blood cultures, in *Prosthetic Heart Valves,* Brewer, L. A., Ed., Charles C Thomas, Springfield, Ill., 1969, 719.

881. **Blakemore, W. S., McGarrity, G. J., Thurer, R. J., Wallace, H. W., MacVaugh, H., III, Coriell, L. L.,** Infection by air-borne bacteria with cardiopulmonary bypass, *Surgery,* 70, 830, 1971.

882. **Carey, J. S. and Hughes, R. K.,** Control of infection after thoracic and cardiovascular surgery, *Ann. Surg. (Chicago),* 172, 916, 1970.

883. **Keown, K. K. and Gilman, R. A.,** Open Heart Surgery: anesthesia and surgical experiences, *J.A.M.A.,* 165, 781, 1957.

884. **Weiss, W. A. and Bailey, C. P.,** Extracorporeal circulation in cardiac surgery, *Anesth. Analg. (Cleveland),* 39, 438, 1960.

885. **Waterworth, P. M., Lockey, E., Berry, E. M., and Pearce, H. M.,** A critical investigation into the antibiotic sterilization of heart valve homografts, *Thorax,* 29, 432, 1974.

886. **Martin, C. M.,** A national bacteremia registry, *J. Infect. Dis.,* 120, 495, 1969.

887. **Alexander, J. W., Fisher, M. W., and MacMillan, B. G.,** Immunological Control of *Pseudomonas* infection in burn patients: a clinical evaluation, *Arch. Surg. (Chicago),* 102, 31, 1971.

888. **Young, L. S., Meyer, R. D., and Armstrong, D.,** *Pseudomonas aeruginosa* vaccine in cancer patients, *Ann. Intern. Med.,* 79, 518, 1973.

889. **McCabe, W. R., Greely, A., DiGenio, T., and Johns, M. A.,** Humoral immunity to type-specific and cross-reactive antigens of gram-negative bacilli, *J. Infect. Dis.,* 128, S284, 1973.

890. **Stamm, W. E., Martin, S. M., and Bennett, J. V.,** Epidemiology of nosocomial infections due to gram-negative bacilli: aspects relevant to development and use of vaccines, *J. Infect. Dis.,* 136, S151, 1977.

891. Center for Disease Control, Isolation Techniques for Use in Hospitals, 2nd ed., DHEW Publ. No. (CDC) 76-8314, U.S. Government Printing Office, Washington, DC, 1975.

892. Health Resources Administration, Minimum Requirements of Construction and Equipment for Hospital and Medical Facilities, U.S. Government Printing Office, Washington, D.C., 1974.

893. **Lowbury, E. J. L., Lilly, H. A., and Bull, J. P.,** Methods for disinfection of hands and operation sites, *Br. Med. J.,* 2, 531, 1964.

894. **Steere, A. C. and Mallison, G. F.,** Handwashing practices for the prevention of nosocomial infections, *Ann. Intern. Med.,* 83, 683, 1975.

895. **Mallison, G. F.,** The inanimate environment in *Hospital Infections,* Bennett, J. V. and Brachman, P. S., Eds., Little, Brown, Boston, 1979, 81.

896. **Kunin, C. M.,** *Detection, Prevention and Treatment of Urinary Tract Infection,* 2nd ed., Lea & Febinger, Philadelphia, 1974.

897. **Stamm, W. E.,** Guidelines for prevention of catheter-associated urinary tract infections, *Ann. Intern. Med.,* 83, 386, 1975.

898. Foley, R., Administration of intravenous therapy: nursing policies, procedures, & techniques, in *Modern IV Practices,* Medical Directions, Chicago, Ill., 1979, 1.

899. Pierce, A. K., Sanford, J. P., Thomas, G. D., and Leonard, J. S., Long-term evaluation of decontamination of inhalation-therapy equipment and the occurrence of necrotizing pneumonia, *N. Engl. J. Med.,* 282, 528, 1970.

900. Center for Disease Control, The control of pulmonary infections associated with tracheostomy, *National Nosocomial Infections Study Report, Second Quarter 1971,* 1972, 14.

901. Pierce, A. K. and Sanford, J. P., Bacterial contamination of aerosols, *Arch. Intern. Med.,* 131, 156, 1973.

902. Duncalf, D., Care of anesthetic equipment and other devices, *Arch. Surg. (Chicago),* 107, 600, 1973.

903. Phillips, I., King, A., Jenkins, S., and Spencer, G., Control of respirator-associated infection due to *Pseudomonas aeruginosa, Lancet,* 2, 871, 1974.

904. Masferrer, R. and DuPriest, M., Six-year evaluation of decontamination of respiratory therapy equipment, *Respir. Care,* 22, 145, 1977.

905. Committee on Hospital Infection, Medical Research Council, Aseptic methods in the operating suite, *Lancet,* 1, 705, 1968.

906. Committee on Control of Surgical Infections of the Committee on Pre- and Post-operative care, American College of Surgeons: manual on control of infection in surgical patients, Attemeier, W. A., Barnes, B. J., Pulaski, E. J., Sandusky, W. R., Burke, J. F., and Clowes, G. A., Eds., Lippincott, Philadelphia, 1976.

907. Maki, D. G., The epidemiology of surgical infection—guidelines for prevention, *J. Surg. Pract.,* 6, 10, 1977.

908. James, L. S., Graven, S. N., Kay, J. L., Korones, S. B., Meyer, H. B., Muirhead, D. M., Jr., Oliver, T. K., Jr., Sinefield, H., Spear, R. L., Sutherland, J. M., Swyer, P. R., Hasselmeyer, E., Knox, E., and Talner, N. S., Skin care of newborns, *Pediatrics,* 54, 682, 1974.

909. Keay, A. J. and Simpson, R. M., Prevention of infection in nurseries for the newborn, *Postgrad. Med. J.,* 53, 583, 1977.

910. Kandall, S. R., Control of bacterial infection in the nursery, *Pediatr. Ann.,* 90, 1976.

911. Bartlett, R. C., Groschel, D. H. M., Mackel, D. C., Mallison, G. F., and Spaulding E. H., Microbiological surveillance, in *Manual of Clinical Microbiology,* 2nd ed., Lennette, E. H., Spaulding, E. H., Truant, J. P., Eds., American Society of Microbiology, Washington, D.C., 1974, 845.

912. Guidelines for peer review, Veterans Administration Ad Hoc Interdisciplinary Advisory Committee on Antimicrobial Drug Usage, Kunin, C. M., Ed., *J.A.M.A.,* 237, 1001, 1977.

913. Stone, H. H., Prophylactic use of antibiotics, *South. Med. J.,* 70 (Suppl. 1), 1, 1977.

914. Maki, D. G. and Schuna, A. A., A study of antimicrobial misuse in a university hospital, *Am. J. Med. Sci.,* 275, 271, 1978.

915. Levine, A. S., Siegel, S. E., Schreiber, A. D., Hauser, J., Preisler, H., Goldstein, I. M., Seidler, F., Simon, R., Perry, S., Bennett, J. E., and Henderson, E. S., Protected environments and prophylactic antibiotics: a prospective controlled study of their utility in the therapy of acute leukemia, *N. Engl. J. Med.,* 288, 477, 1973.

916. Schimpff, S. C., Greene, W. H., Young, V. M., Fortner, C. L., Jepsen, L., Cusack, N., Block, J. B., and Wiernik, P. H., Infection prevention in acute nonlymphocytic leukemia: laminar air flow room reverse isolation with oral, noabsorbable antibiotic prophylaxis, *Ann. Intern. Med.,* 82, 351, 1975.

917. Dietrich, M., Gaus, W., Vossen, J., van der Waaij, D., and Wendt, F., Protective isolation and antimicrobial decontamination in patients with high susceptibility to infection: a prospective cooperative study of gnotobiotic care in acute leukemia patients: clinical results, *Infection,* 5, 107, 1977.

918. Rodriguez, V., Bodey, G. P., Freireich, E. J., McCredie, K. B., Gutterman, J. U., Keating, M. J., Smith, T. L., and Gehan, E. A., Randomized trial of protected environment—prophylactic antibiotics in 145 adults with acute leukemia, *Medicine (Baltimore),* 57, 253, 1978.

919. Lowbury, E. J. L., Babb, J. R., and Ford, P. M., Protective isolation in a burns unit: the use of plastic isolators and air curtains, *J. Hyg.,* 69, 529, 1971.

920. Burke, J. F., Quinby, W. C., Bondoc, C. C., Sheehy, E. M., and Moreno, H. C., The contribution of a bacterially isolated environment to the prevention of infection in seriously burned patients, *Ann. Surg.,* 186, 377, 1977.

921. Jarrett, F., Balish, E., Moylan, J. A., and Ellerbe, S., Clinical experience with prophylactic antibiotic bowel suppression in burn patients, *Surgery,* 83, 523, 1978.

922. Noble, W. C. and Somerville, D. A., Cutaneous populations, in *Microbiology of Human Skin,* Vol. 2 (Series: Major Problems in Dermatology), Rook, A., Ed., W. B. Saunders, London, 1974, 50.

923. Mabieck, C. E., Significance of coagulase-negative staphylococcal bacteriuria, *Lancet,* 2, 1150, 1969.

924. Wallmark, G., Arremark, I., and Telander, B., *Staphylococcus saprophyticus:* a frequent cause of acute urinary tract infection among female outpatients, *J. Infect. Dis.,* 138, 791, 1978.

925. Schoenbaum, S. C., Gardner, P., and Shillito, J., Infections of cereobrospinal fluid shunts: epidemiology, clinical manifestations, and therapy, *J. Infect. Dis.*, 131, 543, 1975.

926. Fitzgerald, R. H., Peterson, L. F., Washington, J. A., II, Van Scoy, R. E., and Coventry, M. B., Bacterial colonization of wounds and sepsis in total hip arthroplasty, *J. Bone Jt. Surg.*, 55-A, 1242, 1973.

927. Hunter, G. and Dandy, D., The natural history of the patient with an infected total hip replacement, *J. Bone Jt. Surg.*, 59-B, 293, 1977.

928. Sabath. L. D., Barrett, F. F., Wilcox, C., and Finland, M., Methicillin resistance of *Staphylococcus aureus* and *Staphylococcus epidermidis, Antimicrob. Agents Chemother.*, 302, 1969.

929. Zaky, D. A., Bentley, D. W., Douglas, R. G., Jr., Biggar, R., Messner, M., and E. Pincus, Prosthetic valve endocarditis (PVE) due to methicillin-resistant *Staphylococcus epidermidis*, Abstracts of the 15th Interscience Conf. Antimicrobial Agents and Chemotherapy, Washington, D.C., September 24-26, 1975.

930. Hammond, G. W. and Stiver, G., Combination antibiotic therapy in an outbreak of prosthetic endocarditis caused by *Staphylococcus epidermidis, Can. Med. Assoc. J.*, 118, 524, 1978.

931. Cluff, L. E., Surveillance as a control system (panel). Statement of moderator, in *Proceedings of the International Conference on Nosocomial Infections*, Brachman, P. S. and Eickhoff, T. C., Eds., American Hospital Association, Chicago, 291.

932. Maki, D. G., The role of surveillance in prevention of hospital-acquired infection (symposium), in *The Role of Surveillance in Prevention of Infection*, Proc. of the Annual Meeting of the Society for Epidemiologic Research, Toronto, Canada, June 17, 1976; *Am. J. Epidemiol.*, 104, 358, 1976.

HOSPITAL ACQUIRED URINARY TRACT INFECTION

Richard A. Garibaldi

INTRODUCTION

Each year, approximately 40 million persons are hospitalized as acute care patients in hospitals in the U.S. It has been estimated that 3.6% of these patients, or 1.26 million persons, develop hospital acquired infections.[1] Of these, the urinary tract is the most frequently involved site of primary infection, accounting for 41% of all hospital acquired infections.[1] Thus, 1.5% of patients hospitalized in this country annually — over 500,000 persons — develop nosocomial urinary tract infections.

The risk of nosocomial urinary tract infections is not evenly distributed among all hospitalized patients. Certain factors are associated with an increased risk of acquisition. Foremost among these risk factors is instrumentation of the genitourinary tract. Urethral instrumentation or catheterization precedes infection in 75 to 100% of cases acquired by hospitalized patients.[2-8] Included among the procedures that predispose to urinary tract infections are certain surgeries such as transurethral prostatic resection, cystoscopy, and urethral dilatation. However, the most important association is the use of indwelling urethral catheters for drainage of the bladder urine.

The risk of acquiring a catheter-associated urinary tract infection is related to the method and duration of catheterization. Between 0.5 and 8% of patients subjected to a single, short-term catheterization will acquire bacteriuria.[9-12] This risk is increased in certain patient populations with diminished host resistance.[5,11,13] However, the risk of acquiring an infection is even greater in patients with long-term indwelling catheters. Prior to the era of closed sterile drainage, 85 to 100% of patients became bacteriuric during their period of catheterization.[2,4,7,8,10,14,15] Now, with closed sterile gravity drainage, rates of infection have been reduced dramatically. Under study conditions, the incidence of infection with properly maintained closed drainage systems has been lowered to less than 10%.[4,16,17] Despite this great reduction in infection rates, even today, 10 to 20% of the estimated 4 million hospitalized patients receiving catheter drainage acquire catheter-associated bacteriuria each year (Table 1).[18,19]

This chapter will review the epidemiology and control of hospital acquired urinary tract infections. Particular stress will be given to the clinical characteristics and consequences of these infections, pathophysiologic considerations, epidemiologic factors such as reservoirs of infection, modes of transmission, and descriptions of endemic and epidemic spread, and methods of prevention and control.

CLINICAL ASPECTS

Signs and Symptoms

In the noncatheterized patient, the symptoms of an acute urinary tract infection include fever, urgency, urinary frequency, dysuria, suprapubic pressure, and sometimes flank pain.[20] The clinical impression of a urinary tract infection is substantiated by a microscopic examination of the urine revealing white blood cells with or without red blood cells; a Gram stain of the unspun urine usually reveals the etiologic agent. The detection of bacteria by Gram stain of unspun urine correlates very well with a bacterial count of greater than 10^5 organisms per milliliter.[2,21,22] The diagnosis may be confirmed by bacteriologic culture of an early morning, midstream urine specimen revealing greater than 10^5 bacteria per milliliter of urine. A colony count of this mag-

Table 1
ESTIMATION OF THE ANNUAL INCIDENCE IN THE U.S. OF CATHETER-ASSOCIATED URINARY TRACT INFECTIONS AND THEIR CONSEQUENCES

Population	%	Number
Patients admitted to acute care hospitals	—	40,000,000
Patients catheterized	10	4,000,000
Catheterized patients who acquire bacteriuria	15	600,000
Bacteriuric patients who become bacteremic	1	6,000
Bacteremic patients who die of sepsis	30	1,800

nitude on a single urine collection is reproducible 80% of the time and suggests a true bacterial colonization of the urine rather than contamination of the specimen with normal urethral flora.[2] Growth of greater than 10^5 organisms per milliliter of urine has been termed "significant" bacteriuria. The presence of significant bacteriuria has been shown to correlate reasonably well with the presence of infection within the urinary tract.[23,24] The documentation of pyuria (greater than five white blood cells per high-powered microscopic field) is not a prerequisite to the diagnosis of urinary tract infection. Approximately 50% of patients with significant bacteriuria have no pyuria,[25,26] and, vice versa, 10 to 30% of patients with pyuria have no bacteriuria.[5,25] Often, patients with significant bacteriuria have neither symptoms nor signs of acute infection.

In the catheterized patient, the diagnosis of a urinary tract infection is even more complex. These patients are usually hospitalized and have an underlying disease condition which may cause fever or other symptoms suggestive of a urinary tract infection, such as low back pain, polyuria, or dysuria. Their underlying illness may also render them susceptible to infections at other sites (such as pneumonia in patients with multiple sclerosis, decubitus ulcers in paraplegics, wound infections in postoperative patients, etc.). Thus, fever may not be a useful indicator of urinary tract infection. Furthermore, the presence of an indwelling draining catheter may obscure symptoms of local bladder inflammation; urinary frequency and dysuria may not be noticed by either the patient or clinician. In these patients, pyuria may occur secondary to a mechanical cystitis caused by irritation of the catheter tip rubbing against the bladder wall, and may not be a reliable indicator of bacterial infection.

In patients with indwelling urethral catheters, bacterial colony counts may also be subject to misinterpretation. In noncatheterized patients, a colony count of greater than 10^5 organisms per milliliter in a midstream urine specimen is needed to separate bacterial contamination from bladder colonization with a reasonable degree of reproducibility. In the catheterized patient, urine specimens are collected by aseptically puncturing the catheter tubing with a needle and syringe to collect urine from the catheter lumen. A properly collected catheter urine specimen is rarely contaminated by meatal or periurethral flora; thus, colony counts of even less than 10^5 organisms per milliliter may reflect bladder colonization. Moreover, lower colony counts would be expected in urine which is continually being drained because bacteria are not permitted to multiply in the urinary bladder. We have found that colony counts of greater than 10^3 organisms per milliliter in catheter aspirates of patients with indwelling urethral catheters are reproducible and may represent bladder colonization.[18]

Definitions of Hospital Acquired Urinary Tract Infection

For purposes of surveillance, the Center for Disease Control has defined nosocomial

Table 2
DEFINITIONS OF URINARY TRACT INFECTION

	Noncatheterized patient	Catheterized patient
Definite	Symptoms Colony count $\geq 10^5$/ml	Symptoms Colony count $\geq 10^3$/ml
Probable	No symptoms Colony count $\geq 10^5$/ml or Symptoms Colony count $\geq 10^4$/ml	No symptoms Colony count $\geq 10^3$/ml
Possible	Symptoms Pyuria or Symptoms Colony count 10^3–10^4/ml (one species) or $\geq 10^5$/ml (two species)	Symptoms Colony count $< 10^3$/ml (one species) or $\geq 10^3$/ml (two species)
Doubtful	± Symptoms Colony count $< 10^3$/ml or more than two species	No symptoms Colony count $< 10^3$/ml or more than two species

urinary tract infection as a urine culture with a colony count of greater than 10^5 organisms per milliliter from a patient without previous manifestations of infection or previous positive culture.[27] The patient may be asymptomatic or symptomatic. Infection is also diagnosed if a patient develops suggestive symptoms and a urinalysis reveals greater than ten white blood cells per high-powered microscopic field. A patient with previously diagnosed bacteriuria who becomes colonized with a new pathogen is also considered to have a new infection. Infection is considered to be nosocomial if the patient had a prior negative urinalysis and/or culture and develops clinical symptoms while hospitalized.

In our hospital, we have subclassified our definition of urinary tract infection to be more specific in our designations (Table 2). In patients without indwelling catheters, infections are categorized as definite, probable, possible, or doubtful. Definite infections are microbiologically confirmed with urine colony counts of greater than 10^5 colonies per milliliter in patients with symptoms of dysuria, urgency, frequency, flank pain, or fever. Probable infections include patients with asymptomatic bacteriuria with greater than 10^5 bacteria per milliliter of urine, or patients with symptoms and greater than 10^4 organisms per milliliter in a single midstream urine collection. Possible infections are diagnosed if the patient is symptomatic and has pyuria with greater than five white blood cells per high-powered microscopic field in unspun urine but no urine culture, or if the patient has symptoms and 10^3 to 10^4 organisms per milliliter urine of a single bacterial species or greater than 10^5 organisms with two species. Doubtful infections are recorded if the urine culture reveals less than 10^3 organisms or more than two species of bacteria in a patient with minimal urinary symptoms. Similarly, in patients with indwelling urethral catheters, definite infections require symptoms and microbiologic confirmation with a urine colony count of greater than 10^3 organisms per milliliter; probable infections are defined by asymptomatic bacteriuria with greater than 10^3 organisms per milliliter; possible infections have symptoms with low urine colony counts (less than 10^3 per milliliter); and doubtful infections are asymptomatic with low colony counts of multiple isolates.

We classify infections as hospital acquired if symptoms occur later than 48 hr after admission or if previously collected urine has revealed no evidence of incubating infection. Cultural surveys have revealed that from 10 to 20% of hospitalized patients have asymptomatic bacteriuria at the time of hospital admission or insertion of an indwelling catheter.[6,8,13,18,19] These patients may develop symptoms of a urinary tract infection with positive cultures during the period of their hospitalization and be counted as hospital acquired infections when actually they harbored the infecting bacterial pathogen prior to hospitalization. In fact, patients with preexistent asymptomatic bacteriuria appear to develop more frequent and more clinically serious urinary tract infections after catheterization than noncolonized patients.[6] Failure to identify asymptomatic bacteriurics may lead to falsely classifying some community acquired infections as hospital acquired.

Consequences of Infection

For most patients with temporary indwelling urethral catheters, the development of catheter-associated bacteriuria is relatively benign and resolves with removal of the catheter, with or without antibiotic therapy. However, urinary catheterization and infection are the predisposing factors most frequently associated with the acquisition of nosocomial Gram-negative bacteremia.[8,28-32] Approximately 40% of cases of Gram-negative rod bacteremia are secondary to urinary tract infections. Prospective studies, using sensitive culture techniques for aerobic and anaerobic bacteria, have reported an 8% incidence of bacteremia following urethral catheterization.[33,34] Patients with preexistent urinary tract infections develop bacteremias more frequently following instrumentation than those who are initially nonbacteriuric. Most episodes of bacteremia at the time of catheterization are transient and not associated with significant morbidity or mortality. However, 2 to 3% of infected, catheterized patients develop clinically significant bacteremias during their periods of catheterization,[1] and 20 to 50% of bacteremic patients die with Gram-negative rod sepsis.[8,29-31] Differences in case/fatality ratios among septic patients cited by various investigators reflect differences in case selection and severity of the underlying disease in the populations studied.

The long-term consequences of catheter-associated infections are more difficult to determine. No studies are avilable which have prospectively evaluated the costs or morbidity of subsequent symptomatic infections following an episode of catheter-associated bacteriuria. Rates of asymptomatic bacteriuria determined several months after removal of the catheter from infected patients have varied widely. Most studies have observed low rates of chronic bacteriuria,[35-37] but one study observed persistent colonization in 60% of patients at 2 and 3 months after catheter removal.[38] The clinical significance of chronic asymptomatic bacteriuria with reference to arterial hypertension, premature delivery and chronic renal failure remains a subject of some controversy.

EPIDEMIOLOGY

As with any type of infection, the epidemiology of nosocomial urinary tract infections involves an intricate interaction between a susceptible host, a virulent organism, and a mechanism by which the host and pathogen are brought together.

The Host

Certain patients are more susceptible than others in acquiring catheter-associated infections. Patients with long-term indwelling catheters are at greater risk than patients subjected to single, in-and-out urethral catheterizations. Patients who are exposed to a single urethral catheterization for purposes of obtaining a urine specimen, for relief of acute obstruction, or for determination of residual urine have a 0.5 to 8% risk of acquiring bacteriuria.[9-12] Single catheterizations performed on patients with underlying problems such as elderly bedridden women, men undergoing urologic procedures, and women undergoing complicated labors and deliveries have a risk between 15 and 30%.[5,11,13] The difference in rates between healthy and debilitated patients may be explained by the fact that debilitated patients are more likely than healthy patients to have urethral colonization with potentially pathogenic Gram-negative bacilli.[39,40] Urethral flora may be mechanically pushed into the urinary bladder during the act of catheter insertion. Bacteria may also be introduced into the bladder at the time of catheterization if the catheter has been inadequately sterilized or is contaminated due to poor aseptic technique.[4,41]

Patients who require longer term indwelling catheterization are at increased risk of acquiring bacteriuria. Overall, approximately 20% of these patients acquire bacteriuria during their periods of catheterization.[18,19] In general, the likelihood of acquiring bacteriuria increases with increasing durations of catheterization. Of patients with indwelling catheters surveyed at 2 days, approximately 15% are bacteriuric; after 10 days of catheterization, approximately 50% of patients are bacteriuric. The average rate of acquisition of bacteriuria by susceptible patients remains constant and varies between 5 and 10% for each day of catheterization.[18] The exact risk of acquiring bacteriuria is influenced greatly by host factors. Female, elderly, and critically ill patients are at greater risk than males, young patients, and patients with less severe underlying illnesses. Females have approximately twice as great a risk of acquiring catheter-associated bacteriuria as males.[18] This is probably attributable to the fact that the shorter female urethra allows perineal or meatal bacteria easier entry into the bladder by migration in the mucous space between the indwelling catheter and urethral wall. In addition, female patients tend to be catheterized for longer durations because they cannot be treated with external condom drainage. However, our studies have shown that the average daily risk of acquiring bacteriuria for females is more than two and one half times that of males — an observation which is independent of duration of catheterization.[18] Thus, anatomic differences between males and females seem to be the most important factor to account for their differences in susceptibility to catheter-associated infection.

Another major risk factor is severity of underlying disease. This risk factor probably accounts, to some degree, for the increased rates of bacteriuria observed for elderly patients and patients with nonsurgical illnesses. In our studies, more than 50% of catheterized patients with rapidly fatal underlying diseases acquired bacteriuria compared with only 21% of patients with nonfatal underlying diseases.[18] Several explanations are possible to explain these differences: (1) Patients with debilitating underlying illnesses may have diminished phagocytic capabilities or depressed immune responsiveness. (2) These patients are more likely to be receiving medications or treatments which may impair host defenses. (3) They may be catheterized for longer periods. (4) Patients with serious underlying diseases are more likely to be colonized with "more pathogenic" hospital flora.[42-46] (5) These patients may be bedridden and have less attention paid to their personal hygiene, thus allowing enteric organisms greater opportunity to colonize the perineal and meatal areas.[47] Colonization of the meatal area with Gram-negative bacilli and/or Enterococci is an important risk factor for subsequent catheter-associated urinary tract infection.[39,48]

The Organisms

Enteric Gram-negative bacilli are the most frequently reported etiologic agents of catheter-associated urinary tract infections. In virtually all studies reporting the relative frequency of various isolates during nonepidemic periods, *E. coli* is the most frequently

Table 3
RELATIVE FREQUENCIES OF
SELECTED PATHOGENS
CAUSING NOSOCOMIAL
URINARY TRACT INFECTIONS

NNIS Program, CDC, 1976

Pathogen	Frequency (%)
Escherichia coli	32
Streptococcus, Group D	14
Proteus — Providencia	10
Pseudomonas aeruginosa	9
Klebsiella spp.	9
Candida spp.	4
Enterobacter spp.	4
Pseudomonas, other spp.	3
Staphylococcus epidermidis	3
Serratia spp.	2
Other pathogens	10

identified organism.[1,18,19] Table 3 lists the frequencies of various urinary pathogens reported to the Center for Disease Control's National Nosocomial Infection Study in 1976.[1] The vast majority of these organisms are derived from the patient's own gastrointestinal tract.

Within the first 48 to 72 hr of hospitalization, normal bacterial flora in the mouth and gastrointestinal tract undergo disruption and alteration. In the mouth, Gram-negative rods acquired from the hospital environment supplant the normal, predominately Gram-positive aerobic and anaerobic flora.[44-46] This change occurs more quickly and completely in patients who are receiving antimicrobics or who are moribund. However, even hospitalized patients now receiving antimicrobics eventually become colonized with resistant organisms.[45,49] It has been shown that fecal flora is also altered by hospitalization and antibiotic therapy.[42,43] In particular, intestinal colonization with resistant strains of *Klebsiella,*[42,50] *Proteus rettgeri,*[26] and certain serotypes of *E. coli*[43] have been demonstrated in the fecal flora of patients receiving antibiotics. Several prospective studies[18,19,42,43,50] and epidemic reports[26,51-53] have shown that catheterized patients receiving antibiotics are more likely to develop urinary tract infections with antibiotic-resistant organisms.

Epidemics of catheter-associated urinary tract infections are often caused by bacteria which are resistant to many commonly prescribed antibiotics. The mechanisms by which bacteria develop resistance has been analyzed in some epidemic investigations. Selective pressures of broad-spectrum antibiotic usage is a major factor in determining the resistance patterns of infecting organisms. Many types of Enterobacteriaceae commonly acquire antibiotic resistance from episomally transferred R-factors. However, transferable resistance of this type cannot always be demonstrated by in vitro mating experiments with epidemic strains.[54] Thus, the selection of antimicrobic-resistant organisms seems to be a result of the ability of resistant bacteria to survive treatment as well as genetic transference of resistance mediated by R-factors.

Antibiotic resistance does not necessarily imply a more severe infection. Many outbreaks with resistant organisms have been associated with a large number of asymptomatic cases.[25,52,55,56] The clinical severity of infection seems to be more related to the severity of the patient's underlying disease rather than to the type of infecting organism.[26,57,58] However, when the host is debilitated, the infection is symptomatic, and

Table 4

RESERVOIRS OF BACTERIA WHICH ARE ASSOCIATED WITH
CATHETER-ASSOCIATED URINARY TRACT INFECTIONS

| | Reservoir | | | |
Organism	Fecal colonization	Other infected patients	Contaminated objects	Common source
Escherichia coli	+ + + +	+	0	0
Klebsiella spp.	+ + +	+ +	+	0
Proteus spp.	+ +	+ + +	+ +	+
Pseudomonas aeruginosa	+	+ +	+ +	+ + +
Serratia spp.	0	+ + + +	0	0

the organism is antibiotic resistant, the possibility of developing bacteremia or death
is increased.[8,29,30,52,59,60]

Reservoirs of Gram-Negative Bacilli

E. coli, Proteus, Klebsiella, and *Enterobacter* species frequently colonize the colon
of man as normal commensals (Table 4).[42] Strains of *E. coli* are present in virtually
all fecal specimens. A close relationship exists between strains or serotypes of organisms found in the gastrointestinal tract and in subsequent or simultaneous catheter-
associated urinary tract infections.[43,47,61,62] Hospital strains of *E. coli* are infrequently
isolated from inanimate objects in the hospital environment.[43]

Klebsiella species can be found in 10 to 20% of fecal specimens before exposure to
the hospital environment.[42,50] Once hospitalized, patients may become intestinally colonized with selected hospital strains of *Klebsiella,* which appear to be more pathogenic
than normal commensal species.[50,52] One study has reported an attack rate of nosocomial *Klebsiella* infection of 45% in patients who become colonized with a specific antibiotic-resistant strain (serotype 8) which was acquired after hospital admission.[50] Thus,
intestinal flora acquired during hospitalization may in certain situations be more pathogenic than normal commensal bacteria.[49,50]

Proteus species are identified in approximately 20% of fecal specimens from newly
admitted or nonhospitalized patients.[26,42,63,64] However, in patients hospitalized on
wards with epidemic *Proteus* infections, 75 to 100% of patients eventually acquire
fecal colonization with the epidemic strain.[26,61,63] *Proteus* species of the same Dienes
type or serotype can usually be isolated from both stool and urine specimens of infected patients;[61,63] however, it is often difficult to determine a sequential or cause-
and-effect relationship. *Proteus* species recovered from contaminated reservoirs in the
hospital environment have also been implicated as sources of epidemic infection.
Cross-infection of patients has been traced to contact with contaminated urinary leg
drainage bags or collecting bottles,[64,65] rectal thermometers,[26] and hand transfer.[53] In
these epidemics, fecal colonization with *Proteus* species has not been identified, and
autoinfection has been considered unlikely.

On the other hand, certain bacteria, such as *Pseudomonas aeruginosa* and *Serratia*
species, do not usually colonize the intestinal tract.[42,51,54,55,66,67] Nevertheless, stool carriage rates for *Pseudomonas aeruginosa* of greater than 20% have been observed in
some hospitalized populations.[67,69] The frequency of isolation of *Pseudomonas* increases with an increasing duration of hospitalization.[60,68,69] In one ward situation
where *Pseudomonas* urinary tract infections were epidemic, more than 50% of patients
were stool carriers and 85% of patients were colonized with *Pseudomonas* organisms

in their rectum, urethra, or perineal areas.[47] In such an epidemic situation, the same strains of *Pseudomonas* were isolated from the urinary tract as from the various sites of colonization. However, in most descriptions of epidemic catheter-associated infections caused by *Pseudomonas aeruginosa,* the major source of infection is environmental.[41,56,67,70] In these situations, incriminated reservoirs of infection have included contaminated urinals, bedpans, germicidals or antiseptic solutions, and urologic instruments.

Intestinal colonization with *Serratia* species is rare and not thought to be an important source for the spread of catheter-associated infections. Interestingly, in several epidemic investigations, few environmental reservoirs of *Serratia* species have been identified.[51,53-55,58,59,71,72] Epidemics of catheter-associated infection caused by *Serratia* have been linked to hospital units in which patients are spatially crowded and under intense antibiotic pressure. In these situations, it is thought that infected patients, per se, act as reservoirs of infection, and bacteria are transmitted via cross-contamination by hospital personnel who passively carry organisms on their hands.[41,54,55,72,73]

Thus, organisms which have been implicated as causes of catheter-associated infections have been found in the hospital environment colonizing patients' gastrointestinal tracts, contaminating items shared among patients, contaminating instruments used for urethral catheterization, and being carried on the hands of personnel. These organisms are usually acquired from the hospital environment and therefore are frequently resistant to commonly used antimicrobic agents. This selection process singles out resistant strains or unusual bacterial species as causes of epidemic spread. Epidemiologic markers of this type are often used to identify sources of infection and modes of transmission in epidemic situations.

Modes of Spread

The major routes for the acquisition of catheter-associated urinary tract infections are autoinfection with patient's own gastrointestinal flora and cross-contamination from items in the hospital environment or common sources (Figure 1). Autoinfection probably accounts for the greatest number of sporadic cases of infection; cross-contamination, however, is responsible for the greatest number of instances of epidemic spread.

The sequence of autoinfection begins with events which alter the normal composition of intestinal flora after exposure to the hospital environment. The exact mechanism by which this modification occurs is not well understood. Bacterial organisms present in mouth flora, selected by the pressures of antimicrobic therapy, may be ingested and colonize the gut; antibiotics may directly eradicate certain commensal bacteria which normally exert antibacterial pressures on more resistant organisms, thereby allowing the more resistant organisms to flourish,[43] or, foods prepared in the hospital environment and contaminated by hospital flora may be ingested and become part of the normal gut flora. Contamination of foods and medicines has been reported with *Pseudomonas aeruginosa, E. coli,* and *Klebsiella* species.[66,74] Salads and other cold foods carry the highest colony counts of bacteria; after ingestion, these organisms have been recovered from stool samples for 2 to 4 days.[69] These intestinal organisms may subsequently colonize the perineal and periurethral areas of catheterized patients.[47] Perineal organisms may then contaminate the indwelling catheter and periurethral mucosa. Immobile and fecally incontinent patients such as paraplegics are particularly susceptible to acquire catheter-associated infections because of virtually constant fecal contamination of their perineal areas. We and others have found that prior colonization of the urethral meatus with enteric Gram-negative bacilli or Enterococci frequently preceded the acquisition of catheter-associated infection.[39,75,76] Urethral bac-

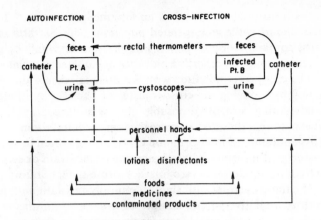

FIGURE 1. Epidemiology of catheter-associated urinary tract infection. (Adapted from Dutton, A. A. C. and Ralston, M., *Lancet,* 1, 115, 1957.)

teria are then able to gain access into the urinary bladder by migrating retrogradely in the mucous space between the urethral mucosa and indwelling catheter.[77]

Cross-contamination of catheter drainage systems occurs when pathogenic bacteria are derived from sources in the hospital environment. Inanimate instruments, utensils, and human vectors have been found to be responsible for introducing pathogenic bacteria into the urinary bladder. The catheter drainage system itself is the most important predisposing factor to the acquisition of nosocomial urinary tract infections by cross-contamination. It may carry organisms into the bladder because it has been improperly sterilized or contaminated with nonsterile solutions;[4,56,70,78,79] or, it may serve as a conduit for the retrograde migration of bacteria in urine within the catheter lumen[80] or in the extralumenal, periurethral mucous space.[77] Cystoscopes and other genitourinary instruments may similarly serve as vectors or conduits for the passage of pathogenic bacteria into the urinary bladder.[4]

In hospital areas where there is a high density of catheterized patients, pathogenic bacteria can be spread from patient to patient by ward personnel acting as vectors for bacterial transfer. Personnel may become colonized with Gram-negative organisms in their mouth, rectum, or other moist areas,[81] or become passive hand carriers without significant colonization.[51] Several investigators have reported that from 30 to more than 50% of randomly tested hospital personnel carry antibiotic-resistant, Gram-negative bacilli on their hands.[52,53,2] In addition, various types of hand lotions have been reported to be contaminated with greater than 10^5 colonies per milliliter of such potential pathogens as *Serratia marcescens, Pseudomonas aeruginosa, Escherchia intermedia, Klebsiella pneumoniae,* and *Enterobacter* species.[83] Pathogenic bacteria, obtained from contacts with contaminated products or from exposures to infected or colonized patients, may be carried passively on the hands of ward personnel. As they move from catheterized patient to catheterized patient, they may deposit bacteria on uninfected drainage systems or contaminate collected urine. These bacteria subsequently are able to migrate into the urinary bladder and cause infection.

The transfer of pathogenic organisms from hospital personnel to patients is not a new discovery. In 1847, Semmelweis made the original observation on the importance of hand contamination in the transmission of infection.[84] Subsequently, others have shown that bacteria can be transferred from one patient to another even in different hospital rooms, with hospital personnel as an intermediary vector.[85] In fact, a community-wide epidemic of catheter-associated infections with *Serratia marcescens* was attributed to cross-contamination of patients in different hospitals by personnel who moved from one hospital to the other.[54] Epidemics of catheter-associated urinary tract infections caused by cross-contamination with *Serratia marcescens* and *Proteus rettgeri* have been curtailed by reducing the cross-transfer of bacteria by reinforcing the importance of handwashing, use of disposable gloves, and geographically separating catheterized patients so that they do not share the same hospital room.[51,53,54,72,86]

Sources of cross-contamination or common exposures can often be found in epidemics of catheter-associated infection in which one particular strain or serotype of bacteria is isolated. Often the epidemic is recognized because the laboratory reports an unusual incidence of enteric bacteria with similar, multiply-resistant antibiotic sensitivity patterns or identifies a relatively large number of isolates of an uncommon bacterial species, such as *Serratia marcescens, Providencia stuartii,* or *Proteus rettgeri.* Whenever a common bacterial isolate is linked with a large number of cases, a common source exposure or cross-contamination should be sought. Common source epidemics have been attributed to contaminated germicidals *(Pseudomonas* species), rectal thermometers or bedpans (*Proteus* species), and urinals, drainage bags, and collection bottles (*Proteus* species). Rarely, a single serotype may predominate in an epidemic presumed secondary to autoinoculation with intestinal organisms.[47,50] In these epidemics, a common source of intestinal colonization such as contaminated foods or medicines should be investigated.

Routes of Bacterial Entry Into the Bladder

Three possible means by which bacteria may enter into the bladder have been identified. These are

1. Inoculation of organisms from the distal urethra or from a contaminated catheter at the time of catheter insertion
2. Retrograde intralumenal spread from the drainage bag reservoir or catheter tubing into the bladder
3. Retrograde migration of bacteria into the bladder outside the catheter lumen in the periurethral mucous sheath

Occasional bacteria may reach the urinary tract via hematogenous or lymphatic spread, but these routes probably account for only a very small minority of catheter-associated infections. It is extremely important to identify the specific routes of bacterial contamination of the bladder because proper understanding of the pathogenesis of infection may lead to successful preventive measures.

The possibility of introducing potentially pathogenic bacteria at the time of catheterization has long been recognized.[4,87] The risks of acquisition of bacteriuria after a single, in-and-out catheterization range between 0.5 and 30%, [2,9-13] the higher rates being found in patients with more severe underlying diseases. Early investigators observed that episodes of catheter-associated bacteriuria occurring within the first 18 hr after catheterization were caused by nonhospital acquired strains.[4] They hypothesized that these infections were caused by the inoculation of urethral organisms into the bladder during catheterization, with subsequent establishment of infection when the catheter was left in place. The distal urethra is frequently colonized with a variety of enteric bacilli and cocci which can cause infection when inoculated into bladder urine.[75,88] Even with thorough cleansing of the meatal area, the anterior aspect of the urethra retains its normal flora.[9] A catheter introduced into the bladder passes through this flora and may contaminate bladder urine. In our studies, we have noted higher rates of bacteriuria in the first 48 hr after catheterization in patients catheterized by less medically trained hospital personnel than those catheterized by physicians or nurses.[18] This observation suggests, but does not prove, that careless technique with catheter insertion may be associated with increased risks of acquisition of bacteriuria. However, we observed no increased rate in the development of catheter-associated bacteriuria on the first or second day following catheterization compared with the average daily rate of catheter-associated infection. This would imply that hospital personnel who use sterile equipment and who have some knowledge of aseptic technique are able to catheterize patients without introducing gross bacterial contamination on most occasions.

The risk of acquiring infection increases the longer the catheter is allowed to remain indwelling.[18,19] There has long been debate over the relative importance of the retrograde spread of bacteria inside the catheter lumen to the urinary bladder vs. the retrograde movement of bacteria extralumenally in the periurethral mucous space. Certainly, in the era of open urinary drainage, the migration of bacteria within the catheter lumen was the most important route of infection. With open drainage, rates of bacteriuria invariably approached 100% after 2 to 4 days of catheterization.[2,4,8] Dukes,[14] in 1928, introduced a "closed" drainage system to decrease the possibility of contamination in the drainage reservoir, and was able to show a marked diminution of catheter-associated infections. However, routine use of closed sterile systems was not advocated in the literature until the 1950s and 1960s.[4,19,41,89-91] With closed drainage, rates of catheter-associated infection have been reduced to approximately 20%.[18,19] Oftentimes, the acquisition of infection can be traced to errors in the maintenance of the closed drainage system.[18] Bacteria may be inadvertently inoculated into the urinary drainage system at several possible sites (Figure 2). The most important of these are the junction between the indwelling catheter and the collection tubing, reflux from the drainage bag reservoir to the catheter tubing, and contamination of the tip of the drainage bag outlet spigot.[92] The catheter-tubing junction is particularly important because it may become disconnected accidentally with patient movement or it may be opened carelessly by hospital personnel for specimen collections or instillation of irrigating solutions.

Once bacteria are introduced into the drainage system, they can migrate with relative ease into the urinary bladder. Studies done in the 1950s showed that stagnant urine was an excellent culture medium and that motile strains of *E. coli* and *Proteus* were able to ascend in a standing column to reach bladder urine.[93] Contaminated urine may also reach the bladder when the drainage bag or catheter tubing are placed above bladder level and urine is allowed to flow back into the bladder. Finally, irrigating solutions which may be instilled by opening the catheter tubing junction may result in contamination of the drainage system and cause bacteria to be washed into the catheterized bladder.[94] Even in hospitals where the concepts of closed sterile drainage are stressed and practiced, catheter-associated infections caused by retrograde, intralumenal spread continue to occur.[18,19,80] In one study, circumstantial evidence for the relative importance of the intralumenal route of infection was obtained by observing that contamination of the drainage bag reservoir usually preceded the development of significant bladder infection.[80] Of 23 patients who developed catheter-associated infections, 20 became bacteriuric 1 to 6 days after the drainage bag reservoir was first noted to be contaminated. In our studies, 17 of 95 patients who acquired catheter-associated bacteriuria were noted to have contaminated bag reservoirs for at least 1 day before the establishment of bacteriuria.[18] Standing columns of urine in the drainage tubing, malpositioned bags, or open connectors were observed in 12 of 17 systems in the period

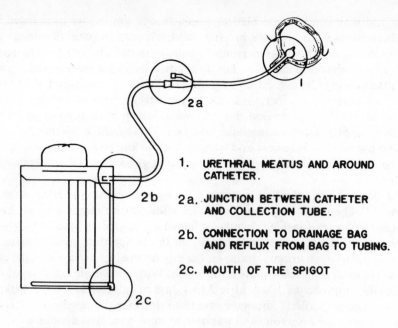

1. **URETHRAL MEATUS AND AROUND CATHETER.**

2a. **JUNCTION BETWEEN CATHETER AND COLLECTION TUBE.**

2b. **CONNECTION TO DRAINAGE BAG AND REFLUX FROM BAG TO TUBING.**

2c. **MOUTH OF THE SPIGOT**

FIGURE 2.   Entry points for bacteria into catheter drainage systems. (1) Extralumenal entry — between catheter and urethral mucosa (2) intralumenal spread: (a) junction between catheter and collecting tube, (b) reflux from drainage bag to collecting tube, (c) drainage spigot. (Adapted from Kunin, C. M., *Prevention and Management of Urinary Tract Infections*, 2nd ed., Lea & Febiger, Philadelphia, 1974. With permission.)

between bag colonization and bacteriuria. Thus, errors in the care of closed sterile drainage seem to play a major role in allowing bacterial entry into the drainage system and permitting retrograde colonization of bladder urine.

The presence of an indwelling catheter also facilitates the extralumenal migration of bacteria into the bladder. In 1956, Kass and Schneiderman,[77] placed *Serratia marcescens* in the periurethral areas of three catheterized, comatose patients and observed bladder colonization 48 to 74 hr later. They concluded that the bacteria migrated into the bladder in the mucous sheath between the catheter and urethral mucosa. We and others have observed that meatal or periurethral colonization with potential urinary tract pathogens predisposes to the subsequent acquisition of catheter-associated bacteriuria.[39,40,48,76] In some epidemic investigations, the epidemic strain has been found in perineal or periurethral cultures of infected patients,[47] or contaminating of the catheter tubing of uninfected patients.[51] The extralumenal spread of bacteria into the bladder might help to explain the observaton that females generally have twice the risk of acquiring catheter-associated infections compared to males. Because the female urethra is shorter than that of males, it may be more easily traversed extralumenally by motile enteric bacilli. This route then, may be a major mode of entry for bacteria to reach the bladder in female patients.

All three routes of bacterial entry into the bladder probably play some role in the pathogenesis of catheter-associated urinary tract infections. The dramatic reduction in rates of infection after the introduction of closed sterile drainage attests to the importance of retrograde intralumenal spread. Intralumenal spread is still observed when breaks in closed sterile drainage occur and catheter urine becomes contaminated. Extralumenal spread may occur even in the presence of properly maintained, closed sterile drainage. One could hypothesize that most cases of autogenous infection occur secondary to the colonization of the periurethral area or drainage tubing with enteric bacilli and that these organisms migrate into the bladder in the periurethral mucous sheath. A wide variety of preventive techniques and/or products have been introduced as adjuncts to closed sterile drainage to limit the entry of bacteria by these routes.

EPIDEMIC PATTERNS

Epidemics of catheter-associated urinary tract infections may go unrecognized in hospitals where there are no active surveillance programs to monitor hospital acquired infections. Epidemic situations can sometimes develop insidiously and are easily overlooked. Routine surveillance monitoring should include a review of bacterial isolates by site from microbiology laboratory records, regular ward rounds, and review of individual patient charts as necessary. Records should be kept regarding the numbers of nosocomial urinary tract infections by service or patient location. These records should include observations such as the bacteriologic identification of the infecting organism, use of indwelling catheterization or genitourinary instrumentation, and listing of patient's major underlying diseases. Denominators should be determined for the calculation of attack rates of infection. Suitable denominators might include the number of admissions or discharges to the particular medical or surgical service or specialty unit over the specific length of time. Monthly or quarterly infection rates should be calculated and reviewed to identify increases in the incidence of infection, clustering of cases, or isolations of unusual bacterial species.

In the nonepidemic situation, sporadic cases of catheter-associated infection are caused most commonly by autoinoculation of organisms colonizing the patient's own intestinal tract. Multiple-antibiotic resistance of infecting organisms is not observed as frequently in this situation as in epidemic situations, particularly in patients who themselves are not receiving antibiotics. In sporadic cases, *E. coli* are implicated most often as causes of infection, reflecting the predominance of this organism in normal stool flora.[42] Although *E. coli* is the most common species identified in sporadic cases, infections may be caused by a wide variety of bacterial species which colonize the gastrointestinal tract.[1,18,19] Cross-contamination also is responsible for some catheter-associated infections in nonepidemic situations;[18,95] however, it is virtually impossible to determine the relative frequency of autoinfection and cross-infection in the absence of epidemic spread.

Frequently, it is difficult to differentiate endemic from epidemic occurrences of catheter-associated infections (Table 5). In nonepidemic periods, approximately 10% of patients hospitalized on general medical or surgical wards acquire catheter-associated bacteriuria in hospitals where closed-sterile drainage is advocated.[18,19] Endemic rates may be greater on certain specialty wards such as intensive care units, urology wards, or rehabilitation areas because of their selected patient populations. Because the background incidence of endemic catheter-associated infections is so high, epidemic increases in rates may not be recognized unless they are identified by formal or informal surveillance activities. Epidemic occurrences are often recognized because (1) the attack rate in a specific hospital area is inordinately high, affecting virtually all catheterized patients, (2) an unusual epidemic species is identified such as *Serratia marcescens, Proteus rettgeri,* or *Providencia stuartii,* or (3) unusual, multiple-antibiotic resistant strains are isolated.

Autoinfection

Epidemics of catheter-associated urinary tract infections have been attributed to three routes of acquisition: autoinfection, cross-infection, and common source expo-

Table 5

EPIDEMIOLOGIC PATTERNS OF CATHETER-ASSOCIATED URINARY TRACT INFECTION

Factor	Endemic pattern	Epidemic patterns		
	Sporadic cases	Autoinfection	Cross-infection	Common source
Characteristics of infecting organism				
Stool flora	+ + + +	+ + +	0	0
"Water bug"	0	0	+	+ + + +
Multiple antibiotic resistance	+	+ + +	+ + + +	+ +
Organisms most frequently isolated	*Escherichia coli* *Enterococci*	*Klebsiella* spp. *Proteus* spp. *Enterobacter* spp.	*Serratia marcescens* *Proteus rettgeri* *Providencia stuartii*	*Pseudomonas* spp.
Reservoir				
GI colonization	+ + + +	+ + + +	0	0
Other colonized patients	+	+ +	+ + + +	0
Environmental contamination	+	+	+ +	+ +
Common source	0	0	+ +	+ + + +
Mode of transmission				
Autoinfection	+ + + +	+ + + +	0	0
Hand contamination of personnel	+	+ +	+ + + +	+
Clustering of patients	+	+ +	+ +	0
Contaminated product	0	0	+ +	+ + + +
Risk factors predisposing to infection				
Long-term indwelling catheter	+ + + +	+ + + +	+ + +	0
Broad-spectrum antibiotics	+	+ + +	+ + + +	0
Type of underlying disease	+ + +	+ + + +	+ + + +	0
Contact with contaminated product	0	0	+ +	+ + + +

sures (Table 5). To date, only one investigation has been able to document autoinfection as the major route of acquisition of epidemic urinary tract infections by demonstrating fecal carriage of the epidemic strain preceding the development of urinary tract infection. In this study, Selden et al.[50] showed that 45% of patients who acquired intestinal colonization with type 8 *Klebsiella* after admission to the hospital developed subsequent urinary tract infection with that organism. Others have identified simultaneous colonization of the stool or perineal area and urinary tract with epidemic strains of *Proteus* species,[61,63] *E. coli*,[43,62,96] *Klebsiella*,[52] *Enterobacter*,[52] and *Pseudomonas aeruginosa*.[47] In these outbreaks, a majority of paired isolates from stool swabs and urinary tract cultures were identical when tested by serotyping, antibiotic resistance patterns, or Dienes testing. On the basis of this observation and a lack of positive cultures from environmental sources, these investigators hypothesized that autoinoculation of intestinal flora into the catheterized urinary tract was the most likely route of transmission. The likelihood that these infections were secondary to autoinoculation was enhanced by the observation that, in these epidemic situations, many different bacterial strains were identified in infected patients rather than a single epidemic strain. However, these authors were unable to show whether stool colonization was actually a cause or a consequence of the urinary tract infection.

One outbreak of catheter-associated infection has been reported which involved spread by both cross-contamination and autoinoculation in the pathogenesis of infection.[26] Improperly cleaned rectal thermometers were implicated as the vehicle of bacterial spread from patient to patient. Contaminated thermometers initiated rectal colonization with epidemic strains of *Proteus mirabilis*. After 2 weeks of hospitalization in the affected unit, more than 90% of all patients were colonized with these strains. Subsequent infection of the catheterized urinary tract in these patients was presumed to be secondary to autoinoculation with fecal bacteria. These observations suggest that selected hospital flora can, on occasion, colonize the intestinal tract of susceptible patients and that these organisms can subsequently be inoculated into and infect the catheterized urinary tract by contiguous spread from the rectum to the urethral meatus or indwelling collection system.

Cross-Infection

Most reported epidemics of catheter-associated urinary tract infection have been attributed to cross-infection (Table 5). In these outbreaks, a single epidemic strain or serotype of bacteria is responsible for a majority of cases. The organisms most frequently implicated in these epidemics are *Serratia marcescens*, *Proteus rettgeri*, and *Providencia stuartii*. Oftentimes, the fact that the organism has an unusual microbiologic designation or a multiply-resistant antibiotic sensitivity pattern serves as an epidemiologic marker.[50-55] In epidemics spread by cross-infection, the implicated pathogen is invariably not found in stool or perineal cultures of infected patients.[3,53,64] Often, however, the epidemic strain is found in environmental cultures, including instruments used in genitourinary surgery,[4,41] urine receptacles,[41,64,67] urinary leg bags,[65] bedpans,[67,97,98] or washcloths.[98] Some of these objects serve as vehicles for the spread of infection. Nonetheless, the most common vectors for the spread of bacteria from one patient to another, or from a contaminated surface to a susceptible patient, are the hands of hospital personnel.[3,41,51,53-55,67] In epidemics of catheter-associated urinary tract infection caused by *Serratia marcescens*, hand transfer has been a major source of cross-infection. In these outbreaks, rectal colonization or colonization of other mucous membranes of patients or personnel is rarely identified, environmental cultures are usually negative, and common source exposures are not found.[51,54,55,72,73] Spread of infection by cross-contamination is suggested by (1) the isolation of single *Serratia* strains of serotypes in a given epidemic, (2) the observation that cases are usually crowded in a designated area with a high density of catheterized patients, and (3) the finding of positive cultures of pooled handwashings of hospital personnel.[51,54,55] With epidemic catheter-associated *Serratia* infections, it is hypothesized that the urinary tracts of patients with symptomatic or asymptomatic infections are the primary reservoirs of bacteria and that organisms are transferred from patient to patient indirectly by passive carriage on the hands of noncolonized personnel. Similarly, passive hand transfer of organisms from patient to patient has been implicated in epidemics of *Proteus rettgeri* and *Providencia stuartii* urinary tract infection.[53,55,57]

Cross-infections can occur in any area of the hospital, but they usually are associated with certain high risk units. Patients in these units are usually grouped into geographically separate areas because they have certain types of underlying diseases which require specialized care. Frequently, the underlying disease predisposes them to genitourinary instrumentation or to chronic urethral catheterization. Thus, paraplegics or spinal cord injury patients in rehabilitation units,[47,53,65,99] stroke or polio patients on neurology services,[25] prostate surgery patients on urology wards,[4,51,67] and critically ill patients in intensive care units[54] are at special risk of acquiring infection. These patients frequently are hospitalized for long durations and receive broad-spectrum antimicrobic therapy at some time during their hospitalization. Use of antibiotics enables antibiotic-resistant organisms to flourish in the hospital environment. Thus, when cross-contaminations with bacteria from environmental sources does occur, it is usually caused by resistant bacteria.

Common Source Infection

Common source exposures responsible for catheter-associated urinary tract infections are of two types: (1) exposures to commonly used items which are contaminated from environmental or patient contacts, and (2) contacts with contaminated products. Cystoscopy equipment, urinals, leg bags, bedpans, and rectal thermometers have been implicated as vehicles of bacterial transmission. Most often, these items are contaminated after having been used by infected patients and inadequately sterilized between uses. Bacteria are transmitted from patient to patient indirectly by contact with the contaminated item. Usually, infected patients themselves are the reservoirs of the epidemic strain and the sources of contamination of the implicated items. Nurses or other hospital personnel may also serve as common sources for the acquisition of catheter-associated urinary tract infections. A nurse who was colonized with the epidemic strain, was implicated as a common source in an epidemic of serious *Proteus mirabilis* infection among patients in a newborn nursery.[81] Hand lotions used by hospital personnel have been found to be frequently contaminated with potential urinary pathogens.[83] These bacteria could be transferred from contaminated hands to catheterized patients in an epidemic situation. However, no epidemics have yet been identified in which a particular nurse or contaminated hand lotion has been a source of epidemic catheter-associated urinary tract infections.

Only a few contaminated products have been identified as common sources of epidemic urinary tract infections.[41,56,70] In each of these epidemics, a germicidal or antiseptic solution used for cleansing either the meatal area or catheter equipment was contaminated with a *Pseudomonas* species. The epidemics were identified by surveillance efforts which detected increased incidences of catheter-associated urinary tract infections caused by the unusual bacterial isolate. In each of these outbreaks, the spread of infection was curtailed by eliminating the contaminated source. Foods or medicines might also serve as common sources for gastrointestinal colonization with an epidemic strain and subsequent autoinfection.[69] However, no outbreaks have yet been attributed to this source.

THE RATIONALE FOR PREVENTION AND CONTROL

Prevention of Infection

In 1958, Beeson[79] was among the first to point out the potential dangers of urinary catheterization in his classic editorial entitled "The Case Against the Catheter". He recommended that catheter use be restricted to times when it was absolutely necessary; he urged physicians to avoid catheterizations and remove indwelling catheters as early as possible. Nonetheless, at times, the catheter is an indispensible adjunct to medical or surgical treatment and must be used. Special precautions must be taken to decrease the risk of developing a catheter-associated infection. The rationale for preventing infection rests upon knowledge of the epidemiology of the spread of bacteria within the hospital environment and routes of bacterial entry into the bladder. Methods to decrease the risks of infection have focused on two areas: (1) prevention of bacterial entry into the urinary bladder, and (2) removal of bacteria from the bladder before infection occurs.[100]

Prevention of Bacterial Entry Into the Bladder

Bacteria can gain entry into the urinary bladder by inoculation at the time of catheter insertion, by retrograde intralumenal spread, and by migration extralumenally in the periurethral mucous sheath. Recommendations to prevent bacterial inoculation at the time of catheterization have included thorough cleansing of the urethral meatus with a germicidal solution, liberal application of an antibacterial lubricant, and meticulous aseptic technique.[4,9,17,91,101] Sterile, disposable urinary instruments and catheters should be used whenever possible; nondisposable items should be thoroughly cleaned and sterilized by heat or ethylene oxide between uses.[4,100] Only trained personnel should be allowed to insert urethral catheters,[18] and the importance of aseptic technique should be reinforced periodically.[102] Some investigators have recommended that special teams be trained to insert and care for indwelling catheters.[101,103]

With indwelling catheters, the major advance in limiting the retrograde intralumenal spread of bacteria into the bladder has been the introduction and implementation of closed sterile gravity drainage.[4,7,17,19,92,100] This technique demands that the drainage system not be disconnected except under strict aseptic precautions, that urine not be allowed to form a standing column, that reflux not occur between drainage bag and catheter tubing or tubing and urinary bladder, and that specimens be collected by aseptic needle puncture of the catheter tubing. All sections of the catheter tubing and drainage bag reservoir are sterile and closed to outside contamination. If any part is contaminated by inappropriate technique, accidental disconnection, or leaks — or is observed to be functioning improperly — it should be replaced with a new system.[19,92,102] It is recommended that the closed system not be irrigated routinely with antibiotic or antiseptic solutions unless urine drainage is impeded by obstruction.[16,102] In controlled studies where continuous irrigation has been used as an adjunct to closed sterile drainage, it has not proven to be efficacious.[94] Catheters with irrigation were disconnected almost twice as often as nonirrigated control systems because they had an extra junction for the instillation of irrigating solutions which could be opened. Breaks in closed sterile drainage were thought to have allowed bacterial entry into irrigated drainage systems and offset any possible beneficial effect of antibiotic suppression.[94]

Other adjuncts to closed sterile drainage have been shown not to have any significant beneficial effect when evaluated prospectively in controlled studies. A variety of types of one-way valves, air-locks, and drip chambers have been introduced to prevent reflux of urine from the drainage bag reservoir to the catheter tubing. Thornton and Andreole[80] suggested that the presence of a nonreflux valve could delay the acquisition of bacteriuria from 1 to 6 days following bag contamination. However, their data showed no overall reduction in the rate of catheter-associated infection, and their observations regarding delayed acquisition were uncontrolled. In a prospective, controlled evaluation of catheter drainage systems, Finkelberg and Kunin[104] observed no differences in rates of bacteriuria among six systems, including some with valves or drip chambers and some without. Another possible adjunct to the maintenance of closed-sterile drainage was introduced by Gibbon[105] in 1958. Using a long, plastic catheter which connected directly to the drainage bottle, he was able to maintain sterile urine for up to 2 weeks in a group of paraplegic patients. Nonetheless, it is generally thought that if closed sterile gravity systems are kept closed and maintained properly, no additional adjuncts are needed to prevent retrograde intralumenal spread of bacteria into the bladder.[92]

Closed sterile drainage does not prevent bacteria from reaching the bladder extralumenally by retrograde spread in the mucous space between the catheter and urethral wall. A number of procedures have been introduced in an attempt to prevent the entry of bacteria by this route. Many of these modifications are based on sound theoretical grounds and have been shown to have some efficacy when open drainage systems were widely used.[4,16,105-107] However, they have resulted in little or no additional reduction in rates of catheter-associated infection when used with closed sterile drainage systems. Kunin and co-workers,[108,109] in prospective studies of closed systems, found no added benefit of antibacterial lubricants or antibacterial substances impregnated in catheters when compared with control systems. Similarly, many investigators have recommended the use of daily or twice-daily meatal care as a logical approach to preventing extralumenal spread of bacteria into the bladder.[92,101,102] However, the efficacy of this recommendation is unproven. In a prospective study, Britt et al.[110] found no decrease in acquired bacteriuria when twice-daily cleansing with a povidone-iodine solution was compared with routine ward care. Other modifications in the technique of catheter care have been suggested but have not yet been subjected to rigorous study, including the use of small bore, siliconized indwelling catheters which might be less traumatic to the urethral mucous,[105] and foam pads to stabilize the catheter as it extends from the urethral meatus which might prevent the catheter from moving in and out of the urethra.[111]

Removal of Bacteria From the Bladder

Signs or symptoms of infection may not be apparent for a variable length of time after bacteria have gained access to the urinary bladder. Infection may be averted if steps are taken to eliminate the contaminating organisms immediately by flushing the bladder or treating the patient with antimicrobic therapy. Some investigators recommend that a moderate diuresis should be induced in all patients with indwelling catheters to promote a constant washout of the urinary tract.[92,101] However, many catheterized patients cannot maintain adequate enough fluid intake or be treated with diuretics to flush out contaminating organisms. In addition, the effectiveness of this recommendation has not yet been evaluated in controlled studies. Contaminating bacteria might also be removed by discontinuing catheterization or by changing the catheter drainage system. Discontinuation of catheterization is often associated with a clearing of bacteriuria with or without antibiotic treatment;[35] changing the contaminated system must be accompanied by concurrent specific antibiotic therapy to be effective in clearing bladder colonization.

Many investigators have studied the efficacy of antibiotic prophylaxis or early treatment in the control of catheter-associated infections. Local instillaton of antibiotics or antibacterial solutions was reported to be effective in reducing rates of catheter-associated infection prior to the widespread use of closed urinary drainage.[8,112] In these studies, continuous infusions of neomycin and polymyxin-B or weak (0.25%) acetic acid were associated with dramatic decreases in infection rates. However, more recent studies of patients who were also receiving closed drainage have not ben able to repeat these observations.[94,113] In a randomized controlled trial of neomycin-polymyxin irrigant, Warren et al.[94] reported no decrease in infection rates, but did observe an increase in antibiotic-resistant isolates in patients who received irrigation. They postulated that irrigation suppressed some bacterial colonization but that administration of the irrigating solution enabled bacterial contamination to occur. Frequently, the contaminating bacteria were resistant to the antibiotics in the irrigating solution. They concluded that irrigation had no ultimate effect on the rate of acquisition of catheter-associated infection and selected a more antibiotic-resistant bacterial population as infecting agents.

Several studies have reported that prophylactic systemic antibiotics also are ineffective in reducing rates of catheter-associated urinary tract infections and select for antibiotic-resistant organisms.[100,114,115] These observations were generally derived from patients who were catheterized for relatively long durations. We observed that antimicrobial agents lowered rates of bacteriuria in patients catheterized for less than 4 days and that this effect was independent of age, sex, and underlying disease.[18] Antibiotics were of no benefit and predisposed to resistant bacteria in patients catheterized for longer than 4 days. Other investigators have also reported that systemic antibiotics may prevent infection in patients catheterized for short periods.[19,116,119] However, routine use of prophylactic therapy is not yet recommended.[102,103,118] The potential benefits of antibiotics are thought to be offset by such factors as antibiotic-resistant infections, adverse toxic or hypersensitivity reactions, unsuspected drug interactions, occurrence of nonurinary infections due to resistant organisms, and further selection of resistant hospital flora.

Early treatment with systemic antibiotics has also been recommended as a potentially effective way of removing bacteria from the colonized bladder.[102,119,120] However, because many instances of catheter-associated bacteriuria occur asymptomatically, daily bacteriologic monitoring of catheter urine would have to be performed to identify colonized patients early and to aid in the selection of specific antimicrobic therapy.[92,119] Although this approach to infection prevention appears sound, its efficacy and liabilities in terms of effect on infection rates, cost, adverse drug reactions, and induction of antibiotic resistance has not yet been studied.

Control of Epidemic Spread

In any epidemic situation, particular attention should be given to the prevention of new infections by rigorous aseptic technique at the time of catheter insertion and careful maintenance of the closed drainage system. In addition, special attempts must be made to diminish reservoirs of the epidemic strain, identify and eliminate common sources, interrupt contact spread, and modify risk factors.[55]

Diminishing the Reservoirs

Epidemiologic surveillance is the keystone to early epidemic recognition and initiation of control measures. Calculation of attack rates of infection by hospital location, service, patient diagnoses, or types of surgery can help to identify occult reservoirs of infection. Sometimes, prospective bacteriologic surveys of high-risk catheterized patients are needed to identify asymptomatic, colonized patients who may themselves be reservoirs of infection. Once symptomatic and asymptomatic cases are identified, an attempt should be made to reveal exposures which may have been common sources of infection. Selected items that are implicated as possible common reservoirs should be cultured, and incriminated items should be removed or sterilized. If hospital personnel are identified as reservoirs of infection, they should be temporarily removed from the high-risk area and given treatment to eliminate colonization with epidemic strain.

If the epidemic investigation determines that the reservoir of infection is colonization of the patient's gastrointestinal or urinary tract, steps should be taken to lessen the magnitude or character of this colonization.[55] Alteration of intestinal flora might be effected by diminishing the general usage of broad-spectrum systemic antimicrobic agents which are responsible for the selection of antibiotic-resistant strains, or by the use of oral, nonabsorbable antimicrobic agents to eradicate the epidemic strain from the intestinal flora. Treatment with urinary antiseptics such as methenamine hippurate, or instillation of antibacterial solutions by continuous irrigation, may suppress urinary colonization when it is not feasible or indicated to treat with systemic agents. Decreasing the magnitude of colonizing bacteria may decrease the likelihood of autoinfection in the case of gastrointestinal flora and cross-infection via hand contamination in the case of urinary tract colonization. However, the effectiveness of these approaches has not yet been tested in an epidemic situation.

Interrupting Contact Spread

The infected or colonized urinary drainage system should be cared for as though it were an open wound.[55] Gloves should always be worn when an infected catheter system is manipulated or perineal area is cleaned. Handwashing should be reemphasized even when gloves are worn. Emphasis and insistence on handwashing is of vital importance to control contact-spread infection.[18,53,55,92] Handwashing facilities must be available and conveniently situated for use of personnel between patient contacts. Appropriate use of handwashing facilities requires both personal motivation and easy access. If patients are grouped in a unit away from handwashing facilities, hospital personnel will soon forget the need for proper hand care. In that situation, two alternatives for epidemic control exist: dispersal of catheterized patients to individual rooms without catheterized roommates, or insistence that personnel wear disposable gloves between patient contacts.[54,86]

Spread of infection among catheterized roommates has been observed in several epidemics of catheter-associated infection.[51,53,86] In fact, the presence of a catheterized roommate who is colonized or infected with the epidemic strain was a critical risk factor for the acquisition of infection in these epidemics. Therefore, it is recommended that, in epidemic situations, patients with indwelling catheters not share the same room unless special precautions are taken. In intensive care units or other open-ward situations, special precautions might include staffing by different nursing personnel or spatial separation to the greatest degree possible.[55,86]

Contacts with contaminated vehicles such as bedpans, rectal thermometers, germicidal solutions, or urinals may also be sources of epidemic spread. These vectors must be identified by epidemiologic investigation and cultural surveys. Once identified, appropriate steps should be taken to break the chain of contact-spread. This process might include eliminating incriminated reservoirs, using disposable equipment, paying stricter attention to aseptic techniques, or reassessing sterilization procedures. In addition, geographic dispersal of high-risk patients away from high-risk areas would help to lessen the likelihood of exposure to common sources of infection.

Modifying Risk Factors

A number of host-risk factors have been identified which predispose patients to the acquisition of catheter-associated bacteriuria. Most of these factors cannot be altered by the attending physician, including such predisposing factors as female sex, old age, or debilitating underlying disease.[18,19] Certain variables, however, are alterable and may be manipulated to contain epidemic spread. Catheter use should be avoided whenever possible; durations of catheterizations should be minimized; techniques of closed, sterile drainage should be flawless; and stratagems of antibiotic usage should be reevaluated. In some situations, use of broad-spectrum agents which induce the emergence of resistant strains should be restricted. In other situations, prophylactic use of certain systemic agents or local irrigants may be justified to eliminate or reduce the quantity of colonizing bacteria. It must be stated, however, that the use of prophylactic antibiotics is still quite controversial[18,19,103] and should be evaluated in a prospective, controlled study.

CONCLUSION

New technologies such as indwelling urethral catheterization predispose to the development of new problems such as catheter-associated infections. Insights into the epidemiology of how these infections are transmitted and acquired have provided rational approaches for infection prevention and control. Over the past 20 years, dramatic decreases have occurred in the rates of catheter-associated infections; but, even today, 20% of catheterized patients acquire infections, and epidemic spread still occurs. At times, errors in the technique of catheter care or personal hygiene are implicated as causes of infection. Innovative approaches including new types of catheters, team approaches to catheter care, educational incentives, and novel antibiotic programs are being evaluated to further reduce the infectious risks of catheterization. Impaired host defenses in some patients and the occasional occurrence of human errors may make it impossible to prevent all catheter-associated infections. However, studies of new approaches to prevent and control this most important cause of hospital acquired infections must be encouraged.

REFERENCES

1. Center for Disease Control, National Nosocomial Infections Study Report, Annual Summary 1976, February 1978.
2. Kass, F. H., Asymptomatic infections of the urinary tract, *Trans. Assoc. Am. Physicians*, 69, 56, 1956.
3. Dutton, A. A. C. and Ralston, M., Urinary tract infection in a male urologic ward, *Lancet*, 1, 115, 1957.
4. Gillespie, W. A., Linton, K. B., Miller, A., and Slade, N., The diagnosis, epidemiology and control of urinary infection in urology and gynaecology, *J. Clin. Pathol.*, 13, 187, 1960.
5. Brumfitt, W., Davies, B. I., and Rosser, F. I., Urethral catheter as a cause of urinary-tract infection in pregnancy and puerperium, *Lancet*, 2, 1059, 1961.
6. Kaitz, A. L. and Williams, E. J., Bacteriuria and urinary-tract infectons in hospitalized patients, *N. Engl. J. Med.*, 262, 425, 1960.
7. Levin, J., The incidence and prevention of infection after urethral catheterization, *Ann. Intern. Med.*, 60, 914, 1964.
8. Martin, C. M., Bookrajian EN, Bacteriuria prevention after indwelling urinary catheterization, *Arch. Intern. Med.*, 110, 209, 1962.

9. **Guze, L. B. and Beeson, P. B.**, Observations on the reliability and safety of bladder catheterization for bacteriologic study of the urine, *N. Engl. J. Med.*, 255, 474, 1956.
10. **Kass, E. H.**, Bacteriuria and diagnosis of infections of the urinary tract with observations on the use of Methionine as a urinary antiseptic, *Arch. Intern. Med.*, 100, 709, 1957.
11. **Turck, M., Goffe, B., and Petersdorf, R. G.**, The urethral catheter and urinary tract infection, *J. Urol.*, 88, 834, 1962.
12. **Turck, M. and Petersdorf, R. G.**, The role of antibiotics in the prevention of urinary tract infections, *J. Chronic Dis.*, 15, 683, 1962.
13. **Lytton, B.**, Urinary infection in cystoscopy, *Br. Med. J.*, 2, 547, 1961.
14. **Dukes, C.**, Urinary infections after excision of the rectum: their cause and prevention, *Proc. R. Soc. Med.*, 22, 259, 1928.
15. **Lunt, R. L., Dutton, W. A. W., Dewhurst, C. J., and Russell, C. S.**, The incidence of infection following gynecological operations, *Lancet*, 1, 1240, 1957.
16. **Desautels, R. E., Walter, C. W., Groves, R. C. and Harrison, J. H.**, Technical advances in the prevention of urinary tract infection, *J. Urol.*, 87, 487, 1962.
17. **Ansell, J.**, Some observations on catheter care, *J. Chronic Dis.*, 15, 675, 1962.
18. **Garibaldi, R. A., Burke, J. P., Dickman, M. L., and Smith, C. B.**, Factors predisposing to bacteriuria during indwelling urethral catheterization, *N. Engl. J. Med.*, 291, 215, 1974.
19. **Kunin, C. M. and McCormack, R. C.**, Prevention of catheter-induced urinary-tract infections by sterile closed drainage, *N. Engl. J. Med.*, 274, 1155, 1966.
20. **Hoeprich, P. D.**, Urethritis and cystitis, in *Infectious Diseases*, Hoeprich, P. D., Ed., Harper & Row, New York, 1977, 428.
21. **Knight, V., Draper, J. W., Brady, E. A., and Attmore, C. A.**, Methenamine mandelate: antimicrobial activity absorption and excretion, *Antibiot. Chemother. Washington, D.C.*, 2, 615, 1952.
22. **Kass, E. H.**, Chemotherapeutic and antibiotic drugs in the management of infections of the urinary tract, *Am. J. Med.*, 18, 764, 1955.
23. **MacDonald, R. A., Levitin, H., Mallory, G. K., and Kass, E. H.**, Relation between pyelonephritis and bacterial counts in urine: autopsy study, *N. Engl. J. Med.*, 256, 915, 1957.
24. **Effersoe, P. and Jensen, E.**, Urinary tract infection vs. bacterial contamination, *Lancet*, 1, 1342, 1963.
25. **Riley, H. D. Jr. and Knight, V.**, Urinary tract infection in paralytic poliomyelitis, *Medicine, (Baltimore)* 37, 281, 1958.
26. **Edebo, L. and Laurell, G.**, Hospital infection of the urinary tract with proteus, *Acta Pathol. Microbiol. Scand.*, 43, 93, 1958.
27. **Garner, J. S., Bennett, J. V., Scheckler, W. E., Maki, D. G., and Brackman, P. S.**, Surveillance of nosocomial infections, *Proc. Inter. Conf. Nosocomial Infections*, Center for Disease Control, Atlanta, August 3-6, 1970, 277.
28. **McCabe, W. R. and Jackson, G. G.**, Gram-negative bacteremia. I. Etiology and ecology, *Arch. Intern. Med.*, 110, 847, 1962.
29. **McCabe, W. R. and Jackson, G. G.**, Gram-negative bacteremia. II. Clinical, laboratory and therapeutic observations, *Arch. Intern. Med.*, 110, 856, 1962.
30. **Freid, M. A. and Vosti, K. L.**, The importance of underlying disease in patients with gram-negative bacteremia, *Arch. Intern. Med.*, 121, 418, 1968.
31. **DuPont, H. L. and Spink, W. W.**, Infections due to gram-negative organisms: an analysis of 860 patients with bacteremia at the University of Minnesota Medical Center, *Medicine (Baltimore)*, 48, 307, 1969.
32. **McGowan, J. E., Jr., Parrott, P. L., and Duty, V. P.**, Nosocomial bacteremia: potential for prevention of procedure-related cases, *J.A.M.A.*, 237, 2727, 1977.
33. **Sullivan, N. M., Sutter, V. L., Carter, W. T., Attebery, H. R., and Finegold, S. M.**, Bacteremia after genitourinary tract manipulation: bacteriological aspects and evaluation of various blood culture systems, *Appl. Microbiol.*, 23, 1101, 1972.
34. **Sullivan, N. M. Sutter, V. L., Mims, M. M., Marsh, V. H., and Finegold, S. M.**, Clinical aspects of bacteremia after manipulation of the genitourinary tract, *J. Infect. Dis.*, 127, 49, 1973.
35. **Cox, C. E. and Hinman, F., Jr.**, Incidence of bacteriuria with indwelling catheter in normal bladders, *J.A.M.A.*, 178, 151, 1961.
36. **Clarke, B. G. and Joress, S.**, Quantitative bacteriuria after use of indwelling catheters: incidence in genito-urinary surgery, *J.A.M.A.*, 174, 1593, 1960.
37. **Tyler, C. W. and Oseasohn, R.**, The relationship of in-lying catheterization to persistent bacteriuria in gynecologic patients, *Am. J. Obstet. Gynecol.*, 86, 998, 1963.
38. **Paterson, M. L., Barr, W., and MacDonald, S.**, Urinary infection after colporrhaphy: its incidence, causation, and prevention, *J. Obstet. Gynaecol. Br. Commonw.*, 67, 394, 1960.

39. Garibaldi, R. A., Burke, J. P., Britt, M. R., Miller, W. A., and Smith, C. B., Urethral colonization and catheter-associated bacteriuria, *N. Engl. J. Med.*, 303, 316, 1980.

40. Shackman, R. and Messent, D., The effect of an indwelling catheter on the bacteriology of the male urethra and bladder, *Br. Med. J.*, 2, 1009, 1954.

41. Pyrah, L. N., Goldie, W., Parsons, F. M., and Raper, F. P., Control of *pseudomonas pyocyanea* infection in a urological ward, *Lancet*, 2, 314, 1955.

42. Rose, H. D. and Schreier, J., The effect of hospitalization and antibiotic therapy on the gram-negative fecal flora, *Am. J. Med. Sci.*, 255, 228, 1968.

43. Winterbauer, R. H., Turck, M., and Petersdorf, R. G., Studies on the epidemiology of *Escherichia coli* infections. V. Factors influencing acquisition of specific serologic groups, *J. Clin. Invest.*, 46, 21, 1967.

44. Johanson, W. G., Pierce, A. K., and Sanford, J. P., Changing pharyngeal bacterial flora of hospitalized patients, *N. Engl. J. Med.*, 281, 1137, 1969.

45. Johanson, W. G., Pierce, A. K., Sanford, J. P., and Thomas, G. D., Nosocomial respiratory infections with gram-negative bacilli, *Ann. Intern. Med.*, 77, 701, 1972.

46. Valenti, W. M., Trudell, R. G., and Bentley, D. W., Factors predisposing to oropharyngeal colonization with gram-negative bacilli in the aged, *N. Engl. J. Med.*, 298, 1108, 1978.

47. Montgomerie, J. Z. and Morrow, J. W., *Pseudomonas* colonization in patients with spinal cord injury, *Am. J. Epidemiol.*, 108, 328, 1978.

48. Bultitude, M. I. and Eykyn, S., The relationship between the urethral flora and urinary infection in the catheterised male, *Br. J. Urol.*, 45, 678, 1973.

49. Kirby, W. M. M., Corpron D. O., and Tanner, D. C., Urinary tract infections caused by antibiotic-resistant coliform bacilli, *J.A.M.A.*, 162, 1, 1956.

50. Selden, R., Lee, S., Wang, W. L. L., Bennett, J. V., and Eickhoff, T. C., Nosocomial *Klebsiella* infections: intestinal colonization as a reservoir, *Ann. Intern. Med.*, 74, 657, 1971.

51. Maki, D. G., Hennekens, C. G., Phillips, C. W., Shaw, W. V., and Bennett, J. V., Nosocomial urinary tract infection with *Serratia marcescens*: an epidemiologic study, *J. Infect. Dis.*, 128, 579, 1973.

52. Noriega, E. R., Liebowitz, R. E., Richmond, A. S., Rubinstein, E., Schaefler, S., Simberkoff, M. S., and Rahal, J. J., Jr., Nosocomial infection caused by gentamicin-resistant, streptomycin-sensitive *Klebsiella*, *J. Infect. Dis.*, 131, 45, 1975.

53. Lindsey, J. O., Martin, W. T., Sonnenwirth, A. C., and Bennett, J. V., An outbreak of nosocomial *Proteus rettgeri* urinary tract infection, *Am. J. Epidemiol.*, 103, 261, 1976.

54. Schaberg, D. R., Alford, R. H., Anderson, R., Farmer, J. J., Melly, M. A., and Schaffner, W., An outbreak of nosocomial infection due to multiple resistant *Serratia marcescens*: evidence of interhospital spread, *J. Infect. Dis.*, 134, 181, 1976.

55. Schaberg, D. R., Weinstein, R. A., and Stamm, W. E., Epidemics of nosocomial urinry tract infection caused by multiple resistant gram-negative bacilli: epidemiology and control, *J. Infect. Dis.*, 133, 363, 1976.

56. Hardy, P. C., Ederer, G. M., and Matsen, J. M., Contamination of commercially packaged urinary catheter kits with the pseudomonad EO-1, *N. Engl. J. Med.*, 282, 33, 1970.

57. Edwards, L. D., Cross, A., Levin, S., and Landau, W., Outbreak of a nosocomial infection with a strain of *Proteus rettgeri* resistant to many antimicrobials *Am. J. Clin. Pathol.*, 61, 41, 1974.

58. Lancaster, L. J., Role of *Serratia* species in urinary tract infections, *Arch. Intern. Med.*, 109, 82, 1962.

59. Davis, J. T., Foltz, E., and Blakemore, W. S., *Serratia marcescens*, a pathogen of increasing clinical importance, *J.A.M.A.*, 214, 2190, 1970.

60. Wilfert, J. N., Barrett, F. F., and Kass, E. H., Bacteremia due to *Serratia marcescens*, *N. Engl. J. Med.*, 279, 286, 1968.

61. Story, P., *Proteus* infections in hospital, *J. Pathol.*, 68, 55, 1954.

62. Schwarz, H., Schirmer, H. K. A., Ehlers, B., and Post, B., Urinary tract infections: correlation between organisms obtained simultaneously from the urine and feces of patients with bacteriuria and pyuria, *J. Urol.*, 101, 765, 1969.

63. deLouvois, J., Serotyping and the Dienes reaction of *Proteus mirabilis* from hospital infections, *J. Clin. Pathol.*, 22, 263, 1969.

64. Kippax, P. W., A study of *Proteus* infections in a male urological ward, *J. Clin. Pathol.*, 10, 211, 1957.

65. Washington, J. A., II, Senjem, D. H., Haldorson, A., Schutt, A. H., and Martin, W. J., Nosocomially acquired bacteriuria due to *Proteus rettgeri* and *Providencia stuartii*, *A.J.C.P.*, 60, 836, 1973.

66. Shooter, R. A., Walter, K. A., Williams, V. R., Horgan, G. M., Parker, M. T., Asheshov, E. H., and Bullimore, J. F., Faecal carriage of *Pseudomonas aeruginosa* in hospital patients, *Lancet*, 2, 1331, 1966.

67. **McLeod, J. W.,** The hospital urine bottle and bedpan as reservoirs of infection by *Pseudomonas pyocyanea, Lancet,* 1, 394, 1958.

68. **Bodey, G. P.,** Epidemiological studies of *Pseudomonas* species in patients with leukemia, *Am. J. Med. Sci.,* 260, 82, 1970.

69. **Shooter, R. A., Cooke, E. M., Gaya, H., Kumar, P., Patel, N., Parker, M. T., Thom, B. T., and France, D. R.,** Food and medicaments as possible sources of hospital strains of *Pseudomonas aeruginosa, Lancet,* 1, 1227, 1969.

70. **Lee, J. C. and Fialkow, P. J.,** Benzalkonium chloride — source of hospital infection with Gram-negative bacteria, *J.A.M.A.,* 177, 708, 1961.

71. **Wheat, R. P., Zuckerman, A., and Ranta, L. A.,** Infection due to chromobacteria, *Arch. Intern. Med.,* 88, 461, 1951.

72. **Allen, S. D. and Conger, K. B.,** *Serratia marcescens* infection of the urinary tract: a nosocomial infection, *J. Urol.,* 101, 621, 1969.

73. **Taylor, G. and Keane, P. M.,** Cross-infection with *Serratia marcescens, J. Clin. Pathol.,* 15, 145, 1962.

74. **Shooter, R. A., Faiers, M. C., Cooke, E. M., Breaden, A. L., and O'Farrell, S. M.,** Isolation of *Escherichia coli, Pseudomonas aeruginosa,* and *Klebsiella* from food in hospitals, canteens, and schools, *Lancet,* 2, 390, 1971.

75. **Cox, C. E.,** The urethra and its relationship to urinary tract infection: the flora of the normal female urethra, *South. Med. J.,* 59, 621, 1966.

76. **Brehmer, B. and Madsen, P. O.,** Route and prophylaxis of ascending bladder infection in male patients with indwelling catheters, *J. Urol.,* 108, 719, 1972.

77. **Kass, E. H., and Schneiderman, L. J.,** Entry of bacteria into the urinary tracts of patients with inlying catheters, *N. Engl. J. Med.,* 256, 556, 1957.

78. **Omland, T.,** Nosocomial urinary tract infections caused by *Proteus rettgeri, Acta Pathol. Microbiol. Scand.,* 48, 221, 1960.

79. **Beeson, P. B.,** Editorial: the case against the catheter, *Am. J. Med.,* 24, 1, 1958.

80. **Thornton, G. F. and Andriole V. T.,** Bacteriuria during indwelling catheter drainage, *J.A.M.A.,* 214, 339, 1970.

81. **Burke, J. P., Ingall, D., Klein, J. O., Gezon, H. M., and Finland, M.,** *Proteus mirabilis* infections in a hospital nursery traced to a human carrier, *N. Engl. J. Med.,* 284, 115, 1971.

82. **Salzman, T. C., Clark, J. J., and Klemm, L.,** Hand contamination as a mechanism of cross infection in nosocomial infection with antibiotic-resistant *Escheria coli* and *Klebsiella-Aerobacter, Antimicrob. Agents Chemother.,* 7, 97, 1967.

83. **Morse, L. J., and Schonbeck, L. E.,** Hand lotions — a potential nosocomial hazard, *N. Engl. J. Med.,* 278, 376, 1968.

84. **Sinclair, W. J.,** *Semmelweis — His Life and His Doctrine,* Sherratt & Hughes, London, 1909, 49.

85. **Williams, R. E. O., Blowers, R., Garrod, L. P. and Shooter, R. A.,** *Hospital Infection: Causes and Prevention,* Lloyd — Luke, London, 1960.

86. **Maki, D. G., Hennekens, C. H., and Bennett, J. V.,** Prevention of catheter-associated urinary tract infection, *J.A.M.A.,* 221, 1270, 1972.

87. **Emmett, J. L.,** Preoperative and postoperative care in transurethral prostatectomy, *Surg. Clin. North Am.,* 20, 1061, 1940.

88. **Helmholz, H. F., Sr.,** Determination of the bacterial content of the urethra: a new method, with results of a study of 82 men, *J. Urol.,* 64, 158, 1950.

89. **Gillespie, W. A.,** Discussion on urinary infections, *Proc. R. Soc. Med.,* 49, 45, 1956.

90. **Kunin, C. M. and McCormack, R. C.,** Prevention of catheter-induced urinary-tract infections by a sterile closed drainage system, *N. Engl. J. Med.,* 274, 1155, 1966.

91. **Desautels, R. E.,** Aseptic management of catheter drainage, *N. Engl. J. Med.,* 263, 189, 1960.

92. **Kunin, C. M.,** Detection, *Prevention and Management of Urinary Tract Infections,* 2nd ed., Lea & Febiger, Philadelphia, 1974.

93. **Weyrauch, H. M. and Bassett, J. B.,** Ascending in an artificial urinary tract, experimental study, *Stanford Med. Bull.,* 9, 25, 1951.

94. **Warren, J. W., Platt, R., Thomas, R. J., Rosner, B., and Kass, E. H.,** Antibiotic irrigation and catheter-associated urinary-tract infections, *N. Engl. J. Med.,* 299, 570, 1978.

95. **Orskov, I.,** Nosocomial infections with *Klebsiella* in lesions of the urinary tract, *Acta Pathol. Microbiol. Scand. Suppl.,* 259, 1952.

96. **Schwartz, H., Schirmer, H. K. A., Post, B., and Ehlers, B.,** Correlation of *Escherichia coli* occurring simultaneously in the urine and stool of patients with clinically significant bacteriuria: serotyping with group-specific O antisera, *J. Urol.,* 101, 379, 1969.

97. **Traub, W. H., Craddock, M. E., Raymond, E. A., Fox, M., and McCall, C. E.**, Characterization of an unusual strain of *Proteus rettgeri* associated with an outbreak of nosocomial urinary-tract infection, *Appl. Microbiol.*, 22, 278, 1971.

98. **Traube, W. H.**, Isolation of an antibiotic-resistant, lactose-fermenting strain of *Proteus rettgeri*, *Experientia*, 26, 437, 1970.

99. **Milner, P. F.**, The differentiation of Enterobacteriaceae infecting the urinary tract, *J. Clin. Pathol.*, 16, 39, 1963.

100. **Sanford, J. P.**, Hospital-acquired urinary-tract infections, *Ann. Intern. Med.*, 60, 903, 1964.

101. **Lindan, R.**, The prevention of ascending, catheter-induced infections of the urinary tract, *J. Chronic Dis.*, 22, 321, 1969.

102. **Stamm, W. E.**, Guidelines for prevention of catheter-associated urinary tract infections, *Ann. Intern Med.*, 82, 386, 1975.

103. **Keresteci, A. G. and Leers, W. D.**, Indwelling catheter infection, *Can. Med. Assoc. J.*, 109, 711, 1973.

104. **Finkelberg, Z. and Kunin, C.**, Clinical evaluation of closed urinary drainage systems, *J.A.M.A.*, 207, 1657, 1969.

105. **Gibbon, N.**, A new type of catheter for urethral drainage of the bladder, *Br. J. Urol.*, 30, 1, 1958.

106. **Mulla, N.**, Indwelling catheter in gynecologic surgery, *Obstet. Gynecol.*, 17, 199, 1961.

107. **McLeod, J. W., Mason, J. M., and Pilley, A. A.**, Prophylactic control of infection of the urinary tract consequent on catheterisation, *Lancet*, 1, 292, 1963.

108. **Butler, H. K. and Kunin, C. M.**, Evaluation of Polymyxin catheter lubricant and impregnated catheters, *J. Urol.*, 100, 560, 1968.

109. **Kunin, C. M. and Finkelberg, Z.**, Evaluation of an intraurethral lubricating catheter in prevention of catheter-induced urinary tract infections, *J. Urol.*, 106, 928, 1971.

110. **Britt, M. R., Burke, J. P., Miller, W. A., Steinmuller, R. A., and Garibaldi, R. A.**, The non-effectiveness of daily meatal care in the prevention of catheter-associated bacteriuria (abstract) 16th Interscience Conf. Antimicrobic Agents and Chemotherapy, Chicago, 141, 1976.

111. **Viant, A. C., Linton, K. B., Gillespie, W. A., and Midwinter, A.**, Improved method for preventing movement of indwelling catheters in female patients, *Lancet*, 1, 736, 1971.

112. **Kass, E. H. and Sossen, H. S.**, Prevention of infection of urinary tract in presence of indwelling catheters, *J.A.M.A.*, 169, 1181, 1959.

113. **Gladstone, J. L., and Robinson, C. G.**, Prevention of bacteriuria resulting from indwelling catheters, *J. Urol.*, 99, 458, 1968.

114. **Petersdorf, R. G., Curtin, J. A., Hoeprich, P. D., Peeler, R. N., and Bennett, I. L.**, A study of antibiotic prophylaxis in unconscious patients, *N. Engl. J. Med.*, 257, 1001, 1957.

115. **Appleton, D. M. and Waisbren, B. A.**, The prophylactic use of chloramphenicol in transurethral resections of the prostate gland, *J. Urol.*, 75, 304, 1956.

116. **Lacy, S. S., Drach, G. W., and Cox, C. E.**, Incidence of infection after prostatectomy and efficacy of cephaloridine prophylaxis, *J. Urol.*, 105, 836, 1971.

117. **Plorde, J. J., Kennedy, R. P., Bourne, H. H., Ansell, J. S., and Petersdorf, R. G.**, Course and prognosis of prostatectomy, *N. Engl. J. Med.*, 272, 269, 1965.

118. **Shapiro, S. R., Santamarina, A., and Harrison, J. H.**, Catheter-associated urinary tract infections: incidence and a new approach to prevention, *J. Urol.*, 112, 659, 1974.

119. **Butler, H. K. and Kunin, C. M.**, Evaluation of specific systemic antimicrobial therapy in patients while on closed catheter drainage, *J. Urol.*, 100, 567, 1968.

120. **Drach, G. W., Lacy, S. S., and Cox, C. E.**, Prevention of catheter-induced post-prostatectomy infection. Effects of systemic cephaloridine and local irrigation with neomycinpolymyxin through closed-drainage catheter system, *J. Urol.*, 105, 840, 1971.

GASTROINTESTINAL INFECTIONS

James M. Hughes and Richard L. Guerrant

ORIENTATION TO NOSOCOMIAL GASTROINTESTINAL INFECTIONS: DEFINITION, FREQUENCY, MORBIDITY, AND MORTALITY

The gastrointestinal tract harbors microbes that outnumber the body's cells. While these microorganisms may be quite important in many nosocomial infections outside the gastrointestinal tract, the focus of this chapter will be upon "outside" invaders of the gastrointestinal tract that usually produce characteristic gastrointestinal symptoms. Aside from a review of host defenses, no attempt will be made to address the gut as a major source of potentially life-threatening, extraintestinal, nosocomial infections.

Available data on the true frequency, morbidity, and mortality associated with nosocomial gastrointestinal infections are limited. Data compiled in the Center for Disease Control (CDC) National Nosocomial Infections Study (NNIS), which included 82 hospitals in 31 states during 1976, indicate that the rate for recognized nosocomial gastrointestinal infection on all services was 1.4 infections per 10,000 patient discharges. The rate varies from a low of 0.1 per 10,000 discharges from the obstetrics service to a high of 4.6 per 10,000 discharges from newborn nurseries, and 6.1 per 10,000 discharges from the pediatric services. The overall nosocomial gastrointestinal infection rate is considerably lower than those for nosocomial urinary tract, surgical wound, respiratory, cutaneous, and primary bloodstream infections and is comparable to the nosocomial central nervous system infection rate.[1]

Salmonella is responsible for less than one nosocomial gastrointestinal infection per 10,000 hospital discharges. *E. coli* are increasingly recognized enteric pathogens. Besides the classically recognized "enteropathogenic serotypes", some strains may produce an enterotoxin or be invasive. Of 161 nosocomial infection outbreaks investigated by CDC from 1956 through 1975, *Salmonella* accounted for 20 (13%) of outbreaks, second in frequency only to *Staphylococcus aureus*.[2] During this period, 17 additional nosocomial gastrointestinal outbreaks were investigated; 12 of these were due to enteropathogenic *E. coli* serotypes and 5 were due to an unrecognized but presumed infectious etiologic agent. These data suggest that, although nosocomial gastrointestinal illness outbreaks may be relatively uncommon, they are easily recognized, cause sufficient morbidity and mortality, or are sufficiently refractory to routine control measures that they are frequently investigated by CDC.

Few data are available on morbidity and mortality associated with nosocomial gastroenteritis. Considerable morbidity may be associated with salmonellosis outbreaks both in newborns and in patients on adult medical and surgical wards. Complications of *Salmonella* bacteremia may occur. In addition, asymptomatic excretion of *Salmonella* may persist for up to a year following neonatal infection;[3] such carriage rarely results in secondary infection in household contacts.[3,4] In a total of 46 *Salmonella* cross-infection outbreaks reported to CDC from both hospitals and custodial institutions, the case-fatality ratio was 4.9%.[5]

In contrast, in the 30 common-vehicle outbreaks reported from the same types of institutions, the case-fatality ratio was 1.8%. The lower case-fatality ratio in common source outbreaks presumably reflects their tendency to involve primarily adult patients and members of hospital staff, while the cross-infection outbreaks frequently involve infants in newborn nurseries, where the disease is more severe. In certain cross-infection outbreaks in nurseries, even higher case-fatality ratios have been reported.[6] Case-fatality ratios in outbreaks caused by enteropathogenic *E. coli* and rotaviruses are generally lower than those for salmonellosis.

Trends in the occurrence and severity of nosocomial gastrointestinal infections, with the increasing complexity of tertiary care over time, are difficult to follow because of changes in reporting habits, diagnostic tools to recognize "new" pathogens, and in the hospital setting itself.

HOST DEFENSES

Gastrointestinal host defenses are of great importance and are often overlooked. In many instances it is necessary to be reminded of the obvious before appropriate prevention and management can be done.

Personal Hygiene

The number of microorganisms ingested is an obvious determinant of whether one acquires a gastrointestinal infection.[7] Most bacterial pathogens, such as *Salmonella, Vibrio cholerae,* or enterotoxogenic *E. coli*, require the ingestion of 10^5 to 10^8 viable organisms to bypass the normal adult host defense mechanisms and cause infection. In contrast, as few as 10 to 100 shigellae, a number that might readily be transmitted by contact, may cause symptomatic infection in a healthy adult. Likewise, in the hospital setting where the host defenses listed below are impaired, such compromised patients may be susceptible to a much smaller inoculum than healthy adults. The additional potential role of food and drink prepared in the hospital in colonizing the gastrointestinal tract of hospitalized patients with "foreign" flora has been well documented.[8]

Gastric Acidity

The normal acidity of the stomach provides a second major barrier to infection with ingested microorganisms. Neutralization of gastric acidity with antacids or bypassing the gastric acid greatly reduces the infectious dose required for several pathogens.[9] Furthermore, patients who are achlorhydric or who have had gastrectomy procedures are at increased risk of acquiring several gastrointestinal infections with increased frequency and severity.[10]

Normal Flora

Comprised of over 99% anaerobic organisms (10^{11}/g), the normal lower intestinal flora is frequently violated and often overlooked as an important host defense mechanism. As in the upper respiratory tract,[11] alteration of the intestinal flora by antimicrobial agents greatly increases the host's susceptibility to colonization or symptomatic infection by "outside invaders". An increased frequency of *Salmonella* infections among Swedish tourists taking a prophylactic antimicrobial agent over those taking no antimicrobial agent demonstrates the importance of normal flora in humans.[12] In experimental animals, normal bacterial flora have been shown to interact synergistically with host immunity to prevent intestinal infections.[13,14] Furthermore, studies by Bohnhoff, Miller, and Martin[15] have demonstrated the protective effect of normal enteric microflora. This natural resistance is related to the normal colonic flora and their toxic, acidic products and reduced environment. In their studies in experimental mice, a single injection of streptomycin eradicated this resistance and reduced the infectious dose of *Salmonella typhimurium* by over 10^5-fold.

Intestinal Motility

The importance of normal intestinal motility in preventing potentially serious intestinal infections is amply demonstrated. Hospitalized patients with severe ulcerative colitis or pseudomembranous enterocolitis may be at increased risk of "toxic megacolon" if their normal intestinal motility was impaired with antimotility drugs. There are isolated reports of dissemination of *Salmonella* infection after opiates were given for a relatively mild gastroenteritis.[16] The potential risk for increasing the severity of an inflammatory process like shigellosis when antimotility agents are given has also been described.[17] These findings, suggesting an important role for normal intestinal motility as a defense against gut infections, are also supported by experimental animal data in which opiates are often used to increase the infection rate with enteric pathogens given to experimental animals.[18]

Specific Immunity

In addition to the above nonspecific factors and many others that are less well understood (such as intestinal mucus and its glycoprotein content), several specific humoral, cell-mediated and phagocytic host defense mechanisms are important in the intestinal tract. Humoral intestinal immunity may be provided by either leakage of circulating IgG or by locally produced IgA.[19,20] Roles for cell-mediated and phagocytic defenses in the intestinal tract are suggested by the normal appearance of lymphocytes and phagocytes in the lamina propria and by the increased efficacy of adjuvant-boosted typhoid immunization.

SYNDROMES OF NOSOCOMIAL ENTERIC INFECTIONS

Noninfectious Causes

An important first step in the diagnosis of a nosocomial gastrointestinal infection is a careful review of the patient's previous history and any current medication or treatment that might cause diarrhea that should not be considered a nosocomial infection. In addition to laxative abuse and indiscriminant antibiotic usage, numerous other pharmacologic agents must be considered as potential causes of diarrhea. Parasympathomimetic agents may cause hypermotility, cramping, abdominal pain, or diarrhea. Xanthine-related phosphodiesterase antagonists such as caffeine or theophylline may be present in analgesic compounds or in dietary or other stimulants and may, in excess, also cause diarrhea. Thyroid hormone or cardiovascular drugs, including digitalis glycosides, quinidine, or ganglionic blockers, may also contribute to gastrointestinal symptoms. Antimetabolites, particularly colchicine and antifolate compounds, have their greatest effect on rapidly dividing intestinal mucosal cells and thus have major gastrointestinal side effects. Numerous osmotically active agents often contribute to diarrhea in the hospitalized patient. In addition to osmotic cathartics (such as magnesium citrate), antacids, special diets, hyperalimentation, and other feeding supplements are commonly complicated by osmotic diarrhea in the hospital.

Endocrine causes of diarrhea include nonbeta cell pancreatic islet tumors, medullary carcinoma of the thyroid, carcinoid tumors, and other tumors associated with increased serum prostaglandins or vasoactive intestinal polypeptide (VIP).[21] Adrenal insufficiency or hypoparathyroidism may also be associated with diarrhea.

A careful evaluation for causes of diarrhea should also include consideration of diabetic neuropathy, gastrointestinal leukemia or lymphoma, uremia, carcinoma, or vasculitic processes such as polyarthritis, lupus, or scleroderma. Mechanical and anatomic derangements such as blind loop syndromes, Hirschsprung's disease, or mechanical partial obstruction by intrinsic or extrinsic mass lesions may cause diarrhea through obstruction to solids or bacterial overgrowth. Congenital or acquired deficiencies of specific enzymes, such as disaccharidases, pancreatic, or bilary enzymes, should be considered as potential causes of diarrhea in hospitalized patients.

Antibiotic-Associated Diarrhea and Pseudomembranous Colitis

Initially recognized as a postoperative complication in the preantibiotic era,[22] pseudomembranous colitis is now considered to be an infectious process. This syndrome has been attributed in some instances to *Staphylococcus aureus*, an organism which has been demonstrated to produce a cell-destroying toxin (cytotoxin) that could theoretically produce mucosal damage.[23,24] In recent years, this syndrome has been increasingly associated with several antimicrobial agents, most notably clindamycin.[25,26] There is a slight predominance of females over males and a greater risk with increasing age. Pseudomembranous colitis has been reported in up to 10% of patients receiving clindamycin. This disease has followed both parenteral and oral clindamycin, and does not appear to be clearly related to either dose or duration of therapy.

While several theories regarding the pathogenesis of antibiotic-associated pseudomembranous colitis have been advanced, including possible viral processes and direct toxic effects, considerable recent evidence incriminates a cytotoxin-producing *Clostridium difficile* infection.[27,28] Furthermore, a potent cytotoxic material can be detected in the stools of patients with pseudomembranous colitis that causes cecal damage and death in a hamster model, and a cell-damaging effect in tissue culture cells.[29-31] This toxin can be neutralized by *C. sordellii* antiserum, but not by specific antisera prepared against other clostridial species.

While diarrhea constitutes a major side effect of several antibiotics, including tetracycline, chloramphenicol, penicillin, ampicillin, lincomycin, and clindamycin, early recognition of the pseudomembranous enterocolitis syndrome that may also be associated with any of these antibiotics is of paramount importance. The presence of fecal leukocytes in the methylene blue preparation of fresh stool specimens may provide a clue of distal colonic inflammation; however, the diagnosis of pseudomembranous enterocolitis is made by the proctoscopic appearance of small (1 to 5 mm) raised whitish-yellow plaques of an exudative "pseudomembrane" that may become confluent over an erythematous intact colonic mucosa.[26]

The vast majority of cases of pseudomembranous colitis will resolve spontaneously if the antibiotic is discontinued early in the course of this complication. If the antibiotic is continued, the disease may persist or progress to a life threatening, toxic state. Occasional cases will arise after the antibiotic has been discontinued. Therapy involves discontinuing the antibiotic and prescribing supportive fluid therapy. Several antimicrobial agents (such as oral vancomycin) and potential toxin binding materials (such as cholestyramine) are under investigation and may offer some promise.

Necrotizing Enterocolitis

Initially recognized as "enteritis necroticans" in post-World War II Germany,[32] and subsequently as "pig-bel" following pork feasts in New Guinea,[33] necrotizing enterocolitis is defined pathologically by segmental gangrene and radiographically by small amounts of gas in the intestinal wall, portal venous system, or peritoneal cavity late in the course of the disease. The commonest nosocomial setting in which necrotizing enterocolitis occurs is in the newborn infant, usually of low birth weight and less than 1 week of age. In association with prematurity, maternal infections during delivery, or umbilical vein exchange transfusion, a newborn may develop abdominal distension, vomiting, or apneic spells. The illness rapidly progresses to bloody diarrhea, intestinal perforation, shock, septicemia, and pneumatosis intestinalis, with a mortality that may exceed 70%.

The pathogenesis of necrotizing enterocolitis appears to involve some type of ischemic mucosal injury that may result from hypoxemia or hypotension. The toxic effects of leached plasticizers from polyvinyl chloride catheters have also been suggested. Several bacteria have been implicated, including *Pseudomonas, Klebsiella, E. coli,* and *Clostridia* species including *C. butyricum* and *C. perfringens* type C (the latter in adults from New Guinea).

Management of necrotizing enterocolitis must include early suspicion and recognition, discontinuance of umbilical catheters or oral feeding, careful supportive parental fluid therapy, and aggressive surgical excision of necrotic bowel if evidenced by pneumatosis intestinalis, peritonitis, or obstruction. Necrotizing enterocolitis appears to be rare in breast-fed infants.

Food Poisoning Syndromes

The syndrome of food poisoning should be included in the differential diagnosis whenever hospitalized patients or hospital staff members develop acute gastrointestinal illness characterized by vomiting or diarrhea. The major clues to the differential diagnosis of food poisoning syndromes are provided by the incubation period of the illness, the presence or absence of vomiting, and the presence or absence of fever.[35] Examination of fresh stool specimens for the presence of polymorphonuclear leukocytes may aid in distinguishing illnesses caused by bacteria which penetrate the intestinal mucosa.[36] Finally, the type of food responsible for an outbreak may suggest the etiologic agent. The major causes of food poisoning and clues to their diagnosis are summarized in Table 1.

For patients who experience nausea and vomiting within 1 hr of eating a meal, the most likely diagnosis is that of chemical food poisoning, which may be caused by various heavy metals including copper, zinc, cadmium, and tin.[37] When the incubation period ranges from 1 to 6 hr and the illness is characterized by nausea and vomiting as well as by diarrhea, staphylococcal food poisoning is by far the most likely diagnosis. However, *Bacillus cereus* may also cause this syndrome,[38] perhaps by a preformed, heat stable toxin analogous to *S. aureus*. When the incubation period is between 8 and 16 hr, and the illness is characterized primarily by abdominal cramps and diarrhea — and fewer than 25% of patients have been vomiting, — the most likely diagnosis is *C. perfringens* food poisoning.[39] On occasion, *B. cereus* may also cause this syndrome.[38] When an outbreak is characterized by fever, abdominal cramps, and diarrhea with an incubation period ranging from 16 to 48 hr, the major etiologic considerations are *Salmonella, Shigella, V. parahaemolyticus,* and invasive *E. coli.* Of these organisms, the most likely cause of a nosocomial outbreak of food poisoning is *Salmonella.* When patients develop illness characterized primarily by fever and abdominal cramps within 16 to 48 hr of a meal, *Yersinia enterocolitica* should be considered in the differential diagnosis. In outbreaks characterized by abdominal cramps and diarrhea with an incubation period ranging from 16 to 72 hr, enterotoxigenic *E. coli, V. parahaemolyticus,* and non-01 strains of *V. cholerae* (nonagglutinable vibrios, noncholera vibrios) should be considered, although none of these are common causes of nosocomial food poisoning outbreaks.

There are obviously exceptions to these general rules. For example, in common source food-borne *Salmonella* or *Shigella* outbreaks, in which the food is heavily contaminated, incubation periods may be as short as 6 hr. In outbreaks of food poisoning, additional etiologic agents should also be considered. *Campylobacter fetus* ssp. *jejuni,* a recently documented cause of food poisoning, causes an illness characterized by fe-

Table 1

DIAGNOSTIC CLUES IN FOOD POISONING OUTBREAKS

Agent	Symptoms[a]	Incubation Periods (Hr)	Fecal leukocytes	Responsible foods
Heavy Metals	V,C, ± D	<1	No	Acidic beverages
Staphylococcus aureus	V,C, ± D	1—6	No	Meats, egg salads, pastries
Bacillus cereus (short-incubation)	V,C, ± D	1—6	No	Fried rice
Clostridium perfringens	C,D	8—16	No	Meats, gravies
Bacillus cereus (long-incubation)	C,D	8—16	No	Meats, vegetables
Salmonella	F, ± V,C,D	16—48	Yes	Meats, eggs, dairy products
Shigella	F, ± V,C,D	16—48	Yes	Egg salads
Vibrio parahaemolyticus	±F, ± V,C,D	16—72	±	Fish, shellfish
Invasive *Escherichia coli*	F, ± V,C,D	16—48	Yes	Cheese[b]
Yersinia enterocolitica	F,C, ± D	16—48	Yes	Milk[b]
Enterotoxigenic *E. coli*	±V,C,D	16—72	No	?
Vibrio cholerae non 0-1 (NCV,[c] NAG[d])	±V,C,D	16—72	No	Shellfish

[a] F, fever; V, vomiting; C, abdominal cramps; D, diarrhea; ±, may be present or absent.
[b] Only one foodborne outbreak reported.
[c] NCV, noncholera vibrio.
[d] NAG, nonagglutinating vibrios

ver, abdominal cramps and diarrhea which may contain gross blood and fecal leuko-cytes.[40,41] The incubation period of this illness ranges from 2 to 7 days.

The laboratory approach to confirmation of the etiology of these various syndromes varies somewhat with the etiologic agent. In general, stool cultures should be obtained from ill individuals. In the case of *Salmonella* and *Shigella* food-borne outbreaks, stool cultures from food handlers may also be indicated. In suspected staphylococcal food poisoning outbreaks, culture of vomitus from ill individuals, and cultures of nose and hands from food handlers preparing the implicated food item may be of value in con-firming the etiology of the outbreak and the mode of contamination of food. Cultures of implicated food would be useful in confirming the source of all common bacterial food-borne pathogens. Finally, cultures of the food preparation environment may be helpful in confirming the source of a *Salmonella* or *V. parahaemolyticus* outbreak.

OUTBREAKS REPORTED IN THE LITERATURE

Antibiotic-Associated Diarrhea and Pseudomembranous Colitis

The reported incidence of pseudomembranous colitis in association with clindamy-cin use has ranged from 0.1 to 10%.[42,43] The latter report (Tedesco et al.[43]) also noted a 24% incidence of diarrhea with clindamycin in patients from St. Louis. Keefe et al.[44] then reported six cases of pseudomembranous colitis (with two deaths) from Portland, Ore. within a period of 6 months in 1974; the rate was thought to be a significant increase over previous experiences with clindamycin use there.[44] After 20 months of "uneventful prior use" of clindamycin in some 488 patients, Kabins[45] reported 9 doc-umented cases among 53 Chicago patients given clindamycin over a 2-month period in the fall of 1974. Four of these nine patients (44%) died. This disease subsequently seemed to disappear almost as quickly as it had appeared in their hospital. Similarly, all six documented cases of pseudomembranous colitis at the University of Virginia Hospital in Charlottesville that were recognized over a 12-month period in 1976 to 1977 occurred in 2 months among patients receiving various antibiotics.[46]

The disparate experiences in prospective studies and the apparent clustering of cases of pseudomembranous colitis in time and location suggest the spread of an infectious agent among patients predisposed by antibiotics, especially clindamycin.

The recent isolation of both a cytotoxin from the stools of most patients with pseu-domembranous colitis and a clindamycin-resistant, cytotoxin-producing organism, *Clostridium difficile*, from patients in Boston[31] and Birmingham, England[29] offer an explanation for the occurrence of pseudomembranous colitis in the patterns suggesting a nosocomial infection in certain high-risk patients. Some strains of this organism, rarely present in stools of normal persons,[47] have been demonstrated to produce a cytotoxin which can cause enterocolitis in experimental hamsters. Furthermore, lower inoculae are required in germ-free animals or in animals whose normal colonic flora is suppressed by antimicrobial agents, including vancomycin.[48] Although antiserum prepared against *C. sordellii* neutralized the cytotoxic effect in vitro and was protective in the experimental hamster model,[49] it is not yet feasible to employ it in the therapy of patients. The extent to which other organisms might produce this or similar cytotox-ins remains to be determined. While vancomycin and other antimicrobial agents ad-ministered orally may be effective, it should be remembered that these same antimicro-bial agents may predispose experimental animals to colitis after they are discontinued. The role of potential toxin binding agents, such as cholestyramine, also remains to be elucidated.

Necrotizing Enterocolitis

While the association of enterocolitis in the New Guinea highlands has been made indirectly with *C. perfringens* type C, reports of temporal and geographic clustering of nosocomial necrotizing enterocolitis in premature neonates have uncommonly implicated bacterial pathogens. Virnig and Reynolds[49a] reported a clustering of neonatal necrotizing enterocolitis cases at the St. Paul's Children's Hospital in Minnesota with five cases occurring over a 19-day period in August, 1971 in their newborn unit. While three of these five premature infants had severe hyaline membrane disease and all had polyethylene umbilical artery catheters, the authors were unable to implicate any bacterial, viral, or fungal pathogens and suggested that "normal bowel flora" might be involved into pathogenesis of necrotizing enterocolitis. They suggested an association with an altered intestinal mucosa by hypoxemic or other toxic damage. Some have implicated certain *E. coli* strains, in a few instances 0111:B4,[50-52] or *Pseudomonas* strains.[53] For the prevention of the illness, some authors have suggested the use of prophylactic nonabsorbable antimicrobial agents;[54] however, this approach remains quite controversial at present.

Book et al.[55] have noted the temporal and geographic clustering of neonatal necrotizing enterocolitis at their Intermountain Newborn Intensive Care Center in Salt Lake City. Over a 4½-year period between 1972 and 1977, they noted temporal clustering of their 74 cases with a significant predominance in summer and fall months. While they were unable to identify any enteric bacterial, enteroviral, or adenoviral pathogens, they felt their nosocomial infection control measures resulted in a significant decrease in the incidence of necrotizing enterocolitis in their unit. Their control measures included careful isolation of all cases, introduction of Iodophor handwashing, and exclusion of personnel from work if they developed an associated gastrointestinal illness (usually 3 to 5 days).

Howard et al.[56] reported an outbreak of necrotizing enterocolitis at the Royal Free Hospital in London among ten neonates in January and February in 1977. While the usual predisposing factors were not present, they indirectly implicated *C. butyricum* in nine of the ten cases by gas-liquid chromatographic studies of the serum. Seven of the nine patients had positive blood cultures for *C. butyricum*, and gas-liquid chromatographic examination of stools revealed a pattern compatible with *C. butyricum* in six of the affected cases. The reservoir and mode of transmission were not identified.

Food Poisoning Syndromes

C. perfringens food poisoning may occur in the hospital setting. From 1971 through 1976 in England and Wales, 82 (27%) of 302 reported *C. perfringens* food-borne outbreaks occurred in hospitals.[57] In one outbreak, 78% of individuals eating a minced ham dish developed *C. perfringens* food poisoning. In this debilitated patient population, two patients developed severe dehydration requiring intravenous fluid replacement, and one patient died. Hospital staff members were not affected, and there was no information suggesting person-to-person transmission. The minced ham dish was mishandled in the kitchen; the primary food handling deficiency was inadequate refrigeration of large hams after cooking. Control measures included correction of suboptimal food handling practices.

Hepatitis A may be food-borne, and outbreaks have occurred in the hospital setting. In one large outbreak affecting only members of the staff of a large hospital, 44 clinical and 22 subclinical cases of hepatitis A occurred.[58] The highest attack rates were in physicians and dietary service personnel, medical technicians, and nursing students.

Investigation revealed that the illness was associated with food served in the hospital cafeteria. Clinical illness was associated with ingestion of sandwiches in the hospital cafeteria. The source of contamination of the sandwiches was not positively identified, but one of two food handlers might have been the source of the infection. In addition, several cases of hepatitis A occurring in the surrounding community were also traced to the hospital cafeteria. Control measures included recommendations that food handlers with symptomatic hepatitis not return to work until at least 2 to 3 weeks after the onset of jaundice and that food handlers with subclinical hepatitis not return to work until 2 to 3 weeks after the peak of serum enzyme levels. The outbreak subsided spontaneously.

Specific Infections
Salmonella

Nosocomial outbreaks of salmonellosis generally fall into one of two epidemiologic patterns (common-source and cross-infection), although features of both may be associated with a single outbreak. One pattern is that of the explosive common-source, food-borne outbreak which may affect many patients and staff members (see chapter entitled ''An Employee Health Service for Infection Control'' section entitled ''Food Handlers'') throughout a hospital or may be confined to a small number of patients exposed to a specific food item. Such outbreaks may be obvious common-source epidemics. For example, in 1973 18 patients developed nosocomial *Salmonella* gastroenteritis following ingestion of eggnog containing raw eggs.[59] The 18 cases had onset of illness over a 6-day period. The association of illness with consumption of eggnog was highly significant. An interesting feature of the outbreak was that person-to-person spread to eight members of the hospital staff and six additional hospitalized patients was documented; therefore, features of both common-source and cross-infection outbreaks were present. The outbreak was controlled following discontinuance of the use of raw eggs in dietary items and isolation of infected patients.

A more subtle outbreak of food-borne salmonellosis occurred over 20 years ago.[60] In the outbreak, five patients developed salmonellosis caused by either *Salmonella oranienburg* (three cases), *S. montevideo* (one case), or *S. senftenberg* (one case) over a 3-month period. Such an outbreak could easily have gone unrecognized because of the multiple serotypes responsible or have gone uninvestigated because of an erroneous assumption that these cases were sporadic and unrelated. However all five of the patients had been fed through a nasogastric tube; their diets were prepared in two separate kitchens. Further investigation revealed that the dried inactive (brewer's) yeast contaminated with the three *Salmonella* serotypes was responsible for the outbreak. The outbreak was controlled following cessation of use of this product.

Food-borne salmonellosis outbreaks may simultaneously affect patients in multiple hospitals. In 1962 and 1963, a large interstate outbreak of nosocomial gastroenteritis affecting patients, medical staff, and employees of 53 hospitals in 13 states was caused by *S. derby*.[61] Investigation revealed that the responsible vehicle was eggs which were eaten either raw or undercooked. Such an outbreak indicates the need for nationwide surveillance of nosocomial enteric infections.

Common-source *Salmonella* outbreaks have also been traced to contaminated diagnostic reagents and medications of animal origin. These epidemics generally have not presented as typical common-source outbreaks, and since the patients are frequently scattered both in place and in time, such outbreaks may not be readily recognized. For example, an interstate outbreak of *S. cubana* infection occurred in 1966.[62-64] Investigation revealed that carmine dye used as a marker to determine gastrointestinal transit time was the vehicle of transmission. The dye was contaminated with *S. cubana* and had been prepared from beetles. Nosocomial outbreaks of salmonellosis have also been traced to pancreatin, pepsin, bile salts, gelatin, vitamins, and extracts of thyroid, adrenal cortex, pancreas, pituitary, liver, and stomach.[65] In these instances, cases of salmonellosis frequently appear to be sporadic; a high index of suspicion is required to document their association with a common vehicle. Examples are provided by recent outbreaks caused by *S. agona* and *S. schwarzengrund* traced to pancreatin prepared from pancreatic glands of pigs.[66,67]

That new vehicles for transmission of nosocomial salmonellosis may continue to appear is suggested by a report of a small outbreak of *S. oslo* gastroenteritis, in which three of five cases were associated with upper gastrointestinal endoscopy.[68] However, the possible contamination of the endoscope was not documented bacteriologically nor was the mechanism of its potential contamination identified. This outbreak was also remarkable for the fact that *S. oslo* was resistant both to chloramphenicol and ampicillin.

Although common-source *Salmonella* infections have generally not occurred in the newborn nursery setting, two reported epidemics traced to contaminated pooled breast milk have occurred. Both were caused by *S. kottbus*. In both instances, the source of contamination was the donor mothers, neither of whom had evidence of intestinal infection or mastitis but both of whom appeared to be asymptomatically excreting *S. kottbus* organisms in breast milk.[69,70]

An additional medical device associated with a common-source nursery salmonellosis outbreak is rubber tubing attached to a suction apparatus. Onset of illness due to *S. worthington* occurred over 15 days. A similar outbreak had occurred in the same nursery 5 weeks previously, but the source of this outbreak was not determined.[71]

The second major epidemiologic pattern of nosocomial salmonellosis outbreaks is that of cross-infection. Such outbreaks have generally occurred in nurseries or on pediatric wards, but have occasionally occurred on adult wards. On occasion, both infants and adults have been involved.[72] Infection is generally introduced into a nursery or ward by an infant recently born to a mother with clinical or asymptomatic salmonellosis,[73,74] or by a child who has acquired his salmonellosis in the community.[75] Such outbreaks typically last at least several months,[75,76] and one lasted for 2 years.[77] In these outbreaks, organisms appear to be spread from person-to-person by hospital staff. On occasion, *Salmonella* had been isolated from the hands of hospital staff members.[78] In other outbreaks, *Salmonella* have been isolated from environmental sources such as dust,[76,79] water in infant bottle warmers,[73,76] delivery room resuscitators,[80] bedside tables and cribs,[78] a thermometer in a wooden holder,[81] and towels.[76] However, the epidemiologic significance of environmental isolates of *Salmonella* in many of these outbreaks has not been clear.

The frequency with which cross-infection outbreaks of salmonellosis occur among adults has been debated.[61,82] However, documentation of nosocomial person-to-person spread following a *Salmonella* food-borne outbreak[59] and an outbreak of ten cases of antibiotic-resistant *S. heidelberg* infection among adults in the absence of evidence for transmission by a common vehicle,[83] suggests that cross-infection can occur among adult patients as well. Such outbreaks are notoriously difficult to control, and enteric isolation of patients and asymptomatic excreters among the patient population is mandatory. In nursery outbreaks, cohorting of infants and staff is frequently required, and, on occasion, the unit may have to be closed to new admissions and thoroughly disinfected after discharge of the last patient.

Shigella

Since the infectious dose for *Shigella* is in the range of 10 to 100 organisms,[84] nosocomial outbreaks of shigellosis might be anticipated to occur with significant frequency. However, nosocomial transmission of *Shigella* is not often documented. In one reported outbreak, one of the twins born to a mother with a history of diarrhea during the 4 weeks prior to delivery developed *Shigella sonnei* diarrhea with onset on day five of life.[85] Stool culture taken from the mother after recognition of the case in the child also yielded *S. sonnei*. In addition, a nurse caring for the infected infant subsequently developed mild diarrhea and had a stool culture positive for *S. sonnei* with the same pattern of multiple antibiotic resistance as the isolate from the mother and infant. This outbreak illustrates the fact that an infected mother may transmit shigellosis to her child during or shortly after delivery and that the potential exists for spread of the infection from infants to staff in the nursery setting.

The role of hospital staff in the transmission of nosocomial shigellosis is further illustrated in an outbreak of nine cases of shigellosis in the infirmary of a custodial institution.[86] That cross-infection occurred is suggested by the relationship of cases to periods of time when the infirmary was understaffed and when nurses worked with patients both with shigellosis and with noninfected individuals. As patients were bedridden, direct person-to-person spread from one patient to another seemed unlikely. Cases were significantly younger and had been hospitalized for a significantly greater period of time than noninfected controls. The epidemic strain in this outbreak was also multiply antibiotic-resistant as a result of heavy antibiotic pressure in this unit.

That the mother is frequently the source of *Shigella* at the time of delivery is further suggested by a report of four nosocomially acquired sporadic cases of shigellosis.[87] Although none of these four mothers was ill with diarrhea at the time of delivery, family members in two cases had diarrhea, and, in one case, the same organism isolated from the infant was also isolated from household contacts. In a review of eight previously reported cases of neonatal shigellosis, *Shigella* was isolated from the stools of six mothers, three of whom had diarrhea at the time of delivery.[87]

That transmission from mother to child at the time of delivery may occur is further illustrated by a sporadic case with onset of a febrile illness unaccompanied by diarrhea on the fourth day of life.[88] *S. sonnei* was isolated from stool, blood, and cerebrospinal fluid in this patient, and subsequently from the child's mother who had no recent history of diarrhea. In addition to fever, the child had listlessness, anorexia, and generalized seizure and jaundice.

In summary, nosocomial transmission of both *S. sonnei* and *S. flexneri* to patients and hospital staff in both nursery and ward settings has been documented.

E. coli

Enteropathogenic E. coli serotypes (EPEC)

Since first recognized by Bray and Beavan[89] in 1945 and Giles and Sangster[90] in Aberdeen, Scotland in 1948, certain serotypes of *E. coli* have been repeatedly recognized in association with outbreaks of diarrhea among hospitalized infants in newborn nurseries. The newborn is uniquely susceptible in this setting, having not yet acquired normal flora or specific immunity; and outbreaks of diarrhea are relatively common, especially in newborn intensive care units, among infants under 4 months of age. With little water and electrolyte reserve, the newborn may quickly develop a life-threatening enteritis with a high mortality.[91] The serotypes that have been associated classically with infantile diarrhea include: 0111:B4, 055:B5, 0127:B8, 0128:B12, 026:B6, 086:B7,

0119:B14, 0125:B15, 0126:B16, 020:B7, 044:K74, 0114, 0142, and 0158. The majority of these "enteropathogenic" *E. coli* serotypes do not produce either the heat-labile or heat-stable type of enterotoxin and are not invasive. However, they are capable of causing diarrhea and an antibody response in human volunteers from whom they can be reisolated.[92] They are relatively infrequently found among healthy infants or adults not exposed to cases, and are different from *E. coli* found with nonenteric infections.

A number of outbreaks of infantile enteritis associated with *E. coli* 0142 have been described by Hone and colleagues[93] from infants' wards in Scotland and Dublin. Among 54 babies with nosocomial diarrhea in a Dublin hospital, 80% were receiving antimicrobial drugs, and diarrhea was associated with a significantly longer hospitalization by 10 days.[93] While the major incriminated pathogen, *E. coli* 0142, was not found among hospital personnel or in the air samples obtained, its isolation from a cot rail and locker top, and the contiguous location of affected patients' wards, suggested possible cross-infection.

Between September, 1972 and March, 1973 another nursery outbreak of gastroenteritis with *E. coli* 0142 occurred among 56 infants admited to contiguous high-risk nurseries at a county general hospital in Arizona.[94] Four diarrhea-associated deaths occurred, and 17 other infants had intractable diarrhea for more than 14 days, often requiring intravenous therapy. The authors implicated persistence of nosocomial cases as the reservoir from a peak of illness in June and July 1972 through to a second peak ending in March and April 1973. There was a significant association with low birth weight, and illnesses occurred most often during the second week of life. The incriminated *E. coli* 0142 was also isolated from the hands of five personnel, suggesting hand transmission of the pathogen. Parenteral antimicrobial agents were ineffective. After triple handwashing with 3% hexachlorophene soap failed to reduce hand carriage or cross-infection, the epidemic disappeared after closure of the nurseries to admissions, 10-day oral colistin therapy of all infants, and use of disposable gloves in all patient care activities. This organism was also demonstrated to cause fluid secretion in infant rabbit loop assays. The potential role of convalescent or asymptomatic carriage and the importance of strict aseptic technique in control of outbreaks of enteropathogenic *E. coli* infection in newborn nurseries has been emphasized.[94,95]

A more insidious, severe prolonged nosocomial illness has been described over 7 months in association with *E. coli* 0114.[96] Finally, new serotypes continue to be recognized in association with epidemic diarrhea in newborn nurseries.[97] It should be remembered that recognition of a nosocomial infantile enteritis outbreak may require monitoring of illnesses that occur after discharge from a relatively brief 2- to 3-day hospitalization at birth. Although direct transmission has not been conclusively documented, several studies indirectly incriminate cross-infection by hand contact as the most probable means of spread of EPEC in nurseries.

Enterotoxigenic E. coli

While enterotoxigenic *E. coli* that produce either the heat-labile or heat-stable type of enterotoxin have been associated in several studies with sporadic diarrhea among young children, relatively few nosocomial outbreaks have been documented in association with enterotoxigenic *E. coli*. One example in 1976 from special care nurseries of a large pediatric hospital in Houston, Texas revealed the association of an ST (heat stable toxin)-producing *E. coli* 078:K80:H12.[98] Some 55 of 205 infants admitted to the special care nurseries over a 7-month period ending in August 1975 developed a diarrheal illness, characterized by nine or more loose stools a day, that was associated only with oral consumption of formula in contrast to those receiving total parenteral nutrition. Although the organism (found in 18 of 25 symptomatic infants) was sensitive to colistin and to gentamicin, neither of these antimicrobial agents were effective in preventing colonization with this organism. The epidemic organism was isolated from several environmental sources, including the walls of the isolettes and washbasins, as well as the formula being fed to one of the infants. However, there was not an increase in absenteeism among personnel caring for ill infants, and it was isolated only from the stools of one nurse and the hands of a second nurse. While there is a suggestion that feedings might have been contaminated while being administered to an infant, the authors were unable to document widespread colonization among hospital personnel to incriminate a reservoir. Of some concern is the observation that the epidemic strain was multiply resistant to several antibiotics and that this drug resistance and enterotoxin production were conjugally transferred together in vitro. This suggests that the indiscriminate use of antibiotics known to promote multiple drug resistance may also promote the acquisition of plasmids encoding for enterotoxigenicity. The epidemic disappeared coincident with grouping of culture-positive infants in a separate nursery at the opposite end of the hospital that was staffed by separate personnel.

Another outbreak occurring over 3 months among 25 babies in the Glasgow Royal Maternity Hospital was associated with a new *E. coli* O group, 159. The organism was also shown to produce the heat-stable type of toxin in tests using the infant mouse assay.[99] Most of these patients were located on one floor, and the authors suggested that cross-infection might have played a role.

Epidemic infantile diarrhea has also been associated with enterotoxigenic organisms that have not been limited to certain serotypes — or even species. An outbreak in a newborn intensive care unit has been associated with transiently enterotoxigenic organisms that represented multiple serotypes of different organisms *(E. coli, Klebsiella,* and *Citrobacter).*[100] This cluster in time and location of multiple strains of transiently enterotoxigenic *Enterobacteriaceae* raises the possibility of transmission of enterotoxigenicity among etiologic strains by plasmids[101] or bacteriophage.[102]

While invasive *E. coli* have been described in association with a widespread foodborne outbreak,[103] invasive *E. coli* do not appear to be common among either sporadic or epidemic diarrhea, and have not been described in nosocomial outbreaks to date.

Yersinia enterocolitica

One nosocomial outbreak of *Y. enterocolitica* enteritis has been reported from Finland.[104] The index case was a young girl admitted to a pediatric surgical ward with fever, abdominal pain, diarrhea, and suspected appendicitis. She did not undergo surgery and, after her clinical status improved, was transferred to a pediatric ward. Within 2 weeks, six cases of *Y. enterocolitica* infection occurred among hospital staff on these two wards. Each infection was caused by *Y. enterocolitica* serotype 9. All but one of the six staff members infected had been working on one of the two wards while the index case was hospitalized on that ward. The sixth staff case had worked with three other staff cases but had had no contact with the index case. In this outbreak, the organism appears to have spread by cross-infection from patient to staff and subsequently possibly among staff members; however, the possibility of a common vehicle among the hospital staff members was not completely excluded. Transmission of the organism apparently ceased spontaneously.

Rotavirus

Nosocomial transmission of rotavirus has been documented on pediatric wards; both epidemics and sporadic cases have been reported. During a 6-week period in Birmingham in 1974, 6 of 26 children (age range, 3 months to 3 years) hospitalized on an orthopedic ward developed acute diarrheal illness (attack rate 23%).[105] All six ill children had rotavirus in their stools; no non-ill children were rotavirus-positive. The illness was mild; diarrhea lasted from 2 to 28 days. The index case developed diarrhea on the day of admission to the ward, having acquired the infection in the community. The mode of transmission was hypothesized to be by cross-infection.

In a 1-month prospective study of nosocomial diarrhea on two pediatric wards during a community rotavirus outbreak in Atlanta, 12 of 60 children developed diarrhea; 10 of these 12 had stools positive for rotavirus (rotavirus attack rate of 17%).[106] The illness was relatively severe and eight of the ten patients were treated for suspected sepsis. Mean duration of illness was 5.4 days. Identifiable risk factors included age (mean age of nosocomial cases, 5 months; mean age of noninfected children at risk, 17 months) and room location; nosocomial transmission occurred significantly more often in a three-bed intermediate care room on one of the wards. No hospital staff members developed documented rotavirus diarrhea during this period, but 4 of 34 nursery personnel did have diarrhea. Although the mode of transmission was not well documented, transmission of rotavirus infection was felt to be due to cross-infection following admission to the ward of community acquired index cases.

In a 1-year prospective study of hospitalized children with gastroenteritis on pediatric wards in Toronto, 385 of 1751 (22%) had rotavirus in stool specimens.[107] The mean age of these patients was 12 months. Of these 385 patients, 75 (10%) developed gastroenteritis more than 7 days after admission and were thought to represent nosocomial infections. Clinical illness in the 385 cases ranged from mild to severe; four deaths occurred. Several small nosocomial outbreaks limited to patients in certain multiple-bed rooms were reported. Although a distinct winter peak of rotavirus illness acquired in the community was noted, this seasonal trend was less apparent for nosocomial cases.

Nosocomial rotavirus infection may cause both outbreaks and endemic diarrheal disease in newborn nurseries. In addition, in contrast to other age groups in which asymptomatic infection with rotavirus infection appears to be rare,[108] asymptomatic infection of neonates is not uncommon.

During a 20-day period in December 1974, an outbreak of diarrheal illness affecting 15 of 32 infants (attack rate 47%) in a neonatal ward (age range, 1 day to 2 months) occurred in Melbourne.[109] Children in two of the three rooms on the ward were affected. Rotaviruses were present in stool specimens from 8 of 15 ill children, and from 3 of 17 nonill children. Six of the seven negative specimens from ill children were obtained after patients had recovered; the disease was felt to be due to rotavirus, although an enteropathogenic *E. coli* serotype (0111:B4) was also isolated from 11 of 15 ill children and 5 of 17 controls. Five of the ill children and two controls had both rotavirus and the EPEC serotype. Symptoms were mild, and all but one child was ill for less than 4 days. The mode of introduction of rotavirus was not identified, but transmission was felt to occur by cross-infection. The outbreak was controlled by closing the ward to new admissions for 18 days.

In several nursery settings where rotavirus was endemic, asymptomatic infection rates ranging from 23 to 92% have been reported. In a 15-month prospective study of diarrhea in a newborn special care nursery in Melbourne, 257 of 913 babies (28%) admitted within 2 hours of birth developed diarrhea.[110] Rotavirus infection was statistically associated with diarrhea; of the 238 babies with diarrhea studied, 127 (53%) had rotavirus in their stools compared with 37 of 105 (35%) controls. The asymptomatic infection rate was 23%. Rotavirus infection was significantly more common in infants of greater than 32 weeks' gestation and showed a peak incidence during the winter months. Infants on pooled and pasteurized expressed breast milk diets had infection rates similar to those who were bottle fed.

In a prospective study of rotavirus infections in six hospital nurseries in Sydney, 304 of 628 (49%) infants had rotavirus in their stools. Only 84 (28%) were ill; the asymptomatic infection rate in this study was 72%.[111] Infection occurred in five of the six nurseries in the study. During outbreaks of diarrheal illness, rotavirus was statistically associated with illness (present in 61% of ill infants and 46% of nonill infants). Rotavirus infection was not documented in infants less than 24 hr of age, and was most frequent in babies between 3 and 6 days of age. No seasonality was apparent.

In a 12-month prospective study in London, 343 of 1056 (32.5%) of 5-day-old infants in newborn nurseries had rotavirus in their stools.[112] Review of the clinical course of infants on one ward revealed that only 15 of 189 (8%) babies excreting rotavirus were ill; the asymptomatic infection rate was 92%. Fifteen of 20 babies (75%) with diarrhea on this ward were rotavirus-positive compared with 174 of 423 (41%) babies without diarrhea; therefore, rotavirus infection was again statistically associated with diarrheal illness. The illness was mild and no infant required specific therapy. A winter peak in rotavirus infection was again noted. The rotavirus infection rate was somewhat lower in breast-fed than in bottle-fed babies, who also excreted higher titers of rotavirus.

In these nursery settings, the modes of introduction and transmission were not well characterized. As asymptomatic infection in adult household contacts of pediatric cases[113] and hospital personnel [114,115] has been documented, it is possible that infants become infected during or shortly after birth from either a maternal or a hospital staff source. Infection may then spread within the nursery either by cross-infection or, alternatively, may be frequently reintroduced, particularly during the winter months.

Echovirus Type 18

Enteroviruses are not well documented causes of nosocomial gastroenteritis. However, one well-documented outbreak of gastroenteritis in newborn infants caused by echovirus type 18 has been reported.[116] During a 1-week period, 12 of 21 (57%) infants in a premature nursery developed mild diarrheal disease. Affected infants occupied all four separate units in the nursery, and infants in incubators were affected as frequently as those in bassinets. Age and weight did not affect the attack rate. Ten of the 12 ill infants had echovirus type 18 cultured from stool specimens; all 12 ill infants had a fourfold or greater rise in antibody titer to echovirus 18. In contrast, none of nine well infants had either a positive stool culture or seroconversion. In addition, 2 of 26 staff members in the nursery had positive stool cultures for echovirus 18. Both also had a fourfold rise in serum antibody titer. Four days after this outbeak ended spontaneously, five babies in a separate infant ward developed a more severe diarrheal illness over a 4-day period. All five of these infants had echovirus type 18 isolated from stool cultures, while none of the ten control infants on that ward had positive cultures (attack rate 33%). Again, all five ill infants had a fourfold rise in antibody titer to the virus. The fact that one of the two nurses from the premature nursery who had had echovirus type 18 in her stool had worked on the ward where the second outbreak occurred 3 days prior to the onset of the outbreak and had handled at least two of the five infected infants, suggested that cross-infection occurred. Both outbreaks ended spontaneously. Follow-up stool cultures on ill infants from both the nursery and ward were negative several weeks after the outbreaks.

Other Organisms

Any infectious agent which may be transmitted by food or water, or spread from one infected patient to another and cause gastroenteritis, may be associated with outbreaks of nosocomial gastrointestinal illness. Recently recognized causes of acute gastrointestinal infections such as *C. fetus* ssp. *jejuni* and parvovirus-like agents may be anticipated to cause outbreaks of nosocomial gastroenteritis, which may be documented by the use of recently developed laboratory techniques.

APPROACH TO AN OUTBREAK

Before initiating an investigation of a possible nosocomial outbreak of gastroenteritis, one must first determine whether a true increase in the rate of a specific infection has occurred. On occasion, such an assessment may be difficult to make. Between 1956 and 1975, 20 of 181 nosocomial outbreaks investigated by the Center for Disease Control were actually "pseudoepidemics".[117] Since 11 of these 20 pseudoepidemics were caused by errors in processing of cultures (contamination of specimens during collection and transport or during laboratory manipulation), laboratory techniques used to identify the etiologic agent should be reviewed. Additional pseudoepidemics were a result of artifacts of a surveillance system, such as failure to distinguish community acquired from hospital acquired infections or changes in the nature or intensity of surveillance. The gastrointestinal tract was the site of suspected infection in four of the pseudoepidemics; two represented surveillance artifacts (community acquired were mistaken for hospital acquired infections), one resulted from an error in clinical diagnosis, and one resulted from contamination of specimens during processing in the laboratory. Once these possibilities have been considered and discarded, the epidemiologic investigation should begin promptly.

The initial stage of the investigation is concerned with identification of cases. Therefore, a case definition must be developed; for example, in an outbreak of diarrheal illness caused by *Salmonella,* a case might be defined as an individual who had diarrhea alone; in that case, a definition of diarrhea, such as three or more liquid stools per day, must also be developed. Alternative case definitions might be abdominal cramps with diarrhea, fever and diarrhea, or a combination of fever, abdominal cramps, and diarrhea. If asymptomatic infections are documented, they may also be included as cases. The initial case definition may need to be modified as additional data are obtained during the investigation.

Once a case definition is developed, the next step is to find all the cases. Case findings should include a review of available surveillance data such as medical and nursing records, data obtained through routine hospital surveillance for nosocomial infections, and microbiology records. In the case of a nosocomial outbreak of gastroenteritis, a review of records of stool cultures submitted to the microbiology laboratory may be of particular value in case finding. Other surveillance techniques that may be used to identify cases who became ill after hospital discharge include telephone surveys of those patients discharged during the epidemic period and a survey of local physicians caring for patients following discharge. Case findings should also include hospital staff. Cases may be identified through personal interviews with staff members, by a questionnaire survey of hospital staff, and by review of employee health records.

Once cases bave been identified, attack rates may be calculated. In addition to an overall attack rate, attack rates by age and sex should be determined.

The next step should be to characterize the cases in terms of time and place. Dates of onset of illness and of positive cultures for the epidemic organism should be tabulated. In this manner, tbe epidemic period may be defined. Ward-specific attack rates may provide a clue to clustering of illness in the hospital. If illness does cluster an assessment should be made to determine whether certain parts of a ward or certain rooms are associated with illness.

At this stage of the investigation, a hypothesis concerning mode of transmission of the etiologic agent should be formulated and subsequently tested. Nosocomial gastroenteritis outbreaks generally fall into one of several epidemiologic patterns. Data collected to this point may provide an important clue to the mode of transmission. The two major epidemic patterns are that of a common-source outbreak and that of a cross-infection outbreak. Common-source food-borne or water-borne outbreaks are typically explosive in onset, short in duration, and characterized by relatively high attack rates, while cross-infection outbreaks are more frequently associated with lower attack rates and a longer epidemic period. In addition, common-source outbreaks more typically involve adults, while cross-infection outbreaks of nosocomial gastroenteritis most frequently involve children in nurseries or pediatric wards. Of 40 cross-infection outbreaks of nosocomial salmonellosis reported to CDC between 1963 and 1972, 15 occurred in nurseries, 14 occurred on pediatric wards, and 11 occurred on other wards.[5] In contrast, 10 of the 11 common-source outbreaks of salmonellosis reported during this same period occurred on adult medical and surgical wards, and only one occurred on a pediatric ward; no outbreaks occurred in infant nurseries. In a total of 46 cross-infection salmonellosis outbreaks in hospitals and custodial institutions reported during this period, the mean number of persons ill was 13. In contrast. in the 30 common-source outbreaks reported, the mean number ill was 89.

Unfortunately, there will be exceptions to these general rules. For example, an outbreak due to a contaminated common-source food served to patients only intermittently may simulate a cross-infection outbreak. In addition, an attack rate in a common-source outbreak may be high, but the total number of patients infected may be small if a contaminated vehicle is served to only a few individuals. An excellent example of this situation is provided by the outbreak due to dried inactive brewer's yeast served in tube feedings.[60] Finally, a common vehicle outbreak may infect children in nurseries or on pediatric wards if the vehicle is one that is distributed only to those individuals; for example, the two nursery outbreaks of salmonellosis due to contaminated breast milk affected only newborn infants in nurseries.[69,70]

Once the hypothesis is formulated, multiple risk factors to which patients may have been exposed must be evaluated. In the case of gastroenteritis outbreaks, pertinent risk factors include prior antibiotic administration, prior administration of antiperistaltic drugs, prior administration of antacids, history of previous gastric surgery or hypochlorhydria or achlorhydria, hospital diet, and diagnostic or other therapeutic agents of animal origin to which a case may have been exposed. In order to evaluate the significance of any of these possible risk factors, a control population must be selected and evaluated for exposure to these same risk factors. If possible, controls should be matched with cases for certain factors affecting host susceptibility, such as duration of hospitalization, nature of recent surgical procedures or underlying disease. The significance of specific exposures may then be reliably assessed.

Control patients may be selected in a variety of ways. If an outbreak is limited to a specific ward and is of relatively short duration all other patients admitted to the ward during the epidemic period may serve as the control group. If an outbreak involves patients on several wards or throughout a hospital, it will not be practical to include all other patients admitted during the epidemic period as controls. In this case, controls should be selected in a systematic manner, such as the previous or the next patient of comparable age and sex admitted to the hospital or ward. A problem may still arise if many of the controls were also exposed to the true risk factor but were only asymptomatically infected.

Laboratory studies to be considered during the course of an investigation include stool or rectal swab cultures and, on occasion, serologic studies involving paired serum samples. Fecal cultures may be of value both in case finding and in confirmation of cases. In small outbreaks of recent onset, it may be desirable to obtain cultures from all patients satisfying the case definition. In larger outbreaks, this approach may be neither practical nor necessary. Cultures from at least some control individuals should be obtained to rule out the possibility of high asymptomatic infection rates associated with the epidemic organism. In nursery salmonellosis outbreaks, throat cultures may also be useful in evaluating colonization with the epidemic strain.[118] Both serotyping and determination of antibiotic sensitivity patterns of selected isolates may be useful in identifying the epidemic strain. Colicin typing may also be useful in this regard in *Shigella* outbreaks. Serologic studies may be of value in nosocomial *Y. enterocolitica, C. fetus* ssp. *jejuni,* enterotoxigenic *E. coli,* and rotavirus nosocomial outbreaks.

Selected cultures of foods, water, or environmental sources may be of value when the epidemiologic data suggest their association with illness. For example, in the *Salmonella* food-borne outbreaks in which a specific food item is implicated, cultures of raw foods and the remaining food item as well as environmental cultures of items such as knives, meat slicers, and cutting boards in the hospital kitchen may be useful. In nursery *Salmonella* outbreaks, selected culturing of environmental sources may also be useful. However, the practice of submitting multiple environmental cultures collected indiscriminately without reference to the epidemiologic data is to be discouraged.

Preliminary data analysis should be initiated as soon as the investigation is begun and continuously updated throughout its course. Data on age, sex, and ward-specific attack rates should be analyzed for statistically significant differences. Attack rates among staff should be compared with attack rates among patients. In the case of a suspected common source outbreak, meal-, food-, and medication-specific attack rates should be analyzed in a manner similar to that indicated in Table 2(a) for food-specific attack rates. When more than one food item or exposure is implicated in a food-borne outbreak, cross-table analysis, as illustrated in Table 2(b), may identify the specific food or exposure responsible for the outbreak involved. In this example, ingestion of both roast beef and Yorkshire pudding was associated with a significantly increased risk of illness. However, both of these items were frequently eaten by the same individual. When cases and controls are separated into two groups according to whether or not roast beef was eaten, it is apparent that the ingestion of Yorkshire pudding did not alter the attack rate in either group, suggesting that the roast beef alone was responsible for the outbreak.

When the exposure to a contaminated vehicle may have occurred several weeks previously, as in a hepatitis A food-borne outbreak, patients and controls may not recall specific food items which they ingested. In this case, food preferences rather than food-specific attack rates should be determined.[58] In outbreaks which appear to be due to cross-infection, exposure of cases and controls to individual members of the medical and nursing staffs should be evaluated in an effort to determine a link between cases. In this analysis, it should be remembered that cross-infection may occur among both patients and staff following a common-source outbreak.[59] In nursery outbreaks, an effort should be made to identify a maternal or staff source of introduction of the infection.

Once the investigation has begun, preliminary control measures may be implemented as soon as available data indicate a likely mode of transmission for the epidemic organism. In the case of a common-vehicle outbreak, the use of a specific food item such as raw eggs used in eggnog may need to be discontinued.[59] In addition, food handlers who are ill or culture-positive for the epidemic organism in association with the outbreak should be given other duties until they become culture-negative. In the

Table 2
USE OF FOOD-SPECIFIC ATTACK RATES AND CROSS-TABLE ANALYSIS TO IDENTIFY FOOD VEHICLE IN A FOOD-BORNE OUTBREAK

a. Food-Specific Attack Rates

Food	Number of persons eating food			Number of persons not eating food		
	Total	Ill	Percent ill	Total	Ill	Percent ill
Roast beef	100	88	88[a]	10	2	20[a]
Yorkshire pudding	80	80	100[b]	30	10	33[b]
Baked potato	95	78	82	15	12	80
Tossed salad	90	74	82	20	16	80
Wine	70	58	82	40	32	80

[a] Fisher's one-tail exact test: $p < 0.01$.
[b] Fisher's one-tail exact test: $p < 0.001$.

b. Cross-Table Analysis

	Number of persons eating roast beef			Number of persons not eating roast beef		
	Total	Ill	Percent ill	Total	Ill	Percent ill
Number eating Yorkshire pudding	75	67	89	5	1	20
Number not eating Yorkshire pudding	25	21	84	5	1	20

Note: Mantel-Haenszel test: roast beef $p < 0.00001$; Yorkshire pudding $p > 0.75$.

case of food-borne salmonellosis outbreaks which may be associated with extensive environmental contamination, disinfection of kitchen utensils and surfaces may be indicated. In both common-vehicle and cross-infection outbreaks, both symptomatic and asymptomatic infected patients should be isolated and placed on enteric precautions. Ill or culture-positive hospital staff may need to be given other duties not involving patient contact until they become culture-negative. Scrupulous hand washing practices must be emphasized and enforced.[119] In addition, particularly in the nursery setting, it may be necessary to initiate cohorting of both patients and staff so that infected infants are cared for only by certain members of the staff, who in turn do not care for uninfected children.

Persistence of an outbreak in the face of the preliminary control measures may indicate the need for more stringent methods, such as closing a nursery or a ward to further admissions followed by aggressive disinfection of the environment after discharge of the last infected patient. Clinical and microbiologic surveillance for additional cases of illness among patients and staff should continue. Both the microbiology laboratory and employee health service are important components of such a surveillance system.

Once an outbreak has ended, a permanent control program should continue in an effort to ensure that practices contributing to a given outbreak are corrected permanently.

Once an investigation is complete, a final report should be prepared, documenting the epidemiologic features of the outbreak, the mode of transmission of the infectious agent, and control measures implemented. This report should be distributed to medical, nursing, microbiology, infection control, and administrative staff and other interested individuals.

Because of the possibility that a nosocomial outbreak of gastroenteritis may be related to a diagnostic reagent, medication, or commercially distributed food, local, state, and national public health authorities should be notified of an outbreak early in the course of the investigation so that surveillance for similar illness in other hospitals may be initiated, if necessary, at the local and state as well as the national level.

FUTURE

Nosocomial gastrointestinal infections, like other nosocomial infections, may be anticipated to continue, causing difficulties for the hospitalized patient until their causes, pathogenesis, reservoirs, and modes of transmission are better understood. It is clear that increased reliance upon antimicrobial agents does not provide the solution to the problem of increasing nosocomial infections, especially in the gastrointestinal tract. Instead, indiscriminant antibiotic use appears to contribute significantly to the problem of nosocomial infections, both because of increased antibiotic resistance and by alteration of the normal flora defense mechanism. We are increasingly forced to recognize previously unsuspected, relatively avirulent organisms as potentially capable of causing life-threatening disease in the suppressed host. Like antimicrobial resistance, virulence factors themselves (such as enterotoxin production and adherence factors) can also be exchanged between bacteria via transmissible genetic material on plasmids — or possibly even bacteriophage. Consequently, our definition of pathogens and approaches to their control require an increasingly open-minded, innovative approach. Having developed an overreliance on antimicrobial agents, we must seek future solutions which require a return to concern about the causes and pathogenesis of nosocomial infectious processes. This means a renewed interest in alteration in normal host defense mechanisms, such as personal hygiene, normal flora, and other natural barriers; and restoring these to the greatest extent possible. It also means that an improved understanding of the epidemiological risk factors and pathogenic mechanisms will be required to develop new means for the control of nosocomial gastrointestinal infections.

REFERENCES

1. Center for Disease Control, National Nosocomial Infections Study Report (NNIS), Annual Summary 1976, U.S. Dept. of Health, Education and Welfare, 1978.
2. Stamm, W. E., Weinstein, R. A., Dixon, R. E., et al., Manuscript in preparation.
3. Szanton, V. L., Epidemic salmonellosis: a 30-month study of 80 cases of *Salmonella oranienburg* infection, *Pediatrics,* 20, 794, 1957.
4. Abrams, I. F., Cochran, W. D., Holmes, L. B., et al., A *Salmonella newport* outbreak in a nursery with a one-year follow-up: effect of ampicillin following bacteriologic failure of response to kanamycin, *Pediatrics,* 37, 616, 1966.
5. Baine, W. B., Gangarosa, E. J., Bennett, J. V., et al., Institutional salmonellosis, *J. Infect. Dis.,* 128, 357, 1973.
6. Rice, P. A., Craven, P. C., and Wells, J. G., *Salmonella heidelberg* enteritis and bacteremia: an epidemic on two pediatric wards, *Am. J. Med.,* 60, 509, 1976.

7. Blacklow, N. R., Dolin, R., Fedson, D. S., DuPont, H. L., Northrup, R. S., Hornick, R. B., and Chanock, A. M., Acute infectious nonbacterial gastroenteritis: etiology and pathogenesis, *Ann. Intern. Med.*, 76, 993, 1972.

8. Shooter, R. A., Faiers, M. C., Cooke, E. M., et al., Isolation of *Escherichia coli, Pseudomonas aeruginosa,* and *Klebsiella* from food in hospitals, canteens, and schools, *Lancet*, 2, 390, 1971.

9. Giannella, R. A., Broitman, S. A., and Zamcheck, N., Influence of gastric acidity on bacterial and parasitic enteric infections: a perspective, *Ann. Intern. Med.*, 78, 271, 1973.

10. Gitelson, S., Gastrectomy, achlorhydria, and cholera, *Isr. J. Med. Sci.*, 7, 663, 1971.

11. Sprunt, K. and Redman, W., Evidence suggesting importance of role of interbacterial inhibition in maintaining balance of normal flora, *Ann. Intern. Med.*, 68, 579, 1968.

12. Mentzing, L. O. and Ringertz, O., *Salmonella* infection in Tourists. II. Prophylaxis against salmonellosis, *Acta Pathol. Microbiol. Scand.*, 74, 405, 1968.

13. Tannock, G. W. and Savage, D. C., Indigenous microorganisms prevent reduction in cecal size induced by *Salmonella typhimurium* in vaccinated gnotobiotic mice, *Infect. Immun.*, 13, 172, 1976.

14. Schrank, G. D., Verwey, W. F.: Distribution of cholera organisms in experimental *Vibrio cholerae* infections: proposed mechanisms of pathogenesis and antibacterial immunity. *Infect. Immun.*, 13:195-203, 1976.

15. Bohnhoff, M., Miller, C. P., Martin, W. R.: Resistance of the mouse's intestinal tract to experimental *Salmonella* infections. *J. Exp. Med.* 120:805-828, 1964.

16. Sprinz, H., Pathogenesis of intestinal infections, *Arch. Pathol.*, 87, 556, 1969.

17. DuPont, H. L. and Hornick, R. B., Adverse effect of lomotil therapy in shigellosis, *J.A.M.A.*, 226, 1525, 1973.

18. Formal, S. B., Abrams, G. D., Schneider, H., and Sprinz, H., Experimental *Shigella* infections. VI. Role of the small intestine in an experimental infection in guinea pigs, *J. Bacteriol.*, 85, 119, 1963.

19. Pierce, N. F. and Reynolds, H. Y., Immunity to experimental cholera. II. Secretory and humoral antitoxin response to local and systemic toxoid administration, *J. Infect. Dis.*, 131, 383, 1975.

20. Pierce, N. F. and Gowans, J. L., Cellular kinetics of the intestinal immune responses to cholera toxoid in rats, *J. Exp. Med.*, 142, 1550, 1975.

21. Said, S. I. and Faloona, G. R., Elevated plasma and tissue levels of vasoactive intestinal polypeptide in the watery-diarrhea syndrome due to pancreatic, bronchogenic, and other tumors, *N. Engl. J. Med.*, 293, 155, 1975.

22. Pettet, J. D., Baggentoss, A. H., and Dearing, W. H., Postoperative pseudomembranous enterocolitis, *Surg. Gynecol. Obstet.*, 98, 546, 1954.

23. Dearing, W. H., Baggenstoss, A. H., and Weed, L. A., Studies on the relationship of *Staphylococcus aureus* to pseudomembranous enteritis and to postantibiotic enteritis, *Gastroenterology*, 38, 441, 1960.

24. Kapral, F. A., O'Brien, A. D., Ruff, P. D., et al., Inhibition of water absorption in the intestine by *Staphylococcus aureus* delta toxin, *Infect. Immun.*, 13, 140, 1976.

25. Reiner, L., Schlesinger, M. J., and Miller, G. M., Pseudomembranous colitis following aureomycin and chloramphenicol, *Arch. Pathol.*, 54, 39, 1952.

26. Tedesco, F. J., Barton, R. W., and Alpers, D. H., Clindamycin-associated colitis, *Ann. Intern. Med.*, 81, 429, 1974.

27. George, W. L., Sutter, V. L., Goldstein, E. J. C., Ludwig, S. L., and Finegold, S. M., Etiology of antimicrobial-agent-associated colitis, *Lancet*, 1, 802, 1978.

28. George, R. H., Symonds, J. M., and Dimock, F., Identification of *Clostridium difficile* as a cause of pseudomembranous colitis, *Br. Med. J.*, 1, 695, 1978.

29. Larson, H. E., Parry, J. V., Price, A. B., et al., Underscribed toxin in pseudomembranous colitis, *Br. Med. J.*, 1, 1246, 1977.

30. Rifkin, G. D., Fekety, F. R., and Silva, J., Jr., Antibiotic-induced colitis implication of a toxin neutralized by *Clostridium sordelli* antitoxin, *Lancet*, 2, 1103, 1977.

31. Bartlett, J. G., Chang, T. W., Gurwith, M., et al., Antibiotic-associated pseudomembranous colitis due to toxin-producing Clostridia, *N. Engl. J. Med.*, 298, 531, 1978.

32. Hansen, K., Jeckeln, E., Jochim J., et al., *Darmbrand-Enteritis Necroticans,* Stuttgart, 1949.

33. Murrell, T. G. C., Roth, L., Egerton, J., et al., Pig-bel: enteritis necroticans, *Lancet*, 1, 217, 1966.

34. Santulli, T. V., Schullinger, J. N., Heird, W. C., Gongaware, R. C., Wigger, J., Barlow, B., Blanc, W. A., and Berdon, W. E., Acute necrotizing enterocolitis in infancy: a review of 64 cases, *Pediatrics*, 55, 376, 1975.

35. Horwitz, M. A., Specific diagnosis of foodborne disease, *Gastroenterology*, 73, 375, 1977.

36. Harris, J. C., DuPont, H. L., and Hornick, R. B., Fecal leukocytes in diarrheal illness, *Ann. Int. Med.*, 76, 697, 1972.

37. Hughes, J. M., Horwitz, M. A., Merson, M. H., et al., Foodborne disease outbreaks of chemical etiology in the United States, 1970-1974, *Am. J. Epidemiol.*, 105, 233, 1977.

38. Terranova, W. and Blake, P. A., *Bacillus cereus* food poisoning, *N. Engl. J. Med.*, 298, 143, 1978.
39. Loewenstein, M. S., Epidemiology of *Clostridium perfringens* food poisoning, *N. Engl. J. Med.*, 286, 1026, 1972.
40. Skirrow, M. B., *Campylobacter* enteritis: a "new" disease, *Br. Med. J.*, 2, 9, 1977.
41. Guerrant, R. L., Lahita, R. G., Winn, W. C., Jr., et al., Campylobacteriosis in man: pathogenic mechanisms and review of 91 bloodstream infections, *Am. J. Med.*, 55, 584, 1978.
42. The Medical Letter, 16, 73, 1974.
43. Tedesco, F. J., Barton, R. W., and Alpers, D. H., Clindamycin-associated colitis: a prospective study, *Ann. Intern. Med.*, 81, 429, 1974.
44. Keefe, E. B., Katon, R. M., Chan, T. T., Melnyk, C. S., and Benson, J. A., Jr., *Pseudomembranous enterocolitis*, resurgence related to newer antibiotic therapy, *West. J. Med.*, 121, 462, 1974.
45. Kabins, S. A., Outbreak of clindamycin-associated colitis, *Ann. Intern. Med.*, 83, 830, 1975.
46. Cunningham, W. and Guerrant, R., unreported observations.
47. Editorial, Colitis following antibiotic therapy due to *Clostridium difficile*, *J.A.M.A.*, 239, 2101, 1978.
48. Larson, H. E., Antibiotic-induced, toxin mediated, clostridial colitis in humans and hamsters, *Clin. Res.*, 26, 322A, 1978.
49. Allo, M., Waskin, H., Rifkin, G., Silva, J., and Fekety, R., Prevention of clindamycin-induced colitis by *Clostridium sordellii* antitoxin, *Clin. Res.*, 26, 389A, 1978.
49a. Virnig, N. L. and Reynolds, J. W., Epidemiological aspects of neonatal necrotizing entercolitis, *Am. J. Dis. Child.*, 128, 186, 1974.
50. McKay, D. G. and Wahle, G. H., Epidemic gastroenteritis due to *Escherichia coli* 0111:B4, *Arch. Pathol.*, 60, 679, 1955.
51. Drucker, M. M., Polliack, A., Yeiven, R., et al., Immunofluorescent demonstration of enteropathogenic *Escherichia coli* in tissue of infants dying with enteritis, *Pediatrics*, 46, 855, 1970.
52. Speer, M. E., Taber, L. H., Yow, M. D., et al., Fulminant neonatal sepsis and necrotizing enterocolitis associated with a "nonenteropathogenic" strain of *Escherichia coli*, *J. Pediatr.*, 89, 91, 1976.
53. Mizrahi, A., Barlow, O., Berdon, W., et al., Necrotizing enterocolitis in premature infants, *J. Pediatr.*, 66, 697, 1965.
54. Egan, E. A. Mantilla, G., Nelson, R. M., et al., A prospective controlled trial of oral kanamycin in the prevention of neonatal necrotizing enterocolitis, *J. Pediatr.*, 89, 467, 1976
55. Book, L. S., Overall, J. L., Herbst, J. J., et al., Clustering of necrotizing enterocolitis: interruption by infection-control measures, *N. Engl. J. Med.*, 297, 984, 1977.
56. Howard, F. M., Flynn, D. M., Bradley, J. M., et al., Outbreak of necrotising enterocolitis caused by *Clostridium butyricum*, *Lancet*, 2, 1099, 1977.
57. Thomas, M., Noah, N. D., Male, G. E., et al., Hospital outbreak of *Clostridium perfringens* food-poisoning, *Lancet*, 1, 1046, 1977.
58. Meyers, J. D., Romm, F. J., Tihen, W. S., et al., Food-borne hepatitis A in a general hospital: epidemiologic study of an outbreak attributed to sandwiches, *J.A.M.A.*, 231, 1049, 1975.
59. Steere, A. C., Hall, W. J., III, Wells, J. G., et al., Person-to-person spread of *Salmonella typhimurium* after a hospital common-source outbreak, *Lancet*, 1, 319, 1975.
60. Kunz, L. J. and Ouchterlony, O. T. B., Salmonellosis originating in a hospital: a newly recognized source of infection, *N. Engl. J. Med.*, 253, 761, 1955.
61. Sanders, E., Sweeney, F. J., Jr., Friedman, E. A., et al., An outbreak of hospital-associated infections due to *Salmonella derby*, *J.A.M.A.*, 186, 984, 1963.
62. Lang, D. J., Kunz, L. J., Martin, A. R., et al., Carmine as a source of nosocomial salmonellosis, *N. Engl. J. Med.*, 276, 829, 1967.
63. Komarmy, L. E., Oxley, M. E., and Brecher, G., Hospital-acquired salmonellosis traced to carmine dye capsules, *N. Engl. J. Med.*, 276, 850, 1967.
64. Eickhoff, T. C., Nosocomial salmonellosis due to carmine, *Ann. Intern. Med.*, 66, 813, 1967.
65. Baine, W. B., Gangarosa, E. J., Bennett, J. V., et al., Institutional salmonellosis, *J. Infect. Dis.*, 128, 357, 1967.
66. Rowe, B. and Hall, M. L. M., *Salmonella* contamination of therapeutic pancreatic preparation, *Br. Med. J.*, 4, 51, 1975.
67. Glencross, E. J. G., Pancreatin as a source of hospital-acquired salmonellosis, *Br. Med. J.*, 2, 376, 1972.
68. Chmel, H. and Armstrong, D., *Salmonella oslo:* a focal outbreak in a hospital, *Am. J. Med.*, 60, 203, 1976.
69. Center for Disease Control, *Salmonella kottbus* meningitis associated with contaminated breast milk, *Morbid. Mortal. Weekly Rep.*, 20, 154, 1971.
70. Ryder, R. W., Crosby-Ritchie, A., McDonough, B., et al., Human milk contaminated with *Salmonella kottbus:* a cause of nosocomial illness in infants, *J.A.M.A.*, 238, 1533, 1977.

71. Ip, H. M. H., Sin, W. K., Chau, P. Y., et al., Neonatal infection due to *Salmonella worthington* transmitted by a delivery-room suction apparatus, *J. Hyg.,* 77, 307, 1976.

72. Datta, N. and Pridie, R. B., An outbreak of infection with *Salmonella typhimurium* in a general hospital, *J. Hyg.,* 58, 229, 1960.

73. Epstein, H. C., Hochwald, A., and Ashe, R., *Salmonella* infections of the newborn infant, *J. Pediatr.,* 38, 723, 1951.

74. Abramson, H., Infection with *Salmonella typhimurium* in the newborn, *Am. J. Dis. Child.,* 74, 576, 1947.

75. Rice, P. A., Craven, P. C., and Wells, J. G., *Salmonella heidelberg* enteritis and bacteremia: an epidemic on two pediatric wards, *Am. J. Med.,* 60, 509, 1976.

76. Mushin, R., An outbreak of gastro-enteritis due to *Salmonella derby, J. Hyg.,* 46, 151, 1948.

77. Hirsch, W., Sapiro-Hirsch, R., Berger, A., et al., *Salmonella edinburg* infection in children: a protracted hospital epidemic due to a multiple-drug-resistant strain, *Lancet,* 2, 828, 1965.

78. Watt, J., Wegman, M. E., Brown, O. W., et al., Salmonellosis in a premature nursery unaccompanied by diarrheal disease, *Pediatrics,* 22, 689, 1958.

79. Bate, J. G. and James, U., *Salmonella typhimurium* infection dust-borne in a children's ward, *Lancet,* 2, 713, 1958.

80. Rubenstein, A. D. and Fowler, R. N., Salmonellosis of the newborn with transmission by delivery room resuscitators, *Am. J. Public Health,* 45, 1109, 1955.

81. Edgar, W. M. and Lacey, B. W., Infection with *Salmonella heidelberg, Lancet,* 1, 161, 1963.

82. MacGregor, R. R. and Reinhart, J., Person-to-person spread of *Salmonella:* a problem in hospitals?, *Lancet,* 2, 1001, 1973.

83. Lintz, D., Kapila, R., Pilgrim, E., et al., Nosocomial *Salmonella* epidemic, *Arch. Intern. Med,* 136, 968, 1976.

84. DuPont, H. L. and Hornick, R. B., Clinical approach to infectious diarrheas, *Medicine (Baltimore),* 52, 265, 1973.

85. Salzman, T. C., Scher, C. D., and Moss, R., Shigellae with transferable drug resistance: outbreak in a nursery for premature infants, *J. Pediatr.,* 71, 21, 1967.

86. Weissman, J. B. and Hutcheson, R. H. Jr., Shigellosis transmitted by nurses, *South. Med. J.,* 69, 1341, 1976.

87. Haltalin, K. C., Neonatal shigellosis: Report of 16 cases and review of the literature, *Am. J. Dis. Child.,* 114, 603, 1967.

88. Whitfield, C. and Humphries, J. M., Meningitis and septicemia due to Shigellae in a newborn infant, *J. Pediatr.,* 70, 805, 1967.

89. Bray, J. and Beavan, T. E. D., Slide agglutination of *Bacterium coli* var. *neapolitanum* in summer diarrhea, *J. Pathol. Bacteriol.,* 60, 395, 1948.

90. Giles, C. and Sangster, G., An outbreak of infantile gastroenteritis in Aberdeen, *J. Hyg.,* 46, 1, 1948.

91. Neter, E., Enteritis due to enteropathogenic *Escherichia coli,* present-day status and unsolved problems, *J. Pediatr.,* 55, 223, 1959.

92. Levine, M. M., Nalin, D. R., Hornick, R. B., et al., *Escherichia coli* strains that cause diarrhea but do not produce heat-labile or heat-stable enterotoxins and are non-invasive, *Lancet,* 1, 1119, 1978.

93. Hone, R., Fitzpatrick, S., Keane, C., et al., Infantile enteritis in Dublin caused by *Escherichia coli* 0142, *Med. Microbiol.,* 6, 505, 1973.

94. Boyer, K. M., Petersen, N. J., Farzaneh, I., Pattison, C. P., Hart, M. C., and Maynard, J. E., An outbreak of gastroenteritis due to *E. coli* 0142 in a neonatal nursery, *J. Pediatr.,* 86, 919, 1975.

95. Kaslow, R. A., Taylor, A., Dweck, H. S., et al., Enteropathogenic *Escherichia coli* infection in a newborn nursery. *Am. J. Dis. Child.,* 128, 797, 1974.

96. Jacobs, S. I., Holzel, A., Wolman, B., et al., Outbreak of infantile gastroenteritis caused by *Escherichia coli* 0114, *Arch. Dis. Child.,* 45, 656, 1970.

97. Rowe, B., Gross, J., Lindop, R., et al., A new *E. coli* O Group 0158 associated with an outbreak of infantile enteritis, *J. Clin. Pathol.,* 27, 832, 1974.

98. Ryder, R. W., Wachsmuth, I. K., Buxton, A. E., Evans, D. G., DuPont, H. L., Mason, E., and Barrett, F. F., Infantile diarrhea produced by heat-stable enterotoxigenic *Escherichia coli, N. Engl. J. Med.,* 295, 849, 1976.

99. Gross, R. J., Rowe, B., Henderson, A., Byatt, M. E., and Maclaurin, J. C., A new *Escherichia coli* O-group, 0159, associated with outbreaks of enteritis in infants, *Scand. J. Infect. Dis.,* 8, 195, 1976.

100. Guerrant, R. L., Dickens, M. D., Wenzel, R. P., et al., Toxigenic bacterial diarrhea: nursery outbreak involving multiple bacterial strains, *J. Pediatr.,* 89, 885, 1976.

101. Skerman, F. J., Formal, S. B., and Falkow, S., Plasmid-associated enterotoxin production in a strain of *Escherichia coli* isolated from humans, *Infect. Immun.,* 5, 622, 1972.

102. Takeda, Y. and Murphy, J., Bacteriophage conversion of heat-labile enterotoxin in *Escherichia coli,* *J. Bacteriol.,* 133, 172, 1978.

103. Marier, R., Wells, J. G., Swanson, R. C., Callahan, W., and Mehlman, I. J., An outbreak of enteropathogenic *Escherichia coli* foodborne disease traced to imported french cheese, *Lancet,* 2, 1376, 1973.

104. Toivanen, P., Olkkonen, L., Toivanen, A., et al., Hospital outbreak of *Yersinia enterocolitica* infection, *Lancet,* 1, 801, 1973.

105. Flewett, T. H., Bryden, A. S., and Davies, H., Epidemic viral enteritis in a long-stay children's ward, *Lancet,* 1, 4, 1975.

106. Ryder, R. W., McGowan, J. E., Jr., Hatch, M. H., et al., Reovirus-like agent as a cause of nosocomial diarrhea in infants, *J. Pediatr.,* 90, 698, 1977.

107. Middleton, P. J., Szymanski, M. T., and Petric, M., Viruses associated with acute gastroenteritis in young children, *Am. J. Dis. Child.,* 131, 733, 1977.

108. Editorial, Rotaviruses of man and animals, *Lancet,* 1, 257, 1975.

109. Bishop, R. F., Hewstone, A. S., Davidson, G. P., et al., An epidemic of diarrhoea in human neonates involving a reovirus-like agent and 'enteropathogenic' serotypes of *Escherichia coli, J. Clin. Pathol.,* 29, 46, 1976.

110. Cameron, D. J. S., Bishop, R. F., Veenstra, A. A., et al., Noncultivable viruses and neonatal diarrhea: fifteen-month survey in a newborn special care nursery, *J. Clin. Microbiol.,* 8, 93, 1978.

111. Murphy, A. M., Albrey, M. B., and Crewe, E. B., Rotavirus infections of neonates, *Lancet,* 2, 1149, 1977.

112. Chrystie, I. L., Totterdell, B. M., and Banatvala, J. E., Asymptomatic endemic rotavirus infections in the newborn, *Lancet* 1, 1176, 1978.

113. Kapikian, A. Z., Kim, H. W., Wyatt, R. G., et al., Human reovirus-like agent as the major pathogen associated with "winter" gastroenteritis in hospitalized infants and young children, *N. Engl. J. Med.,* 294, 965, 1976.

114. von Bonsdorff, C. H., Hovi, T., Makela, P., et al., Rotavirus associated with acute gastroenteritis in adults, *Lancet,* 2, 423, 1976.

115. Kim, H. W., Brandt, C. D., Kapikian, A. Z., et al., Human reovirus-like agent infection: occurrence in adult contacts of pediatric patients with gastroenteritis, *J.A.M.A.,* 238, 404, 1977.

116. Eichenwald, H. F., Ababio, A., Arky, A. M., et al., Epidemic diarrhea in premature and older infants caused by Echo virus type 18, *J.A.M.A.,* 166, 1563, 1958.

117. Weinstein, R. A. and Stamm, W. E., Pseudoepidemics in hospital, *Lancet,* 2, 862, 1977.

118. Szmuness, W., Infections hospitalieres par *Salmonella enteritidis* chez les enfants, *Rev. Hyg. Med. Soc.,* 13, 531, 1965.

119. Steere, A. C. and Mallison, G. F., Handwashing practices for the prevention of nosocomial infections, *Ann. Intern. Med.,* 83, 683, 1975.

CHOOSING THE CORRECT STATISTICAL TESTS

Stanley M. Martin

INTRODUCTION

The analysis of nosocomial infection data can take any of several paths depending upon the study objectives, the hypothesis to be tested, and the available data. This chapter presents methods that are applicable to certain common hypothesis-testing situations encountered in the investigation of nosocomial infection outbreaks. These methods can apply as well to studies of the association of certain factors with the occurrence of nosocomial infections. The purpose here is to acquaint the reader with several significance tests and to indicate when they can be used as analysis tools. It is not within the scope of the chapter to provide the theoretical basis or rationale for each test or to include all tests; instead, for this purpose, appropriate references are provided.

Certain characteristics of the data must be defined in order to select the proper statistical test. For example, tests that are appropriate for attribute data may not apply to measurement data; similarly, procedures applicable to independent samples may not be pertinent to paired samples. This chapter presents statistical tests for independent samples and tests that apply to paired samples. These are separated further into methods appropriate for attribute data and measurement data.

Data collected on nosocomially infected patients and hospitalized, not-infected patients can generally be considered as either attributes or measurements. Attributes commonly examined include such factors as the presence of those procedures which penetrate, are inserted, or are attached to the patient, and exposure to certain surgical procedures, trauma, other infected patients or staff, and other environmental factors (e.g., use or nonuse of antibiotics) that can predispose the patient to nosocomial infection. Attribute data also include observations on patient characteristics such as sex and specific diagnoses or conditions (e.g., diabetes, cirrhosis, alcoholism, etc.). Measurement data, on the other hand, are data giving size, age, temperature, volume, dosage level, etc. recorded for each patient in the infected and not-infected groups. The investigator may be interested in determining whether a particular attribute is associated with nosocomial infection, or interest may lie in deciding whether the group of patients with nosocomial infection had a longer or shorter average exposure to a suspected infection source, tended to weigh more or less (e.g., in the nursery), or had a different level of some measurable body substance (e.g., Blood Urea Nitrogen — [BUN]) than the not-infected group. The data must be examined to decide whether the variables are measurements or attributes when attempting to find a valid test of significance.

In addition to decisions about which tests are valid, decisions about which of several valid tests is "better" for a particular situation include considerations of power and efficiency; a treatment of this subject is given by Siegel.[1] The power of a test is its probability of rejecting the null hypothesis, i.e., the hypothesis of no difference, when it is false; in other words it is the ability of a test to detect a real difference. A general rule can be briefly stated that the power of tests which are based upon more underlying assumptions is greater than the power for corresponding tests which require fewer assumptions. The investigator confronted with data from which he wishes to test a hypothesis must then examine the nature of the data to determine whether t-tests or other parametric tests (i.e., tests which require assumptions about the parameters of the population from which the sample was drawn) are appropriate. These parametric tests which depend upon more rigid assumptions, (e.g., that the data were selected from normally distributed populations) are desirable when one considers power. Commonly, however, nosocomial infection data are such that specification of the parent distribution can be difficult and the assumption of normality can be inappropriate. The distribution-free, or nonparametric procedures (i.e., tests which do not require assumptions about the population parameters) provide adequate methods for most hypothesis tests performed on nosocomial infection data and do not require the investigator to make unrealistic assumptions about the parent distributions. Furthermore, satisfactory power can usually be obtained from these tests.

When a parametric procedure is judged inappropriate, one might wish to know, before collecting the data — reviewing patient charts or other records, interviewing physicians, or examining patients — what increase in sample size would be necessary in order to achieve comparable power with a nonparametric test that could be obtained if a corresponding parametric test were appropriate. The relative sample-size requirements for tests to achieve comparable power are known as efficiency determinations. Consistent with fewer assumptions underlying the nonparametric tests, these tests are generally less efficient than their corresponding parametric tests. Therefore, thought should be given to including more infected and not-infected patients in the study in order to increase the power associated with a particular nonparametric test.

The decision as to whether to employ parametric or nonparametric tests can be guided by considering the following argument. First, parametric tests offer more power; therefore, these tests should be favored, if the data meet the underlying assumptions. For example, the t-test requires that the observations be chosen from populations that are normally distributed and that the observations be independent. Second, suitable "transformations" of the data can be used so that underlying assumptions of the parametric test are met. Some statistical analyses use the logarithm, square root, arc sine, or other transformations[2,3] to "normalize" a distribution or to make variances constant. However, the interpretation of significance tests from these transformed data can present problems, and some debate[4] remains over the meaning of significance determined from transformed data. The suitability of a particular transformation should be evaluated for the particular data by examining how well the transformation achieved its intended purpose. If necessary assumptions are not met and suitable transformations are not utilized, one should then proceed to an appropriate nonparametric test.

Study designs to provide data for hypothesis tests are not discussed in detail here, but some comments concerning the value of two independent samples vs. two matched samples must be presented. Many areas of medical research effectively utilize independent samples for comparing means or proportions. However, studies of nosocomial infection problems usually must take into account hospital and patient risk factors which could predispose certain patients to a higher risk of infection and confuse the analysis of variables suspected to be the cause of infection. Care must be taken in the analysis or study design to remove the unequal effects of these factors on the two study groups. Some statistical methods, (e.g., the Mantel-Haenszel Procedure[5]) include techniques to adjust or "fix" certain variables which otherwise would confound or interfere with the variable of interest. On the other hand, the study itself can be designed to remove their effect and allow the variable of interest to be studied without the hidden influence of these confounding variables. This usually requires appropriate matching of patients from the not-infected group with patients in the infected group for variables such as hospital service, primary diagnosis, surgical procedures, other underlying illness, or certain preceding therapeutic factors which can place the patient at higher or lower risk to nosocomial infection. Furthermore, matching can be benefi-

Table 1
HYPOTHETICAL BUN DETERMINATIONS ON 30 INFECTED AND 30 NOT-INFECTED HOSPITALIZED PATIENTS

Not infected			Infected		
20	13	17	13	18	23
19	18	18	14	20	17
15	12	21	14	16	18
11	17	10	19	15	16
13	16	17	14	15	15
14	16	11	25	18	18
18	15	10	22	25	16
21	15	16	14	14	17
15	13	18	19	23	16
13	12	17	24	21	16

cial on certain demographic characteristics such as age and sex. A discussion of matching and its effect on design efficiency in retrospective studies is presented by Mietti-nen.[6] Further consideration of retrospective study designs can be found in papers by Cornfield and Haenszel[7] and Miettinen.[8]

TWO INDEPENDENT SAMPLES

Measurements

First considered as an example are two independent samples of hypothetical BUN determinations from patients hospitalized during a given time period on the General Medicine Service of a single hospital — a sample from 30 patients with *Proteus mirabilis* urinary tract infection (UTI) and a sample from 30 not-infected patients. The populations of interest are BUN determinations from all infected patients and all not-infected patients from this hospital, service, and time period. Inferences made from samples of these populations are limited to these populations. Suppose the charts of all patients admitted to the General Medicine Service during the first 3 months of 1978 were separated into two groups—those indicating *Proteus mirabilis* UTI and those not indicating *Proteus mirabilis* UTI. Then, utilizing a random number table, a random sample of 30 charts was selected from each group. Among the data abstracted from the chart, the BUN determinations in Table 1 were recorded for each patient.

Suppose also that the investigator was interested in determining for General Medicine Service whether the mean BUN for infected patients was the same as the mean BUN for not-infected patients. This hypothesis can be written as

$$H_O: \mu_I = \mu_{NI}$$

$$H_A: \mu_I \neq \mu_{NI}$$

where μ_I and μ_{NI} are the mean BUN values for all infected and not-infected patients, respectively, who were in the hospital at that time, and H_o and H_A are the null and alternative hypotheses. The t-test for two independent samples, assuming equal variances, is appropriate and for the null hypothesis can be written as

$$t = \frac{\bar{x}_I - \bar{x}_{NI}}{s_{(\bar{x}_I - \bar{x}_{NI})}}$$

where $\bar{x}_I$ and $\bar{x}_{NI}$ are the means from the samples of infected and not-infected patients, and where

$$s_{(\bar{x}_I - \bar{x}_{NI})}$$

is the standard error of the difference between the means. It is assumed that the investigator decided upon type 1 and type 2 errors during the design phase of the study. The type 1 error is defined as the probability of rejecting the null hypothesis, H_o, when in fact H_o is true. Stated differently, this is the probability of saying that the two means are different when they are the same. On the other hand, the type 2 error is the probability of accepting the null hypothesis when it is false. This may be stated differently as the probability of concluding that the two means are the same, when they actually are different. For this example, it is assumed that the type 1 error, α, was set at 0.05. The t-statistic is calculated as follows:

1. The variance of the difference between means is estimated by

$$s^2_{(\bar{x}_I - \bar{x}_{NI})} = \frac{(n_I - 1)s^2_I + (n_{NI} - 1)s^2_{NI}}{(n_I + n_{NI} - 2)} \times \left(\frac{1}{n_I} + \frac{1}{n_{NI}} \right)$$

where n_I and n_{NI} are the sample sizes of infected and not-infected patients, respectively,

$$s^2_{NI} = \frac{\sum_{i=1}^{n_{NI}} (x_{NI_i} - \bar{x}_{NI})^2}{n_{NI} - 1} = 9.689 \qquad s^2_I = \frac{\sum_{i=1}^{n_I} (x_{I_i} - \bar{x}_I)^2}{n_I - 1} = 12.695$$

$$\bar{x}_{NI} = \frac{\sum_{i=1}^{n_{NI}} x_{NI_i}}{n_{NI}} = 15.37 \qquad \bar{x}_I = \frac{\sum_{i=1}^{n_I} x_{I_i}}{n_I} = 17.83$$

Then

$$s^2_{(\bar{x}_I - \bar{x}_{NI})} = \frac{(30 - 1)(12.695) + (30 - 1)(9.689)}{(30 + 30 - 2)} \times \left(\frac{1}{30} + \frac{1}{30} \right) = 0.746$$

and

$$s_{(\bar{x}_I - \bar{x}_{NI})} = \sqrt{s^2_{\bar{x}_I - \bar{x}_{NI}}} = 0.864$$

2. Then "t" is calculated as follows:

$$t = \frac{17.83 - 15.37}{0.864}$$

$$= 2.86$$

3. The decision to accept or reject the null hypothesis is made by comparing the calculated value of t with the tabulated value,

$$\pm t \left(\frac{\alpha}{2}, n_I + n_{NI} - 2df \right)$$

for the two-tailed test. When the calculated value of t is greater than

$$t \left(\frac{\alpha}{2}, n_I + n_{NI} - 2df \right)$$

or less than

$$-t \left(\frac{\alpha}{2}, n_I + n_{NI} - 2df \right)$$

the null hypothesis is rejected. For this example,

$$t = 2.86 > t \left(\frac{\alpha}{2}, n_I + n_{NI} - 2df \right) = 2.00$$

and the null hypothesis is rejected.

A more conservative and less powerful nonparametric test procedure can be used to test a similar hypothesis about the means. For example, the Wilcoxon Rank Sum Test[9] can be used to test the hypothesis that the BUN samples came from two populations having the same means. This test is not based upon the BUN measurements directly; instead, the observations are ranked from one to $n_I + N_{NI}$ with the smallest observation receiving a rank of one. Note that the samples are temporarily combined during the ranking procedure, but are separated again when the ranking is finished. Situations frequently occur as in the BUN data in which some observations are tied. When ties occur, each of the ties is assigned the average of the ranks that would have been assigned to these observations if they had not been tied. For example, patients numbered 24 and 27 of Table 1 each had BUN measurements of ten. These two observations occupy the positions for ranks 1 and 2; therefore they are each assigned the average of these two ranks, $(1 + 2/2) = 1.5$. The next higher observations are those corre-

Table 2

RANKED HYPOTHETICAL BUN DETERMINATIONS FOR 30 INFECTED AND 30 NOT-INFECTED HOSPITALIZED PATIENTS

Not infected			Infected		
Number	BUN	Rank	Number	BUN	Rank
1	20	50.5	1	13	9
2	19	48	2	14	14.5
3	15	21	3	14	14.5
4	11	3.5	4	19	48
5	13	9	5	14	14.5
6	14	14.5	6	25	59.5
7	18	42.5	7	22	55
8	21	53	8	14	14.5
9	15	21	9	19	48
10	13	9	10	24	58
11	13	9	11	18	42.5
12	18	42.5	12	20	50.5
13	12	5.5	13	16	28.5
14	17	35.5	14	15	21
15	16	28.5	15	15	21
16	16	28.5	16	18	42.5
17	15	21	17	25	59.5
18	15	21	18	14	14.5
19	13	9	19	23	56.5
20	12	5.5	20	21	53
21	17	35.5	21	23	56.5
22	18	42.5	22	17	35.5
23	21	53	23	18	42.5
24	10	1.5	24	16	28.5
25	17	35.5	25	15	21
26	11	3.5	26	18	42.5
27	10	1.5	27	16	28.5
28	16	28.5	28	17	35.5
29	18	42.5	29	16	28.5
30	17	35.5	30	16	28.5

sponding to patients numbered 4 and 26. The BUN measurements for these two patients are also tied and are each assigned the average of the next two available ranks, $(3 + 4/2) = 3.5$. The observations of Table 1 are now presented in Table 2 with their appropriate ranks.

The sum of the ranks assigned to the smaller sample is determined and compared with the tabulated values provided by Wilcoxon et al.[10] Since the two samples in this example are of equal size, the sum of ranks from either the infected group or the not-infected group could be used. The sum of ranks for the not-infected group is 757.5, which is less than the tabulated lower value, 783, for a two-sided test at the 0.05 significance level. The conclusion, then, is that the mean BUN from the sample of not-infected patients is not the same as the mean BUN from the sample of infected patients.

Although the BUN data have been used to demonstrate the Wilcoxon Rank Sum Test, Wilcoxon and Wilcox[9] pointed out the problems with this test when a large number of ties are present. They indicated that the effect of many ties is to reduce the ability of the test to detect a difference at some specified level of significance.

Attributes

It is seldom that measurement data such as the BUN observations collected during the course of investigation of a nosocomial infection outbreak are useful in determining the source of the outbreak. Attribute data are more commonly collected to determine which factors are probably associated with the outbreak. For example, *Staphylococcus aureus* surgical wound infections in patients whose surgical procedures were performed by the same surgeon or who were exposed to the same paramedical person, *Proteus mirabilis* urinary tract infections among catheterized patients, and *Enterobacter cloacae* infection among patients receiving intravenous fluids, can be studied by determining the attack rates among patients with or without the suspected factor. Otherwise, samples of infected and not-infected patients can be selected and the proportions having the attribute (exposed to the factor) determined in each group.

Suppose, as in the example of BUN measurements, that samples of infected and not-infected patients from the same service are separately selected to study the possible association of infection with indwelling urinary catheters. The observations can be summarized in a 2 × 2 table for analysis as follows: The hypothesis to be tested is that infection is independent of catheters. An obvious reaction to these data is that a higher proportion of infected patients (0.77) than not-infected patients (0.17) were catheterized. Several tests are available for testing this hypothesis. However, Fisher[11] presented an exact test which with modern calculating equipment should be the test of choice for the above design and hypothesis. A simple approximation by chi-square can be used when the sample sizes are adequate and when the expected number calculated for each cell is of sufficient size. Some disagreement has evolved regarding these two values; Ostle[12] has indicated expected values of three or greater are acceptable, while Snedecor and Cochran[13] have warned against using chi-square when the total sample size, $n_I + n_{NI}$, is less than 20, or when the total sample size is between 20 and 40 with one or more expected numbers as small as 5. The exact test is applicable regardless of these criteria and can be programmed on many programmable "pocket" calculators. If the exact test is programmed, it should be chosen above the chi-square test in situations similar to that of Table 3. The exact test and the chi-square approximation are presented here to provide both the method of choice and a suitable alternative for use in the absence of adequate calculating equipment.

The 2 × 2 table giving results of observations on infection and urinary catheterization is "generalized" in Table 4 for presenting formulas applicable to results from other similarly designed studies.

The null and alternative hypotheses may be stated as

$$H_O: P_I = P_{NI}$$

$$H_A: P_I \neq P_{NI}$$

where P_I is the proportion of the infected population which has the attribute, and where P_{NI} is the proportion of the not-infected population which has the attribute. These are population proportions which are estimated from the two samples by $p_I = (a/a + b)$ and $p_{NI} = (c/c + d)$. Ostle[12] presents the exact probability of observing a particular p_I and p_{NI}, assuming that H_o is true and the marginal totals are fixed, by

$$P = \frac{(a + b)! \, (c + d)! \, (a + c)! \, (b + d)!}{a! \, b! \, c! \, d! \, N!}$$

Maxwell[14] states this probability in a slightly different way as the probability of a particular set of values of a, b, c, and d. The meanings of these two expressions of the probability, however, are equivalent. In order to test the hypothesis, H_o, the sum

Table 3
HYPOTHETICAL NUMBER
OF PATIENTS INFECTED
OR NOT INFECTED AND
PRESENCE OR ABSENCE
OF CATHETERS

	Catheter		
Patient	Yes	No	Total
Infected	23	7	30
Not infected	5	25	30
Total	28	32	60

Table 4
GENERAL 2 × 2 TABLE FOR TWO
INDEPENDENT SAMPLES

	Attribute		
Patient	Present	Absent	Total
Infected	a	b	a + b
Not infected	c	d	c + d
Total	a + c	b + d	a + b + c + d = N

of the probability for the observed data and the probabilities for values of p_I and p_{NI} which differ more than the observed values is obtained. Substituting the observed values from Table 3 into the formula for P, the probability associated with that particular set of values is determined by

$$P_0 = \frac{30! \times 30! \times 28! \times 32!}{23! \times 7! \times 5! \times 25! \times 60!} = 2.797 \times 10^{-6}$$

Next, values of p_I and p_{NI} which are more discrepant than the observed values are determined by successively changing the values of a, b, c, and d in the table of observed values, while keeping the marginal totals fixed, until each table having an associated probability which is no larger than the probability associated with the observed data is determined and its probability calculated. Detailed explanations for determining these tables are given in several statistical textbooks — for example Siegel[1] and Maxwell.[14] One such arrangement for the data of Table 3 is shown in Table 5, from which the second probability is calculated by substituting the new values of a, b, c, and d into the formula for P.

$$P_1 = \frac{30! \times 30! \times 28! \times 32!}{24! \times 6! \times 4! \times 26! \times 60!} = 1.569 \times 10^{-7}$$

This process is continued until the probabilities have been calculated for all more divergent data arrangements.

Table 5
THE SECOND MOST DIVERGENT ARRANGEMENT OF THE DATA FROM TABLE 3

| | Catheter | | |
Patient	Yes	No	Total
Infected	24	6	30
Not infected	4	26	30
Total	28	32	60

Referring to the data of Table 3, the calculated probabilities are

$$P_0 = \frac{30! \times 30! \times 28! \times 32!}{23! \times 7! \times 5! \times 25! \times 60!} = 2.797 \times 10^{-6}$$

$$P_1 = \frac{30! \times 30! \times 28! \times 32!}{24! \times 6! \times 4! \times 26! \times 60!} = 1.569 \times 10^{-7}$$

$$P_2 = \frac{30! \times 30! \times 28! \times 32!}{25! \times 5! \times 3! \times 27! \times 60!} = 5.578 \times 10^{-9}$$

$$P_3 = \frac{30! \times 30! \times 28! \times 32!}{26! \times 4! \times 2! \times 28! \times 60!} = 1.149 \times 10^{-10}$$

$$P_4 = \frac{30! \times 30! \times 28! \times 32!}{27! \times 3! \times 1! \times 29! \times 60!} = 1.174 \times 10^{-12}$$

$$P_5 = \frac{30! \times 30! \times 28! \times 32!}{28! \times 2! \times 0! \times 30! \times 60!} = 4.194 \times 10^{-17}$$

$$P = P_0 + P_1 + P_2 + P_3 + P_4 + P_5 = 0.00000296$$

The sum of these probabilities, P, is the probability for obtaining the observed data or arrangements of the data which are more discrepant than the observed data in the direction of $p_I > p_{NI}$. Tables should also be constructed for data arrangements which are at least as different as the observed data in the direction of $p_I < p_{NI}$ in order to test the hypothesis, $H_0: P_I = P_{NI}$. When the sample sizes of the infected and not-infected groups are equal, as is the case for the data of Table 3, the probabilities for data arrangements in the second direction are equal to the probabilities for arrangements in the first direction. Therefore, the computation for this example can be completed by simply multiplying the probability for one direction by two. The exact test probability then becomes $P = 0.00000592$. When P is compared with $\alpha = 0.05$, the null hypothesis, $H_0: P_I = P_{NI}$, is rejected. That is, the two attributes, infection and catheter, are not judged to be independent.

The chi-square approximation can be used to test these data — note that $n_I + n_{NI} = 60$, and the smallest expected value is $(28/60) \times 30 = 14$. The test is calculated simply from the computational formula as follows:

$$\chi^2 = \frac{N\left(\left|\ ad - bc\ \right| - \frac{N}{2}\right)^2}{(a + b)\ (c + d)\ (a + c)\ (b + d)}$$

$$= \frac{60\left(\left|\ 23 \times 25 - 7 \times 5\ \right| - \frac{60}{2}\right)^2}{28 \times 32 \times 30 \times 30}$$

$$= \frac{15606000}{806400}$$

$$= 19.35$$

This value of chi-square is compared with the tabulated value of chi-square with one degree of freedom to test the hypothesis of independence of the two attributes. Assuming that $\alpha = 0.05$ is the chosen significance level, the tabulated $\chi^2_{(0.05, 1df)}$ is 3.84, and the hypothesis is rejected.

TWO MATCHED SAMPLES

Infections in hospitalized patients only occasionally can be studied by independent case and control groups. More frequently, the controls which are selected for comparison must be carefully matched on several subtle but critical variables, such as those mentioned earlier, to avoid confounding the variable of interest. The significance tests which follow are applicable to data from matched samples.

Measurements

Suppose the BUN observations from Table 1 were collected not as stated before but via a design that selected a matched, not-infected patient for each infected patient. A suitable control for each infected patient would be a not-infected patient of similar age, sex, and time of hospitalization, located on the same service, perhaps one who had experienced the same surgical procedure, and who had the same primary diagnosis. The hypothesis that the mean BUN for infected patients was the same as the mean BUN for not-infected patients for this sample design can again be tested by a t-test; however, this is the t-test for paired observations. The data to be used to test the hypothesis are now arranged in Table 6 to show the pairing. The table presents BUN observations for each member of the pair and the difference between observations for each pair. The test is based upon the distribution of differences, which is assumed to be normal. The hypothesis of no difference between mean BUN levels for the data of Table 6 can be tested as follows:

$$t = \frac{\bar{d}}{s_{\bar{d}}}$$

where

$$\bar{d} = \frac{\sum\limits_{i=1}^{n} d_i}{n} = -2.47 \qquad s_{\bar{d}} = \sqrt{\frac{\sum\limits_{i=1}^{n} (d_i - \bar{d})^2}{n\ (n - 1)}} = 0.897$$

and n = number of pairs. Then t = $(-2.47/0.897) = -2.75 < t_{(0.05, 29df)} = -2.04$, and the hypothesis that the two means are equal is rejected.

Attributes

Studies of factors associated with nosocomial infections commonly require the matched-pair design, as in the above example; additionally, these studies usually involve determinations of attributes. Tests are now presented that can be applied in these situations. Hypothetical data from Tables 6 and 7 are used to illustrate the methodology for these tests. Table 7 indicates the presence or absence of indwelling urinary catheters for infected patients and their matched controls with matching based upon the same criteria as in the previous BUN example. The presence of a catheter is indicated by "1", while "0" indicates the absence of a catheter. Table 8 presents the general method for summarizing the results of paired observations. This table counts pairs rather than single observations, and hypothesis tests are based only upon the pairs in which the members of the pair exhibited different outcomes. Thus, these tests utilize only cells b and c and exclude cells a and d. All the observations from Table 7 are summarized in this way in Table 9. The test excludes the four pairs in which both members of the pair were catheterized and the six pairs in which neither member of the pair was catheterized. The pairs remaining, then, are the single pair in which the infected patient was not catheterized, while the matched, not-infected patient was catheterized, and 19 pairs in which the infected patients were catheterized while their matched, not-infected patients were not catheterized. The effective sample size for the test is 20.

The sign test is an exact test which uses only the sign of the difference in each pair and does not take into account the size of the difference. Therefore, this test is applicable to both the paired BUN data and the paired catheter data. The test requires that the observations be paired and that the measurements within each pair have some directional relationship to each other, i.e., higher, lower, or equal. As might be expected with its broad applicability, the sign test is not very efficient when compared to other tests which take size of differences into account. Siegel,[1] Snedecor and Cochran,[13] and others discuss this test and compare its efficiency with other tests which might be applied. Even though it is among the less powerful tests, its simplicity and validity for a wide range of data can allow large sample sizes to be taken so that adequate power is achieved. The test is based upon the assumption that when the sign of the difference between members of each pair is taken, the number of pluses should equal the number of minuses, if the observed variable is unrelated to either of the two groups. For the data of Table 7 one would expect as many not-infected patients as infected patients to have been catheterized, if in fact catheterization were unrelated to infection. The effective number of pairs (i.e., untied pairs) from the table is 20; thus if the attributes are unrelated, one would expect to have observed ten infected patients catheterized while their not-infected matches were not catheterized, and ten infected patients not catheterized while their not-infected matches were catheterized. The exact probability of observing a given number or fewer of pluses and minuses is determined from

$$P = \sum_{x=0}^{c} \frac{N!}{x! \, (N-x)!} \, (0.5)^x \, (1 - 0.5)^{N-x}$$

Table 6
HYPOTHETICAL BUN LEVELS FOR MATCHED INFECTED AND NOT-INFECTED PATIENTS

Pair number	Not infected	Infected	Difference (d)	Pair number	Not infected	Infected	Difference (d)
1	20	16	4	16	16	19	−3
2	19	18	1	17	15	13	2
3	15	25	−10	18	15	14	1
4	11	23	−12	19	13	24	−11
5	13	15	−2	20	12	15	−3
6	14	15	−1	21	17	17	0
7	18	18	0	22	18	22	−4
8	21	17	4	23	21	18	3
9	15	14	1	24	10	16	−6
10	13	14	−1	25	17	14	3
11	13	21	−8	26	11	19	−8
12	18	16	2	27	10	20	−10
13	12	18	−6	28	16	16	0
14	17	23	−6	29	18	14	4
15	16	16	0	30	17	25	−8

Table 7
PRESENCE OF INDWELLING URINARY CATHETER IN MATCHED INFECTED AND NOT-INFECTED PATIENTS

Pair number	Not infected	Infected	Pair number	Not infected	Infected
1	0	1	16	0	1
2	0	0	17	0	0
3	0	1	18	1	1
4	1	0	19	0	1
5	0	1	20	0	1
6	0	1	21	1	1
7	1	1	22	0	1
8	0	0	23	0	1
9	0	1	24	0	0
10	0	1	25	0	1
11	0	1	26	0	1
12	0	0	27	0	1
13	0	0	28	0	1
14	0	1	29	0	1
15	1	1	30	0	1

Table 8
GENERAL 2 × 2 TABLE FOR TWO MATCHED SAMPLES (TABULATION OF PAIRS OF PATIENTS)

Infected patients — attribute present?	Not-infected patients — attribute present?		
	Yes	No	Total
Yes	a	b	a + b
No	c	d	c + d
Total	a + c	b + d	N

Table 9
SUMMARIZATION OF THE DATA
FROM TABLE 7

Infected	Not infected		
	Catheter	No catheter	Total
Catheter	4	19	23
No catheter	1	6	7
Total	5	25	30

where c is the smaller of the number of pluses or minuses, and N is the number of untied pairs. This is the sum of the binomial probabilities for values from 0 through the number observed, assuming that the pluses and minuses should occur with equal frequency. For the example of infection and catheterization this probability is

$$P = \sum_{x=0}^{1} \frac{20!}{x!\,(20-x)!}\,(0.5)^x\,(1-0.5)^{20-x}$$

In order to illustrate the calculations, the terms of the summation are given below:

$$P_0 = \frac{20!}{0!\,(20-0)!}\,(0.5)^0\,(0.5)^{20} = (1)\,(1)\,(0.5)^{20} = 0.000000954$$

$$P_1 = \frac{20!}{1!\,(20-1)!}\,(0.5)^1\,(0.5)^{19} = (20)\,(0.5)\,(0.5)^{19} = 0.000019073$$

$$P = \sum_{x=0}^{1} \frac{20!}{x!\,(20-x)!}\,(0.5)^x\,(1-0.5)^{20-x} = 0.000020027$$

The two-tailed test probability is obtained by multiplying this probability by two to obtain $P = 0.000040054$. When P is compared to $\alpha = 0.05$, the null hypothesis is rejected in favor of the alternative.

A second procedure which is frequently used in testing attribute data from paired samples was introduced by McNemar.[15] McNemar's test, like other tests of paired data, is based on those pairs in which the members are untied with respect to the observation variable. The test is a chi-square test, but not the ordinary chi-square as presented earlier. In fact, a frequent error in the analysis of paired data is the application of the ordinary chi-square test as though the two samples were independent. The formula given below includes a continuity correction which is discussed in most elementary statistics textbooks — for example, Snedecor and Cochran[13] and Ostle.[12]

$$\chi^2 = \frac{(|b-c|-1)^2}{b+c}$$

The observations from Table 9 are again used to illustrate the test procedure. From this table b = 19 and c = 1, so that

$$\chi^2 = \frac{(\,|\,19-1\,|\,-1)^2}{19+1}$$

$$= \frac{(18-1)^2}{20}$$

$$= \frac{289}{20}$$

$$= 14.45$$

This chi-square is greater than the tabulated chi-square with one degree of freedom and $\alpha = 0.05$ ($\chi^2_{(0.05, 1df)} = 3.84$), and the hypothesis that catheterization is not associated with infection is rejected in favor of the alternative hypothesis that the two factors are associated. Because the ordinary chi-square (which requires that the observations be independent) is commonly misused for paired data, I again emphasize that matched samples by definition do not meet the assumption of independence required by the ordinary chi-square. Therefore, chi-square for independent samples is not appropriate for matched samples, and one should seek a test such as the McNemar test or sign test which takes the matching into account.

Although the sign test is applicable to data such as the BUN determinations of Table 6, this test ignores information about the size of the differences. It can be beneficial in instances involving observations of a higher order than simple determination of higher, lower, etc. to use a test which takes into account some measure of how much higher, how much lower, etc. for each pair. Certainly, the paired t-test takes into account both the sign and the size of differences for each pair, but this test requires the normality assumption, which can be inappropriate. In this case suitable alternative nonparametric tests are available. Recall that the Wilcoxon Rank Sum Test was used to illustrate a nonparametric test alternative to the t-test for independent samples. The Wilcoxon Signed Rank Test[9] is a good alternative to the t-test for matched pairs. This test is based upon ranks which indicate size, and signed differences which give direction. The paired BUN determinations from Table 6 are used below to illustrate the procedure for testing the hypothesis that infected and not-infected patients were drawn from populations having the same mean BUN.

The first step of the procedure is to take the differences in each pair including the sign of the difference (Table 10). Next, the absolute values of these differences are ranked assigning the smallest difference a rank of 1, the largest difference a rank of N, and nonzero differences of the same magnitude an identical rank, which is the average of the ranks that would have been used for these differences, if they were untied. Table 10 illustrates the ranking; note that this ranking of the absolute values from lowest to highest excludes consideration of sign. Signs are restored to the ranks after the ranking is complete. Consider in the table, the five differences which have the value +1 and −1. For purposes of ranking, −1 and +1 are given the same ranks. These are determined by finding the average of the ranks that would have been assigned if the five were untied. If these were not tied, ranks 1, 2, 3, 4, and 5 would be assigned, giving an average of

$$\frac{1+2+3+4+5}{5} = \frac{15}{5} = 3$$

Table 10

RANKING METHOD FOR THE WILCOXON SIGNED RANK TEST USING BUN LEVELS FOR MATCHED INFECTED AND NOT-INFECTED PATIENTS

Pair number	Not infected	Infected	Difference	Rank	Signed rank
1	20	16	+ 4	14.5	+ 14.5
2	19	18	+ 1	3	+ 3
3	15	25	−10	23.5	−23.5
4	11	23	−12	26	−26
5	13	15	− 2	7	− 7
6	14	15	− 1	3	− 3
7	18	18	0	—	—
8	21	17	+ 4	14.5	+ 14.5
9	15	14	+ 1	3	+ 3
10	13	14	− 1	3	− 3
11	13	21	− 8	21	−21
12	18	16	+ 2	7	+ 7
13	12	18	− 6	18	−18
14	17	23	− 6	18	−18
15	16	16	0	—	—
16	16	19	− 3	10.5	−10.5
17	15	13	+ 2	7	+ 7
18	15	14	+ 1	3	+ 3
19	13	24	−11	25	−25
20	12	15	− 3	10.5	−10.5
21	17	17	0	—	—
22	18	22	− 4	14.5	−14.5
23	21	18	+ 3	10.5	+ 10.5
24	10	16	− 6	18	−18
25	17	14	+ 3	10.5	+ 10.5
26	11	19	− 8	21	−21
27	10	20	−10	23.5	−23.5
28	16	16	0	—	—
29	18	14	+ 4	14.5	+ 14.5
30	17	25	− 8	21	−21

Therefore, the differences for pairs numbered 2, 6, 9, 10, and 18 are each ranked 3. In the final ranking step, the sign of each difference is also given to its rank; for example, the pairs numbered 2, 9, and 18 are assigned ranks of +3 while pairs numbered 6 and 10 are assigned ranks of −3. The next larger difference, −2 and +2, for pairs numbered 5, 12, and 17 are assigned ranks in a similar way beginning with the next unused rank, 6, and determining the average rank that would be used if the three differences were untied. This average is

$$\frac{6 + 7 + 8}{3} = \frac{21}{3} = 7$$

The ranking continues in this manner until the pair having the highest difference (pair number 4) is assigned a rank of 26. The column headed "Signed rank" contains these ranks with their appropriate signs.

Finally, the negative ranks and positive ranks are separately summed, and the absolute value of the smaller of the two, T, is compared with the critical value in order to make a decision about the hypothesis. The two sums for the BUN example, ignoring the signs, are (1) sum of positive ranks — 14.5 + 3 + 14.5 + 3 + 7 + 7 + 3 + 10.5

+ 10.5 + 14.5 = 87.5; (2) sum of negative ranks — 23.5 + 26 + 7 + 3 + 3 + 21 + 18 + 18 + 10.5 + 25 + 10.5 + 14.5 + 18 + 21 + 23.5 + 21 = 263.5.

Tables of critical values for the Signed Rank Test were provided by Wilcoxon et al.[10] and have been partially reproduced in several textbooks that present the test. Referring to Wilcoxon's tables with n = 26 and α = 0.05 significance level, the critical value, T_o, for the smaller of the two sums is 98. The hypothesis that the two samples of BUN levels were taken from populations having the same means is rejected, since T = 87.5 < T_o = 98.

DISCUSSION

The procedures presented are limited to the testing of hypotheses from two matched samples. Methods[16-18] are available for testing hypotheses about the association of an attribute or factor with infection when two or more not-infected patients are matched to each infected patient.

Many liberties have been taken in this chapter to present a selected list of statistical tests and to make general statements in some instances. At least in part, this approach is based on some knowledge of the usual characteristics of data collected about nosocomial infections. Statistical texts on methodology of significance testing should be expected to state assumptions and details of theory, whereas for the specific purpose of testing data on nosocomial infections, experience with these data has been used to select the tests for each situation without presenting the justifications. The issue of one-tailed vs. two-tailed tests has not been raised. For consistency, two-tailed tests were used to illustrate the test procedures; however, many investigations of the association of certain factors with nosocomial infections appropriately use one-tailed tests. One would suspect, for example, that the association of indwelling urinary catheters with nosocomial infections would be in the direction of more infected patients than not-infected patients having catheters, thus suggesting a one-tailed test. The statement of the hypothesis and the use of a one-tailed or two-tailed test are discussed in most elementary statistics texts.

The following flow chart (Figure 1) may help the reader find appropriate test procedures. Note that other tests that were not discussed in this chapter can be added in appropriate blocks as necessary. Siegel[1] provides a more complete chart which identifies appropriate conditions for application of these and other tests.

These discussions of appropriate tests have purposely avoided the crucial question about the approach to analyzing nosocomial infection data. While methods are presented for hypothesis tests that apply to certain study designs and hypotheses, this chapter should not be taken as an argument for always using a statistical test instead of some other approach to understanding what the data say. A common sense interpretation of descriptive statistics, hypothesis test results, or estimation procedures must ultimately be used to communicate the message clearly.

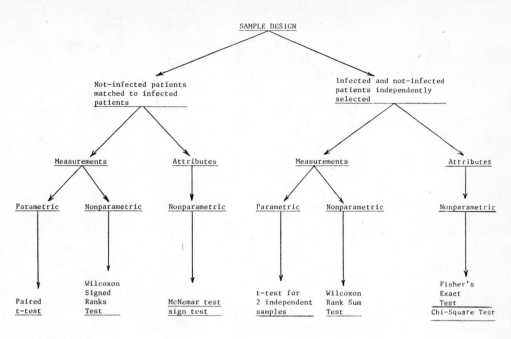

FIGURE 1. Diagram for selecting appropriate statistical tests for nosocomial infection data.

REFERENCES

1. Siegel, S., *Nonparametric Statistics for the Behavioral Sciences,* McGraw-Hill, New York, 1956.
2. Bartlett, M. S., The use of transformations, *Biometrics,* 3, 39, 1947.
3. Steel, G. D. and Torrie, J. H., *Principles and Procedures of Statistics,* McGraw-Hill, New York, 1960.
4. Feinstein, A. R., *Clinical Biostatistics,* C. V. Mosby, St. Louis, 1977, 66.
5. Mantel, N. and Haenszel, W., Statistical aspects of the analysis of data from retrospective studies of disease, *J. Natl. Cancer Inst.,* 22, 719, 1959.
6. Miettinen, O. S., Matching and design efficiency in retrospective studies, *Am. J. Epidemiol.,* 91(2), 111, 1970.
7. Cornfield, J. and Haenszel, W., Some aspects of retrospective studies, *J. Chronic Dis.,* 11, 523, 1960.
8. Miettinen, O. S., The matched pairs design in the case of all-or-none responses, *Biometrics,* 24, 339, 1968.
9. Wilcoxon, F. and Wilcox, R. A., *Some Rapid Approximate Statistical Procedures,* American Cyanamid Co., Pearl River, N.Y., 1964.
10. Wilcoxon, F., Katti, S. K., and Wilcox, R. A., *Critical Values and Probability Levels for the Wilcoxon Rank Sum Test and the Wilcoxon Signed Rank Test,* American Cyanamid Co. and Florida State University, 1963.
11. Fisher, R. A., *Statistical Methods for Research Workers,* Oliver and Boyd, Edinburgh, Scotland, 1950.
12. Ostle, B., *Statistics in Research,* Iowa State University Press, Ames, Iowa, 1954.
13. Snedecor, G. W. and Cochran, W. G., *Statistical Methods,* Iowa State University Press, Ames, Iowa, 1968.
14. Maxwell, A. E., *Analysing Qualitative Data,* Methuen & Company Ltd., London, 1971, 23.
15. McNemar, Q., *Psychological Statistics,* John Wiley & Sons, New York, 1955.
16. Cochran, W. G., The comparison of percentages in matched samples, *Biometrika,* 37, 256, 1950.
17. Miettinen, O. S., Individual matching with multiple controls in the case of all-or-none responses, *Biometrics,* 25, 339, 1969.
18. Pike, M. C. and Morrow, R. H., Statistical Analysis of Patient-Control Studies in Epidemiology, Factor Under Investigation an All-or-None Variable, *Br. J. Prev. Soc. Med.,* 24, 42, 1970.

DESIGNING A STUDY TO ANSWER INFECTION-CONTROL QUESTIONS

Timothy R. Townsend

INTRODUCTION

Many persons who have neither performed studies nor done research, regard such activities as being limited to very special people working in laboratories or large research-oriented institutions. As with most skills, performing studies or doing research is a learned activity; few, if any, persons are "born" to be investigators. The purpose of this chapter is to guide the nonresearch-oriented person through the steps necessary to design, perform, and publish the results of a study. It is hoped that through this step-by-step introduction to the performance of studies, persons who have never felt they could initiate such undertakings would be encouraged to do quality research, particularly since many such individuals are in constant contact with a vast untapped reservoir of clinical experience. Obviously, everything that one would need to know to become a competent investigator cannot be covered in a single chapter of a book, but the major steps can be outlined briefly, and the reader is encouraged to seek specialized information, as needed, from other textbooks and articles.

DETERMINING THE QUESTION

The first step in performing a study, and often the most difficult one for the inexperienced investigator, is to determine what specific question the study is supposed to answer. If one thinks about his everyday work as an infection-control practitioner, it should be obvious that questions arise frequently for which there are no good answers. Some examples of these questions might be: Since there were six patients with *Serratia marcescens* bacteremia in the intensive care unit in the past month and all had intravascular pressure monitoring devices in use, could the devices be the source of the bacteremia? Does daily meatal care reduce or increase the risk of Foley bladder catheter-associated urinary tract infections? Should anesthesia and respiratory therapy equipment be sterilized or just disinfected between patient use?

There are two very important points that the investigator must consider when determining the question to be answered by the study. First, the investigator must decide whether the question is an important one. A study designed to determine whether an iodophor ointment which is manufactured by company "A" should be used around the entry site of an indwelling vascular catheter as opposed to one manufactured by company "B" may not be nearly so important a study as to whether an ointment should be used at all. Second, the investigator must focus the question in such a way that it is sufficiently precise. The question as to whether anesthesia and respiratory therapy equipment needs to be sterilized or disinfected might be too general. This particular question might be very difficult to answer, whereas a more precise question would be whether there was a greater incidence of postoperative pneumonia following use of ethylene oxide sterilized anesthesia equipment compared to glutaraldehyde disinfected equipment. The investigator who fails to ask whether the question is precise and manageable in terms of finding a reasonable answer may find the study nearly impossible to perform.

SELECTING THE TYPE OF STUDY

There are four basic types of studies that are generally used to answer questions pertaining to infection-control problems: descriptive studies, retrospective or case-control studies, prospective observational studies, and propsective experimental studies. The type of study selected is often determined by the specific question the investigator wishes to have answered by the study.

If an investigator is interested in a particular disease or event and wishes to determine the characteristics or attributes of patients who have that disease or who have suffered that event, a descriptive study might be most appropriate. For example, if one is interested in examining the hospital's experience with nosocomial *Serratia marcescens* bacteremia, then all cases of such disease occurring within any particular period of time would be collected, and characteristics or attributes such as age, sex, location within the hospital, underlying disease, etc. would be recorded. The most commonly occurring attribute, such as location in an intensive care unit, may give some clue as to the pathogenesis of the disease process. This type of study design is usually chosen when an investigator is not testing a particular hypothesis but is searching for clues to associations between a disease and various traits common to those with the disease.

If an investigator observes that several attributes are common to patients with a particular disease and wishes to find out which attribute or attributes are most strongly associated with a particular disease, a retrospective case-control study might be performed. Retrospective or case-control studies determine the attributes or risk factors associated with a particular disease or event by contrasting the occurrence of those factors in a group of patients with the disease or event with those who do not have the disease or event. For example, if it was noted that many cases of nosocomial *Serratia marcescens* bacteremia had occurred among patients on the surgical service in the intensive care unit and a number of characteristics, such as exposure to various personnel and invasive devices, were common to most of the cases, then the investigator would compare attributes (age, sex, exposure to personnel, devices, etc.) among two groups of patients: all patients with *Serratia marcescens* nosocomial bacteremia in the intensive care unit and all patients without *Serratia marcescens* nosocomial bacteremia in the intensive care unit. In this situation it may be noticed that *Serratia marcescens* nosocomial bacteremia was strongly associated with the use of an intravascular pressure-monitoring device.

If an investigator has developed a hypothesis that a particular attribute is important in the pathogenesis of an infection and wishes to determine whether there is a difference in the rate of occurrence of the infection in a group of patients in whom the attribute is present compared to a group of patients in whom it is not present, then a prospective observational study might be most appropriate. In a prospective observational study, patients in whom the disease has not manifested itself are selected and grouped according to whether a particular attribute under study is present or not. The patients are then observed for a period of time to determine how many with the particular attribute develop the disease or event being studied. For example, if an indwelling intravascular pressure-monitoring device is thought to be important in the pathogenesis of *Serratia marcescens* nosocomial bacteremia, then patients admitted to an intensive care unit who are free from bacteremia at the initiation of the study would be grouped according to whether they had such a monitoring device used or not. The patients in each group would be observed over a period of time to see whether there was any difference in the rate of occurrence of nosocomial *Serratia marcescens* bacteremia.

Prospective experimental studies are quite similar to prospective observational studies except that in the former the investigator chooses which patients will have the particular attribute under study. In the preceding example of a prospective observational study of nosocomial *Serratia marcescens* bacteremia, the investigator did not choose which patients were to use intravascular pressure-monitoring devices. That choice was made by the various physicians caring for the patients. In contrast, in a prospective experimental study, the investigator would make the choice as to which patients were to receive the intravascular monitoring device.

ASCERTAINING PREVIOUS EXPERIENCE

After deciding the precise question to be answered by the study and choosing the best study design suited to answer the question, one should ascertain whether the question has previously been asked, answered, and the results published. The first step in this process would be to read about the particular subject of the study in textbooks, journals, or other articles in the literature. Textbooks are often several months to a year or so out of date by the time that they are published, so one should not rely on these sources of information to provide the most up-to-date information. Journals and other articles in the current literature are an excellent source of information because the question pertinent to the study is usually well-defined, and precise and other literature bearing on the same subject is often quite well reviewed. The *Index Medicus* which may be found in some libraries is organized in such a manner that it is very easy to find which books, periodicals, and articles have been published on a certain subject. In addition to the *Index Medicus,* some libraries have computer search facilities that will print out the sources of information available on a variety of given topics. If the *Index Medicus* or computer search facilities are not available in a particular library, it may be that these resources can be made available through an interlibrary loan service. The National Library of Medicine at the National Institutes of Health in Bethesda, Md. may be of great assistance to an investigator in terms of either providing resource information directly, or indicating where it may be available. Finally, one resource that may be particularly valuable to an investigator seeking information on previous research in a particular area, is an established investigator or expert who has done research on the subject.

STUDY FEASIBILITY

Once an investigator has clearly chosen the subject matter to be studied, the best type of study, and has obtained a thorough knowledge of the material that has been published on the subject, he must determine whether it is feasible to carry out the study. A major factor in determining the feasibility of a study is the time necessary to do the study. Prospective studies generally take longer to perform than do descriptive or case-control studies.

Both the particular question that the investigator is studying and the type of study design chosen, will greatly influence the amount of time needed to complete the study. If an investigator wished to study postoperative wound infections following cholecystectomies and only three or four cholecystectomies were performed monthly at this hospital, a prospective study may take years before a sufficient number of patients had been studied so that adequate conclusions could be drawn.

An additional component in determining whether a particular study is feasible is the number of personnel that may be available to an investigator to assist in the performing of the study. A variety of factors may influence the number of personnel needed in any particular study: type of study design, number of patients included in the study, nature and amount of data sought from each patient, etc. If medical records were to be used as the information source for a certain descriptive study, an investigator may want to gather the data needed for the study from a small sample of records prior to initiating the study. As a result, he might be able to estimate the amount of time needed to abstract all study patients' records and determine the number of personnel required to complete the task within the particular time limits established to perform the study.

Probably the largest factor in determining the feasibility of any study is money. Estimates of the amount of money needed to perform a particular study usually can be made only after the needs in terms of time, personnel, and equipment have been estimated. Methods for obtaining money for studies is beyond the scope of this chapter; however, a suggested reading list is provided at the end of this chapter, where excellent articles and books on this subject are presented. Generally, prospective studies are more expensive than case-control or descriptive studies, but the particular question addressed by the study is usually a major factor in cost. An investigator, when contemplating performing a study, should consider the possibility of collaborating with other investigators and thereby possibly performing a better study with less expenditure of time, personnel, and money on the part of any one collaborator.

It is obvious that this phase of planning a study involves a great deal of "playing with figures". An investigator may wish, for example, to study the incidence of postoperative pneumonia in two groups of patients: one in which ethylene oxide sterilization was used for the anesthesia equipment and the other in which the equipment was disinfected with 2% glutaraldehyde. After developing a rough estimate of the time, personnel, and financial needs to perform a prospective, experimental study, he may realize that he did not have the resources to carry out the study. However, he was able to determine that within the past year his particular hospital had switched from using 2% glutaraldehyde to ethylene oxide for disinfecting/sterilizing anesthesia equipment. By refiguring time, personnel, and money, he was able to determine that a descriptive study was quite feasible. Quite possibly the descriptive study might not be the definitive or ideal study to answer the question, but the descriptive study might provide information that was not available in the literature at that time. Just because the ideal or definitive study cannot be performed is no reason to ignore the question. Each investigator must attempt to do the least expensive study that will provide the best answer to the question.

ETHICAL CONSIDERATIONS

There are a number of ethical considerations that must be taken into account when performing research. An investigator performing a retrospective study using patients' records must be aware that the patients' right to privacy must be protected. Some institutions have very stringent rules and regulations regarding access to patient records, whereas other institutions may not have such a policy. Generally, the administrator or the medical records librarian is the person charged legally with the custody of medical records, so these individuals should be consulted prior to the initiation of a study utilizing these sources of information. Likewise, special permission may be needed if other sources of data such as birth records, death certificates, or hospitalization cost records are utilized.

In addition to these ethical considerations regarding the right of privacy which are common to most retrospective studies, prospective studies often present other types of ethical problems. Prospective studies in which the patient is required to make a choice — to participate or not to participate in the study or to have a procedure performed or a specimen obtained — must make provisions for obtaining the informed consent of the patient. The concept of informed consent is constantly undergoing redefinition in the U.S. today. Most institutions have a legal adviser who is aware of the current requirements for obtaining informed consent. These persons may be a very valuable resource for an investigator contemplating a prospective study.

Prospective experimental studies, by virtue of the fact that patients enrolled in the study are receiving an attribute such as a drug, a device, or other type of treatment, present very difficult ethical considerations. Some element of danger to the patient is inherent in such types of studies because the possible outcomes or side effects that may be associated with a particular assigned attribute may be unknown and conceivably could cause significant morbidity or mortality. Accordingly, an investigator contemplating such a study should take several steps to clarify the ethical considerations implicit in the study. There should be a thorough search of the literature to confirm that there are no data available that indicate that one of the attributes that will be assigned to patients is better or worse than any other assigned attribute. If there is a suggestion from the literature that one attribute is better or worse, it may be unethical to subject patients to that particular attribute. If, on the other hand, there are no data available as to whether one attribute is better than the other, then the investigator might want to discuss the situation with physicians who will be referring patients into the study to see if they would have any reservations about assigning any particular patient to any of the proposed study groups. This is very important, because, as will be discussed later (see "Study Designs — Prospective Experimental Studies"), an investigator wants to avoid having patients entered into the study who will later be withdrawn. The physicians who will be referring patients into the study should be fully informed as to the ranges of outcomes and side effects due to the particular attribute(s) under study. A particularly vexing problem concerning prospective experimental studies is what to do if during the study it becomes obvious that one particular study group, receiving a certain treatment or other attribute, is experiencing a far worse outcome than other groups. There are several ways that this problem can be approached, none of which are entirely satisfactory. The investigator may "blind" the trial such that neither the patient nor the persons evaluating the patient are aware of what attribute had been assigned to that particular patient. In this situation it is not until the analysis of the data is completed that the impact of the ethical situation is realized. This technique merely delays — but does not eradicate — the ethical problem. A modification of this technique would be for the investigator, prior to the onset of the study, to choose specified time intervals during the study to do a preliminary analysis of the data, and, if significant differences are noted, stop the study. The problem with this technique is that very often the investigators are dealing with very small numbers early in the study, and sequential evaluations, one of which on a random basis may be significant, may be totally misleading.

STUDY DESIGNS

Once an investigator has precisely defined the question for which he seeks an answer, generally determined what type of study would be best suited to answer this question, ascertained whether the study had been done previously, and considered whether the study is feasible and ethical, the next step is the actual design of the study. In this section each of the four basic study designs will be discussed in some detail, and they are arranged in a sequence whereby the simplest is presented first and the most complex last. Principles discussed in relation to each study design are particularly applicable to that study design but may also be applicable to other study designs as well.

Descriptive Studies
Descriptive studies describe the attributes found among patients with similar diseases

or events, and the frequency of occurrence of any one particular attribute provides clues that a possible association exists between the attribute and the disease or event. The initial step in designing a descriptive study involves defining the particular disease or event. If an investigator wished to study the attributes of patients with postoperative wound infections, it would be necessary to define what a postoperative wound infection was. There are a variety of ways in which postoperative wound infections have been defined, such as: pus at the incision site; a certain number of millimeters of erythema around an incision site; the presence of induration; the presence of pus, erythema, and induration, or combinations thereof; any clinical diagnoses by the attending physician, etc. The definition of the disease should be simple, precise, and sufficiently refined so that there is little confusion in determining which patients to include and which patients to exclude.

After determining the definition of the disease or event, the next step is to decide which attributes are to be examined. Some of the most common attributes examined are the patient's age, sex, race, service, location within the hospital, and underlying disease. The purpose of a descriptive study is to examine a number of attributes, one or more of which may be associated with a particular infection. The investigator, however, should be aware that the more attributes that are examined the greater the amount of personnel, time, and — possibly — money, will be needed for the study. It is important for the investigator to be discriminative and creative in selecting the attributes for study. A thorough review of the pertinent literature and good common sense in terms of biological interrelationships will be of great help in choosing the attributes.

The accuracy of the sources of information from which the study data are collected should be determined by the investigator. Medical records of hospitalized patients may be an adequate source of such information as the results of a laboratory test, but may be totally inaccurate in terms of providing information regarding a drug allergy history. Direct questioning of patients, either by a self-administered questionnaire or by direct interview, may be a good source of certain information. However, data derived from this method may be subject to considerable error. Patients may either forget or intentionally withhold certain information, or may be confused by the question, particularly if the questionnaire is poorly designed, and thereby give erroneous answers. Direct interview of patients has its own hazards in addition to those just mentioned. The interviewer, either by variations in inflections in his voice or in his facial expressions, may give emphases that influence a patient's response. If an investigator chooses to use the interview technique, it may be worthwhile to have the interviewers undergo special training.

Once an investigator has decided what data will be collected and has some measure of the accuracy of those data, it may be important to go through a "dummy" analysis. By developing fictitious data, the investigator is able to evaluate a number of possible results that he can expect from the study. In doing this preliminary analysis, it will be easy for the investigator to evaluate whether his data base is adequate. By thinking through the results of the study, he may find certain pieces of information that were not collected that should have been, or certain pieces of information that were collected, may need to be collected in a different manner. In addition, the investigator may become aware that certain data being collected are totally superfluous to the results of the study and therefore need not be collected at all. The basic format for analyzing data in a descriptive study is shown in Table 1. The important information is found in the far right-hand column, which shows the percent of patients with a particular attribute. Those attributes that are most common to patients with a particular disease or event are those most likely to be associated with a particular disease or event.

Table 1
AN EXAMPLE OF DATA
ORGANIZATION: A DESCRIPTIVE
STUDY OF *SERRATIA
MARCESCENS* IN AN INTENSIVE
CARE UNIT

Attribute	Number of patients possessing attribute/ number of patients	Percent
Sex		
Male	10/20	50
Female	10/20	50
Age (in years)		
<40	1/20	5
41—50	2/20	10
51—60	7/20	35
>60	10/20	50
Surgical service	19/20	95
IPMD[a] exposure	18/20	90

[a]   Intravascular pressure-monitoring device.

Since firm statistical associations usually cannot be made from data from descriptive studies, the numbers of patients enrolled in these types of studies is less critical than in other types of study designs. The size of a particular descriptive study is often determined by factors beyond the investigator's control. The frequency of occurrence of the disease or event is one of the major determinants of the size of a study.

Considerable caution should be exercised in interpreting the data from a descriptive study. Too often, investigators will overinterpret the association between one or more attributes and the disease or event being studied. If a single attribute is associated with the disease or event, then one can develop a hypothesis regarding cause and effect that must be tested by further study. If, on the other hand, two or more attributes are associated with a particular disease or event, several possibilities for interpretation exist. There may be an association between the two attributes. For example, if the results of a particular study indicated that nosocomial bacteremia was associated with patients with severe underlying illness and was also associated with patients located in an intensive care unit, the independent (secondary) association between patients with severe underlying illness and their location in intensive care units may be so strong that a descriptive study may not be able to distinguish the relative importance of any one attribute. Another possibility for interpretation may be that there is no one attribute that has a cause-and-effect relationship and that two or more attributes must be present in order for the disease or event to occur. If both severe underlying disease and location in an intensive care unit have a strong association with nosocomial bacteremia, it may be that both attributes are necessary for the occurrence of the disease. On the other hand, each of the two attributes may contribute to the occurrence of the disease independently, but to a lesser degree than when both are present and working in tandem. In this situation, further study may be necessary to sort out the relative strengths of the various associations.

Retrospective or Case-Control Studies

Retrospective or case-control studies are used to determine the attributes or risk factors associated with a particular disease or event by contrasting the occurrence of those factors in a group of patients with the disease or event with those not having the disease or event. Case-control studies may be helpful in determining which of many attributes appears to be associated with a particular disease or event. Occasionally however, a single hypothesis is tested using this study design. In this situation, only a single attribute is examined for its association with a particular disease or event. If a particular descriptive study had shown that all patients in an intensive care unit who developed *Serratia marcescens* bacteremia had been exposed to an intravascular pressure-monitoring device, then the following hypothesis could be tested: Is the use of intravascular pressure-monitoring devices significantly associated with *Serratia marcescens* bacteremia in intensive care unit patients? To test this hypothesis, an investigator might perform a retrospective or case-control study in which all patients with *Serratia marcescens* bacteremia occurring in the intensive care unit were compared to a group of patients with similar characteristics in the intensive care unit who did not have bacteremia. The frequency with which intravascular pressure-monitoring devices were used in these two populations would then be compared. In order to perform this type of study, five basic steps must be considered: selection of cases, selection of controls, sources of information, analysis of information, and interpretation of information.

Selection of Cases

As in descriptive studies, the initial step in selecting cases is to establish a case definition. Diagnostic criteria should be clear and reproducible. In the event that it seems nearly impossible to clearly define the case, one can resolve the problem by providing several case definitions. Once the study is completed, one can examine the association of various attributes with the groups of cases that were defined differently. If strong associations are found only for cases defined a particular way, those cases may then define the "standard diagnostic criteria" that may be useful in future studies. If an investigator were studying the association between the use of a particular type of suture and the occurrence of postoperative wound infections, he might define cases of postoperative wound infection in the following manner: pus at the incision site, a positive wound culture, or a clinical diagnosis of infection made by the attending surgeon. If cases were grouped according to each definition and analyzed separately for their association with the particular type of suture, the investigator might have found the strongest association existed only for cases of postoperative wound infections that were defined as "pus at the incision site".

Once a case definition has been determined, an investigator should make every attempt to find all patients that fit that case definition. Depending on the particular study, one should consider all possible methods of detecting cases. If an investigator were studying cases of bacteremia, the searching of patients' medical records following discharge would not be a very efficient method of finding cases because laboratory reports of positive blood cultures might either be lost, enroute from the laboratory to the chart, or misfiled in the wrong chart. A better method might be to examine the records of the microbiology laboratory looking for positive blood culture results. Similarly, the best method of finding patients who might have postoperative wound infections would be the operating room log book that lists every patient undergoing surgery.

Lastly, the population from which the cases will be drawn should be defined. In most instances this population will be defined by the nature of the study. When studying the association between the use of intravascular pressure-monitoring devices and *Serratia marcescens* nosocomial bacteremia in patients in an intensive care unit, it is obvious that the population from which cases would be drawn would be the intensive care unit. In other situations the population may be not so obvious, so it may be advisable for an investigator, once cases have been selected, to characterize cases according to a number of attributes such as patient location, type of surgery, underlying disease, etc. to make sure that neither extraneous cases have been included nor previously undetected cases excluded.

Selection of Controls

A control group is a group of individuals that do not have the disease or event being studied and yet reflect the characteristics of the population from which the cases were drawn. Ideally, controls should not differ from cases (except that they do not have the infection) in any way that might affect the frequency of attributes that may be associated with the disease. In other words, cases and controls must be representative of the same population or, if the cases are selected in any way, the controls must have the same selection factors applied. For example, if the cases are patients with bacteremia in an intensive care unit, controls should be nonbacteremia patients in the intensive care unit. If, however, most cases are surgical patients (selection factor), then controls must have the same selection factors applied, e.g., nonbacteremic surgical patients in the intensive care unit. As noted in the preceding section ("Selection of Cases"), it may be useful to characterize cases prior to doing a case-control study, so that the attributes determined in this characterization process will help find an appropriate control group. A patient's service designation is frequently used as a selection factor for both cases and controls in studies of hospital populations. However, an investigator should be familiar with the various types of bias that may be introduced when service is used as a selection factor. Different hospitals, particularly large referral hospitals, may have totally different patient populations on different services. If a particular neurosurgeon has an unusually good reputation and many of his patients are referrals from a wide geographic area, patients on the neurosurgery service may be of higher socioeconomic status, different racial characteristcs, or of a different age composition to other services. Such bias must be carefully noted and taken into account when selecting controls.

Attributes such as age, sex, race, socioeconomic status, and coexisting diseases may influence the frequency with which a particular disease occurs in a population. Insofar as possible, these attributes should occur with similar frequency among cases and controls.

Once the population from which controls are to be selected has been determined, the investigator must decide whether to use the entire population as controls or to select only a sample from the population. The size and nature of the particular study will strongly influence the choice of which method is used. If the study is small, there may be no choice but to use the entire population. If, for example, one were studying bacteremia in an intensive care unit and during the study period there were only five patients with bacteremia and ten without bacteremia, it would probably be reasonable to use all ten nonbacteremic patients as controls. However, in order for an entire population to serve as controls, the same sources of information should be used for both cases and the entire control population. This is often a problem in hospital studies in which medical records are used as the source of information and may not be available for all cases and controls.

Instead of using the entire population as the control population, the investigator may select controls from the population using a variety of sampling techniques. Although sampling techniques are important — and a good study can be ruined by poor sampling techniques — one should be aware that if the population from which the controls are to be selected has been carefully chosen, any good sampling technique will probably serve adequately. Excellent sampling of a poorly chosen control population probably is as erroneous as poor sampling of an excellent control population.

Sampling techniques generally fall into three categories: random, systematic, and paired. Only a brief discussion of these types of sampling techniques will be presented, and if further details are sought, either a statistician's assistance or one of the many books on biostatistics or sampling methods may be of help to the reader.

A random sample is one in which each patient in the population has an equal chance of being selected. Usually each individual in the population is given a number. Then, using a table of random numbers (or other random number generating techniques), one selects certain numbers. Patients numbered accordingly are the ones that are selected. The number of controls selected depends on the number of cases and the size of the control population. Generally the number selected will equal the number of cases or will be two — or occasionally three — times the number of cases.

A systematic sample is one in which the control population is sequentially numbered; then every other, or every tenth, hundredth, etc., is chosen as the control. As long as the order in which the population is sequentially numbered is random and not biased by some attribute affecting the population (e.g., a particular surgeon who only operates on certain days so his patients might appear in the population with a repetitive periodicity), then each patient has an equal chance of being chosen. Since bias may be present that may be inapparent to the investigator, the systematic sampling technique should be used only in special circumstances, and then it may be best to have a statistician's expert advice.

A major advantage of the random or systematic sampling technique is that findings can be generalized to the entire population from which the sample was derived. However, a word of caution is offered about using the random or systematic technique: the investigator should be sure that each patient in the population has an equal chance of being chosen. If a patient is readmitted to a hospital, he may be listed in the population twice, thereby giving that patient a greater chance of being chosen. There are techniques for avoiding these biases, and a statistician's advice should be sought in these situations.

A paired sample is one in which controls are selected from the population because of some temporal or geographic relationship to the case. For example, a control selected for a bacteremic case in an intensive care unit might be the first nonbateremic patient occupying the bed next to the case. This technique is used when it is impractical to enumerate totally the population from which controls are selected, which is necessary when random or systematic sampling is used. The criteria for pairing must be rigidly adhered to; otherwise, bias may be introduced. Before setting criteria, all possible complications of the selecting process must be considered and managed in a uniform manner. An investigator must make provision for a situation, for example, where the patient with bacteremia was in a single room and a control had to be selected by some other uniform mechanism.

Paired sampling can be further refined using matched-paired cases and controls or by using a stratified sample. A stratified sample requires knowledge of attributes of the entire control population to be sampled, which negates one of the major advantages of the paired sample technique. For this reason it is rarely used. Matched-paired sampling is relatively difficult to do well and usually requires a statistician's assistance. The reader is referred to several available biostatistic textbooks for further information on matched-paired sampling.

Sources of Data

In most studies pertaining to infection control problems, the medical record is the primary source of information from which attributes of cases and controls are determined. Other sources of information should not be overlooked, and often the particular question for which an answer is being sought by the study might direct the investigator to other sources of information. If an investigator wished to study the occurrence of postoperative wound infections following a certain operative procedure, the operating log book might indicate not only the population from which cases are derived but also that from which the controls might be selected. Additional information relative to these cases and controls might be kept in other operating room records such as the surgeon's office records or the records of the head nurse in the operating room (e.g., operating room personnel assignments that indicate who may have been in particular operating rooms during certain procedures).

Once all possible sources of information relative to cases and controls are determined, it should be documented that the same completeness of data are available for both cases and controls. It is not necessary for all data to be available for all cases and all controls, but it is recommended that deficiencies in the data be minimized and equally distributed among cases and controls. If operating room personnel exposure data is available for nearly all cases but is missing for over half of the controls, it may be difficult to put a great deal of credibility in the results of an analysis of that particular attribute. Not only should an investigator be aware of possible differences in the completeness of the data base for cases and controls, but he should also be aware of possible differences in the accuracy of the data base for the two groups of study patients.

Analysis of Data

The format used to analyze data in retrospective case-control studies involves comparing the frequency of occurrence of attributes, suspected of having an association with the disease or event being studied, among the cases and among the controls (Table 2). The attributes may be discrete or grouped. Discrete attributes may be, for example, exposure to surgeon A, surgeon B, etc. An example of grouped attributes might be the duration of exposure to a particular intravenous fluid: 0 to 12 hr, 13 to 24 hr, etc.

Organizing data in this format allows the investigator to list the attributes suspected of being associated with the particular disease or event, determine the frequency of occurrence of each attribute among the cases and among the controls, and determine the difference in frequency of occurrence between the two groups. It is this difference in the frequency of occurrence of a particular attribute that lends strength to the association between the particular attribute and the disease or event. The previous chapter discusses the various statistical tests that can be applied to data generated by retrospective case-control studies. In general, these tests are used to calculate the probability that a difference in the occurrence of a particular attribute among cases and controls, as great or greater than the one observed, might be due to chance alone, if, in fact, there is no relationship between the attribute and the disease or event in question.

If a statistically significant difference has been found in the occurrence of a particular attribute among cases and controls, two additional analyses should be performed: the first analysis examines whether the difference noted can be explained by a secondary association between the attribute and some other attribute that is associated with the disease or event; the second analysis should determine the magnitude of the risk of the attribute associated with the disease or event.

A thorough knowledge of the disease or event under study will aid the investigator in determining if secondary associations are confounding the statistically significant association discovered in the study. An example of a secondary association might be

Table 2
AN EXAMPLE OF DATA ORGANIZATION: A RETROSPECTIVE CASE-CONTROL STUDY OF POSTOPERATIVE WOUND (POW) INFECTIONS ASSOCIATED WITH A PARTICULAR SURGEON

Attribute[a]	Number of patients infected (cases)	Number of patients not infected (controls)	Total
A	5	2	7
B	1	12	13
Total	6	14	20

[a] Attribute A, surgery performed by surgeon A; attribute B, surgery performed by surgeons B, C, D, etc.

Table 3
AN EXAMPLE OF A SECONDARY ASSOCIATION CONFOUNDING A CASE-CONTROL STUDY: A STUDY OF FOLEY CATHETER-RELATED URINARY TRACT INFECTIONS (UTI)

Duration of use of Foley catheter	Number of infections (UTI)	
	Cases	Controls
0—24 hr	1	0
25—48 hr	2	1
49—72 hr	3	2
73—96 hr	8	4
>96 hr	9	6

as follows: if one were studying nosocomial urinary tract infections and found a statistically significant association with a particular manufacturer's Foley catheter (cases) compared to another manufacturer's catheter (controls), but, on further analysis it was found that among cases the length of time that the catheter was in use was twice as long as among controls, one would have a secondary association (duration of catheterization and infection) that was confounding the study. Secondary associations need not totally ruin a study, but since they are difficult to deal with, they should be minimized by careful thought and planning prior to starting a study. Secondary associations can often be identified by studying the distribution of the unsuspected association factors separately within subgroups of both the cases and the controls. If the duration of catheterization is grouped as shown in Table 3, it is evident that the longer the catheterization, the more infections in both cases and controls, even though the number of infections in cases might be significantly more than in controls. This observation will warn the investigator of possible secondary associations. There are statistical manipulations that can be used to handle secondary associations; the most commonly employed is adjustment. This technique should only be attempted by an investigator who is completely familiar with its use, and even then it is wise to have the advice of a statistician.

The magnitude or strength of the association between an attribute and the particular disease is measured by calculating the estimated relative risk or odds ratio. Retrospec-

Table 4
AN EXAMPLE OF CALCULATING
AN ODDS RATIO: A STUDY OF
BACTEREMIA ASSOCIATED WITH
I.V. FLUID USE

Attribute[a]	Cases (bacteremic)	Controls (nonbacteremic)
X	8 (a)	2 (b)
Y	2 (c)	2 (d)

$$\text{Odds Ratio} = \frac{a \times d}{c \times b} = \frac{8 \times 2}{2 \times 2} = \frac{16}{4} = 4$$

[a] Attribute X, exposure to i.v. fluid manufactured by X; attribute Y, no exposure to i.v. fluid manufactured by X.

tive or case-control studies cannot directly measure the magnitude of the risk unless all cases and the entire control population are studied. Prospective studies, however, can directly measure the magnitude of the risk, and the term used in that situation is "relative risk". Odds ratios are good approximations of the magnitude of the risk. An example of the method of calculating an odds ratio is shown in Table 4. An odds ratio is an approximation of incidence of the disease or event among exposed patients divided by the incidence among nonexposed patients. The theory behind odds ratio calculations is beyond the scope of this book, and interested readers should consult a biostatistics textbook.

Interpretation of Data

In order to interpret the results of a retrospective or case-control study reliably, one should be certain the following questions concerning study design are satisfactorily answered: Were the cases representative of cases of the disease in general? Was the control group representative of the population from which the cases came? Were data pertinent to cases and controls accurate and complete? Was the analysis sufficiently rigorous to detect statistical differences and to suggest probable associations?

In addition to the above factors concerning good study design, there are other factors that should be considered in interpreting the results of retrospective or case-control studies. Are the findings, in general, in accordance with other studies on the subject? If no other studies exist that are similar, are the results of the study logical, based on the known biology of the disease?

Finally, the ultimate purpose of doing a retrospective or case-control study is to try to find or confirm an association between an attribute and a disease. The question of whether this association constitutes "proof" of a cause-and-effect relationship is difficult to answer: a statistically significant association found in a retrospective case control study may be sufficient proof for some individuals, whereas others may insist that proof can only be established by doing a prospective experimental study. Very few infection-control questions have been approached using an experimental study design, and often the only data available about a certain disease are those from case-control studies. In situations where only a case-control study is feasible, the responsibility rests with the investigator to design the very best study that is feasible so as to establish the strongest "proof" possible.

Prospective Observational Studies

In prospective observational studies, the investigator selects a group of individuals in whom the disease or event being studied has not occurred. He then groups the individuals according to certain attributes and observes them for a period of time to determine how many of those with a particular attribute develop the infection being studied. Usually a hypothesis exists concerning the association between the particular attribute and the disease. For example, an association between nosocomial bacteremia and the use of an intravascular pressure-monitoring device may have been noticed from a descriptive or a case-control study of patients with bacteremia. In the descriptive or case-control study, the cases were defined by virtue of their developing bacteremia first; then their exposure to various risk factors was examined. In contrast, in a prospective observational study, the two groups of patients — one that is exposed to intravascular pressure-monitoring devices and one not exposed to such devices — are first defined, then observed for a period of time for the development of bacteremia.

Selection of Study Groups

The selection of study groups in prospective observational studies shares many of the problems discussed earlier for descriptive and for retrospective or case-control studies. In addition to these problems, an investigator selecting groups of patients for a prospective observational study has difficulties peculiar to this type of study design. First, the investigator must determine the scope of the population to be studied: a broad general population or a narrow specific population. If an investigator was studying the relationship between nosocomial bacteremia and the use of intravascular pressure-monitoring devices, he must decide whether to study the occurrence of bacteremia following the use of such devices in the entire hospital population or only in patients in intensive care units. The particular hypothesis being tested may help decide which population is the most appropriate to study, but, as often happens, the option of studying either a general population or a narrow but, highly exposed population will present itself.

A major problem encountered in studying a general population is that the population often must be subdivided according to degree of exposure. If, for example, intravascular pressure-monitoring devices are used for patients undergoing cardiac catheterization, for patients in an intensive care unit, and for patients undergoing major surgery, it is obvious that each type of use involves different types of patients, and the devices are used for somewhat different lengths of time in each general category of use. Another difficulty in performing such studies in broad-based populations is that large numbers of patients may need to be followed, which will require more resources in terms of time, personnel, and money, although the frequency of the occurrence of the disease or event will determine these numbers.

A major advantage, however, of broad-based population studies is that the results have wide applicability. If an investigator had chosen the entire hospital population to study the relationship between nosocomial bacteremia and the use of intravascular pressure-monitoring devices, he could generalize his results to the entire hospital rather than limiting them to one subgroup, such as intensive care unit patients.

If an investigator chooses to study the broad-based population, two pertinent pieces of information must be obtained from study patients. First, data must be collected that will allow the investigator to classify patients into subgroups based on exposure to the attribute or factor under study. Second, data must be collected in such a way that the investigator can determine whether patients, both those with and those without the attribute, are similar with respect to age, sex, race, etc., or any variable that might be secondarily associated with the disease under study. This second point is very important because any exclusion of patients for lack of being able to obtain data from them may seriously bias the study. If an investigator is unable to obtain certain data on a large segment of the study population, the question arises as to whether the "missing" patients are different from those that are "found". For example, if the entire hospital population was being studied to determine the relationship between nosocomial bacteremia and the use of intravascular pressure-monitoring devices and the investigator was unable to obtain data from a large number of patients from the cardiac catheterization subgroup due to the fact that these patients were discharged from the hospital the day following their procedure, a significant bias may be introduced into the study. This bias may be that relatively "mild" bacteremia would be missed and that a disproportionately large number of bacteremia cases in the study would be more clinically "severe" because the other two subgroups (intensive care unit and major surgery patients) contributed more to the numbers of affected cases than they should have.

There are both advantages and disadvantages to selecting a narrow-based or highly exposed population for study. Major advantages to studying this type of population might be that very little subgrouping may be needed, and, depending upon the particular disease being studied, the numbers of patients required for study may be fewer than if a general population were used. A notable disadvantage, however, is that the narrower the scope of the population studied the less widely applicable the results. A study of bacteremia associated with intravascular pressure-monitoring devices used in patients undergoing open heart surgery may be limited in its applicability since factors common to patients with open heart procedures (e.g., suture material or other foreign bodies in or on the endocardium) may alter their susceptibility to "low level" bacteremia.

In broad-based population studies, the entire nonexposed group of patients serves as the comparison group to the exposed patients whereas in some narrow-based population studies, there may be a need to select a comparison group. This need arises when all or nearly all patients either possess or are exposed to the attribute being studied. If, for example, an investigator is studying the relationship between nosocomial bacteremia and the use of intravascular pressure-monitoring devices and if the only patients in whom such devices are used are those undergoing cardiac catheterization (and the device is used in every such patient), a special comparison group must be selected. Two types of comparison groups may be used: a general population or a selected population. When a general population is used for comparison, the observed rate of occurrence of a particular disease in that group is compared with the rate of occurrence in the study group. This type of comparison is used only when the rates of occurrence are quite different. If the usual rate of occurrence of nosocomial bacteremia in a particular hospital was 5 per 1000 admissions and the rate of bacteremia following the use of intravascular pressure-monitoring devices was 200 per 1000 admissions, assuming the characteristics of the two populations were reasonably comparable, one might be able to demonstrate a significant association between the attribute and the disease. The use of a selective comparison group has many of the same difficulties in selection that one finds when selecting controls in a retrospective or case-control study, in that the comparison group should not differ from cases in any way that might affect the frequency of attributes that may have a cause-and-effect relationship to the disease. Similar methods of sampling and controlling bias in the comparison group would be used in this situation as in a retrospective or case-control study.

Determination of Outcome

Regardless of the method of selection of the population, determining the outcome (follow-up) of patients is necessary in a prospective observational study. Defining a case of a particular disease has been mentioned earlier in relation to descriptive and case-control study designs, and many of the problems outlined in those sections are applicable to defining a case in a prospective observational study. There is, however, an additional problem in this respect that is unique to prospective studies. Since patients, when they enter the study, are free of the disease being studied and become defined only as a case at some point during the follow-up or observation period, the frequency of assessment of the study population to determine which patients have become cases is an important aspect in defining a case in prospective studies. Obviously, one would want to assess the population neither so infrequently that cases would be missed nor so frequently that erroneous cases would be included.

The particular disease being studied usually will determine the frequency of assessment of the study population.

Prior to initiating a prospective study, the investigator must decide what constitutes the observation or follow-up period. A certain percent of nosocomial infections do not become apparent until the patient has been discharged from the hospital, and the particular site infected often determines the frequency with which these types of infections occur: urinary tract infections may occur frequently following discharge from the hospital whereas bloodstream infections may not. In most prospective studies of nosocomial infections, the follow-up period consists of the remaining portion of the hospitalization following exposure to or identification of the particular attribute under study. This limitation of the follow-up period may bias the results to a varying degree, depending on the particular disease being studied.

An investigator must be aware of observer bias in determining outcomes in the study population. Ideally, the person who assigns study patients to the various subgroups according to attributes or exposures should not be the person who assesses the patients to determine their outcome. This type of study is often called a "blind" or "single blind" study ("double blind" study in which the patient as well as the observer does not know the attribute or exposure will be discussed in a succeeding section). "Blind" techniques usually increase the cost and numbers of personnel needed for a study but are usually worth it. Another technique that can be used to manage observer bias is to attempt to measure the amount of bias and try to correct for it during the analysis of the study or try to prove the bias was insignificant in terms of the outcome of the study. In addition, an investigator can attempt to handle bias by defining what constitutes a case in as objective a manner as possible in such a way that there is no judgment required on the part of the observer.

Analysis of Data

The format used to analyze data in a prospective observational study involves deriving a rate of occurrence of a specified outcome among various subgroups in the study population (Table 5). As in retrospective or case-control studies, the attributes may either be discrete or grouped.

Organizing data in this manner allows the investigator to visualize which of possibly many attributes being studied is associated with the highest (or lowest) rate of occurrence of disease in the study population. Those attributes demonstrating the highest rates are the most strongly associated with the occurrence of the disease or event under study. The numerator of the rate is the number of outcomes or events, and the denominator is a quantitative measure of the population at risk. In most studies concerning nosocomial infection control problems, the numerator is the number of infections and the denominator is the number of patients at risk. Instead of using the number of patients at risk as the denominator, another convenient method of quantitating risk is to use patient-days or some other similar measure of person-time such as patient-weeks, etc. This technique is useful, particularly when the time of observation is not

Table 5
A SAMPLE OF DATA ORGANIZATION: A PROSPECTIVE
OBSERVATIONAL STUDY OF BACTEREMIA FOLLOWING
INTRAVASCULAR PRESSURE-MONITORING DEVICE USE

Attribute[a]	Patients Developing Bacteremia	Patients not developing bacteremia	Total patients	Infection rate[b] (%)
A	8	32	40	20
B	2	38	40	5

[a] Attribute A, exposure to device; attribute B, no exposure to device.
[b] Number of outcomes (bacteremia) per number of patients at risk.

uniform for all patients. Person-time is calculated as follows: if 5 persons are exposed to some risk factor for 4 days, then 20 person-days (5 × 4) of exposure occurred, which is the same as 4 persons exposed for 5 days; if 2 persons are exposed for 10 days then 20 person-days (2 × 10) of exposure also occurred; etc. The assumption is that the degree of risk was uniform over the time period considered. If risk changes over the time period, there are ways of adjusting for this, and the reader is referred to one of the epidemiology textbooks listed at the end of this chapter for a complete discussion of this technique. Person-time at risk is a very useful tool. However, in order to apply statistical tests to such data, very sophisticated analytic techniques are needed. Without these techniques, the strength of association derived from the data must be based on inspection, logic, and goodness of fit with known biological phenomena.

The strength of the association between a particular attribute and the occurrence of a disease or event can be measured in two ways: relative risk and attributable risk. Relative risk can be measured directly in prospective studies and is expressed as the ratio of the rates of occurrence of the disease or event in two subgroup populations. Table 6 shows an example of the calculation of a relative risk. The rates for more than two attributes can be compared using relative risk by comparing each to an overall rate or by comparing each to the rate for one particular attribute of interest. For example, if the rate of infection among patients with the attribute "manufacturer X Foley catheter" was 3% and this manufacturer's brand of catheter is the "standard" brand, the rates of infection among those using brands A, B, C, etc., could each be compared to the "standard" to determine the magnitude of the risk associated with the other brands relative to brand X.

Attributable risk is the absolute incidence (rate of occurrence) of the disease among patients with a particular exposure or other attribute that can be attributed to that exposure. Attributable risk is calculated by subtracting the rate of occurrence of the disease or event found in one subgroup from that of another subgroup (Table 7). When more than two attributes are being studied, attributable risk can be derived for each attribute in a similar fashion to that described above for relative risk.

Interpretation of Data

As can be seen from Tables 6 and 7, where the same data were subjected to both relative risk and attributable risk analysis, two totally different results were noted. The two types of analyses permit us to examine data from two different viewpoints, and depending upon the type of information we are seeking from the data, one or both analyses may be used. Relative risk, in general, tends to give information concerning the extent to which a particular attribute or attributes are related in a cause-and-effect manner to the disease or event in question. In general, attributable risk gives informa-

Table 6

AN EXAMPLE OF CALCULATING RELATIVE RISK: A STUDY OF
BACTEREMIA FOLLOWING EXPOSURE TO INTRAVASCULAR
PRESSURE-MONITORING DEVICES

Attribute[a]	Patients developing bacteremia	Patients not developing bacteremia	Total patients	Infection rate[b] (%)	Relative risk[c]
A	8	32	40	20	
B	2	38	40	5	4

[a] Attribute A, exposure to device; attribute B, no exposure to device.
[b] Number of infected patients per number of patients at risk.
[c] A ratio of rates: 20/5 = 4.

Table 7

AN EXAMPLE OF CALCULATING ATTRIBUTABLE RISK: A STUDY OF
BACTEREMIA FOLLOWING EXPOSURE TO INTRAVASCULAR PRESSURE-
MONITORING DEVICES

Attribute[a]	Patients developing bacteremia	Patients not developing bacteremia	Total patients	Infection rate (%)	Attributable risk
A	8	32	40	20[b]	
B	2	38	40	5	15

[a] Attribute A, exposure to device; attribute B, no exposure to device.
[b] Number of infected patients per number of patients at risk.
[c] A difference of rates: 20 − 5 = 15.

Table 8

AN EXAMPLE OF THE COMPARISON OF RELATIVE
RISK AND ATTRIBUTABLE RISK: A STUDY OF
BACTEREMIA FOLLOWING I.V. FLUID USE

Exposure[a]	Infection rate: nonexposed	Infection rate: exposed	Relative risk	Attributable risk
A	0.8	2.0	2.50	1.2
B	0.6	0.8	1.33	0.2
C	0.4	0.5	1.25	0.1
D	0.2	0.8	4.00	0.6

[a] Exposure of patients to different manufacturers' I.V. fluids, brand A, brand B, etc.

tion concerning the proportion of risk of the disease or event that is contributed by a particular attribute. Table 8 demonstrates how these two analyses permit different interpretations of data. If one is attempting to determine which of four intravenous fluids from four different companies is most strongly associated with bacteremia, one would examine relative risk and find, in this example, company D's I.V. fluid most strongly associated with a risk of bacteremia. If, on the other hand, one wanted to know, for brand D, how much risk of bacteremia is attributable to the use of brand D, one would note that only 0.6 (infections per 100 patients exposed) was attributable to that brand. In contrast, for brand A, 1.2 (infections per 100 patients exposed) were attributable to the use of that I.V. fluid. In terms of the "public health problem" created by the use of brand A compared to brands B, C, etc., brand A is a major contributor whereas in terms of the "cause and effect" between the use of I.V. fluids in this hypothetical study, brand D is the one with a significant association.

There is an additional technique an investigator may use to determine the proportion of the risk attributable to the particular exposure. To do this, the attributable risk is divided by the rate of occurrence of the event among the exposed patients.

It is important for an investigator to learn how to use relative risk and attributable risk to interpret data from prospective studies. A more thorough discussion of these techniques may be found in several good epidemiology textbooks, and it is recommended that unless an investigator is thoroughly familiar with these techniques a statistician's assistance should be sought.

Prospective Experimental Studies

Prospective experimental studies are very similar in design to prospective observational studies except that rather than classifying patients according to the attribute already possessed by the patient, the investigator selects patients free of the disease or event being studied and allocates them to groups; each group then is assigned a different attribute. The patients are then observed for a period of time to see what influence the assigned attribute has on the occurrence of a particular disease or event under study. This study design is also referred to as a "clinical trial", an "intervention study", or a "treatment trial". Many of the principles of study design discussed in the preceding section concerning prospective observational studies apply to prospective experimental studies. However, these latter types of studies are sufficiently different in design that considerable additional skill is necessary for an investigator to adequately perform such a study. This discussion will be limited to some of those additional characteristics found in experimental studies, and no attempt will be made to include all characteristics which separate these two types of studies. In addition, some principles discussed in this section might be applicable to prospective observational studies or to retrospective or case-control studies. Experimental studies are sufficiently complex, costly, and demanding of an investigator's time that a team approach is often used. That team might include investigators from cooperating institutions since the number of observations needed for a valid study might not be possible in any one institution or hospital.

Size of the Study Population

Early in the planning stage of a prospective experimental study the decision must be made as to the number of patients that will be needed to be studied. Obviously the investigator wants a sufficient number of patients entered into each study group so that if the outcomes are different in different study groups, he can be confident that the difference is due to the assigned attribute and not due to chance alone. Conversely, if there is no difference, he wants to be confident that, indeed, no real difference exists. In order to determine how many patients must be entered into a study, the investigator must first estimate the number of expected outcomes. Statistical testing for significant differences is based on outcomes, not numbers of patients entered into the study. If the numbers of outcomes needed in two study groups of patients were 40 and 60, for example, to show statistical significance, then it would not matter statistically if these 100 total outcomes came from 200 or 2000 patients who had been entered into the study.

Since statistical testing for significant differences is based on the number of outcomes, the next logical step in planning the size of the study population is to determine how large a difference between outcomes in different study groups must be observed to distinguish whether one assigned attribute is better, worse, or the same as the other attribute or attributes. An investigator needs to estimate how much of a difference in outcome might be expected between the study groups because it is on this estimate that the entire size of the study is based. Suppose, for example, an investigator was trying to determine whether antibiotic ointment applied to the site of an indwelling vascular catheter prevented subsequent bacteremia or not and he estimated that using the ointment would prevent 25% of bacteremias. In order to have an even chance of detecting a difference or not missing a difference of this magnitude, he would have to enter enough patients such that 200 bacteremias would occur: 75 or fewer in the ointment group, 125 or more in the nonointment group.[1] If, on the other hand, he estimated that the ointment would reduce the bacteremia rate by two thirds, then only 20 bacteremias (7 or fewer in the ointment group and more than 13 in the nonointment group) need occur. In general, the greater the difference in outcomes associated with particular attributes, the fewer the number of outcomes that must occur to allow an investigator to be confident that at least an even chance of showing statistical significance exists.

It is understandable that it might be difficult to carry out such a study as given in the previous example. First, it may be unlikely that a bacterial ointment will prevent one fourth, let alone two thirds, of bacteremias; second, even if it did prevent one fourth, in order to study 200 bacteremias one would have to enter 20,000 patients with intravascular catheters into the study, assuming a bacteremia rate of 1% — certainly a formidable task even for a multihospital study.

Method of Assigning Attributes

Once the numbers of patients in this study have been determined, some technique must be devised to allocate the patients into groups to which the attributes being studied will be assigned. The most common method of assigning attributes is to use the random allocation technique. Randomization is based on the principle that each patient entering the study has an equal chance (if so desired by the investigator) of being assigned to a particular study group. Unequal randomization to achieve study groups of different sizes is used in special circumstances, the details of which are beyond the scope of this book. The desired end result of the randomization technique is that each study group will be composed of patients with similar characteristics (age, sex, disease status, etc.). Although the randomization process maximizes the chances that the groups will be as similar as possible, it is the investigator's responsibility to demonstrate that the randomization process worked. Therefore, he must actually determine the characteristics of the groups under study and prove that they are indeed similar. There are many techniques available for performing the randomization process, the easiest being the use of a table of random numbers. If two subgroups of patients are desired, then, as patients are entered into the study, they are assigned to group 1 if the next number in the column of numbers in the random number table is an odd digit, and they are assigned to group 2 if it is an even digit. This technique is occasionally subject to error on the part of the investigator or the person making the assignment of patients into the study groups and more sophisticated techniques are available.

There is some debate as to whether stratification of patients according to characteristics (e.g., age, sex, underlying disease, etc.) should occur at the time of randomization or at the end of the study when the data are analyzed. Arguments for stratification at randomization are that the data are recorded without any bias based on outcome, that data are not subject to error due to poor memory or other retrospective data-retrieval mechanisms, and that adverse effects from the assigned attribute that may be present in only one subgroup of patients will be more easily recognized and the study terminated. Arguments for stratification at analysis are that with good statistical techniques, stratification can be handled retrospectively, provided adequate data for characterizing patients were obtained at entry into the study, and that entry stratification unnecessarily complicates administrative aspects of the study.

Closely related, at least in terms of planning a study, to allocating patients to study groups is what to do with patients who are ineligible for study because either they are originally excluded from the study for a variety of reasons, or once into the study, voluntarily or involuntarily withdraw or somehow are lost during the follow-up portion of the study. If an investigator was comparing the incidence of urinary tract infection associated with two different types of Foley bladder catheters (brand X and brand Y), an example of exclusion would be a patient who appeared to need a Foley catheter but, before getting the patient registered into the study and randomized to receive a particular catheter, the patient's physician decided a Foley catheter was unnecessary. This situation presents no problem for the study because no bias is introduced into the study population. On the other hand, suppose the patient was entered into the study but instead of receiving one of the study catheters, the patient received brand Z by mistake. This situation in which the patient would be required to withdraw from the study may seriously bias the study. There are several techniques that can be used to handle the problem of patient withdrawal from the study: tightly control the study so mistakes are not made; make sure the correct attribute has been assigned before entering the patient into the study; or treat all such withdrawals as if they were exclusions who had never entered the study. An example of a patient lost to follow-up during a study might be: after 5 days into the study, a patient in the brand X catheter group had his catheter inadvertently replaced with a nonstudy catheter, brand Z. This situation may bias the study, particularly if it happens more frequently in one subgroup compared to another. If it happens rarely and with equal frequency in all subgroups, it probably causes little problem. In any case, it is acceptable to use the data, collected for such lost patients, that were obtained prior to their loss from the study. These patients are treated as if they ended their study period at the time that they were lost.

Analysis and Interpretation of the Data

Data from a prospective experimental study are analyzed and interpreted in a manner similar to that described earlier for prospective observational studies. However, there are some additional techniques of analysis that are particularly useful for experimental studies.

When the duration of exposure to a risk factor or attribute is important and, rather than use person-time as the denominator in calculating rates of occurrence of the particular outcome (which may require very sophisticated statistical analyses), a relatively simple technique can be used for analysis. This technique compares the risk of a particular outcome caused by a certain duration of exposure to one attribute with the risk caused by a certain duration of exposure to another attribute. This technique is called the "log rank test" or "Mantel-Haenszel Test". The principle of the log rank test is that on a particular day following exposure to two attributes — for example, A and B — the numbers of outcomes occurring on that day should be proportional to the number of patients in group A and group B, assuming that when an outcome occurs, the patient to whom it occurs is "removed" from the study group. For example, if 200 patients had been randomized to groups A (100 patients) and B (100 patients), and by day 5, 25 outcomes had occurred in group A and 50 outcomes had occurred in group B, 75 patients would be remaining in group A and 50 patients in group B. On day 6, the number of outcomes that one would predict should occur, assuming attributes A and B have equal influence (risk) in causing the outcome, would be proportional to the number of patients at risk in each group (A/B = 75/50 = 3/2: three outcomes in group A for every two outcomes in group B). In other words, if the risk due to attribute A is equal to the risk due to attribute B in terms of causing the particular outcome, we should expect 3/2 more outcomes in this group since there are 3/2 times the number of patients in group A. If, however, attributes A and B are not equal in terms of risk and on day 6, instead of three outcomes in group A for every two in group B, six outcomes in group A were observed for every two in group B, it would be obvious that the observed ratio had deviated considerably from the ratio. From these observations it is apparent that if one compares the expected ratio of outcomes on any particular day following exposure to an observed ratio, one can apply standard statistical tests to determine if a difference exists. The details of the calculations necessary to perform a log rank test are beyond the scope of this book, but a simplified explanation with sample calculations are available to the nonstatistician.[2]

EXECUTION OF THE STUDY

Once the study has been conceived and designed, the next step is the execution of the study. Early in this phase of the study it may be advisable to set up a reasonable timetable indicating when various study activities are to be initiated and completed. The time necessary to perform a study will vary depending upon the study design and the particular question being studied. A timetable should be based on an honest estimate of the actual time needed to complete all phases of the study because it is on this timetable that resources, including money, equipment, and people, will be allocated. Many investigators have had the unhappy experience of coming to the end of a 2-year study with only half the number of patients studied and no more money available. Although it may be impossible to avoid all mistakes in estimating time needed to perform the study, there are several measures that can be taken to reduce the risk of mistakes. A "study within a study" (pilot study) may be useful in avoiding such errors. First, for example, during a prospective observational study of bacteremia in which 200 patient outcomes are needed, it may be advisable to perform a quick descriptive study of the same population to determine how long it might take for 200 bacteremias to occur. Often the extra time and effort needed to do this additional study will pay off in avoiding costly errors. Another use of a timetable in avoiding mistakes is that a timetable permits the investigator to visualize the many different activities needed to perform the study. By visualizing these activities, more efficient use of time can be realized. Generally speaking, the more people that are involved in the study such as technicians, clerks, etc., the more important a timetable becomes for making efficient use of time.

During a study's design phase, an investigator should give some thought to the data collection form that will be used to record the patient-based data in the study. In many institutions, data collection forms, particularly those on which patient-based data are recorded, are quasi-legal documents and often the forms must be approved by a human studies committee or some other similar organization. As was noted in an earlier section on ethical considerations, a consent form may be needed depending on the type of study and type of patient-based data collected. The two forms, consent and data collection, should be considered a functional unit in terms of medical/legal issues. It is always wise to check with a human studies committee before a final draft of the data form and consent form are completed to make sure they are acceptable. Designing the data collection form will help an investigator to focus on what information should or should not be collected. Extraneous data that either will not be analyzed, cannot be related to an attribute under study, or is not a possible confounding variable, does not need to clutter up a data form. The decision of what to include is often a difficult one, and many investigators err on the side of collecting too much information. Too much extraneous information may increase cost and time needed to perform the study or may increase the risk of inaccuracies in the data, due to confusion or fatigue among the data collectors. One often hears the argument that "while the study population is available, as much information as possible should be collected from them, because important information might be missed." The most logical answer to that argument is that if the information that was not collected was so important, it should have been brought to mind before starting the study; if it was not discovered to be important until the study was finished — and it really is important — it may be worth repeating the study, taking the new information into account.

If automatic data processing is used to store and analyze data, it is wise to get professional assistance in designing the data collection form so it can be compatible with the particular type of data processing equipment which will be used. In addition, it is wise to pretest the data collection form, simulating as close as possible the manner in which it will be used. If, for example, medical records are to be the information source, the data collection form should be arranged in such a manner that data can be abstracted from the chart without having to search first the front part of the chart, then the back, then the front, etc.

Except for prospective experimental studies in which some mechanisms should be devised for analyzing data and stopping the study if intolerably adverse effects are affecting one study group, the investigator should avoid the temptation to analyze data before the study is finished. Analyzing data on the first few patients may consciously or unconsciously influence an investigator and introduce bias that may affect the manner in which the remainder of the data collection and analysis of the study are performed. It seems illogical to take the trouble to determine the number of events or outcomes in a study population that will maximize the chance of finding a statistically significant difference and then to ignore those efforts and the rationale behind those efforts, running the risk of drawing conclusions on a totally inadequate sample. If, on the other hand, an investigator wishes to begin analyzing data in order to work out the "bugs" in the analysis process (e.g., the computer program if automatic data processing is used for data analysis), either "dummy" data or data from a pilot study should be used instead of data from the first few patients in the present study.

Both before and during the execution of a study, an investigator should attempt to think of all possible problems that may arise during the study and develop a plan as to how to handle each problem before it happens. For example, if one is performing a retrospective or case-control study using medical records as the information source and one or more of the medical records is lost or otherwise not available, the investigator should plan ahead for that possibility so that inappropriate decisions are not made when the problem arises. Alternative sources of information, the assignment of personnel associated with the study to the medical records department in order to increase the intensity of the search for a particular lost record, or direct interview of the patient may be more rational alternatives rather than dropping the patient from the study. The number of potential problems that can arise during a study may seem to be infinite, but an investigator should be able to identify most by simply examining the function of every person, place, or object involved in the study and determining what possibly could go wrong with the study if that particular person, place, or object should fail to operate properly. Illness and death among personnel involved in the study, accidents, and automatic data processing equipment failure are some examples of various problems that could arise during the study. Probably 99% of the problems one can think of will not happen during the study, but one can increase the odds against failure of the study for technical reasons by some forethought and planning.

PUBLICATION OF RESULTS

Once the study has been completed and the results determined often the final problem the investigator must deal with is whether to publish the study or not. There is no easy answer to this question, but if the study has been well done in that the question the study addressed was an important one, the literature pertinent to this subject thoroughly researched, proper study design and analysis used, and the study executed well, then it is reasonable to assume that the study should at least be considered for publication.

If the investigator is convinced that the study should be considered for publication, there are several steps that are usually followed in order to accomplish that goal.

First, the investigator may want to share the results with a trusted colleague who may give helpful suggestions regarding the manner in which the study might be prepared for publication. In addition, this colleague's advice whether to publish or not may be sought. It is often helpful at this stage to have an "outside" opinion — the opinion of a person famiiar with the subject under study but one who has not been intimately involved with the study.

Second, the format of publication should be determined. Most studies are submitted to journals, but other avenues might be considered such as oral presentation at a scientific meeting, compendiums of recent studies concerning a particular subject, review articles and newsletters or magazines published by special interest groups, or the lay press. Since most studies are submitted to journals, the remainder of this discussion of publishing the results of the study will be directed at that format although the principles discussed may apply to other formats.

Third, the particular journal to which the manuscript will be submitted should be selected. Here again, consultation with trusted colleagues familiar with the subject under study may be helpful, particularly those with previous publishing experience. One factor to be considered in selecting a journal is the general readership of a journal. Some, like the *New England Journal of Medicine,* have broad readership among physicians and other health care workers, while others, like the *Journal of Pediatrics,* are read primarily by persons with a particular interest. If the study being considered for publication has wide applicability, it is advisable to submit the manuscript to a journal with a broad readership, whereas if the study applies, for example, only to infants, a pediatric journal may be more appropriate.

Fourth, once a journal has been selected, the manuscript should be arranged so as to conform to that particular journal style. Most journals have an "instruction for authors" publication that details the publication style to be used, and these instructions usually can be obtained either from the journals' editorial office or the publisher. Several sources may be available to investigators in terms of assistance in preparing the final manuscript. Textbooks and local college courses on writing style, as well as colleagues experienced in publishing, may be helpful in this area.

Finally, the finished manuscript is submitted to the journal and generally the editor will provide all necessary instructions — or at least be available for inquiries if needed. It is important to point out that it is considered unethical to submit the same or similar manuscript to another journal until the first journal has rejected the manuscript. If the journal is a "refereed" journal (submitted articles are reviewed by independent experts), the manuscript will be sent to reviewers. The reviewers will recommend to the editor of the journal either to accept the manuscript for publication, accept it if certain indicated revisions are done, or reject it. If the manuscript is accepted, which rarely happens, it usually will appear as an article in the journal in a few months, depending upon the editor's discretion. If revisions are necessary, the manuscript is returned to the investigator, who may either revise and resubmit it, or withdraw it from consideration, and, if desired, submit it to a different journal upon notification in writing to the original journal (this latter option may not be a particularly advisable practice). Upon completing revisions, the manuscript is returned to the editor for final acceptance, and, if accepted — as usually happens if the revisions are acceptable — publication usually will occur within several months. If the journal is not a "refereed" journal, the editor or editorial board will serve the function outlined above for "refereed" journals, and the procedure may be modified somewhat.

The goal of publishing the results of a study is to share the investigator's experience with the medical-scientific community. The medical-scientific community is interested not only in important questions but answers to those questions. Those answers should come from well-conceived, well-designed, and well-executed studies which are well presented in an accessible, acceptable forum. As long as these basic concepts are kept in mind, there is no reason that any member of the medical-scientific community cannot participate in the exchange of common experience.

SUGGESTED READING

Brown, B. W. and Hollander, M., *Statistics, A Biomedical Introduction,* John Wiley & Sons, New York, 1977.

Schor, S., *Fundamentals of Biostatistics,* G. P. Putnam's Sons, New York, 1968.

Colton, T., *Statistics in Medicine,* Little, Brown, Boston, 1974.

Lilienfeld, A. M., *Foundations of Epidemiology,* Oxfrd University Press, New York, 1976.

Fox, J. P., Hall, C. E., and Elueback, L. R., *Epidemiology, Man and Disease,* Macmillan, New York, 1970.

Hillman, H. and Abrabonel, K., *The Art of Winning Foundation Grants,* Vanguard Press, New York, 1975.

White, V. P., *Grants — How To Find Out About Them and What To Do Next,* Plenum Press, New York, 1975.

McGowan, J. E., Research proposals — guidelines to dueling for dollars, *Assoc. Pract. Infect. Control J.,* 4, 6, 1976.

REFERENCES

1. Petro, R., Pike, M. C., Armitage, P., Breslow, N. E., Cox, D. R., Howard, S. V., Mantel, N., McPherson, K., Petro, J., and Smith, P. G., Design and analysis of randomized clinical trials requiring prolonged observation of each patient. I. Introduction and design, *Br. J. Cancer,* 34, 610, 1976.

2. Petro, R., Pike, M. C., Armitage, P., Breslow, N. E., Cox, D. R., Howard, S. V., Mantel, N., McPherson, K., Petro, J., and Smith, P. G., Design and analysis of randomized clinical trials requiring prolonged observation of each patient. II. Analysis, *Br. J. Cancer,* 35, 7, 1977.

Resources for the Infection Control Practitioner

THE LOCAL HEALTH DEPARTMENT

Joel L. Nitzkin

Local health departments in the U.S. vary widely in size, range of services, quality of service, and expertise. The variation is so great that each community hospital is best advised to get to know its local health department. A few telephone calls and an occasional invitation for health department staff to meet with the infection control committee can provide remarkable insight into the range and quality of services the Department has to offer and whether the Department is likely to be of help or hindrance in dealing with epidemics of nosocomial infection and medicolegal problems.

Almost all local health departments provide communicable disease control services and environmental surveillance. Very few are directly involved in health facility licensure, inspection, or reimbursement. Only 2% of all local health departments are involved in any way in health personnel registration.[1] Local health departments may or may not provide laboratory services.

It is critical to understand that the term "health department" when used in the hospital environment almost always refers to the State Health Department and usually refers to the regulatory or funding role of the State Health Department or sophisticated laboratory services usually available at the state level. Community hospital contact with local health departments is usually limited to management of reportable communicable diseases, provision of limited ambulatory care services, birth certificates, death certificates, and inspection of hospital kitchens.

The quality of a local health department's communicable disease control program can often be judged on the basis of whether it is law-enforcement or service in tone. A department demanding reports solely on the basis of a legal requirement and providing no meaningful feedback is apt to have minimal service capacity and little or no ability to provide technical assistance in the management of nosocomial or community-based outbreaks. With this type of local department, one should learn whom to contact at the state health department for advice. A department requesting communicable disease reports to help prevent the spread of communicable diseases, quoting the law as a reference that enables such reporting not to be a breach of medical confidence, and provides periodic tabulations of locally reportable diseases, is likely to be an excellent source of help in working up nosocomial outbreaks and providing advice and consultation of substantial value in preventing medicolegal complications which might otherwise result from outbreaks of nosocomial infection. Local health department involvement in the investigation and control of an outbreak is an excellent means of demonstrating that the hospital has done everything possible to halt the spread of infection. With a skilled health department staff, this can often be done without publicity or fanfare, and with extra protection to the public image of the hospital if news of the outbreak leaks to the media.

The local health department is often the best source or consultation regarding the diagnosis, treatment, and management of tuberculosis, dark-field microscopy for diagnosis of syphilis, and community investigation and follow-up of case reports of almost any communicable disease.

The specific infectious disease problems with which a health department frequently deals and has experience is illustrated in the form of the Communicable Disease Report for the year ending December 26, 1980 for the Monroe County Department of Health (Table 1). Vaccine-preventable tuberculosis and sexually transmissible diseases are generally diseases with specific programs aimed at investigation and control. The enteric

Table 1
COMMUNICABLE DISEASE REPORT FOR WEEK 52 — WEEK ENDING DECEMBER 26, 1980[a]

Disease category	Disease	This week	This month	Year to date 1980	Year to date 1979	Year to date 1978
Vaccine	Measles	0	0	25	4	20
preventable	Mumps	0	0	2	3	5
disease	Pertussis	0	0	7	8	1
	Polio	0	0	0	0	0
	Rubella[b]	0	0	6(4)	12(51)	15
Tuberculosis	Tuberculosis, pulmonary	0	6	44	46	50
	Tuberculosis, other	0	0	9	18	9
	Atypical, mycobacteriosis	0	0	0	1	1
Sexually	Syphilis, infectious	1	5	93	46	79
transmissible	Syphilis, other	0	3	28	15	36
	Gonorrhea	91	353	3796	3935	4746
	Nongonococcal urethritis	11	88	1400	1537	1455
	Herpes genitalis	2	7	130	131	155
	Venereal warts	3	14	111	79	72
Enteric and	Salmonella	2	9	91	53	39
systemic viral	Shigella	1	12	77	23	89
	Food poisoning, other	0	0	37	41	109
	Hepatitis, infectious and other	0	3	71	37	80
	Hepatitis B	1	4	50	46	40
	Infectious mononucleosis	5	28	498	585	441
CNS and	Encephalitis	0	0	3	2	1
systemic bacterial	Meningitis, aseptic	0	4	21	18	22
	Meningococcal disease	0	0	2	1	4
	H. Influenza Type B disease	0	2	19	17	15
	Meningitis, bacterial, other	0	2	5	5	9
Bugs and bites	Animal bites	7	24	995	883	1116
	Animal rabies	0	0	2	2	0
	Head lice	3	65	517	108	3
	Pubic lice	0	9	166	140	142
	Scabies	3	15	111	97	62

CUMULATIVE TOTALS FOR OTHER DISEASES

	1980	1979	1978		1980	1979	1978
Amebiasis	0	1	0	Leptospirosis	0	0	0
Chickenpox (11)	435	226	473	Lymphogranuloma venerum	2	0	1
Cholera	0	0	0	Malaria	2	1	2
Clonorchiasis	0	1	0	Psittacosis	1	0	1
Coccidiomycisis	0	1	0	Rabies	0	0	0
Enterobiasis	0	6	0	Reye's syndrome	2	1	0
Giardiasis	0	2	16	Ringworm	18	51	0
Hepatitis B (asym)	1	0	2	Rocky Mt. spotted fever	0	0	1
Herpes zoster	1	0	1	Strep lab reports (5)	400	349	6725
Hospital infection	4	0	0	Toxoplasmosis	0	1	1
Legionnaire's disease	6	4	2	Trichinosis	0	0	1
Leprosy	1	0	0	Typhoid	0	3	1
Kawasaki disease	2	0	0	Congenital Rubella synd.	2	0	0
Campylobacter fetus	15	0	0				

Note: This report reflects the number of cases which have been investigated and/or confirmed by the health department and whose report cards have been forwarded to the State Health Department. It does not reflect the actual number of cases reported by doctors, clinics, hospitals, etc., for the particular week mentioned above.

Table 1 (continued)
COMMUNICABLE DISEASE REPORT FOR WEEK 52 — WEEK ENDING DECEMBER 26, 1980[a]

reflect the actual number of cases reported by doctors, clinics, hospitals, etc., for the particular week mentioned above.

[a] Monroe County Department of Health, 111 Westfall Road, Rochester, N.Y., 14602.

[b] Parenthesis after rubella indicate the number of rubella cases in college campus residents.

and systemic viral diseases are diseases of concern to the sanitation and water supply sections of the health department and are frequently investigated to rule out the possibility of environmental common sources. Infectious mononucleosis is included in the list because of the frequency with which it appears in the differential diagnosis of hepatitis or leptospirosis.

Central nervous system and systemic bacterial diseases have two elements of concern. One of these is the possible need for postexposure chemoprophylaxis of contacts exposed to meningococcal disease. The other is the consideration of possible mosquito control activities which may be required in response to reports of arthropod airborne encephalitis. The "bugs and bites" category deals with rabies control, school health concerns, and diseases which may be seen with some frequency in the venereal disease clinic.

Of the diseases listed on the bottom of the form, the provision of free streptococcal throat cultures is a common activity, time-honored, but of relatively little value in terms of public health activities directed at the control of rheumatic fever. Typhoid is the disease which health departments probably have the greatest expertise in dealing with, with most of the work being directed at the case reports of suspect typhoid, reported on the basis of typhoid agglutination studies in persons with other diseases who had previously received typhoid vaccine. Typhoid remains in many jurisdictions a disease frequently reported, frequently investigated, but seldom confirmed.

Health departments see hospitals and clinics as their eyes and ears within the community. Hospitals are usually the major source of communicable disease reports and other types of morbidity information which tell departmental staff what problems are occurring, the effectiveness of current departmental programming, and what priorities should be set for future action. Hospitals can also help the local health department by providing informal input on community problems which might not otherwise come to the attention of department staff, particularly problems concerning changes in attitude by physicians, patients, and other health providers concerning the role of government in health care delivery. Finally, in developing a spirit of mutual support, most local health departments are dependent at least to some degree on financial support from local city or county government. If hospitals support health department requests for increased staff and improvements in service in areas of mutual interest to the hospitals and department, the local health department can sometimes be of great value in improving communications and securing more favorable action from state regulatory and funding agencies.

With well over a thousand local health departments in the U.S., it is difficult to provide additional information of a general nature which is likely to be accurate and of specific interest to infection control staff. There is simply no substitute for getting to know key staff within the local health department and no better way to get to know them than by inviting them to speak and meet with an infection control committee meeting or at a meeting of the community-wide infection control group.

REFERENCES

1. **Miller, C. A., Brooks, E. F., DeFriese, G. H., Gilbert, B., Jain, S. C., and Kavaler, F.,** A survey of local health departments and their directors, *Am. J. Public Health,* 67, 931, 1977.

THE STATE HEALTH DEPARTMENT

Grayson B. Miller, Jr. and Robert S. Jackson

Hospital acquired infections have not been a traditional concern for most state health departments. The Center for Disease Control (CDC) was the first government agency to become interested in nosocomial infections through its practice of offering epidemic aid to the states. After numerous investigations of hospital associated outbreaks of infectious diseases, it became obvious that nosocomial infections were important economically as well as a significant source of morbidity and mortality. As a result of the increased understanding developed through these early CDC investigations, most State Health Departments now consider hospital acquired infections to be an important area of responsibility. As the focus of epidemiology has widened during the last two decades, most state health departments have devoted more resources to the investigation and control of nosocomial infections.

The State Health Department serves as the most competent source of epidemiologic advice and assistance available in most states and is responsible for the investigation, control, and prevention of disease which occurs within the state. Most State Health Departments have an organizational unit directed by a trained public health epidemiologist specifically assigned to fulfilling this responsibility. The public health epidemiologist and his staff have investigated numerous nosocomial outbreaks; they have a unique knowledge of the hospital and the special problems of infection control there as well as the relationship of the hospital to the community's health. Only with this perspective can seemingly insignificant pieces of information from several hospitals be correlated into the recognition of a community or statewide problem. The epidemiologist working in the State Health Department is available for consultation with hospitals, will often participate in the investigation of hospital outbreaks through his staff and the staffs of local health departments, and frequently acts as a liaison between a hospital and other state or federal health authorities whose knowledge and resources might be helpful in solving the problem at hand.

The epidemiologist can frequently assist a hospital in obtaining specialized laboratory services when the situation requires them for the investigation and/or control of a hospital infection problem. Examples of these specialized laboratory services include identification of unusual pathogens, serotyping of *Salmonella* organisms and bacteriophage typing of staphylococci. The State Health Department may be the only source of training, other than the CDC, available for hospital employees. Although the availability and content of such training varies from state to state, your state or a neighboring state may offer training sufficient to meet your hospital's needs. The State Health Department also stands as a resource for many diverse problems ranging from vermin control to the protection of the hospital's water supply to arranging for the follow-up of certain patients through the local health departments.

As previously mentioned, the prevention and control of infectious diseases and other diseases of public health importance are prime responsibilities of the State Health Department. In meeting these responsibilities and in protecting the community's health, the State Health Department depends upon private physicians and hospitals to report cases of disease through the local health departments. Although physicians are required to report certain diseases in every state, few states require hospitals to report nosocomial outbreaks or cases of community acquired disease. Voluntary reporting by hospitals would increase the state and local health departments' abilities to deal with community health problems by improving their knowledge of what is happening in the community. Disease reporting, although traditionally limited to infectious diseases, has been expanded in some states to include at least potential occupational and toxic substances exposures. The reporting of diseases by local physicians and hospitals is the basic element in developing and maintaining an adequate statewide disease surveillance system. After collection, the data can be assembled and analyzed with the underlying purpose of attempting to control and prevent certain diseases and, thereby, to protect the health of the community.

In the following appendix, the reader will note an alphabetical listing of states and territories with accompanying addresses and phone numbers of state and territorial epidemiologists.

APPENDIX

Listing of addresses and phone numbers of the state and territorial epidemiologists.

State Health Department
State Office Building
Montgomery, Alabama 36130
(205) 832-7275

State Department of Health and Social Services
Room 222, MacKay Building
338 Denali Street
Anchorage, Alaska 99501
(907) 272-7534

State Department of Health Services
State Health Building
1740 West Adams Street
Phoenix, Arizona 85007
(602) 255-1200

State Department of Health
4815 West Markham Street
Little Rock, Arkansas 72201
(501) 661-2242

State Department of Health Services
2151 Berkeley Way
Berkeley, California 94704
(415) 540-2566

State Department of Health
4210 East 11th Avenue
Denver, Colorado 80220
(303) 320-8333, Ext. 3100

State Department of Health
79 Elm Street
Hartford, Connecticut 06115
(203) 566-5475

State Department of Health and Social Services
Division of Public Health
Jesse Cooper Building
Capitol Square
Dover, Delaware 19901
(302) 736-4745

Community Health and Hospital Admin.
1875 Connecticut Avenue, N.W.
Washington, D.C. 20009
WATS direct 202-673-6758

Department of Health and Rehabilitative Services
Health Program Office, Epidemiology
Room 113, Building 1
1323 Winewood Boulevard
Tallahassee, Florida 32301
(904) 488-2905

State Department of Human Resources
Division of Physical Health
47 Trinity Avenue, S.W.
Atlanta, Georgia 30334
(404) 656-4767

State Department of Health
P. O. Box 3378
Honolulu, Hawaii 96801
(808) 548-5985

State Department of Health and Welfare
Statehouse
Boise, Idaho 83720
(208) 334-4164

State Department of Public Health
535 West Jefferson
Springfield, Illinois 62761
(217) 782-3948

State Board of Health
1330 West Michigan Street
Indianapolis, Indiana 46206
(317) 633-8422

Robert Lucas State Office Building
State Department of Health
Des Moines, Iowa 50319
(515) 281-4914

State Department of Health and Environment
Forbes AFB, Building 740
Topeka, Kansas 66620
(913) 862-9360, Ext. 481

State Department for Human Resources
Bureau for Health Services
275 East Main Street
Frankfort, Kentucky 40621
(502) 564-4935

State Department of Health and Human Resources
Office of Health Services and Environmental Quality
P.O. Box 60630
325 Loyola Avenue
New Orleans, Louisiana 70160
(504) 568-5005

State Department of Human Services
Bureau of Health
221 State Street
Augusta, Maine 04333
(207) 289-3201

State Department of Health and Mental Hygiene
201 West Preston Street
Baltimore, Maryland 21201
(301) 383-2605

State Department of Public Health
600 Washington Street
Boston, Massachusetts 02111
(617) 727-2688

State Department of Public Health
Bureau of Disease Control and Lab. Services
P. O. Box 30035
Lansing, Michigan 48909
(517) 373-1396

State Department of Health
717 Delaware Street, S.E.
Minneapolis, Minnesota 55440
(612) 296-5414

State Board of Health
Felix J. Underwood Building
2423 N. State Street
Jackson, Mississippi 39205
(601) 354-6650

State Department of Social Services
Division of Health
1511 Christy Drive
Jefferson City, Missouri 65102
(314) 751-2713, Ext. 286

State Department of Health and Environmental Sciences
W. F. Cogswell Building
Helena, Montana 59601
(406) 449-2645

State Department of Health
301 Centennial Mall South
P. O. Box 95007
Lincoln, Nebraska 68509
(402) 471-2939

State Department of Human Resources
Division of Health
Capitol Complex, Room 200
505 East King Street
Carson City, Nevada 89710
(702) 885-4800

State Department of Health and Welfare
Division of Public Health
Health and Welfare Building, Hazen Drive
Concord, New Hampshire 03301
(603) 271-1110, Ext. 4476

State Department of Health
John Fitch Plaza
P. O. Box 1540
Trenton, New Jersey 08625
(609) 292-4046

New Mexico Health and Environment Department
Health Services Division
P. O. Box 968
Sante Fe, New Mexico 87503
(505) 827-5671, Ext. 246

State Department of Health
Tower Building, Empire State Plaza
Albany, New York 12237
(518) 474-3186

Department of Health, City
125 Worth Street
New York, New York 10013
(212) 566-8214

State Department of Human Resources
Division of Health Services
225 North McDowell Street
P. O. Box 2091
Raleigh, North Carolina 27602
(919) 733-3421

State Department of Health
State Capitol
Bismarck, North Dakota 58505
(701) 224-2376

State Department of Health
246 North High Street
Columbus, Ohio 43215
(614) 466-4643

State Department of Health
Division of Epidemiology
1000 N.E. Tenth Street
Oklahoma City, Oklahoma 73152
(405) 271-4060

Department of Human Resources
State Health Division
1400 S. W. Fifth Avenue
Portland, Oregon 97201
(503) 229-5792

State Department of Health
Division of Epidemiology
P. O. Box 90
Harrisburg, Pennsylvania 17120
(717) 787-3350

State Department of Health
75 Davis Street
Providence, Rhode Island 02908
(401) 277-2362

State Department of Health and Environmental Control
J. Marion Sims Building
2600 Bull Street
Columbia, South Carolina 29201
(803) 758-7970

State Department of Health
Joe Foss Building
Pierre, South Dakota 57501
(605) 773-3357

Communicable Disease Control
522 R. S. Gass State Office Building
Ben Allen Road
Nashville, Tennessee 37216
(615) 741-7247

State Department of Health
1100 West 49th Street
Austin, Texas 78756
(512) 458-7207

State Department of Social Services
Division of Health
Room 460, 150 West North Temple
P. O. Box 2500
Salt Lake City, Utah 84110
(801) 533-6129

State Department of Health
60 Main Street
Burlington, Vermont 05401
(802) 862-5701, Ext. 246

State Department of Health
Room 701, The James Madison Building
109 Governor Street
Richmond, Virginia 23219
(804) 786-6261

Department of Social and Health Services
Health Services Division, Epidemiology Section
1409 Smith Tower
Seattle, Washington 98104
(206) 464-6461

State Department of Health
151 11th Avenue
South Charleston, West Virginia 25303
(304) 348-5358

State Department of Health and Social Services
Division of Health
Box 309
Madison, Wisconsin 53701
(608) 266-1251

State Department of Health and Social Services
Division of Health and Medical Services
Hathaway Building
Cheyenne, Wyoming 82002
(307) 777-7951

Department of Public Health and Social Services
Government of Guam
P. O. Box 2816
Agana, Guam 96910
734-9057 or 9916
Overseas Operator: 734-9901
(Cable or telegram, only; mailgram service not available.)

Director, Preventive Health Division
Department of Health, Edificio "A"
Call Box 70184
San Juan, Puerto Rico 00936
(809) 751-6289
(Cable or telegram, only; mailgram service not available.)

Department of Public Health and Environmental Services
Commonwealth of the Northern Mariana Islands
Saipan, Mariana Islands 96950
Cable Address: HICOTT SAIPAN
(Cable or telegram, only; mailgram service not available.)

Department of Medical Services
Division of Public Health
Government of American Samoa
LBJ Tropical Medical Center
Pago Pago, American Samoa 96799
633-4606
(Cable or telegram, only; mailgram service not available.)

Virgin Islands Department of Health
P. O. Box 1442
St. Thomas, V.I. 00802
(809) 774-1321
(Cable or telgram, only; mailgram service not available.)

THE CENTER FOR DISEASE CONTROL

Julia S. Garner

BACKGROUND

The Center for Disease Control (CDC) is a principal public health agency of the federal government and has a major responsibility for programs to control and prevent human disease. Originally charged with responsibility for infectious disease control, its responsibilities have gradually enlarged to encompass a large number of noninfectious diseases as well. As a result, in 1970 its name was changed from Communicable Disease Center to Center for Disease Control.*

Unlike most federal agencies, the headquarters for CDC is not located in Washington, but in Atlanta, Ga. The facilities consist primarily of classrooms, offices, and laboratories; there are no facilities for patient care at CDC. Most of the laboratories are housed in separate buildings connected by a series of passageways. For example, a separate building is used for virology, and another for mycology, parasitology, and bacteriology. Moreover, a separate maximum containment laboratory has recently been completed for work with highly contagious exotic diseases such as Lassa fever, Marburg virus, Ebola virus disease, and the South American hemorrhagic fevers, all caused by class 4 viruses that are endemic in many parts of the world. Many of these laboratories are restricted areas, and entrance to them requires up-to-date immunization for the diseases being worked on therein; therefore, they are not generally open to the public. In addition, CDC has other installations in the Atlanta area and has field stations in other areas of the country.

CDC employs almost 4000 persons; about half of them work in the Atlanta area. In addition to those assigned to field stations, others are working on projects of interest to CDC at state and local health departments, and some are stationed abroad for variable periods carrying out special programs. Because CDC is engaged in such a wide range of activities, it requires the services of highly specialized professional and technical men and women in medical and related fields. Many of these are nationally and internationally recognized as experts in their fields. Most of these experts work in a very specialized area often dealing exclusively with one type of disease or activity. Therefore, when trying to obtain information from these experts, it is important that inquiries, particularly letters, reach the appropriate organizational unit; otherwise, considerable delays can occur. Thus, answers to urgent questions may best be obtained by telephone. Moreover, emergency telephone coverage is always available.

ORGANIZATIONAL STRUCTURE

Administratively, CDC is organized by bureaus of specialized interest. Some of the bureaus provide specific services of interest to those concerned with hospital infection control.

The Bureau of Epidemiology is responsible for surveillance, epidemic investigation and control of most communicable diseases, including hospital infections, and, in addition, has active epidemiologic programs for a number of chronic diseases such as cancer, birth defects, diabetes, and arthritis. A program in family planning evaluation

---

* This chapter was written before CDCs most recent reorganization, which was proposed in 1980 and is still in progress. Despite changes in organizational structures and titles, the various functions of CDC as described in this chapter are expected to continue.

has been active in studying demographic trends, complications associated with various contraceptive methods, and morbidity associated with abortions.

The Bureau of Health Education provides leadership and direction to a comprehensive national health education program for the prevention of disease, disability, premature death, and undesirable and unnecessary health problems, and serves as a clearing house on health education in general.

The Bureau of Laboratories serves as a national and world reference center for bacteriology, mycology, parasitology, virology, and other laboratory methods for identifying most communicable and a number of noninfectious diseases. Through state and local health departments, clinical practitioners submit specimens for reference identification or confirmation. One of its major tasks is the development of improved laboratory methods, as well as evaluation of methods proposed by others. An increasingly important function of this bureau is evaluation of commercial clinical laboratories under the provisions of the Laboratory Licensure and Development Act, enacted in 1967. This bureau also provides consultation, training, and informational services in laboratory techniques and laboratory management.

The Bureau of State Services is responsible for evaluating and controlling vaccine-preventable diseases, venereal diseases, and tuberculosis; and for environmental health activities for urban rat control and childhood lead-based paint poison prevention. Working with state and local health departments, this bureau provides both funds and technical support for most of the nation's immunization programs — for example, immunization against childhood diseases such as measles, poliomyelitis, and rubella, as well as immunization against influenza.

The Bureau of Training provides home study materials and conducts courses at CDC and elsewhere, relating to epidemiology and communicable disease control. This bureau also provides consultation regarding training to state and local health departments, health care facilities, and others involved in communicable disease control and some chronic disease problems.

The activities of the remaining two bureaus, Smallpox Eradication and Tropical Diseases, are primarily those of international health. Through these bureaus, CDC personnel have been intimately involved in the world-wide effort to eradicate smallpox and control malaria.

Two services out of the Office of the Center Director are of general interest to those concerned with hospital infection control. The first, the Office of Information, organizes and administers the CDC public information program. During large outbreaks, particularly those of national importance, the Office of Information, rather than the bureau conducting the investigation, usually assists the press and the public concerning the investigation. In addition to these activities, general information concerning CDC can be obtained from this office. The second office of general interest is the Office of International Services, which plans, organizes, and administers programs of specialized experience for foreign health workers. This office also provides for the reception and orientation of foreign visitors to the CDC; therefore, any foreign health worker seeking to visit the CDC or seeking to take CDC courses should contact this office rather than one of the bureaus.

Specific programs in hospital infection control, with the exception of training, are organized within the Bureau of Epidemiology. For the past two decades, CDC epidemiologists have assisted state health departments and hospitals in the investigations of epidemics occurring in hospitals. From these investigations a number of recommendations have been derived that are widely accepted by hospitals and incorporated into their routine practices. In addition, the Bureau of Epidemiology has studied alternative methods for surveillance of nosocomial infections, and the methods recommended by

CDC have been widely adopted. When major problems in hospital infection control are recognized, whether they are responsible for epidemic disease or not, CDC epidemiologists often attempt to define their causes and find solutions through epidemiologic or laboratory field study. For example, CDC epidemiologists are currently directing the SENIC Project, the Study of the Efficacy of Nosocomial Infection Control Programs, to study the approaches to hospital infection control which have been practiced in the past several years to determine which ones offer the most effectiveness for the least cost.

Within the Bureau of Epidemiology, several organizational units are involved in various areas of hospital infection control. Some of these are involved extensively in hospital infection control because of their expertise in surveillance, prevention, and control of hospital infection in general, whereas others are involved only when the pathogen causing the problem occurs in the hospital rather than the community and expertise about the pathogen and its epidemiology are required. The organizational unit in the Bureau of Epidemiology that is concerned exclusively with hospital infection control is the Hospital Infections Branch of the Bacterial Diseases Division. This branch provides consultation on control of hospital acquired infections, assists in development of effective surveillance systems, conducts prospective epidemiologic and laboratory studies of endemic infection problems in institutions, provides epidemiologic and laboratory assistance in investigating outbreaks of nosocomial infections, formulates guidelines for hospital infection control, and participates in training hospital personnel in the epidemiology and control of nosocomial infections. The Hospital Infections Branch is also responsible for the development and implementation of the National Nosocomial Infections Study (NNIS), a collaborative surveillance program of hospital infections in approximately 80 acute-care institutions throughout the U.S.

Another organizational unit in the Bureau of Epidemiology with expertise in an area of much concern to those involved in infection control in health care facilities is the Hepatitis Laboratories Division. Rather than being located in Atlanta, this division is located in Phoenix, Ariz. and conducts clinical, field, and laboratory investigations on viral hepatitis and dialysis-associated diseases; develops and evaluates methods for diagnosis, prevention, and control of these diseases; and conducts a national surveillance program for viral hepatitis. This division also provides epidemic aid and other assistance to state and local health departments for the investigation of nosocomial outbreaks of hepatitis and dialysis-associated diseases, and serves as a World Health Organization Collaborating Center for Reference and Research on Viral Hepatitis.

The Parasitic Diseases Division, also of the Bureau of Epidemiology, conducts clinical, field, and laboratory investigations of parasitic diseases, such as *Pneumocystis carinii* pneumonia, giardiasis, scabies, and toxoplasmosis. Moreover, the Viral Diseases Division, also of the Bureau of Epidemiology, conducts surveillance of enteric, neurotropic, respiratory, and other viral diseases. These divisions also provide epidemic aid and consultation upon request to state and local health departments, other federal agencies, medical centers, and research institutions.

In addition to the Bureau of Epidemiology, other bureaus within CDC have expertise and provide services in areas pertaining to hospital infection control. The Tuberculosis Control Division of the Bureau of State Services provides guidelines for prevention of tuberculosis transmission in hospitals and for tuberculosis control programs for hospital employees. Moreover, both the Bureau of Laboratories and the Bureau of Training conduct training courses pertaining to nosocomial infection control. The courses are described later in this chapter.

SPECIFIC SERVICES FOR HOSPITAL INFECTION CONTROL

The following is presented to inform infection-control personnel, infection-control committee members, and others involved in nosocomial infection control about how to utilize specific CDC services for hospital infection control.

Guidelines for Hospital Infection Control

Various guidelines that hospitals may use in approaching surveillance, prevention, and control of hospital acquired infections have been formulated by CDC. These, and a limited selection of guidelines formulated by others, some in collaboration with CDC, are available from the Hospital Infections Branch. These include guidelines for surveillance of nosocomial infections, insertion and care of various catheters and pressure-monitoring devices, tracheostomy care, hand washing, microbiologic sampling, and sterilization. Guidelines for the role of the laboratory and the employee health service in nosocomial infection control are also available. Because the facilities and resources vary between hospitals, these guidelines are not necessarily applicable for all hospitals. Nevertheless, single copies of a particular guideline or a general packet of guidelines are available by writing the Center for Disease Control, Attention: Hospital Infections Branch, Atlanta, Ga. 30333.

Guidelines for isolation are contained in the Center for Disease Control *Isolation Techniques for Use in Hospitals.,* however, this manual is not available from CDC. It must be purchased from the Government Printing Office, Public Documents Section, Superintendent of Documents, Washington, D.C. 20402. The telephone number for Order and Information Clerks is (202) 783-3238. The price of the manual is $3.25 per copy. The correct Superintendent of Documents Stock Number (017-023-00094-2) must be specified and the exact amount of money — check or money order made payable to Superintendent of Documents — submitted. Otherwise, the order will not be processed.

Consultation on Hospital Infection Control

When the above-mentioned guidelines cannot answer questions concerning nosocomial infections, medical and nurse epidemiologists and other health professionals are available for consultation. However, it is important to realize the limits of this consultation.

Statistical data on nosocomial infections available from CDC are limited to those reported from the 80 hospitals that collaborate with the Hospital Infections Branch in the National Nosocomial Infections Study (NNIS). Hospitals submitting data to NNIS, although geographically distributed throughout the U.S., may not constitute a representative sample of all U.S. hospitals. Moreover, the data from NNIS are generally limited to data about rates of infection by site, pathogen, service, and type of hospital.

The CDC does not routinely test and compare different brands of commercially distributed patient care products, equipment, or disinfectants to determine which product is superior to another; therefore, CDC cannot recommend brand names or products. Occasionally, an epidemiologic investigation of a problem will implicate a particular brand or a product as the source or in the transmission of disease. When this occurs, this information is disseminated by an article in the CDC *Morbidity and Mortality Weekly Report,* in scientific journal articles, or through press releases from the CDC Office of Information.

With these limitations in mind, letters and telephone inquiries concerning policies and procedures to prevent hospital acquired infections in general, and those caused by bacterial diseases in particular, should be directed to Center for Disease Control, Attention: Hospital Infections Branch, Atlanta, Ga. 30333, telephone (404) 329-3406. Letters and telephone inquiries about nosocomial viral hepatitis and dialysis-associated diseases should be directed to the Hepatitis Laboratories Division, Bureau of Epidemiology, CDC, 4402 North Seventh Street, Phoenix, Ariz. 85014, telephone (602) 241-2665. If another office at CDC is involved in research on the subject of an inquiry, the inquiry can be forwarded to that office by either of the above.

Assistance for Investigating Hospital Epidemics

Medical epidemiologists, microbiologists, statisticians, and others from the Bureau of Epidemiology, in cooperation with other staff personnel at CDC, investigate outbreaks of hospital acquired infections. State health departments can usually provide assistance for investigating hospital epidemics; therefore it is worthwhile to establish a relationship with state and local health departments. Small outbreaks or outbreaks involving diseases in which the epidemiology and methods of control are well understood may not require an on-site investigation; when this occurs, assistance in the form of telephone consultation and literature may be adequate. However, if follow-up conversation indicates that the problem is continuing or if the problem represents an unusual event, pathogen, product, or procedure, then an on-site investigation may be conducted if the hospital requests it, and if local and state health officials endorse CDC's assistance. CDC is responsible for coordinating investigations involving disease problems of interstate significance and is especially interested in participating in investigations that may relate to such problems. Moreover, investigations of outbreaks in federal institutions traditionally have been principal responsibilities of CDC. Nosocomial outbreaks caused by bacterial pathogens or involving commercially distributed product are usually investigated by the Hospital Infections Branch. However, certain bacterial diseases, especially those related to enteric diseases, meningococcal, or Legionnaries' disease, causing nosocomial outbreaks, may be investigated in collaboration with the Enteric Diseases Branch and the Special Pathogens Branch also located in the Bacterial Diseases Division, Bureau of Epidemiology. Nosocomial outbreaks caused by viral hepatitis or those that are dialysis-associated, are investigated by the Hepatitis Laboratories Division. Nosocomial outbreaks of other viral and parasitic diseases are usually investigated by their respective divisions in collaboration with the Hospital Infections Branch. Telephone numbers for epidemic assistance are

Bacterial Diseases Division	(404) 329-3684
Enteric Diseases Branch	(404) 329-3753
Hospital Infections Branch	(404) 329-3406
Special Pathogens Branch	(404) 329-3687
Hepatitis Laboratories Division	(602) 241-2665
Parasitic Diseases Division	(404) 329-3676
Viral Diseases Division	(404) 329-3786

Dissemination of Current Information

Information of current interest to those concerned with hospital infection control is often featured in the *Morbidity and Mortality Weekly Report* (MMWR). This report, published weekly by CDC, contains epidemiologic notes and reports of interesting cases or outbreaks, environmental hazards, contaminated commercially distributed products, and other public health problems of current interest to hospital and other health care workers; and statistical summaries of specified notifiable diseases. The Recommendations of the Public Health Service Advisory Committees on Immunization Practices are published in the MMWR when changes in recommendations have been made. For specific information concerning the MMWR, contact Center for Disease Control, Attention: Editor, *Morbidity and Mortality Weekly Report,* Atlanta, Ga. 30333. Send mailing list additions, deletions, and address changes to Center for Disease Control, Attention: Distribution Services Section, MASO, 1-SB-36, Atlanta Ga. 30333.

Training Health Professionals in Hospital Infection Control

Medical and nurse epidemiologists from the Hospital Infections Branch and others in the Bureau of Epidemiology having responsibility for nosocomial infection control, participate in training activities conducted by CDC, professional associations and organizations, and health care facilities. Because responsibilities for epidemic investigations and field studies take precedence over involvement in training, CDC epidemiologists are not always available to fill training requests. An effort is made to be available, however, for national and large regional meetings on nosocomial infection control or related subjects. Letters concerning requests for a Hospital Infections Branch speaker for nosocomial infection control should be directed to Center for Disease Control, Attention: Chief, Hospital Infections Branch, Atlanta, Ga. 30333. Requests for speakers on other aspects of nosocomial infection should be referred to other persons at CDC.

Courses for Hospital Infection Control

As previously mentioned, the Bureau of Training and Bureau of Laboratories at CDC offer courses that may assist infection-control personnel in hospital infection control.

Bureau of Training Courses

Of particular interest is the Bureau of Training's course "Surveillance, Prevention, and Control of Hospital Associated Infections". This course is designed primarily for hospital infection control nurses. Others are admitted by special arrangement. The course provides participants with an understanding of the magnitude and complexity of the existing problems in nosocomial infections. Principles and methods of epidemiology, a review of microbiology, as well as the principles and applications of aseptic practice, make up the core of the curriculum. Emphasis is placed on surveillance systems, clinical aspects of infection, prevention and control of cross-infection, isolation, the total environment, laboratory support, and certain administrative aspects of infection-control implementation. Six months' experience in an infection-control position is a prerequisite for admission to the course. Further information about this course or applications for the course can be obtained by writing Center for Disease Control, Attention: Hospital Infections Training, Instructional Services Division, Bureau of Training, Atlanta, Ga. 30333, telephone (404) 262-6665.

Bureau of Laboratories Courses

The Bureau of Laboratories offers two courses of interest to hospial infection control personnel. "Microbiology of the Hospital Environment" offers a summary of contemporary thought on the microbiologic aspects of the hospital environment. It examines the animate and inanimate environment, introduces practical working tools of microbiologic assay techniques, and covers the fundamentals of methodology for environmental control. This 4-day course is offered several times a year. It is primarily designed for hospital personnel who have professional responsibilities in environmental control. However, nurses, physicians, microbiologists, sanitarians, and other infection-control committee members may attend.

The second course of interest, "Clinical Microbiology in Control of Nosocomial Infections," consists of lectures and discussions on the microbiologic aspects of control of nosocomial infections. Course contents include currently accepted laboratory diagnostic procedures for the major etiologic agents and introduction to epidemic investigations and epidemiologic aspects of nosocomial infections. This 5-day course is offered several times a year. Training and/or experience in microbiology or epidemiology is a prerequisite for attending this course. Further information about these courses or applications can be obtained by writing Center for Disease Control, Attention: Registrar, Bureau of Laboratories, Building 3, Room B-12, Atlanta, Ga. 30333, telephone (404) 329-3837.

Surveillance Reports

Surveillance reports on approximately two dozen topics are prepared by CDC; subjects range from abortion to veterinary public health. The following two are of particular interest to those concerned with hospital infection control.

National Nosocomial Infections Study Report — Annual summaries of infections from the National Nosocomial Infections Study (NNIS) hospitals are compiled and analyzed and published in NNIS reports. In addition to containing surveillance data, they also contain epidemiologic notes and reports, methods of prevention and control of nosocomial infections, and laboratory aspects in the control of nosocomial infections. For specific information concerning the content of NNIS reports, contact Center for Disease Control, Attention: National Nosocomial Infections Study, Bureau of Epidemiology, Atlanta, Ga. 30333.

Hepatitis Surveillance Report — This report is produced by the Hepatitis Laboratories Division, Bureau of Epidemiology, CDC, which serves as the World Health Organization Collaborating Center for Reference and Research on Viral Hepatitis. These reports contain data on morbidity trends, recent outbreaks of special interest, laboratory notes, recommendations for sterilization and disinfection of objects and equipment exposed to hepatitis virus, and the latest recommendations of the Public Health Service Advisory Committee on Immunization Practices for hepatitis. Specific information about the Hepatitis Surveillance Report can be obtained from Viral Hepatitis Surveillance Activity, Hepatitis Laboratories Division, Bureau of Epidemiology, CDC, 4402 North Seventh Street, Phoenix, Ariz. 85014.

Mailing list additions, deletions, and address changes for these and other surveillance reports should be sent to Center for Disease Control, Attention: Distribution Services Section, MASO, 1-SB-36, Atlanta, Ga. 30333.

In summary, various services are available from CDC for infection-control personnel, infection-control committee members, and others involved with control of nosocomial infections. Many of these services are also available from state health departments and other organizations and associations. Therefore, it is important for those with responsibilities for nosocomial infection control to establish a relationship with their state health department and to familiarize themselves with the services available from organizations and associations such as the American Hospital Association, the American Society for Microbiology, the Association for Practitioners in Infection Control (APIC), and others.

Table 1
CONTACTS AND TELEPHONE NUMBERS FOR MAJOR TYPES OF INQUIRIES

Advice and consultation	Contact	Telephone number
General nosocomial infection control Guidelines Isolation techniques Speakers for conferences Epidemic assistance[a]	Hospital Infections Branch CDC Atlanta, Ga. 30333	(404)329-3406
Hepatitis and dialysis-associated diseases	Hepatitis Laboratory Division CDC 4402 North Seventh Street Phoenix, Ariz. 85014	(602)241-2665
Training Infection control nurses	Hospital Infections Training Instructional Services Division Bureau of Training CDC Atlanta, Ga. 30333	(404)262-6665
Microbiologists	Registrar Bureau of Laboratories CDC Atlanta, Ga. 30333	(404)329-3837
International visitors	Office of International Services CDC Atlanta, Ga. 30333	(404)329-3336
Publications *Morbidity and Mortality Weekly Report* *National Nosocomial Infections Study Report* *Hepatitis Surveillance Report*	Distribution Services Section, 1-SB-36 CDC Atlanta, Ga. 30333	(404)329-3219
Isolation Techniques for Use in Hospitals[b]	Government Printing Office Public Documents Section Superintendent of Documents Washington, D.C. 20402	(202)783-3238

[a]   State health departments are also available for epidemic assistance.
[b]   Must be ordered from the Government Printing Office — not CDC.

If the services of CDC are desired, the official mailing address is

Center for Disease Control
Attention: (List appropriate bureau, office, or laboratory)
Atlanta, Ga. 30333

The telephone number is (404) 329-3311 for the information operator. Otherwise, direct dialing to the appropriate office or laboratory is preferred. Contacts and telephone numbers for major inquiries are listed in Table 1.

ASSOCIATION FOR PRACTITIONERS IN INFECTION CONTROL

Karen J. Axnick
and
Carole De Mille

HISTORY

The role of the infection control nurse, first conceptualized and implemented in Great Britain, was introduced in the U.S. in 1963. In the ensuing 15 years, the discipline of infection control has emerged from a variety of professional backgrounds to become a strong component of quality patient care.

As the number of practitioners swelled, the twofold need for communication and education found expression in the organizational efforts of Claire Coppage, R.N., MPH, of the Center for Disease Control. In April 1972, a steering committee composed of 20 nurses met in North Carolina; the foundation for a multidisciplinary, international infection control organization was laid.

ORGANIZATION

The Association for Practitioners in Infection Control (APIC) is a nonprofit organization composed of over 5000 members and governed by an elected Board of nine directors and six officers. Membership, which is open to all individuals involved in or concerned with infection control activities, reflects the multidisciplinary nature of the infection control spectrum. While the predominant member category is registered nurses, there are also physicians, microbiologists, and medical technologists as principal support groups. All 50 states and 18 foreign countries are represented.

The purpose of the Association "... To improve patient care by serving the needs and aims common to all disciplines who are united by infection-control activities ..." is addressed at both national and local levels for both individual and group membership.

OBJECTIVES

The fulfillment of the Association's purpose is achieved through activities implemented under the following, primary objectives.

To Initiate and Develop Effective Communication
American Journal of Infection Control

The official publication of the Association has undergone a dramatic metamorphosis since its inception as the *APIC Newsletter*. Now published quarterly, the *American Journal of Infection Control* represents a major voice for infection control practitioners (ICPs) of all professional backgrounds. Original manuscripts reporting research findings and comprehensive review articles are complemented by book, current periodical, and audiovisual material reviews, educational and professional opportunities, innovations in infection control programs, and official communiques and reports of the Association.

Local Chapters

While the Journal and other activities have enhanced a strong, national identity, the strength of the Association is rooted in the membership at the local level. Chapter status, first bestowed in 1975, has been granted to over 50 local infection control groups. Regular meetings in major metropolitan areas provide practitioners with the opportunity to exchange information, to raise issues, and to air concerns with their colleagues.

To Support the Development of Education Programs Designed to Assist the Practitioner in Gaining Proficiency
Annual Conference

Since 1975, an annual, international conference has been designed and implemented to address the educational needs of both the novice and the expérienced ICP. Well attended by over one third of the membership, these meetings create a stimulating milieu in which members can gain new insights and update skills. Topics have included overviews of nosocomial infections, microbiology, virology, and communication skills; epidemiology and surveillance methodologies; high-risk patient populations and therapeutic modalities; antibiotic utilization and review. In direct response to the growth and development of the discipline, the conferences have given increasing emphasis to the presentation of original papers concerning hospital infection control, hospital epidemiology, and nosocomial infectious diseases. The compilation of this valuable information in published proceedings and professionally recorded tapes has contributed significantly to the increasing body of infection control literature.

Education Committee

The APIC Education Committee also recognizes the pressing need for ongoing educational opportunities. To this end, regional educational conferences are encouraged through the provision of core objectives and basic curricula outlines as well as seed funds to initiate planning and implementation of 1-day seminars. These workshops are available for a variety of infection control concerns:

· Extended care facilities
· Microbiology
· Education of the adult learner
· Surgical wounds
· Antimicrobials

Starter Kit

The novice ICP seeking assistance in this new role can now obtain a "Starter Kit". Developed as a concise resource for the beginner, the kit contains basic information concerning the role of the ICP, surveillance methodology, the Infection Control Committee, laboratory aspects, and accreditation standards. These materials are complemented by references and reprints addressing the consultative process, hepatitis, employee health programs, hospital infection control manuals, and outbreak investigation.

Certification

The paucity of standardized educational programs to prepare qualified practitioners in this new health care speciality is well recognized. As a positive step toward formal, academic credentials, the APIC Board is studying the need for certification of APIC members. An opinion survey taken at the 1978 national business meeting underlined the priority of this issue by the membership. Subsequently, methodologies and tools for certification are being pursued.

To Support the Development of Effective and Rational Infection-Control Programs in Health Care Facilities

Position Paper

Concern over the multiplicity of role definitions and responsibilities for ICPs was first voiced at a meeting of the American Hospital Association's Advisory Committee on Infections Within Hospitals in 1974. Over the next 4 years, multiple drafts of an APIC position paper received critical analysis and review. The final document outlining the necessary expertise of the practitioner and scope of an infection control program was endorsed by 96% of the voting members in May 1978.

Interorganizational Communication

APIC has established a strong profile in cooperative efforts with other organizations and agencies relating to infection control. Members currently participate in the Committee on Infections Within Hospitals of the American Hospital Association, the Board of Directors of the National Foundation of Infectious Diseases (NFID), and the Federation of Nursing Specialities in conjunction with the American Nurses Association. Additionally, good rapport is maintained with the Center for Disease Control, the Joint Commission on Accreditation of Hospitals, and the American Society for Microbiology.

To Encourage Standardization and Critical Evaluation of Infection-Control Practices

The Association, in maintaining that the goal of improved patient care is shared by professionals in a variety of settings has established a Committee of Public Relations to enhance communication with industrial representatives. In this vein, educational and commercial exhibits were initiated at the 1977 national educational conference. This provides the membership with the opportunity to review currently available products and equipment.

APIC has also coordinated several multidisciplinary meetings to address the controversies surrounding sterilization and disinfection of endoscopic equipment. Guidelines endorsed by the manufacturers and members of a variety of health care disciplines have been prepared for dissemination to appropriate professional organizations.

To Promote Quality Research Practices and Procedures Related to Infection Control

Through the generosity of several corporations, APIC has been able to offer modest scholarship funds in support of investigations to evaluate existing or to develop new infection control practices in microbiology and patient care.

SUMMARY

APIC offers a unique opportunity for colleagues in infection control to develop a broad communication and educational system bridging many professional disciplines. Further information for individual memberships and chapter locations may be obtained by writing to:

National Offices
Association for Practitioners in Infection Control
Route 2, 359 Milwaukee Avenue
Half Day, Ill. 60069

Index

INDEX